Study Guide and Procedure Checklist Manual for

Kinn's The Medical Assistant

An Applied Learning Approach

Fourteenth Edition

Brigitte Niedzwiecki, MSN, RN, RMA
Medical Assistant Program Director & Instructor
Chippewa Valley Technical College
Eau Claire, Wisconsin

Julie Pepper, BS, CMA (AAMA)
Medical Assistant Instructor
Chippewa Valley Technical College
Eau Claire, Wisconsin

P. Ann Weaver, MSEd, MT (ASCP)
Medical Assisting Instructor
Chippewa Valley Technical College
Eau Claire, Wisconsin

ELSEVIER

ELSEVIER

3251 Riverport Lane
St. Louis, Missouri 63043

Study Guide and Procedure Checklist Manual for
Kinn's The Medical Assistant, Fourteenth Edition

ISBN: 978-0-323-60869-5

ISBN: 978-0-323-60869-5

Printed in the United States of America

Last digit is the print number: 9 8 7 6 5 4 3 2 1

Working together
to grow libraries in
developing countries

www.elsevier.com • www.bookaid.org

To the Student

This study guide was created to help you to achieve the objectives of each chapter in your text and establish a solid base of knowledge in medical assisting. Completing the exercises in each chapter in this guide will help reinforce the material studied in the textbook and learned in class.

STUDY HINTS FOR ALL STUDENTS

Ask Questions!

There are no stupid questions. If you do not know something or are not sure about it, you need to find out. Other people may be wondering the same thing but are too shy to ask. The answer could be a matter of life or death for your patient. That is certainly more important than feeling embarrassed about asking a question.

Chapter Objectives

At the beginning of each chapter in the textbook are learning objectives that you should have mastered by the time you have finished studying that chapter. Write these objectives in your notebook, leaving a blank space after each. Fill in the answers as you find them while reading the chapter. Review to make sure your answers are correct and complete. Use these answers when you study for tests. You should also do this for separate course objectives that your instructor has listed in your class syllabus.

Vocabulary

At the beginning of each chapter in the textbook are vocabulary terms that you will encounter as you read the chapter. These terms are in bold type the first time they appear in the chapter.

Summary of Learning Objectives

Use the Summary of Learning Objectives at the end of each chapter in the textbook to help you review for exams.

Reading Hints

As you read each chapter in the textbook, look at the subject headings to learn what each section is about. Read first for the general meaning and then reread parts you did not understand. It may help to read those parts aloud. Carefully read the information given in each table and study each figure and its legend.

Concepts

While studying, put difficult concepts into your own words to determine whether you understand them. Check this understanding with another student or the instructor. Write these concepts in your notebook.

Class Notes

When taking lecture notes in class, leave a large margin on the left side of each notebook page and write only on right-hand pages, leaving all left-hand pages blank. Look over your lecture notes soon after each class while your memory is fresh. Fill in missing words, complete sentences and ideas, and underline key phrases, definitions, and concepts. At the top of each page, write the topic of that page. In the left margin, write the key word for that part of your notes. On the opposite left-hand page, write a summary or outline that combines material from the textbook and the lecture. These can be your study notes for review.

Study Groups

Form a study group with other students so that you can help one another. Practice speaking and reading aloud. Ask questions about material you find unclear. Work together to find answers.

ADDITIONAL STUDY HINTS FOR ENGLISH AS A SECOND LANGUAGE (ESL) STUDENTS

Vocabulary

If you find a nontechnical word you do not know (e.g., drowsy), try to guess its meaning from the sentence (e.g., with electrolyte imbalance, the patient may feel fatigued and drowsy). If you are not sure of the meaning or if it seems particularly important, look it up in the dictionary.

Vocabulary Notebook

Keep a small alphabetized notebook or address book in your pocket or purse. Write down new nontechnical words you read or hear along with their meanings and pronunciations. Write each word under its initial letter so you can find it easily, as with a dictionary. For words you do not know or words that have a different meaning in medical assisting, write down how each word is used and how it is pronounced. Look up the meanings of these words in a dictionary or ask your instructor or first-language buddy (see the following section). Then write the different meanings or uses that you have found in your book, including the medical assisting meaning. Continue to add new words as you discover them.

First-Language Buddy

English as a second language (ESL) students should find a first-language buddy—another student who is a native speaker of English and who is willing to answer questions about word meanings, pronunciations, and culture. Maybe, in turn, your buddy would like to learn about your language and culture; this could be useful for his or her medical assisting career.

Contents

Competency Checklist

Student Name: _____

Admission Cohort: _____

Graduation Date: _____

Competency	Procedure	Date	Grade / Pass	Initial
I. Anatomy & Physiology				
I.P.1.a. Measure and record: blood pressure	Procedure 20.8 Procedure 39.1			
I.P.1.b. Measure and record: temperature	Procedures 20.1 to 20.5			
I.P.1.c. Measure and record: pulse	Procedures 20.6, 20.7 Procedure 39.1			
I.P.1.d. Measure and record: respirations	Procedure 20.7			
I.P.1.e. Measure and record: height	Procedure 20.10			
I.P.1.f. Measure and record: weight	Procedure 20.10 Procedure 43.2			
I.P.1.g. Measure and record: length (infant)	Procedure 43.2			
I.P.1.h. Measure and record: head circumference (infant)	Procedure 43.1			
I.P.1.i. Measure and record: pulse oximetry	Procedure 20.9			
I.P.2.a. Perform: electrocardiography	Procedure 26.1			
I.P.2.b. Perform: venipuncture	Procedures 47.1 to 47.3			
I.P.2.c. Perform: capillary puncture	Procedure 47.4 Procedure 49.4			
I.P.2.d. Perform: pulmonary function testing	Procedures 40.1, 40.2			
I.P.3. Perform patient screening using established protocols	Procedures 31.1 to 31.3			
I.P.4.a. Verify the rules of medication administration: right patient	Procedures 30.1, 30.7 to 30.10 Procedures 31.4 to 31.7 Procedure 40.3			
I.P.4.b. Verify the rules of medication administration: right medication	Procedures 30.1 to 30.10 Procedures 31.4 to 31.7 Procedure 40.3			

Competency	Procedure	Date	Grade / Pass	Initial
I.P.4.c. Verify the rules of medication administration: right dose	Procedures 30.1 to 30.10 Procedures 31.4, 31.5, 31.7 Procedure 40.3			
I.P.4.d. Verify the rules of medication administration: right route	Procedures 30.1 to 30.10 Procedures 31.4 to 31.7 Procedure 40.3			
I.P.4.e. Verify the rules of medication administration: right time	Procedures 30.1 to 30.10 Procedures 31.4, 31.5, 31.7 Procedure 40.3			
I.P.4.f. Verify the rules of medication administration: right documentation	Procedures 30.1, 30.7 to 30.10 Procedures 31.4 to 31.7 Procedure 40.3			
I.P.5. Select proper sites for administering parenteral medication	Procedures 30.7 to 30.10			
I.P.6. Administer oral medications	Procedure 30.1			
I.P.7. Administer parenteral (excluding IV) medications	Procedures 30.7 to 30.10			
I.P.8. Instruct and prepare a patient for a procedure or a treatment	Procedures 25.7, 25.8 Procedures 26.1, 26.2 Procedures 31.1 to 31.7 Procedures 35.1 to 35.7 Procedures 36.2 to 36.4 Procedures 40.1 to 40.3 Procedures 42.1, 42.2			
I.P.9. Assist provider with a patient exam	Procedures 21.3 to 21.10 Procedures 31.1 to 31.4 Procedure 38.1 Procedure 42.1 Procedures 43.1, 43.2 Procedure 44.1			
I.P.10. Perform a quality control measure	Procedure 34.3 Procedure 45.1 Procedure 46.4 Procedures 48.3, 48.7 Procedures 49.3, 49.4			
I.P.11.a. Obtain specimens and perform: CLIA-waived hematology test	Procedures 48.2 to 48.4			
I.P.11.b. Obtain specimens and perform: CLIA-waived chemistry test	Procedures 48.6, 48.7			
I.P.11.c. Obtain specimens and perform: CLIA-waived urinalysis	Procedures 46.1 to 46.3, 46.5, 46.7, 46.8			
I.P.11.d. Obtain specimens and perform: CLIA-waived immunology test	Procedures 49.2 (collection only), 49.3, 49.4			

Competency	Procedure	Date	Grade / Pass	Initial
I.P.11.e. Obtain specimens and perform: CLIA-waived microbiology test	Procedures 49.1 (collection only), 49.2 (collection only), 49.3 (perform test only)			
I.P.12. Produce up-to-date documentation of provider / professional level CPR	*(From outside agency)*			
I.P.13.a. Perform first aid procedures for: bleeding	Procedure 27.5			
I.P.13.b. Perform first aid procedures for: diabetic coma or insulin shock	Procedure 27.1			
I.P.13.c. Perform first aid procedures for: fractures	Procedure 27.5			
I.P.13.d. Perform first aid procedures for: seizures	Procedure 27.3			
I.P.13.e. Perform first aid procedures for: shock	Procedure 27.6			
I.P.13.f. Perform first aid procedures for: syncope	Procedure 27.5			
I.A.1. Incorporate critical thinking skills when performing patient assessment	Procedure 27.2 Procedure 34.1			
I.A.2. Incorporate critical thinking skills when performing patient care	Procedure 26.1 Procedures 47.1 to 47.3			
I.A.3. Show awareness of a patient's concerns related to the procedure being performed	Procedure 26.1 Procedure 47.5			
II. Applied Mathematics				
II.P.1. Calculate proper dosages of medication for administration	Procedure 29.1 Procedure 30.1			
II.P.2. Differentiate between normal and abnormal test results	Procedure 46.4, 46.5 Procedure 48.7 Procedures 49.3, 49.4			
II.P.3. Maintain lab test results using flow sheets	Procedure 45.1 Procedures 49.3, 49.4			
II.P.4. Document on a growth chart	Procedures 43.1, 43.2			
II.A.1. Reassure a patient of the accuracy of the test results	Procedure 46.9			
III. Infection Control				
III.P.1. Participate in bloodborne pathogen training	Procedure 19.1			

Competency	Procedure	Date	Grade / Pass	Initial
III.P.2. Select appropriate barrier/personal protective equipment (PPE)	Procedure 19.3 Procedures 30.7 to 30.10 Procedures 47.1 to 47.4 Procedures 49.2 to 49.4			
III.P.3. Perform hand washing	Procedure 19.2			
III.P.4. Prepare items for autoclaving	Procedure 24.1			
III.P.5. Perform sterilization procedures	Procedure 24.2			
III.P.6. Prepare a sterile field	Procedures 25.3, 25.4, 25.6			
III.P.7. Perform within a sterile field	Procedures 25.3, 25.4, 25.6			
III.P.8. Perform wound care	Procedures 25.6, 25.7			
III.P.9. Perform dressing change	Procedure 25.7			
III.P.10.a. Demonstrate proper disposal of biohazardous material: sharps	Procedures 30.7 to 30.10 Procedures 47.1 to 47.4 Procedure 49.4			
III.P.10.b. Demonstrate proper disposal of biohazardous material: regulated wastes	Procedures 47.1 to 47.4 Procedures 49.2 to 49.4			
III.A.1. Recognize the implications for failure to comply with Center for Disease Control (CDC) regulations in healthcare settings	Procedure 25.7			
IV. Nutrition				
IV.P.1. Instruct a patient according to patient's special dietary needs	Procedure 23.1			
IV.A.1. Show awareness of patient's concerns regarding a dietary change	Procedure 23.1			
V. Concepts of Effective Communication				
V.P.1.a. Use feedback techniques to obtain patient information including: reflection	Procedures 2.1, 2.2, 2.4 Procedure 21.1			
V.P.1.b. Use feedback techniques to obtain patient information including: restatement	Procedures 2.1, 2.2, 2.4 Procedure 21.1			
V.P.1.c. Use feedback techniques to obtain patient information including: clarification	Procedures 2.1, 2.2, 2.4 Procedure 21.1			
V.P.2. Respond to nonverbal communication	Procedures 2.1 to 2.4 Procedure 21.2			
V.P.3. Use medical terminology correctly and pronounced accurately to communicate information to providers and patients	Procedure 21.1			

Competency	Procedure	Date	Grade / Pass	Initial
V.P.4.a. Coach patients regarding: office policies	Procedure 9.3			
V.P.4.b. Coach patients regarding: health maintenance	Procedures 34.2, 34.4 Procedure 38.1 Procedure 41.1 Procedure 42.2			
V.P.4.c. Coach patients regarding: disease prevention	Procedure 22.1			
V.P.4.d. Coach patients regarding: treatment plan	Procedures 35.1 to 35.7			
V.P.5.a. Coach patients appropriately considering: cultural diversity	Procedure 42.2			
V.P.5.b. Coach patients appropriately considering: developmental life stage	Procedure 22.1 Procedure 34.2 Procedure 35.5 Procedure 41.1 Procedure 42.2			
V.P.5.c. Coach patients appropriately considering: communication barriers	Procedure 22.1 Procedure 35.6			
V.P.6. Demonstrate professional telephone techniques	Procedure 8.1			
V.P.7. Document telephone messages accurately	Procedure 8.2			
V.P.8. Compose professional correspondence utilizing electronic technology	Procedures 7.1 to 7.5			
V.P.9. Develop a current list of community resources related to patients' healthcare needs	Procedure 22.2			
V.P.10. Facilitate referrals to community resources in the role of a patient navigator	Procedure 22.2			
V.P.11. Report relevant information concisely and accurately	Procedure 8.2 Procedure 21.1			
V.A.1.a. Demonstrate: empathy	Procedures 2.1 to 2.4 Procedure 21.1 Procedure 44.1			
V.A.1.b. Demonstrate: active listening	Procedures 2.1 to 2.4 Procedure 21.1			
V.A.1.c. Demonstrate: nonverbal communication	Procedures 2.1 to 2.4 Procedure 21.1			
V.A.2. Demonstrate the principles of self-boundaries	Procedure 21.1			

Competency	Procedure	Date	Grade / Pass	Initial
V.A.3.a. Demonstrate respect for individual diversity including: gender	Procedure 2.1			
V.A.3.b. Demonstrate respect for individual diversity including: race	Procedure 2.2			
V.A.3.c. Demonstrate respect for individual diversity including: religion	Procedure 2.3			
V.A.3.d. Demonstrate respect for individual diversity including: age	Procedure 2.4			
V.A.3.e. Demonstrate respect for individual diversity including: economic status	Procedure 2.4			
V.A.3.f. Demonstrate respect for individual diversity including: appearance	Procedures 2.1 to 2.4			
V.A.4. Explain to a patient the rationale for performance of a procedure	Procedure 25.7			
VI. Administrative Functions				
VI.P.1. Manage appointment schedule using established priorities	Procedures 9.1, 9.2, 9.4			
VI.P.2. Schedule a patient procedure	Procedure 9.5			
VI.P.3. Create a patient's medical record	Procedures 10.1, 10.4			
VI.P.4. Organize a patient's medical record	Procedures 10.2, 10.4			
VI.P.5. File patient medical records	Procedures 10.2, 10.4, 10.5			
VI.P.6. Utilize an EMR	Procedure 10.2			
VI.P.7. Input patient data utilizing a practice management system	Procedures 10.1, 10.2			
VI.P.8. Perform routine maintenance of administrative or clinical equipment	Procedure 11.2 Procedure 26.1 Procedure 45.4 Procedure 48.1			
VI.P.9. Perform an inventory with documentation	Procedures 11.1, 11.3			
VI.A.1. Display sensitivity when managing appointments	Procedures 9.2, 9.4, 9.5			
VII. Basic Practice Finances				
VII.P.1.a. Perform accounts receivable procedures to patient accounts including posting: charges	Procedure 16.1			

Competency	Procedure	Date	Grade / Pass	Initial
VII.P.1.b. Perform accounts receivable procedures to patient accounts including posting: payments	Procedures 16.1, 16.3			
VII.P.1.c. Perform accounts receivable procedures to patient accounts including posting: adjustments	Procedure 16.3			
VII.P.2. Prepare a bank deposit	Procedure 16.4			
VII.P.3. Obtain accurate patient billing information	Procedure 9.2 Procedure 16.2			
VII.P.4. Inform a patient of financial obligations for services rendered	Procedure 15.6 Procedure 16.2			
VII.A.1. Demonstrate professionalism when discussing patient's billing record	Procedures 15.2, 15.6 Procedure 16.2			
VII.A.2. Display sensitivity when requesting payment for services rendered	Procedures 15.2, 15.6 Procedure 16.2			
VIII. Third Party Reimbursement				
VIII.P.1. Interpret information on an insurance card	Procedure 12.1 Procedure 15.1			
VIII.P.2. Verify eligibility for services including documentation	Procedure 12.2 Procedure 15.6			
VIII.P.3. Obtain precertification or preauthorization including documentation	Procedure 12.2 Procedure 15.3			
VIII.P.4. Complete an insurance claim form	Procedure 15.4			
VIII.A.1. Interact professionally with third party representatives	Procedure 15.2			
VIII.A.2. Display tactful behavior when communicating with medical providers regarding third party requirements	Procedure 15.2			
VIII.A.3. Show sensitivity when communicating with patients regarding third party requirements	Procedure 15.2			
IX. Procedural and Diagnostic Coding				
IX.P.1. Perform procedural coding	Procedures 14.1, 14.2			
IX.P.2. Perform diagnostic coding	Procedure 13.1			
IX.P.3. Utilize medical necessity guidelines	Procedure 15.5			

Competency	Procedure	Date	Grade / Pass	Initial
IX.A.1. Utilize tactful communication skills with medical providers to ensure accurate code selection	Procedure 14.3			
X. Legal Implications				
X.P.1. Locate a state's legal scope of practice for medical assistants	Procedure 3.2			
X.P.2.a. Apply HIPAA rules in regard to: privacy	Procedure 4.1			
X.P.2.b. Apply HIPAA rules in regard to: release of information	Procedure 4.2			
X.P.3. Document patient care accurately in the medical record	Procedure 21.1 Procedures 22.1, 22.2 Procedures 25.6 to 25.8 Procedures 26.1, 26.2 Procedures 27.1 to 27.6 Procedures 30.1, 30.7 to 3.10 Procedures 31.4 to 31.7 Procedures 34.1 to 34.4 Procedures 35.1 to 35.7 Procedures 36.1, 36.4 Procedure 38.1 Procedure 39.1 Procedures 40.1 to 40.4 Procedure 41.1 Procedure 42.2 Procedures 43.1, 43.2			
X.P.4.a. Apply the Patient's Bill of Rights as it relates to: choice of treatment	Procedure 3.1			
X.P.4.b. Apply the Patient's Bill of Rights as it relates to: consent for treatment	Procedure 3.1			
X.P.4.c. Apply the Patient's Bill of Rights as it relates to: refusal of treatment	Procedure 3.1			
X.P.5. Perform compliance reporting based on public health statutes	Procedure 4.3			
X.P.6. Report an illegal activity in the healthcare setting following proper protocol	Procedure 4.4			
X.P.7. Complete an incident report related to an error in patient care	Procedure 4.5			
X.A.1. Demonstrate sensitivity to patient rights	Procedure 3.1 Procedure 4.1			
X.A.2. Protect the integrity of the medical record	Procedures 10.1 to 10.3			

Competency	Procedure	Date	Grade / Pass	Initial
XI. Ethical Considerations				
XI.P.1. Develop a plan for separation of personal and professional ethics	Procedure 5.1			
XI.P.2. Demonstrate appropriate response(s) to ethical issues	Procedure 5.2			
XI.A.1. Recognize the impact personal ethics and morals have on the delivery of healthcare	Procedure 5.1, 5.2			
XII. Protective Practices				
XII.P.1.a. Comply with: safety signs	Procedure 45.3			
XII.P.1.b. Comply with: symbols	Procedure 45.3			
XII.P.1.c. Comply with: labels	Procedure 45.3			
XII.P.2.a. Demonstrate proper use of: eyewash equipment	Procedure 45.2			
XII.P.2.b. Demonstrate proper use of: fire extinguishers	Procedure 11.6			
XII.P.2.c. Demonstrate proper use of: sharps disposal containers	Procedure 30.2, 30.3, 30.5, 30.7 to 30.10 Procedure 47.1 to 47.4 Procedure 49.4			
XII.P.3. Use proper body mechanics	Procedure 11.4 Procedure 21.3			
XII.P.4. Participate in a mock exposure event with documentation of specific steps	Procedure 11.5			
XII.P.5. Evaluate the work environment to identify unsafe working conditions	Procedure 11.4 Procedure 45.3			
XII.A.1. Recognize the physical and emotional effects on persons involved in an emergency situation	Procedure 11.5			
XII.A.2. Demonstrate self-awareness in responding to an emergency situation	Procedure 11.5			

The Professional Medical Assistant and the Healthcare Team

CAAHEP Competencies	Assessments
V.C.12. Define patient navigator	Workplace Application – 2
V.C.13. Describe the role of the medical assistant as a patient navigator	Workplace Application – 2
VIII.C.4. Define a patient-centered medical home (PCMH)	Skills and Concepts – J. 1
X.C.1. Differentiate between scope of practice and standards of care for medical assistants	Skills and Concepts – C. 1
X.C.2. Compare and contrast provider and medical assistant roles in terms of standard of care	Skills and Concepts – C. 2
V.C.11. Define the principles of self-boundaries	Skills and Concepts – K. 2
ABHES Competencies	**Assessments**
1. General Orientation a. Describe the current employment outlook for the medical assistant	Skills and Concepts – A. 1, 2
b. Compare and contrast the allied health professions and understand their relation to medical assisting	Skills and Concepts – H. 1-19
c. Describe and comprehend medical assistant credentialing requirements, the process to obtain the credential and the importance of credentialing	Skills and Concepts – D. 1
d. List the general responsibilities and skills of the medical assistant	Skills and Concepts – A. 3
5. Human Relations f. Demonstrate an understanding of the core competencies for Interprofessional Collaborative Practice i.e. values/ethics; roles/responsibilities; interprofessional communication; teamwork	Skills and Concepts – J. 2
g. Partner with health care teams to attain optimal patient health outcomes	Skills and Concepts – K. 1
h. Display effective interpersonal skills with patients and health care team members	Skills and Concepts – K. 1
i. Demonstrate cultural awareness	Skills and Concepts – B. 1

ABHES Competencies	Assessments
8. Clinical Procedures i. Identify community resources and Complementary and Alternative Medicine practices (CAM)	Skills and Concepts – G. 3

VOCABULARY REVIEW

Using the word pool on the right, find the correct word to match the definition. Write the word on the line after the definition.

Group A

1. Adhering to ethical standards or right conduct standards
_____

2. The way an individual perceives and processes information to learn new material _____

3. To learn or memorize beyond the point of proficiency or immediate recall _____

4. The process of sorting patients to determine medical need and the priority of care _____

5. A person who identifies patients' needs and barriers, then assists by coordinating care and identifying community and healthcare resources to meet the needs _____

6. How an individual internalizes new information and makes it his or her own _____

7. A learning device (e.g., an image, a rhyme, or a figure of speech) that a person uses to help him or her remember information
_____

8. Meticulous, careful _____

9. How an individual looks at information and sees it as real
_____

10. The process of thinking about new information to create new ways of learning _____

11. Harmful _____

12. Conduct expected of a reasonably prudent person acting under similar circumstances; it falls below the standards of behavior established by law for the protection of others against unreasonable risk of harm _____

Word Pool
- patient navigator
- detrimental
- integrity
- conscientious
- triage
- negligence
- perceiving
- processing
- learning style
- reflection
- overlearn
- mnemonic

Group B

1. A group of diverse medical and healthcare systems, practices, and products that are not generally considered part of conventional medicine. Some are used in combination with conventional medicine and others are used instead of conventional medicine

   _____

2. Emotional or mental condition with respect to cheerfulness or confidence _____

3. A system of medical practice that treats disease by the use of remedies such as medications and surgery to produce effects different from those caused by the disease under treatment

   _____

4. Dependable, able to be trusted _____

5. The process by which something becomes harmful or unusable through contact with something unclean

   _____

6. The ability to determine what needs to be done and take action on your own _____

7. A form of healing that considers the whole person (i.e., body, mind, spirit, and emotions) in individual treatment plans

   _____

8. A concept of care that involves health professionals and volunteers who provide medical, psychological, and spiritual support to terminally ill patients and their loved ones

   _____

9. Behavior toward others; outward manner

   _____

10. The constant practice of considering all aspects of a situation when deciding what to believe or what to do

    _____

11. An important point or group of statistical values that, when evaluated, indicates the quality of care provided in a healthcare facility _____

Word Pool
- critical thinking
- contamination
- allopathic
- holistic
- complementary and alternative medicine (CAM)
- hospice
- indicators
- demeanor
- initiative
- reliable
- morale

ABBREVIATIONS

Write out what each of the following abbreviations stands for.

1. CAAHEP _____

2. CAM _____

3. EHR _____

4. ECG _____

5. CLIA _____

6. OSHA _____

7. IV _____

8. AAMA _____

9. CEU _____

10. AMT _____

11. NHA _____

12. MD _____

13. DO _____

14. OMT _____

15. DC _____

16. NP _____

17. RN _____

18. PA _____

19. IDS _____

20. ED _____

21. PCMH _____

22. AHRQ _____

23. HHS _____

24. IT _____

SKILLS AND CONCEPTS
Answer the following questions. Write your answer on the line or in the space provided.

A. Responsibilities of the Medical Assistant

1. According the U.S. Bureau of Labor Statistics, employment opportunities for medical assistants is expected to grow _____ through _____.

2. List factors for the expected growth in job opportunities for medical assistants._____

   _____

   _____

   _____

   _____

   _____

   _____

3. List five clinical and five administrative skills that are part of the job description for an entry-level medical assistant.

Clinical skills include: _____

_____

_____

_____

_____

_____

Administrative skills include: _____

_____

_____

_____

_____

_____

B. Characteristics of Professional Medical Assistants

1. What methods can the medical assistant use to treat others with courtesy and respect? _____

_____

_____

_____

_____

_____

C. Scope of Practice and Standards of Care for Medical Assistants

1. What is the difference between scope of practice and standards of care? _____

_____

_____

_____

_____

_____

2. Describe the difference between standard of care for a provider and a medical assistant._____

_____

_____

_____

_____

_____

3. Identify five practices that are beyond the scope of practice of medical assistants._____

_____

_____

_____

_____

_____

D. Professional Medical Assisting Organizations, Credentials, and Continuing Education

1. What are some of the differences between the AAMA and AMT? What credentials can be granted by each?

_____

_____

_____

_____

_____

_____

2. Is the NHA involved in medical assistant program curriculum development or accreditation? What service does this company provide?

_____

_____

_____

_____

_____

_____

E. How to Succeed as a Medical Assistant Student

1. Choose three study skills from your reading and describe how you think they will help you learn.

   _____

   _____

   _____

   _____

   _____

2. What test-taking strategies might help you improve your scores?_____

   _____

   _____

   _____

3. Describe what it means to be a critical thinker. _____

   _____

   _____

   _____

   _____

   _____

F. The History of Medicine

1. Describe how the profession of medical assisting began. Why are medical assistants defined as *multi-skilled* healthcare workers?

   _____

   _____

   _____

   _____

G. Medical Professionals

1. _____ physicians, or DOs, complete requirements similar to those for MDs to graduate and practice medicine.

2. _____ provide direct patient care services under the supervision of licensed physicians and are trained to diagnose and treat patients as directed by the physician.

3. Identify five complementary and alternative medicine therapies. _____

    . _____

    _____

    _____

    _____

    _____

4. Explain the role of the hospitalist. _____

    _____

    _____

    _____

    _____

    _____

H. Allied Health Professionals

Match the following descriptions with the appropriate healthcare occupation.

1. _____ Provides services such as injury prevention, assessment, and rehabilitation

2. _____ Is qualified to implement exercise programs designed to reverse or minimize debilitation and enhance the functional capacity of medically stable patients

3. _____ Practices medicine under the direction and responsible supervision of a medical doctor or doctor of osteopathy

4. _____ Performs diagnostic examinations and therapeutic interventions of the heart or blood vessels, both invasive and noninvasive

5. _____ Assists licensed pharmacists by performing duties that do not require the expertise of a pharmacist

6. _____ Assists in developing and implementing the anesthesia care plan

7. _____ Helps to improve patient mobility, relieve pain, and prevent or limit permanent physical disabilities

8. _____ Helps patients use their leisure in ways that enhance health, functional abilities, independence, and quality of life

9. _____ Identifies patients who have hearing, balance, and related ear problems

10. _____ Integrates and applies the principles from the science of food, nutrition, biochemistry, food management, and behavior to achieve and maintain health

11. _____ Evaluates, treats, and manages patients of all ages with respiratory illnesses and other cardiopulmonary disorders

12. _____ Evaluates disorders of vision, eye movement, and eye alignment

13. _____ Performs routine and standardized tests in blood center and transfusion services

14. _____ Uses equipment that produces sound waves, resulting in images of internal structures

15. _____ Uses the nuclear properties of radioactive and stable nuclides to make diagnostic evaluations of the anatomic or physiologic conditions of the body

16. _____ Helps prepare patients for surgery and maintain the sterile field in the surgical suite, making sure all members of the surgical team follow sterile technique

17. _____ Assists in helping patients compensate for loss of function

18. _____ Performs diagnostic testing on blood, body fluids, and other types of specimens to assist the provider in arriving at a diagnosis

19. _____ Provides medical care to patients who have suffered an injury or illness outside the hospital setting

a. audiologist
b. diagnostic cardiovascular technologist
c. therapeutic recreation specialist
d. physical therapist
e. pharmacy technician
f. dietetic technician
g. anesthesiology assistant
h. blood bank technology specialist
i. diagnostic medical sonographer
j. kinesiotherapist
k. occupational therapist
l. orthoptist
m. physician assistant
n. surgical technologist
o. respiratory therapist
p. athletic trainer
q. medical technologist
r. emergency medical technician
s. nuclear medicine technologist

I. Types of Healthcare Facilities

1. Hospitals are classified according to the type of care and services they provide to patients. Describe the three different levels of hospitalized care.

    a. _____

    _____

    _____

    _____

    b. _____

    _____

    _____

    _____

    c. _____

    _____

    _____

    _____

J. The Healthcare Team

1. Define a patient-centered medical home (PCMH) and its five core functions and attributes. _____

    _____

    _____

    _____

    _____

    _____

    _____

    _____

2. Define teamwork in your own words._____

    _____

    _____

    _____

    _____

    _____

K. Professionalism as a Team Member

1. Summarize three obstructions to professionalism.

   a. _____

   _____

   _____

   _____

   b. _____

   _____

   _____

   _____

   c. _____

   _____

   _____

   _____

2. Define the principles of self-boundaries. How do they relate to the field of medical assisting? _____

   _____

   _____

   _____

   _____

   _____

   _____

   _____

3. Describe four time-management techniques medical assistants can use in the healthcare environment to meet the demands of a busy practice.

   a. _____

   b. _____

   c. _____

   d. _____

CERTIFICATION PREPARATION

Circle the correct answer.

1. The first national organization formed for medical assistants was the
    a. CAAHEP.
    b. ABHES.
    c. AMT.
    d. **AAMA.**

2. Which healthcare professional is trained to practice medicine under the supervision of a physician?
    a. Medical technologist
    b. Paramedic
    c. Medical assistant
    d. **Physician assistant**

3. The allied health specialist who performs ultrasound diagnostic procedures under the supervision of a physician is called a(n)
    a. cytotechnologist.
    b. **diagnostic medical sonographer.**
    c. electroneurodiagnostic technologist.
    d. perfusionist.

4. A method of prioritizing patients so that the most urgent cases receive care first is called
    a. case management.
    b. accreditation.
    c. **triage.**
    d. quality control.

5. The health professional who provides basic patient care services, including diagnosing illnesses and prescribing medications, is a
    a. **nurse practitioner.**
    b. nurse anesthetist.
    c. licensed practical nurse.
    d. vocational nurse.

6. One factor is absolutely true about all practicing medical assistants—they are not independent practitioners. Whether certified or not, regardless of length of training or experience, every medical assistant must practice under the direct supervision of a physician or other licensed practitioner (e.g., nurse practitioner or physician assistant).
    a. **Both statements are true.**
    b. Both statements are false.
    c. The first statement is true; the second is false.
    d. The first statement is false; the second is true.

7. Which mind maps would display the cause and effect of events?
    a. Spider map
    b. Fishbone map
    c. **Chain-of-events map**
    d. Cycle map

8. Which is *not* part of critical thinking?
    a. Sorting out conflicting information
    b. Weighing your knowledge about the information
    c. Deciding on a reasonable belief or action
    d. **Incorporating personal beliefs**

9. Deciding which tasks are most important is called
    a. modification.
    b. teaching.
    c. **prioritizing.**
    d. procrastinating.

10. Which statement about professionalism is true?
    a. It must be practiced at all times in the workplace.
    b. It can lead to wage increases and promotions.
    c. Unacceptable behavior is detrimental to the medical assistant's career.
    d. **All of the above are true.**

WORKPLACE APPLICATIONS

1. You are employed by a primary care physician who is investigating the possibility of forming a PCMH with other practitioners and allied health professionals in the community. Refer to the Department of Health and Human Services PCMH Resource Center at http://pcmh.ahrq.gov/. Research the meaning of PCMH and review the research that supports the PCMH model of care. What did you learn? Share this information with your class. *PCMH means - Patient - Centered Medical Home. It provides comprehensive, coordinated, patient - entered primary care.*

2. What does it mean to operate as a patient navigator? Why are medical assistants who are skilled in both administrative and clinical areas ideally suited to help patients navigate complex healthcare systems? How could you help the patient described below? *It means they help patients navigate through the system. She will help patient to make appointment and describe everything.*

    Mrs. Kate Glasgow is an 82-year-old patient in the family practice where you work. Mrs. Glasgow recently suffered a mild cerebrovascular accident (CVA) and her son is trying to help coordinate her care. Mrs. Glasgow does not understand when or how to take her new medications, she is concerned about whether her health insurance will cover the cost of frequent clinic appointments and assistive devices, she doesn't understand how to prepare for magnetic resonance imaging (MRI) the provider ordered, and she dislikes having to comply with getting blood drawn every week.

3. Martin Smith is a patient who always disrupts the clinic. He constantly complains about everything from the moment he enters until the moment he leaves. Karen is at the desk when he arrives to check out and pay his bill. When she tells him that he has a previous balance from a claim that his insurance did not pay, he argues that Karen filed the claim incorrectly. Karen is not in charge of filing insurance claims and did not handle any part of the claim in question. How can she be courteous to this patient? *Karen is an employee. So she follow his Superiority Orders. She need to take over the work of Angela. It might be hurt Angela. But she has no choice.*

INTERNET ACTIVITIES

1. Choose one of the early medical pioneers discussed in this chapter and research him or her using the internet. After conducting the research, create a poster presentation, a PowerPoint presentation, or write a paper and present the results of your research to the class.

2. Research professionalism requirements for other health professions. Talk about the ways that those requirements are similar to or different from those of a medical assistant. Compare professionalism in the healthcare industry to that in other professions, such as law enforcement or education. Talk about why medical professionalism is so critical.

Therapeutic Communication

CAAHEP Competencies	Assessment
V.C.1. Identify styles and types of verbal communication	Skills and Concepts – D. 1, 4-9; Certification Preparation – 2
V.C.2. Identify types of nonverbal communication	Skills and Concepts – C. 2-5; Certification Preparation – 1
V.C.3. Recognize barriers to communication	Skills and Concepts – D. 21 a-h; Certification Preparation – 3
V.C.4. Identify techniques for overcoming communication barriers	Skills and Concepts – D. 22 a-h; Certification Preparation – 4
V.C.5. Recognize the elements of oral communication using a sender-receiver process	Skills and Concepts – D. 2-3
V.C.14.a. Relate the following behaviors to professional communication: assertive	Skills and Concepts – D. 9 a-e, 10
V.C.14.b. Relate the following behaviors to professional communication: aggressive	Skills and Concepts – D. 6 a-e
V.C.14.c. Relate the following behaviors to professional communication: passive	Skills and Concepts – D. 5 a-e
V.C.15. Differentiate between adaptive and non-adaptive coping mechanisms	Skills and Concepts – E. 6-8; Certification Preparation – 5; Internet Activities – 4
V.C.18.a. Discuss examples of diversity: cultural	Skills and Concepts – B. 1
V.C.18.b. Discuss examples of diversity: social	Skills and Concepts – B. 2
V.C.18.c. Discuss examples of diversity: ethnic	Skills and Concepts – B. 3
V.A.3.a. Demonstrate respect for individual diversity including: gender	Procedure 2.1
V.A.3.b. Demonstrate respect for individual diversity including: race	Procedure 2.2
V.A.3.c. Demonstrate respect for individual diversity including: religion	Procedure 2.3
V.A.3.d. Demonstrate respect for individual diversity including: age	Procedure 2.4
V.A.3.e. Demonstrate respect for individual diversity including: economic status	Procedure 2.4

CAAHEP Competencies	Assessment
V.A.3.f. Demonstrate respect for individual diversity including: appearance	Procedure 2.1, 2.2, 2.3, 2.4
V.P.1.a. Use feedback techniques to obtain patient information including: reflection	Procedure 2.1, 2.2, 2.4
V.P.1.b. Use feedback techniques to obtain patient information including: restatement	Procedure 2.1, 2.2, 2.4
V.P.1.c. Use feedback techniques to obtain patient information including: clarification	Procedure 2.1, 2.2, 2.4
V.P.2. Respond to nonverbal communication	Procedure 2.1, 2.2, 2.3, 2.4
V.A.1.a. Demonstrate: empathy	Procedure 2.1, 2.2, 2.3, 2.4
V.A.1.b. Demonstrate: active listening	Procedure 2.1, 2.2, 2.3, 2.4
V.A.1.c. Demonstrate: nonverbal communication	Procedure 2.1, 2.2, 2.3, 2.4
V.C.17.a. Discuss the theories of: Maslow	Skills and Concepts – E. 1, 2 a-e; Certification Preparation – 8-9; Internet Activities – 3
V.C.17.b. Discuss the theories of: Erikson	Skills and Concepts – D. 23, 24 a-i; Certification Preparation – 6
V.C.17.c. Discuss the theories of: Kübler-Ross	Skills and Concepts – D. 25, 26 a-e; Certification Preparation – 7
V.C.11. Define the principles of self-boundaries	Skills and Concepts – D. 27
X.C.10.c. Identify: Americans with Disabilities Act Amendments Act (ADAAA)	Skills and Concepts – F. 1

ABHES Competencies	Assessment
5. Human Relations a. Respond appropriately to patients with abnormal behavior patterns	Skills and Concepts – E. 4
b. Provide support for terminally ill patients 1) Use empathy when communicating with terminally ill patients	Procedure 2.4
b. 2) Identify common stages that terminally ill patients experience	Skills and Concepts – D. 25, 26 a-e
e. Analyze the effect of hereditary and environmental influences on behavior	Skills and Concepts – E. 1-3
i. Display effective interpersonal skills with patients and health care team members	Procedure 2.1, 2.2, 2.3, 2.4

6. Describe aggressive communicators.

   a. Description of communication: _____

   _____

   _____

   b. Nonverbal communication behaviors used: _____

   _____

   _____

   c. How they may feel: _____

   _____

   _____

   d. How others may feel with this behavior: _____

   _____

   _____

   e. Based on what you learned about this type of communicator, how would you professionally communicate with this type of person?

   _____

   _____

7. Describe passive-aggressive communicators.

   a. Description of communication: _____

   _____

   _____

   b. Nonverbal communication behaviors used: _____

   _____

   _____

   c. How they may feel: _____

   _____

   _____

   d. How others may feel with this behavior: _____

   _____

   _____

e. Based on what you learned about this type of communicator, how would you professionally communicate with this type of person?

_____

_____

8. Describe manipulative communicators.

a. Description of communication: _____

_____

_____

b. Nonverbal communication behaviors used: _____

_____

_____

c. How they may feel: _____

_____

_____

d. How others may feel with this behavior:_____

_____

_____

e. Based on what you learned about this type of communicator, how would you professionally communicate with this type of person?

_____

_____

9. Describe assertive communicators.

a. Description of communication: _____

_____

_____

b. Nonverbal communication behaviors used: _____

_____

_____

c. How they may feel: _____

_____

_____

   d.   How others may feel with this behavior:_____

   _____

   _____

   e.   Based on what you learned about this type of communicator, how would you professionally com-
        municate with this type of person?

        _____

        _____

10. What type of communicator should a medical assistant strive to become? Explain why this type of com-
    municator is important in a healthcare setting.

    _____

    _____

    _____

11. What are the advantages of using therapeutic communication in a healthcare setting?_____

    _____

    _____

    _____

12. Describe the difference between active listening and passively hearing what the speaker is saying.

    _____

    _____

    _____

13. List four nonverbal behaviors that can be used during active listening. _____

    _____

    _____

14. Describe open questions or statements and identify when to use them with patients._____

    _____

    _____

    _____

15. Describe closed questions or statements and identify when to use them with patients._____

    _____

    _____

    _____

16. _____ allows the listener to get additional information.

17. _____ or _____ means to reword or rephrase a statement to check the meaning and interpretation.

18. _____ allows the listener to recap and review what was said.

19. _____ allows time to gather thoughts and answer questions.

20. _____ means to put words to the person's emotional reaction, which acknowledges the person's feelings.

21. For each description below, identify the type of barrier to communication.

   a. Noise, lack of privacy, temperature: _____

   b. Fear and anxiety related to being judged by the healthcare professional or the inability to explain personal feelings: _____

   c. Unable to read or write: _____

   d. Hunger, pain, anger, tiredness: _____

   e. Unable to see written communication: _____

   f. Unable to hear verbal communication: _____

   g. Functioning at a lower age level: _____

   h. English is not the patient's primary language: _____

22. Describe ways the medical assistant can help overcome barriers to communication.

   a. Internal distractions: _____

   _____

   _____

   b. Visual impairment: _____

   _____

   _____

   c. Hearing impairment:_____

   _____

   _____

   d. Environmental distractions:_____

   _____

   _____

   e. Illiteracy: _____

   _____

   _____

    f.   Non-English–speaking:_____

        _____

        _____

    g.   Intellectual disability: _____

        _____

        _____

    h.   Emotional distraction:_____

        _____

        _____

23. Discuss how Erikson's theory of psychosocial developmental relates to communicating with patients.

    _____

    _____

    _____

24. Discuss Erikson's psychosocial developmental stages. Your answers should include the goals of the stage and one communication tip for that stage.

    a.   Trust versus Mistrust: _____

        _____

        _____

        _____

    b.   Autonomy versus Shame and Doubt: _____

        _____

        _____

        _____

    c.   Initiative versus Guilt:_____

        _____

        _____

        _____

    d.   Industry versus Inferiority: _____

        _____

        _____

        _____

e.   Identity versus Role Confusion: _____

_____

_____

_____

f.   Intimacy versus Isolation:_____

_____

_____

_____

g.   Generativity versus Stagnation: _____

_____

_____

_____

h.   Ego Integrity versus Despair: _____

_____

_____

_____

25.   Discuss how Kübler-Ross's theory relates to communicating with patients. _____

_____

_____

_____

26.   Describe the following stages of Kübler-Ross's theory.

a.   Denial: _____

_____

_____

b.   Anger: _____

_____

_____

c.   Bargaining: _____

_____

_____

     d. Depression: _____

                 _____

                 _____

     e. Acceptance:_____

                 _____

                 _____

27. Based on the principles of personal boundaries, describe three ways communication with patients differs from communication with family and friends.

_____

_____

_____

_____

_____

_____

_____

_____

_____

E. Understanding Behavior

1. Describe Maslow's Hierarchy of Needs theory._____

_____

_____

_____

_____

_____

2. For the following descriptions, identify the level of need according to Maslow's theory.

    a. Includes air, food, drink, shelter, and warmth: _____

    b. Includes friendship and intimacy: _____

    c. Includes protection form the elements and security: _____

    d. Includes knowledge, curiosity, and understanding: _____

    e. The appreciation of and search for beauty and balance: _____

    f. Includes self-esteem and achievement: _____

    g. The need to realize one's potential: _____

    h. These needs are met by helping others achieve their very best: _____

3. Describe how understanding Maslow's theory can help a medical assistant. _____

_____

_____

4. Why do people use defense mechanisms? _____

_____

_____

5. Identify the defense mechanism based on the following descriptions.

    a. Completely rejects the information: _____

    b. The person comes up with various explanations to justify his or her response:
        _____

    c. Transfers the emotion toward one person to another person or thing: _____

    d. Simply forgets something that is bad or hurtful: _____

6. Describe the difference between adaptive (healthy) coping mechanisms and maladaptive (nonadaptive or unhealthy) coping mechanisms.

    _____

    _____

    _____

7. List four adaptive coping mechanisms._____

    _____

    _____

8. List four maladaptive coping mechanisms. _____

    _____

    _____

F. Closing Comments

1. Discuss the impact of the Americans with Disabilities Act Amendments Act (ADAAA) in relationship to communication barriers in healthcare.

    _____

    _____

    _____

    _____

    _____

2. Discuss three ways that healthcare providers can meet their federal obligation for accommodating patients with communication disabilities.

_____

_____

_____

CERTIFICATION PREPARATION
Circle the correct answer.

1. What is a type of nonverbal communication?
   a. Body language
   b. Oral communication
   c. Email
   d. Letter

2. What is a type of verbal communication?
   a. Written message
   b. Oral communication
   c. Email
   d. All of the above

3. Hunger, pain, anger, and tiredness are considered which type of barrier to communication?
   a. Environmental distractions
   b. Internal distractions
   c. External distractions
   d. Hearing impairment

4. What is a way to overcome environmental distractions?
   a. Help make the patient comfortable.
   b. Use audio recording and large-print materials.
   c. Provide privacy for patients.
   d. Use pictures and models.

5. What is a maladaptive coping mechanism?
   a. Passive-aggressive behavior
   b. Drug and alcohol use
   c. Denial
   d. All of the above

6. Erikson's theory places a 4-year-old child in which developmental stage?
   a. Trust versus Mistrust
   b. Autonomy versus Shame and Doubt
   c. Initiative versus Guilt
   d. Industry versus Inferiority

7. According to Kübler-Ross, when a person feels sadness, fear, and uncertainty, he is in which stage of grief?
   a. Denial
   b. Anger
   c. Bargaining
   d. Depression

8. Which level of Maslow's Hierarchy of Needs includes protection from the elements, security, and stability?
   a. Physiologic needs
   b. Safety needs
   c. Love and belongingness needs
   d. Esteem needs

9. Which level of Maslow's Hierarchy of Needs includes knowledge, curiosity, understanding, and exploration?
   a. Cognitive needs
   b. Aesthetic needs
   c. Self-actualization needs
   d. Transcendence needs

10. A person is using which defense mechanism when she reverts to an old, immature behavior to express her feelings?
    a. Denial
    b. Repression
    c. Regression
    d. Displacement

WORKPLACE APPLICATIONS

1. When Christi was doing her orientation, she observed Sally rooming patients. With the patient seated in the room, Sally stood near the patient collecting the patient's information. She smiled occasionally as she talked with the patient. Christi noticed Sally had poor posture and yawned several times during the patient interview. At times, Sally used appropriate light touch with the patient and used small hand gestures. Describe the positive nonverbal behaviors that Christi observed.

    _____

    _____

    _____

    _____

2. Using #1 above, list the negative and closed nonverbal behaviors that Christi observed. For each type of negative behavior, indicate the correct positive and open behavior that should have been used.

    _____

    _____

    _____

3. Christi is following Samantha during orientation as they work with a Hmong provider. Most of the patients are Hmong. Describe specific cultural differences with nonverbal behaviors that would apply to the Hmong community.

    _____

    _____

    _____

INTERNET ACTIVITIES

1. Using online resources, research a specific culture different than your own. Create a poster presentation, a PowerPoint presentation, or write a paper summarizing your research. Include the following points in your project:
    a. Description of the culture (e.g., origin, typical family structure)
    b. Culture, beliefs, religion, and ethnic customs that influence healthcare discussions, treatments, and care
    c. Beliefs that impact verbal and nonverbal communication

2. Using online resources, research four cultures different than your own. Focus your research on cultural beliefs that impact communication in the healthcare environment. Create a poster presentation, a PowerPoint presentation, or write a paper summarizing your research. Include tips for a medical assistant to remember when working with a patient from each of the cultures.

3. Research Maslow's Hierarchy of Needs. Create a poster presentation, a PowerPoint presentation, or write a paper summarizing the theory and describe its importance to medical assistants. Cite two appropriate references used.

4. Research adaptive (healthy) and maladaptive (nonadaptive, unhealthy) coping mechanisms. Create a list of eight adaptive and eight maladaptive coping mechanisms. Discuss the importance of using adaptive coping mechanisms. Cite two appropriate references used.

Procedure 2.1   Use Feedback Techniques and Demonstrate Respect for Individual Diversity: Gender and Appearance

Name _____   Date _____   Score _____

Tasks: Use feedback techniques (e.g., reflection, restatement, and clarification) to obtain patient information. Respond to nonverbal communication. Communicate respectfully with patients with individual diversity related to gender and appearance. Demonstrate empathy, active listening, and nonverbal communication.

Background: When working with a transgender patient, ask the patient privately which pronouns the person prefers. Make sure to add this information into the patient's health record for future reference.

Scenario: You are rooming Crystal Green. You can see that she has expertly applied her makeup, has long red fingernails, long blonde hair, and is wearing three-inch heels. You are surprised to see that her birth gender is male. This is the first time you have roomed a transgender patient. You are uncomfortable in this situation because you have strong personal beliefs that birth gender should be maintained throughout a person's life.

Directions: Role-play the scenario with a peer, who will be the patient. You need to obtain a brief medical history on this patient (e.g., chief complaint [the main reason for the visit], allergies, the pregnancy history, and the current medications). Your peer (patient) should make up any information required. Use feedback techniques to obtain her information and respond to her nonverbal communication. Demonstrate empathy, active listening, and nonverbal communication.

Equipment and Supplies:
- Patient health record
- Rooming form (optional)
- Pen

Standard: Complete the procedure and all critical steps in _____ minutes with a minimum score of 85% within two attempts (*or as indicated by the instructor*).

Scoring: Divide the points earned by the total possible points. Failure to perform a critical step, indicated by an asterisk (*), results in grade no higher than an 84% (*or as indicated by the instructor*).

Time: Began_____   Ended_____   Total minutes: _____

Steps	Possible Points	Attempt 1	Attempt 2
1. Greet the patient. Identify yourself. Verify the patient's identity with full name and date of birth. Explain the procedure in a manner that is understood by the patient. Answer any questions the patient may have on the procedure.	10		
2. Demonstrate respect for the patient. *(Refer to the Affective Behaviors Checklist – **Respect** and the Grading Rubric)*	15*		
3. Using appropriate closed and open questions and statements, obtain the patient's chief complaint (main reason for the visit), allergies, pregnancy history, and current medications. Document the information in the health record or rooming form.	10		
4. Use feedback techniques, including reflection, restatement, and clarification as information is obtained.	10*		

5.	Respond to the patient's nonverbal communication by using feedback techniques (e.g., reflection). If the patient's nonverbal communication is interpreted differently than the patient's oral statements, clarify the information with the patient.	**10***		
6.	Use active listening skills. *(Refer to the Affective Behaviors Checklist –* ***Active Listening*** *and the Grading Rubric)*	**15***		
7.	Use professional, positive nonverbal communication behaviors. *(Refer to the Affective Behaviors Checklist –* ***Nonverbal Communication*** *and the Grading Rubric)*	**15***		
8.	Demonstrate empathy by listening to the patient and learning about his or her experiences and concerns. *(Refer to the Affective Behaviors Checklist –* ***Empathy*** *and the Grading Rubric)*	**15***		
	Total Score	**100**		

Affective Behavior	**Affective Behaviors Checklist** *Directions: Check behaviors observed during the role-play.*					
	Negative, Unprofessional Behaviors	**Attempt**		**Positive, Professional Behaviors**	**Attempt**	
Respect		**1**	**2**		**1**	**2**
	Rude, unkind, fake/false attitude, disrespectful, impolite, unwelcoming			Courteous, sincere, polite, welcoming		
	Unconcerned with person's dignity; brief, abrupt			Maintained person's dignity; took time with person		
	Unprofessional verbal communication; inappropriate questions			Professional verbal communication		
	Negative nonverbal behaviors, poor eye contact			Positive nonverbal behaviors, proper eye contact		
	Other:			Other:		
Active Listening	Biased, offensive			Remained neutral		
	Interrupted			Refrained from interrupting		
	Did not allow for silence or pauses			Allowed for periods of silence		
	Negative nonverbal behaviors (rolled eyes, yawned, frowned, avoided eye contact)			Positive nonverbal behaviors (smiled, nodded head, appropriate eye contact)		
	Distracted (looked at watch, phone)			Focused on patient, avoided distractions		
	Other:			Other:		

Nonverbal Communication	Muffled voice; too fast or slow of rate; too loud or too soft; unaccepting tone			Clear voice with moderate rate and volume; varying pitch; accepting or neutral tone		
	Incorrectly pronounced words; used words the person did not understand (e.g., medical terminology, generational phrases)			Correctly pronounced words; used words person can understand		
	Stood while patient was sitting; slouching, lack of poised posture			Was at the same position of the patient; had a poised posture		
	Frowned, lack of proper eye contact, inappropriate touch			Smiled, maintained proper eye contact, used light touch on hand when appropriate		
	Other:			Other:		
Empathy	Did not listen to patient's responses			Listened to patient; learn about patient		
	Lack of respect and support demonstrated			Showed respect and support		
	Lack of therapeutic communication techniques used			Used therapeutic communication techniques		
	Negative nonverbal behaviors (e.g., positioning, frowning, poor eye contact)			Positive nonverbal behaviors (e.g., at the same level as patient, smiled, good eye contact)		
	Other:			Other:		

Grading Rubric for the Affective Behaviors Checklist *Directions: Based on checklist results, identify the points received for the procedure checklist. Indicate how the behaviors demonstrated met the expectations.*		**Points for Procedure Checklist**	**Attempt 1**	**Attempt 2**
Does not meet Expectation	• Response lacked respect, active listening, professional nonverbal communication, and/or empathy. • Student demonstrated more than 2 negative, unprofessional behaviors during the interaction.	0		
Needs Improvement	• Response lacked respect, active listening, professional nonverbal communication, and/or empathy. • Student demonstrated 1 or 2 negative, unprofessional behaviors during the interaction.	0		
Meets Expectation	• Response was respectful and empathetic. Demonstrated active listening, professional nonverbal communication. No negative, unprofessional behaviors observed. • More practice is needed for behavior to appear natural and for student to appear comfortable and at ease.	15		

Occasionally Exceeds Expectation	• Response was respectful and empathetic. Demonstrated active listening, professional nonverbal communication. No negative, unprofessional behaviors observed. • At times student appeared comfortable and at ease; but more practice is needed for behavior to become natural and consistent with a professional medical assistant.	15		
Always Exceeds Expectation	• Response was respectful and empathetic. Demonstrated active listening, professional nonverbal communication. No negative, unprofessional behaviors observed. • Student's behaviors appeared natural and comfortable. Behaviors are consistent with a professional medical assistant.	15		

Comments

CAAHEP Competencies	**Step(s)**
V.A.3.a. Demonstrate respect for individual diversity including: gender	2
V.A.3.f. Demonstrate respect for individual diversity including: appearance	2
V.P.1.a. Use feedback techniques to obtain patient information including: reflection	4, 5
V.P.1.b. Use feedback techniques to obtain patient information including: restatement	4
V.P.1.c. Use feedback techniques to obtain patient information including: clarification	4
V.P.2. Respond to nonverbal communication	5
V.A.1.a. Demonstrate: empathy	8
V.A.1.b. Demonstrate: active listening	6
V.A.1.c. Demonstrate: nonverbal communication	7
ABHES Competencies	**Step(s)**
5.i. Display effective interpersonal skills with patients and health care team members	Entire role-play

Procedure 2.2   Use Feedback Techniques and Demonstrate Respect for Individual Diversity: Race

Name _____ Date _____ Score _____

Tasks: Use feedback techniques (e.g., reflection, restatement, and clarification) to obtain patient information. Respond to nonverbal communication. Communicate respectfully with patients with individual diversity related to race. Demonstrate empathy, active listening, and nonverbal communication.

Background: When working with an interpreter, allow time for the person to translate the information to the patient. Also, focus on the patient and do not look at the interpreter when speaking to the patient.

Scenario: You are rooming Maria Hernandez. She is always late for her appointments, and today she was 20 minutes late. She also does not speak English and you need to use a Spanish interpreter for the visit. You are uncomfortable in this situation because you have not worked with an interpreter before. You are also feeling rushed because she was late for her appointment.

Directions: Role-play the scenario with two peers. One peer is the patient and the other peer is the interpreter. While acting as the interpreter, the information can be repeated in English. You need to obtain a brief medical history on this patient (e.g., chief complaint [the main reason for the visit], allergies, the pregnancy history, and current medications). The peer (patient) should make up any information required. Use feedback techniques to obtain her information and respond to her nonverbal communication. Demonstrate empathy, active listening, and nonverbal communication.

Equipment and Supplies:
- Patient health record
- Rooming form (optional)
- Pen

Standard: Complete the procedure and all critical steps in _____ minutes with a minimum score of 85% within two attempts (*or as indicated by the instructor*).

Scoring: Divide the points earned by the total possible points. Failure to perform a critical step, indicated by an asterisk (*), results in grade no higher than an 84% (*or as indicated by the instructor*).

Time: Began _____ Ended _____ Total minutes: _____

Steps	Possible Points	Attempt 1	Attempt 2
1. Greet the patient. Identify yourself. Verify the patient's identity with full name and date of birth. Explain the procedure in a manner that is understood by the patient. Answer any questions the patient may have on the procedure.	10		
2. Demonstrate respect for the patient. (*Refer to the Affective Behaviors Checklist – **Respect** and the Grading Rubric*)	15*		
3. Using appropriate closed and open questions and statements, obtain the patient's chief complaint (main reason for the visit), allergies, pregnancy history, and current medications. Document the information in the health record or rooming form.	10		
4. Use feedback techniques including reflection, restatements, and clarification as information is obtained.	10*		

5.	Respond to the patient's nonverbal communication by using feedback techniques (e.g., reflection). If the patient's nonverbal communication is interpreted differently than the patient's oral statements, clarify the information with the patient.	**10***		
6.	Use active listening skills. *(Refer to the Affective Behaviors Checklist –* ***Active Listening*** *and the Grading Rubric)*	**15***		
7.	Use professional, positive nonverbal communication behaviors. *(Refer to the Affective Behaviors Checklist –* ***Nonverbal Communication*** *and the Grading Rubric)*	**15***		
8.	Demonstrate empathy by listening to the patient and learning about his or her experiences and concerns. *(Refer to the Affective Behaviors Checklist –* ***Empathy*** *and the Grading Rubric)*	**15***		
	Total Score	**100**		

Affective Behavior	**Affective Behaviors Checklist** *Directions:* Check behaviors observed during the role-play.					
Respect	**Negative, Unprofessional Behaviors**	**Attempt**		**Positive, Professional Behaviors**	**Attempt**	
		1	**2**		**1**	**2**
	Rude, unkind, fake/false attitude, disrespectful, impolite, unwelcoming			Courteous, sincere, polite, welcoming		
	Unconcerned with person's dignity; brief, abrupt			Maintained person's dignity; took time with person		
	Focused on the interpreter; rushed the conversation; did not give the patient and interpreter time to talk			Focused on the patient; gave adequate time for the patient and interpreter to respond		
	Unprofessional verbal communication; inappropriate questions			Professional verbal communication		
	Negative nonverbal behaviors, poor eye contact			Positive nonverbal behaviors, proper eye contact		
	Other:			Other:		
Active Listening	Biased, offensive			Remained neutral		
	Interrupted			Refrained from interrupting		
	Did not allow for silence or pauses			Allowed for periods of silence		
	Negative nonverbal behaviors (rolled eyes, yawned, frowned, avoided eye contact)			Positive nonverbal behaviors, smiled, nodded head, appropriate eye contact		
	Distracted (looked at watch, phone)			Focused on patient, avoided distractions		
	Other:			Other:		

Nonverbal Communication	Muffled voice; too fast or slow of rate; too loud or too soft; unaccepting tone			Clear voice with moderate rate and volume; varying pitch; accepting or neutral tone		
	Incorrectly pronounced words; used words the person did not understand (e.g., medical terminology, generational phrases)			Correctly pronounced words; used words person can understand		
	Stood while patient was sitting; slouching, lack of poised posture			Was at the same position as the patient; had a poised posture		
	Frowned, lack of proper eye contact, inappropriate touch			Smiled, maintained proper eye contact, used light touch on hand when appropriate		
	Other:			Other:		
Empathy	Did not listen to patient's responses			Listened to patient; learned about patient		
	Lack of respect and support demonstrated			Showed respect and support		
	Lack of therapeutic communication techniques used			Used therapeutic communication techniques		
	Negative nonverbal behaviors (e.g., positioning, frowning, poor eye contact)			Positive nonverbal behaviors (e.g., at the same level as patient, smiled, good eye contact)		
	Other:			Other:		

Grading Rubric for the Affective Behaviors Checklist *Directions: Based on checklist results, identify the points received for the procedure checklist. Indicate how the behaviors demonstrated met the expectations.*		**Points for Procedure Checklist**	**Attempt 1**	**Attempt 2**
Does not meet Expectation	• Response lacked respect, active listening, professional nonverbal communication, and/or empathy. • Student demonstrated more than 2 negative, unprofessional behaviors during the interaction.	0		
Needs Improvement	• Response lacked respect, active listening, professional nonverbal communication, and/or empathy. • Student demonstrated 1 or 2 negative, unprofessional behaviors during the interaction.	0		
Meets Expectation	• Response was respectful and empathetic. Demonstrated active listening, professional nonverbal communication. No negative, unprofessional behaviors observed. • More practice is needed for behavior to appear natural and for student to appear comfortable and at ease.	15		

Occasionally Exceeds Expectation	• Response was respectful and empathetic. Demonstrated active listening, professional nonverbal communication. No negative, unprofessional behaviors observed. • At times student appeared comfortable and at ease; but more practice is needed for behavior to become natural and consistent with a professional medical assistant.	15		
Always Exceeds Expectation	• Response was respectful and empathetic. Demonstrated active listening, professional nonverbal communication. No negative, unprofessional behaviors observed. • Student's behaviors appeared natural and comfortable. Behaviors are consistent with a professional medical assistant.	15		

Comments

CAAHEP Competencies	**Step(s)**
V.A.3.b. Demonstrate respect for individual diversity including: race	2
V.A.3.f. Demonstrate respect for individual diversity including: appearance	2
V.P.1.a. Use feedback techniques to obtain patient information including: reflection	4, 5
V.P.1.b. Use feedback techniques to obtain patient information including: restatement	4
V.P.1.c. Use feedback techniques to obtain patient information including: clarification	4
V.P.2. Respond to nonverbal communication	5
V.A.1.a. Demonstrate: empathy	8
V.A.1.b. Demonstrate: active listening	6
V.A.1.c. Demonstrate: nonverbal communication	7
ABHES Competencies	**Step(s)**
5.i. Display effective interpersonal skills with patients and health care team members	Entire role-play

Procedure 2.3 Demonstrate Respect for Individual Diversity: Religion and Appearance

Name _____ Date _____ Score _____

Tasks: Respond to nonverbal communication. Communicate respectfully with patients with individual diversity related to religion and appearance. Demonstrate empathy, active listening, and nonverbal communication.

Background: The Sikh religion was founded in Northern India. Sikhs believe in one God, the equality of men and women, justice, and community service. Turbans and kachera are worn at all times for religious reasons. Turbans or scarves cover the uncut hair. If the turban or scarf needs to be removed, an alternative head covering should be provided. The turban or scarf should be treated with respect. Placing it on the floor or near shoes would be a sign of disrespect. Kachera are undershorts/undergarments and at least one leg is to remain in the kachera at all times.

Scenario: You are preparing a patient for an examination. The patient is Sikh. The provider always wants the patient to completely undress, wear a gown, and be seated on the exam table before she comes into the room. You are uncomfortable in this situation because you have never worked with a patient who is Sikh.

Directions: Role-play the scenario with a peer. Instruct the peer (patient) how to prepare for the examination. Respond to the patient's nonverbal communication. Demonstrate empathy, active listening, and nonverbal communication.

Equipment and Supplies:
- Gown and drape sheet (optional)
- Exam table (optional)

Standard: Complete the procedure and all critical steps in _____ minutes with a minimum score of 85% within two attempts (*or as indicated by the instructor*).

Scoring: Divide the points earned by the total possible points. Failure to perform a critical step, indicated by an asterisk (*), results in grade no higher than an 84% (*or as indicated by the instructor*).

Time: Began_____ Ended_____ Total minutes: _____

Steps	Possible Points	Attempt 1	Attempt 2
1. Greet the patient. Identify yourself. Verify the patient's identity with full name and date of birth. Explain the procedure (undressing) in a manner that is understood by the patient. Answer any questions the patient may have on the procedure.	20		
2. Demonstrate respect for the patient. (*Refer to the Affective Behaviors Checklist – **Respect** and the Grading Rubric*)	15*		
3. Respond to the patient's nonverbal communication by using feedback techniques (e.g., reflection). If the patient's nonverbal communication is interpreted differently than the patient's oral statements, clarify the information with the patient.	20*		
4. Use active listening skills. (*Refer to the Affective Behaviors Checklist – **Active Listening** and the Grading Rubric*)	15*		
5. Use professional, positive nonverbal communication behaviors. (*Refer to the Affective Behaviors Checklist – **Nonverbal Communication** and the Grading Rubric*)	15*		
6. Demonstrate empathy by listening to the patient and learning about his or her experiences and concerns. (*Refer to the Affective Behaviors Checklist – **Empathy** and the Grading Rubric*)	15*		
Total Score	100		

Affective Behavior	Affective Behaviors Checklist *Directions:* Check behaviors observed during the role-play.					
Respect	**Negative, Unprofessional Behaviors**	**Attempt**		**Positive, Professional Behaviors**	**Attempt**	
		1	**2**		**1**	**2**
	Rude, unkind, fake/false attitude, disrespectful, impolite, unwelcoming			Courteous, sincere, polite, welcoming		
	Unconcerned with person's dignity; brief, abrupt			Maintained person's dignity; took time with person		
	Unprofessional verbal communication; inappropriate questions			Professional verbal communication		
	Negative nonverbal behaviors, poor eye contact			Positive nonverbal behaviors, proper eye contact		
	Other:			Other:		
Active Listening	Biased, offensive			Remained neutral		
	Interrupted			Refrained from interrupting		
	Did not allow for silence or pauses			Allowed for periods of silence		
	Negative nonverbal behaviors (rolled eyes, yawned, frowned, avoided eye contact)			Positive nonverbal behaviors, smiled, nodded head, appropriate eye contact		
	Distracted (looked at watch, phone)			Focused on patient, avoided distractions		
	Other:			Other:		
Nonverbal Communication	Muffled voice; too fast or slow of rate; too loud or too soft; unaccepting tone			Clear voice with moderate rate and volume; varying pitch; accepting or neutral tone		
	Incorrectly pronounced words; used words the person did not understand (e.g., medical terminology, generational phrases)			Correctly pronounced words; used words person can understand		
	Stood while patient was sitting; slouching, lack of poised posture			Was at the same position of the patient; had a poised posture		
	Frowned. Lack of proper eye contact. Inappropriate touch.			Smiled. Maintained proper eye contact. Used light touch on hand when appropriate.		
	Other:			Other:		

Empathy	Did not listen to patient's responses			Listened to patient; learned about patient		
	Lack of respect and support demonstrated			Showed respect and support		
	Lack of therapeutic communication techniques used			Used therapeutic communication techniques		
	Negative nonverbal behaviors (e.g., positioning, frowning, poor eye contact)			Positive nonverbal behaviors (e.g., at the same level as patient, smiled, good eye contact)		
	Other:			Other:		

Grading Rubric for the Affective Behaviors Checklist *Directions: Based on checklist results, identify the points received for the procedure checklist. Indicate how the behaviors demonstrated met the expectations.*		**Points for Procedure Checklist**	**Attempt 1**	**Attempt 2**
Does not meet Expectation	• Response lacked respect, active listening, professional nonverbal communication, and/or empathy. • Student demonstrated more than 2 negative, unprofessional behaviors during the interaction.	0		
Needs Improvement	• Response lacked respect, active listening, professional nonverbal communication, and/or empathy. • Student demonstrated 1 or 2 negative, unprofessional behaviors during the interaction.	0		
Meets Expectation	• Response was respectful and empathetic. Demonstrated active listening, professional nonverbal communication. No negative, unprofessional behaviors observed. • More practice is needed for behavior to appear natural and for student to appear comfortable and at ease.	15		
Occasionally Exceeds Expectation	• Response was respectful and empathetic. Demonstrated active listening, professional nonverbal communication. No negative, unprofessional behaviors observed. • At times student appeared comfortable and at ease; but more practice is needed for behavior to become natural and consistent with a professional medical assistant.	15		
Always Exceeds Expectation	• Response was respectful and empathetic. Demonstrated active listening, professional nonverbal communication. No negative, unprofessional behaviors observed. • Student's behaviors appeared natural and comfortable. Behaviors are consistent with a professional medical assistant.	15		

Comments

CAAHEP Competencies	Step(s)
V.A.3.c. Demonstrate respect for individual diversity including: religion	2
V.A.3.f. Demonstrate respect for individual diversity including: appearance	2
V.P.2. Respond to nonverbal communication	3
V.A.1.a. Demonstrate: empathy	6
V.A.1.b. Demonstrate: active listening	4
V.A.1.c. Demonstrate: nonverbal communication	5
ABHES Competencies	**Step(s)**
5.i. Display effective interpersonal skills with patients and health care team members	Entire role-play

Procedure 2.4 Use Feedback Techniques and Demonstrate Respect for Individual Diversity: Age, Economic Status, and Appearance

Name _____ Date _____ Score _____

Tasks: Use feedback techniques (e.g., reflection, restatement, and clarification) to obtain patient information. Respond to nonverbal communication. Communicate respectfully with patients with individual diversity related to age, economic status, and appearance. Demonstrate empathy, active listening, and nonverbal communication.

Scenario: You are rooming Mr. Abraham Black (79 years old), who has recently been diagnosed with dementia. He likes to talk about things that happened long before you were born, and you are not interested in those events. He also has a hard time hearing your questions and you frequently repeat questions. Mr. Black has poor personal hygiene. His clothes are dirty and torn. He has an unpleasant body odor. Mr. Black tells you he can't afford to eat if he buys his medications. He doesn't believe in government programs and refuses to take "handouts." You have worked with Mr. Black in the past and have heard this all before numerous times. You would prefer to work with the younger generation and with patients who have better hygiene.

Directions: Role-play the scenario with a peer, who will be the patient. You need to obtain a brief medical history on this patient (e.g., chief complaint [the main reason for the visit], allergies, and the current medications). The peer (patient) should make up any information required. Use feedback techniques to obtain his information and respond to his nonverbal communication. Demonstrate empathy, active listening, and nonverbal communication.

Equipment and Supplies:
- Patient health record
- Rooming form (optional)
- Pen

Standard: Complete the procedure and all critical steps in _____ minutes with a minimum score of 85% within two attempts (*or as indicated by the instructor*).

Scoring: Divide the points earned by the total possible points. Failure to perform a critical step, indicated by an asterisk (*), results in grade no higher than an 84% (*or as indicated by the instructor*).

Time: Began_____ Ended_____ Total minutes: _____

Steps	Possible Points	Attempt 1	Attempt 2
1. Greet the patient. Identify yourself. Verify the patient's identity with full name and date of birth. Explain the procedure in a manner that is understood by the patient. Answer any questions the patient may have on the procedure.	10		
2. Demonstrate respect for the patient. (*Refer to the Affective Behaviors Checklist – **Respect** and the Grading Rubric*)	15*		
3. Using appropriate closed and open questions and statements, obtain the patient's chief complaint (main reason for the visit), allergies, and current medications. Document the information in the health record or rooming form.	10		
4. Use feedback techniques including reflection, restatement, and clarification as information is obtained.	10*		

5.	Respond to the patient's nonverbal communication by using feedback techniques (e.g., reflection). If the patient's nonverbal communication is interpreted differently than the patient's oral statements, clarify the information with the patient.	**10***		
6.	Use active listening skills. *(Refer to the Affective Behaviors Checklist – **Active Listening** and the Grading Rubric)*	**15***		
7.	Use professional, positive nonverbal communication behaviors. *(Refer to the Affective Behaviors Checklist – **Nonverbal Communication** and the Grading Rubric)*	**15***		
8.	Demonstrate empathy by listening to the patient and learning about his or her experiences and concerns. *(Refer to the Affective Behaviors Checklist – **Empathy** and the Grading Rubric)*	**15***		
	Total Score	**100**		

Affective Behavior	Affective Behaviors Checklist *Directions: Check behaviors observed during the role-play.*					
Respect	**Negative, Unprofessional Behaviors**	**Attempt**		**Positive, Professional Behaviors**	**Attempt**	
		1	**2**		**1**	**2**
	Rude, unkind, fake/false attitude, disrespectful, impolite, unwelcoming			Courteous, sincere, polite, welcoming		
	Unconcerned with person's dignity; brief, abrupt			Maintained person's dignity; took time with person		
	Unprofessional verbal communication; inappropriate questions			Professional verbal communication		
	Negative nonverbal behaviors, poor eye contact			Positive nonverbal behaviors, proper eye contact		
	Other:			Other:		
Active Listening	Biased, offensive			Remained neutral		
	Interrupted			Refrained from interrupting		
	Did not allow for silence or pauses			Allowed for periods of silence		
	Negative nonverbal behaviors (rolled eyes, yawned, frowned, avoided eye contact)			Positive nonverbal behaviors (smiled, nodded head, appropriate eye contact)		
	Distracted (looked at watch, phone)			Focused on patient, avoided distractions		
	Other:			Other:		

Nonverbal Communication	Muffled voice; too fast or slow of rate; too loud or too soft; unaccepting tone			Clear voice with moderate rate and volume; varying pitch; accepting or neutral tone			
	Incorrectly pronounced words; used words the person did not understand (e.g., medical terminology, generational phrases)			Correctly pronounced words; used words person can understand			
	Stood while patient was sitting; slouching, lack of poised posture			Was at the same position of the patient; had a poised posture			
	Frowned. Lack of proper eye contact. Inappropriate touch.			Smiled. Maintained proper eye contact. Used light touch on hand when appropriate.			
	Other:			Other:			
Empathy	Did not listen to patient's responses			Listened to patient; learned about patient			
	Lack of respect and support demonstrated			Showed respect and support			
	Lack of therapeutic communication techniques used			Used therapeutic communication techniques			
	Negative nonverbal behaviors (e.g., positioning, frowning, poor eye contact)			Positive nonverbal behaviors (e.g., at the same level as patient, smiled, good eye contact)			
	Other:			Other:			

Grading Rubric for the Affective Behaviors Checklist *Directions: Based on checklist results, identify the points received for the procedure checklist. Indicate how the behaviors demonstrated met the expectations.*	**Points for Procedure Checklist**	**Attempt 1**	**Attempt 2**
Does not meet Expectation <ul><li>Response lacked respect, active listening, professional nonverbal communication, and/or empathy.</li><li>Student demonstrated more than 2 negative, unprofessional behaviors during the interaction.</li></ul>	0		
Needs Improvement <ul><li>Response lacked respect, active listening, professional nonverbal communication, and/or empathy.</li><li>Student demonstrated 1 or 2 negative, unprofessional behaviors during the interaction.</li></ul>	0		
Meets Expectation <ul><li>Response was respectful and empathetic. Demonstrated active listening, professional nonverbal communication. No negative, unprofessional behaviors observed.</li><li>More practice is needed for behavior to appear natural and for student to appear comfortable and at ease.</li></ul>	15		

Occasionally Exceeds Expectation	• Response was respectful and empathetic. Demonstrated active listening, professional nonverbal communication. No negative, unprofessional behaviors observed. • At times student appeared comfortable and at ease; but more practice is needed for behavior to become natural and consistent with a professional medical assistant.	15		
Always Exceeds Expectation	• Response was respectful and empathetic. Demonstrated active listening, professional nonverbal communication. No negative, unprofessional behaviors observed. • Student's behaviors appeared natural and comfortable. Behaviors are consistent with a professional medical assistant.	15		

Comments

CAAHEP Competencies	Step(s)
V.A.3.d. Demonstrate respect for individual diversity including: age	2
V.A.3.e. Demonstrate respect for individual diversity including: economic status	2
V.A.3.f. Demonstrate respect for individual diversity including: appearance	2
V.P.1.a. Use feedback techniques to obtain patient information including: reflection	4, 5
V.P.1.b. Use feedback techniques to obtain patient information including: restatement	4
V.P.1.c. Use feedback techniques to obtain patient information including: clarification	4
V.P.2. Respond to nonverbal communication	5
V.A.1.a. Demonstrate: empathy	8
V.A.1.b. Demonstrate: active listening	6
V.A.1.c. Demonstrate: nonverbal communication	7
ABHES Competencies	**Step(s)**
5.i. Display effective interpersonal skills with patients and health care team members	Entire role-play

Legal Principles

CAAHEP Competencies	Assessment
X.C.1. Differentiate between scope of practice and standards of care for medical assistants	Skills and Concepts – G. 2
X.C.2. Compare and contrast provider and medical assistant roles in terms of standard of care	Skills and Concepts – D. 12
X.C.4. Summarize the Patient Bill of Rights	Skills and Concepts – F. 1
X.C.5. Discuss licensure and certification as they apply to healthcare providers	Skills and Concepts – G. 1 a-c
X.C.6. Compare criminal and civil law as they apply to the practicing medical assistant	Skills and Concepts – C. 2-9
X.C.7.a. Define: negligence	Vocabulary Review – G. 3; Skills and Concepts – D. 7
X.C.7.b. Define: malpractice	Vocabulary Review – G. 4; Skills and Concepts – D. 9
X.C.7.c. Define: statute of limitations	Vocabulary Review – G. 5; Certification Preparation – 2
X.C.8.a. Describe the following types of insurance: liability	Vocabulary Review – G. 11
X.C.8.b. Describe the following types of insurance: professional (malpractice)	Vocabulary Review – G. 12-13
X.C.8.c. Describe the following types of insurance: personal injury	Vocabulary Review – G. 14
X.C.13.a. Define the following medical legal terms: informed consent	Vocabulary Review – G. 20
X.C.13.b. Define the following medical legal terms: implied consent	Vocabulary Review – G. 18; Certification Preparation – 10
X.C.13.c. Define the following medical legal terms: expressed consent	Vocabulary Review – G. 19; Certification Preparation – 10
X.C.13.d. Define the following medical legal terms: patient incompetence	Vocabulary Review – G. 15
X.C.13.e. Define the following medical legal terms: emancipated minor	Vocabulary Review – G. 16
X.C.13.f. Define the following medical legal terms: mature minor	Vocabulary Review – G. 21; Certification Preparation – 8

CAAHEP Competencies	Assessment
X.C.13.g. Define the following medical legal terms: subpoena duces tecum	Vocabulary Review – G. 9; Certification Preparation – 6
X.C.13.h. Define the following medical legal terms: respondeat superior	Vocabulary Review – G. 17; Certification Preparation – 9
X.C.13.i. Define the following medical legal terms: res ipsa loquitur	Vocabulary Review – G. 10; Skills and Concepts – C. 26
X.C.13.j. Define the following medical legal terms: locum tenens	Vocabulary Review – G. 22; Certification Preparation – 7
X.C.13.k. Define the following medical legal terms: defendant-plaintiff	Vocabulary Review – G. 1-2
X.C.13.l. Define the following medical legal terms: deposition	Vocabulary Review – G. 8
X.C.13.m. Define the following medical legal terms: arbitration-mediation	Vocabulary Review – G. 6-7; Skills and Concepts – D. 21; Certification Preparation – 1
X.P.1. Locate a state's legal scope of practice for medical assistants	Procedure 3.2
X.P.4.a. Apply the Patient's Bill of Rights as it relates to: choice of treatment	Procedure 3.1
X.P.4.b. Apply the Patient's Bill of Rights as it relates to: consent for treatment	Procedure 3.1
X.P.4.c. Apply the Patient's Bill of Rights as it relates to: refusal of treatment	Procedure 3.1
X.A.1. Demonstrate sensitivity to patient rights	Procedure 3.1
ABHES Competencies	**Assessment**
4. Medical Law and Ethics c. Follow established policies when initiating or terminating medical treatment	Skills and Concepts – E. 7
4.d. Distinguish between employer and personal liability coverage	Vocabulary Review – G. 12-14 Skills and Concepts – D. 29
4.f. Comply with federal, state, and local health laws and regulations 1) Define the scope of practice for the medical assistant within the state where employed	Procedure 3.2
4.f.2) Describe what procedures can and cannot be delegated to the medical assistant and by whom within various employment settings	Skills and Concepts – G. 3 a-f

21. Describe the two types of alternative dispute resolution. _____

_____

_____

22. What is a summary judgment and why is it used? _____

_____

_____

23. Describe the four "Ds" or four elements that must be proven in malpractice cases. _____

_____

_____

_____

24. Briefly describe the stages of a civil lawsuit. _____

_____

_____

_____

25. Discuss the difference between an expert witness and a fact witness. _____

_____

_____

_____

26. Describe *res ipsa loquitur* and when it is used. _____

_____

_____

_____

27. _____ are large payments made to the plaintiff by the defendant, meant to punish the defendant.

28. _____ are a monetary payment for losses suffered.

29. Describe general liability or commercial liability insurance. _____

_____

_____

30. _____ are monetary payments for emotional pain and anguish.

31. A(n) _____ covers for claims that are made during the policy year, whereas _____ covers claims for lawful acts that occurred during the policy year.

E. Contracts

1. Describe the difference between implied contracts and expressed contracts._____

   _____

2. Describe the statute of frauds and give three types of contracts to which it applies. _____

   _____

   _____

3. Describe the five elements required for a legally binding contract. _____

   _____

   _____

   _____

4. Name three conditions related to competency and capacity that would invalidate a contract._____

   _____

5. Name four benefits of becoming an emancipated minor. _____

   _____

   _____

6. List three reasons providers terminate the provider-patient relationship. _____

   _____

   _____

7. Describe the process of terminating the provider-patient relationship._____

   _____

   _____

   _____

8. Providers can be charged with _____ if they do not follow the proper termination procedure.

9. How can a medical assistant protect the provider from charges of patient abandonment? _____

   _____

   _____

10. List three ways breach of contract can occur in healthcare. _____

   _____

   _____

   _____

11. List the seven elements that must be present for informed consent. _____

_____

_____

_____

12. List five types of patients who can give informed consent. _____

_____

_____

13. List four types of patients who cannot give informed consent. _____

_____

_____

14. Describe the medical assistant's role in informed consent. _____

_____

_____

F. Patient's Bill of Rights

1. Summarize the Patient's Bill of Rights. _____

_____

_____

_____

_____

2. A patient refuses an injection of medication ordered by the provider. Describe the steps that need to be followed by the medical assistant.

_____

_____

_____

_____

G. Practice Requirements

1. Describe the licensure and certification for the following healthcare professionals:

    a. Doctor of medicine (MD) and doctor of osteopathy (DO): _____

_____

b. Physician assistant (PA):_____

_____

c. Nurse practitioner (NP): _____

_____

d. Medical assistant (MA): _____

_____

e. Registered nurse (RN) and licensed practical nurse (LPN): _____

_____

2. Differentiate between the scope of practice and standard of care for medical assistants._____

_____

_____

_____

3. For the following activities, identify if the medical assistant could be delegated (assigned) by the provider to do the activity. Write "yes" on the line if the medical assistant could be delegated the activity. Write "no" on the line if the medical assistant could not do the activity.

a. Prepare the informed consent paperwork. _____

b. Discuss the procedure with the patient for the informed consent. _____

c. Prepare waived laboratory testing. _____

d. Answer phone calls. _____

e. Prescribe medications for the patient's condition. _____

f. Diagnose the patient's condition. _____

CERTIFICATION PREPARATION
Circle the correct answer.

1. Which is a type of alternative dispute resolution where the final decision is legally binding?
    a. Dereliction
    b. Mediation
    c. Arbitration
    d. Summary judgment

2. Which varies by state and indicates the length of time legal action can be taken after an event has occurred?
    a. *Res judicata*
    b. *Res ipsa loquitur*
    c. Release of tortfeasor
    d. Statute of limitations

3. Which is a negligent act classification that means the person failed to act when he or she had a legal duty to act?
    a. Misfeasance
    b. Nonfeasance
    c. Malpractice
    d. Malfeasance

4. Which type of defense involves the defendant admitting wrongdoing and the defense attorney introduces facts that support the defendant's conduct?
    a. Denial defense
    b. Comparative defense
    c. Technical defense
    d. Affirmative defense

5. Which is not one of the "Ds" of negligence?
   a. Duty of care
   b. Dereliction
   c. Deposition
   d. Damages

6. Which is a legal document ordering a person to bring the plaintiff's health record to court?
   a. Subpoena
   b. *Subpoena duces tecum*
   c. *Res ipsa loquitur*
   d. Statute of limitations

7. Which is a physician or advanced-practice professional temporarily contracted to provide healthcare services when a facility has a vacancy, vacation, or a leave of absence?
   a. Telemedicine
   b. Injunction
   c. *Respondeat superior*
   d. *Locum tenens*

8. A person younger than the age of adulthood who demonstrates the maturity to make a personal healthcare decision and can give informed consent for treatment is called a(n)
   a. mature minor.
   b. emancipated minor.
   c. incompetence.
   d. *respondeat superior*.

9. Which means "let the master answer;" thus, the employer/provider is legally responsible for the wrongful actions or lack of actions of the employees if done within the scope of employment?
   a. Tortfeasor
   b. *Res ipsa loquitur*
   c. *Respondeat superior*
   d. *Res judicata*

10. _____ consent is inferred based on signs or conduct of the patient, whereas _____ is given either by the spoken or written word.
    a. Implied; informed
    b. Informed; expressed
    c. Implied; expressed
    d. Expressed; informed

WORKPLACE APPLICATIONS

1. Cara was just graduating from a medical assistant program and decided to take out a professional liability insurance policy. She wants a policy that she can stop paying at retirement and will still be covered for past situations. Describe what type of policy she should purchase.

   _____

   _____

   _____

   _____

2. Dr. Smith and Dr. Brown are family practice providers who trained at the same college. Dr. Smith practices in Los Angeles, CA and Dr. Brown practices in Bayfield, WI (a city of 475 people). Would the standard of care be the same for these two family practice providers? Explain your answer.

   _____

   _____

   _____

3. Jane is a medical assistant who works with Dr. Walden. She identifies herself as "Dr. Walden's nurse" to patients. Discuss how this might impact the standard of care.

_____

_____

4. Ken Thomas was notified by a medical supplier that the mesh that was used for his hernia surgery was faulty. They paid Ken a monetary compensation after Ken signed a release to give up the right to sue the company in the future. Five years later, Ken had to go through surgery to remove the mesh. Ken wanted to sue the company for his pain and suffering. What technical defense would be used to prevent the lawsuit? Discuss this technical defense.

_____

_____

_____

5. Bella, a new CMA, is working with a patient who is undergoing minor surgery. The provider explained the procedure and stepped out of the room. She needs to get the informed consent form signed. When she asks the patient if she has any questions before signing, the patient states she does. How should Bella handle this situation?

_____

_____

_____

INTERNET ACTIVITIES

1. Using the internet, find a local healthcare facility that has their Patient's Bill of Rights posted online. Create a poster presentation or a PowerPoint presentation summarizing the areas addressed in the facility's Patient's Bill of Rights.

2. Using online resources, research how an MD and/or DO can renew his or her license in your state. Write a brief summary of what is required to renew a medical doctor's license in your state. Cite the website(s) used.

3. Credentialed medical assistants need to maintain their credentials through continuing education. Using online resources, identify two sites that offer continuing education for medical assistants. Briefly summarize your findings and cite the websites used.

Procedure 3.1 Apply the Patient's Bill of Rights

Name _____ Date _____ Score _____

Tasks: Apply the patient's bill of rights in scenarios related to choice of treatment, consent for treatment, and refusal of treatment. Demonstrate sensitivity to patient rights.

Scenario 1 (Choice of treatment): Julia Berkley (DOB 7/5/1992) was a patient of Dr. Angela Perez during her entire pregnancy. Julia is experiencing some complications. Dr. Perez explained the choices Julia had for delivery. She stated with the complications, a C-section may be the best option. You are working with Dr. Perez and prepared the consent form for the C-section. You go into the exam room to have Julia sign the consent form. As you discuss the form, Julia tells you that she is fearful of a C-section and wants a vaginal delivery.

Scenario 2 (Consent for treatment): Ken Thomas (DOB 10/25/61) saw Jean Burke N.P. before leaving on a week-long trip out of the country. He is leaving in 3 days and wants a hepatitis A vaccine injection. The area he is traveling to has a high risk for hepatitis A. Jean Burke orders immunoglobulin for Ken, which will provide immediate protection against hepatitis A. You prepare the injection and enter the exam room. As you are telling Ken about the side effects of the medication, he asks, "What is immunoglobulin?" You reply that it is a sterile medication made of antibodies from blood. Ken states that he is a Jehovah's Witness and cannot receive blood products.

Scenario 3 (Refusal of treatment): Aaron Jackson (DOB 10/17/2011) was in for his well-child check. His records indicate that he is due for his first varicella vaccine. You bring the Varicella (Chickenpox) Vaccine VIS (vaccine information statement) and the Vaccine Authorization form to the exam room. As you start discussing the vaccine, Aaron's mother, Patricia, interrupts you and tells you she is not interested in having Aaron get his chickenpox vaccine.

Equipment and Supplies:
- Patient health records
- Patient's Bill of Rights (Figure 3.3)
- General Procedure Consent form (Figure 3.4)
- Varicella (Chickenpox) VIS (available at www.cdc.gov)
- Vaccine Authorization form (Figure 3.5)

Standard: Complete the procedure and all critical steps in _____ minutes with a minimum score of 85% within two attempts (*or as indicated by the instructor*).

Scoring: Divide the points earned by the total possible points. Failure to perform a critical step, indicated by an asterisk (*), results in grade no higher than an 84% (*or as indicated by the instructor*).

Time: Began_____ Ended_____ Total minutes: _____

Steps:	Point Value	Attempt 1	Attempt 2
1. Review the Patient's Bill of Rights. Apply the Patient's Bill of Rights as you role-play each of the three scenarios.	**10***		
2. Using Scenario #1, role-play the situation with a peer. You are the medical assistant. Demonstrate how a medical assistant should handle the situation. Apply the Patient's Bill of Rights to the situation by remembering the rights of the patient. a. Show sensitivity to the patient by being respective and professional. *(Refer to the Checklist for Affective Behaviors.)*	**10***		
b. Ask the patient if she has any questions about the procedures. Let the provider know if the patient has questions.	**10**		
c. Ask the patient what she would like to do. Based on her answer, follow up as necessary.	**10***		
d. Using the health record, document the patient's decision and the name of the provider notified.	**5**		
3. Using Scenario #2, role-play the situation with a peer. You are the medical assistant. Demonstrate how a medical assistant should handle the situation. Apply the Patient's Bill of Rights to the situation by remembering the rights of the patient. a. Show sensitivity to the patient regarding his right to refuse. Be accepting of his beliefs and his refusal. *(Refer to the Checklist for Affective Behaviors.)*	**10***		
b. When the patient refuses the medication, be respectful in your body language and words. Notify the provider.	**10***		
c. Using the health record, document the patient's decision and the name of the provider notified.	**5**		
4. Using Scenario #3, role-play the situation with a peer. You are the medical assistant. Demonstrate how a medical assistant should handle the situation. Apply the Patient's Bill of Rights to the situation by remembering the rights of the patient. a. Show sensitivity to the mother of the patient by being respectful and professional. *(Refer to the Checklist for Affective Behaviors.)*	**10***		
b. Ask the mother if she has any questions about the vaccine. Let the provider know if the mother has questions.	**5**		
c. Ask the mother what she would like to do. Based on her answer, follow up as necessary.	**10***		
d. Using the health record, document the mother's decision and the name of the provider notified.	**5**		
Total Points	**100**		

Checklist for Affective Behaviors

Affective Behavior	Directions: Check behaviors observed during the role-play.					
Sensitivity	**Negative, Unprofessional Behaviors**	**Attempt**		**Positive, Professional Behaviors**	**Attempt**	
		1	**2**		**1**	**2**
	Poor eye contact			Proper eye contact		
	Distracted; not focused on the other person			Focuses full attention on the other person		
	Judgmental attitude; not accepting attitude			Nonjudgmental, accepting attitude		
	Fails to clarify what the person verbally or nonverbally communicated			Uses summarizing or paraphrasing to clarify what the person verbally or nonverbally communicated		
	Fails to acknowledge what the person communicated			Acknowledges what the person communicated		
	Rude, discourteous			Pleasant and courteous		
	Disregards the person's dignity and rights			Maintains the person's dignity and rights		
	Other:			Other:		

Grading for Affective Behaviors		**Point Value**	**Attempt 1**	**Attempt 2**
Does not meet Expectation	• Response lacked sensitivity. • Student demonstrated more than 2 negative, unprofessional behaviors during the interaction.	**0**		
Needs Improvement	• Response lacked sensitivity. • Student demonstrated 1 or 2 negative, unprofessional behaviors during the interaction.	**0**		
Meets Expectation	• Response was sensitive; no negative, unprofessional behaviors observed. • More practice is needed for behavior to appear natural and for student to appear comfortable and at ease.	**10**		
Occasionally Exceeds Expectation	• Response was sensitive; no negative, unprofessional behaviors observed. • At times student appeared comfortable and at ease; but more practice is needed for behavior to become natural and consistent with a professional medical assistant.	**10**		
Always Exceeds Expectation	• Response was sensitive; no negative, unprofessional behaviors observed. • Student's behaviors appeared natural and comfortable. Behaviors are consistent with a professional medical assistant.	**10**		

Documentation – Scenario 1

Documentation – Scenario 2

Documentation – Scenario 3

Comments

CAAHEP Competencies	Steps
X.P.4.a. Apply the Patient's Bill of Rights as it relates to: choice of treatment	1, 2 a-d
X.P.4.b. Apply the Patient's Bill of Rights as it relates to: consent for treatment	1, 3 a-c
X.P.4.c. Apply the Patient's Bill of Rights as it relates to: refusal of treatment	1, 4 a-d
X.A.1. Demonstrate sensitivity to patient rights	2 a, 3 a, 4 a

Procedure 3.2   Locate the Medical Assistant's Legal Scope of Practice

Name _____ Date _____ Score _____

Tasks: Locate the legal scope of practice for a medical assistant practicing in your state. Summarize the scope of practice.

Equipment and Supplies:
• Computer and printer with word processing software and internet access

Standard: Complete the procedure and all critical steps with a minimum score of 85% within two attempts (*or as indicated by the instructor*).

Scoring: Divide the points earned by the total possible points. Failure to perform a critical step, indicated by an asterisk (*), results in grade no higher than an 84% (*or as indicated by the instructor*).

Steps:	Point Value	Attempt 1	Attempt 2
1. Using the internet, search for the medical assistant's scope of practice in your state. Read the scope of practice for your state.	20		
2. Using the word processing software, create a short paper summarizing the medical assistant's scope of practice. Address the following points: a. Can medical assistants give injections? If so, what type of injections? b. Can medical assistants give oral, topical, and/or inhaled medications? c. Can medical assistants calculate drug dosages? d. What is the medical assistant's role with prescriptions? e. Describe additional duties that a medical assistant can legally do in your state. f. Include the website address(es) you used for this paper. *Note:* If your instructor does not provide you with different guidelines for the paper, follow these. Create at least a one-page paper, using double line spacing and a 10-12 point font. Margins should be 1" for all sides.	70		
3. After completing the paper, proofread it. Use correct spelling, punctuation, sentence structure, and capitalization. Make any changes required. Based on your instructor's directions, submit the paper to the instructor.	10		
Total Points	100		

Comments

CAAHEP Competencies	Step(s)
X.P.1. Locate a state's legal scope of practice for medical assistants	Entire procedure
ABHES Competencies	**Step(s)**
4.f.1 Define the scope of practice for the medical assistant within the state where employed	Entire procedure

Healthcare Laws

CAAHEP Competencies	Assessment
X.C.3. Describe components of the Health Information Portability & Accountability Act (HIPAA)	Skills and Concepts – B. 2-7, 13-14; Certification Preparation – 4-7; Workplace Application 1 a-d, 2-3
X.C.7.d. Define: Good Samaritan Act(s)	Skills and Concepts – C. 16-18; Certification Preparation – 1
X.C.7.e. Define: Uniform Anatomical Gift Act	Skills and Concepts – C. 21; Certification Preparation – 2
X.C.7.h. Define: Patient Self Determination Act (PSDA)	Skills and Concepts – C. 19; Certification Preparation – 1
X.C.7.i. Define: risk management	Skills and Concepts – D. 28
X.C.9. List and discuss legal and illegal applicant interview questions	Skills and Concepts – D. 20-22; Certification Preparation – 9
X.C.10.a. Identify: Health Information Technology for Economic and Clinical Health (HITECH) Act	Skills and Concepts – B. 15-17
X.C.10.b. Identify: Genetic Information Nondiscrimination Act of 2008 (GINA)	Skills and Concepts – B. 18-19, D. 19
X.C.10.c. Identify: Americans with Disabilities Act Amendments Act (ADAAA)	Skills and Concepts – D. 23; Certification Preparation – 10
X.C.11.a. Describe the process in compliance reporting: unsafe activities	Skills and Concepts – D. 24
X.C.11.b. Describe the process in compliance reporting: errors in patient care	Skills and Concepts – D. 29
X.C.11.c. Describe the process in compliance reporting: conflicts of interest	Skills and Concepts – D. 11-12
X.C.11.d. Describe the process in compliance reporting: incident reports	Skills and Concepts – D. 25-27
X.C.12.a. Describe compliance with public health statutes: communicable diseases	Skills and Concepts – D. 2 a-d
X.C.12.b. Describe compliance with public health statutes: abuse, neglect, and exploitation	Skills and Concepts – D. 5-7; Workplace Application – 4
X.C.12.c. Describe compliance with public health statutes: wounds of violence	Skills and Concepts – D. 3-4

CAAHEP Competencies	Assessment
X.C.13.n. Define the following medical legal terms: Good Samaritan laws	Skills and Concepts – C. 16-18
X.P.2.a. Apply HIPAA rules in regard to: privacy	Procedure 4.1
X.P.2.b. Apply HIPAA rules in regard to: release of information	Procedure 4.2
X.P.5. Perform compliance reporting based on public health statutes	Procedure 4.3
X.P.6. Report an illegal activity in the healthcare setting following proper protocol	Procedure 4.4
X.P.7. Complete an incident report related to an error in patient care	Procedure 4.5
X.A.1. Demonstrate sensitivity to patient rights	Procedure 4.1

ABHES Competencies	Assessment
4. Medical Law and Ethics b. Institute federal and state guidelines when: 1) Releasing medical records or information	Procedure 4.1, 4.2
4.b.2) Entering orders in and utilizing electronic health records	Procedure 4.3
4.e. Perform risk management procedures	Procedure 4.5
4.f. Comply with federal, state, and local health laws and regulations as they relate to healthcare settings	Procedure 4.1, 4.2, 4.3, 4.4
4.h. Demonstrate compliance with HIPAA guidelines, the ADA Amendments Act, and the Health Information Technology for Economic and Clinical Health (HITECH) Act	Procedure 4.1, 4.2

3. Describe how a provider complies with the public health statutes related to wounds of violence.

   _____

   _____

4. Typically, statutes related to wounds of violence require what types of wounds to be reported?

   _____

5. Describe how a provider complies with the public health statutes related to abuse, neglect, and exploitation of children.

   _____

   _____

6. Describe how a provider complies with the public health statutes related to abuse, neglect, and exploitation of the elderly and dependent adults.

   _____

   _____

7. How does a provider handle domestic abuse situations? _____

   _____

   _____

   _____

8. When a patient is having unusual side effects from a vaccine, the provider or patient/family can file a report to the _____.

9. The _____ created the National Vaccine Injury Compensation Program that provides compensation for children injured by childhood vaccines.

10. A(n) _____ or corporate compliance is a program within a business that detects and prevents violations of state and federal laws.

11. Describe what is meant by *conflict of interest*. _____

    _____

12. Describe the process of compliance reporting related to conflicts of interest. _____

    _____

13. The _____ prohibits intentionally receiving or giving anything of value to get referrals or generate federal healthcare program business.

14. The _____ prohibits a person from submitting false or fraudulent Medicare or Medicaid claims for payment.

15. The _____ prohibits a healthcare provider from referring a Medicare patient for services to a facility in which the provider or the provider's immediate family has a financial relationship.

16. The _____ prohibits intentionally defrauding any healthcare benefit program.

17. Describe how the medical assistant should address workplace violations. _____

_____

_____

18. The _____ prohibits employment discrimination based on color, race, gender, religion, or national origin.

19. The Genetic Information Nondiscrimination Act of 2008 prohibits employment discrimination based on the _____.

20. Describe four interview topics that can put a facility at risk for discrimination lawsuits. _____

_____

_____

_____

21. List three legal interview questions. _____

_____

_____

_____

22. List three illegal interview questions. _____

_____

_____

_____

23. Describe the Americans with Disabilities Act Amendments Act (ADAAA). _____

_____

_____

24. Describe the process in compliance reporting for unsafe activities. _____

_____

_____

25. Name four reasons to complete an incident report. _____

_____

_____

26. What is an incident report and what are its purposes? _____

_____

_____

27. Describe the process in compliance reporting related to incident reports. (When completing an incident report, describe three points a medical assistant should remember.)

_____

_____

_____

28. Define *risk management*. _____

_____

29. The wrong medication was given to the patient. Describe the process in compliance reporting with errors in patient care.

_____

_____

_____

CERTIFICATION PREPARATION
Circle the correct answer.

1. Which state law provides legal protection for those assisting an injured person during an emergency?
   a. Uniform Anatomical Gift Act
   b. Good Samaritan Act
   c. Patient Self-Determination Act
   d. GINA

2. Which act makes organ donation easier?
   a. Uniform Determination of Death Act
   b. National Organ Transplant Act
   c. Uniform Anatomical Gift Act
   d. Patient Self-Determination Act

3. Which act requires most healthcare institutions to inform patients of their rights to make decisions and the facility's policies about advance directives?
   a. Uniform Determination of Death Act
   b. National Organ Transplant Act
   c. Uniform Anatomical Gift Act
   d. Patient Self-Determination Act

4. Which HIPAA standard requires healthcare facilities, insurance companies, and others need to protect patient information that is electronically stored and transmitted?
   a. Standard 1 related to transactions and code sets
   b. Standard 2 related to the Privacy Rule
   c. Standard 3 related to the Security Rule
   d. Standard 4 related to unique identifiers

5. Which means individually identifiable health information stored or transmitted by covered entities or business associates?
   a. Permission
   b. PHI
   c. Covered entities
   d. Limited data set

6. Under HIPAA, healthcare providers, health (insurance) plans, and claims clearinghouses must transmit PHI electronically. What are they called?
   a. Covered entities
   b. PHI
   c. Business associates
   d. Permission

7. Under HIPAA, which is a reason for releasing or disclosing patient information?
   a. De-identify
   b. Business associates
   c. PHI
   d. Permission *(circled)*

8. Which psychotherapy notes are held at a higher level of confidentiality?
   a. Prescriptions for medications treating mental health disorders
   b. Results of the clinical tests related to mental health disorders
   c. Types and frequency of treatments ordered for mental health disorders
   d. What the patient said during the session and the provider's analysis of the statements and the situation *(circled)*

9. Which question is illegal during an interview?
   a. "Are you eligible to work in this state?"
   b. "Can you perform the essential job functions of a medical assistant with or without reasonable accommodation?"
   c. "When did you move to the United States?" *(circled)*
   d. "Can you work on weekends?"

10. Which act expanded the meaning and interpretation of the definition of disability and included people with cancer, diabetes, attention-deficit/hyperactivity disorder, learning disabilities, and epilepsy?
    a. ADA
    b. OSHA
    c. ADAAA *(circled)*
    d. Stark Law

WORKPLACE APPLICATIONS

1. The billing department supervisor at Walden-Martin Family Medical Clinic wants to hire ACE Coders to assist with the billing processes. Answer the following questions using this scenario.

   a. Who is the covered entity? _Billing department supervisor_

   b. Who is the business associate? _ACE coders_

   c. What must be in done before the business associate obtains patient information? _Medical office must execute a written agreement to handle PHI in accordance with HIPPA._

   d. Can the business associates have unlimited access to all patient information? Explain why or why not.
   Business associates don't see patients but they maintain or access to PHI

2. Mrs. Smith asked Bella to call and talk with her daughter, Rosie. Mrs. Smith wanted Bella to tell Rosie the results of her blood test. Mrs. Smith stated that Rosie was a nurse and would understand the information. Can Bella give Mrs. Smith's information to Rosie? If not, what could be done so Rosie could get the information?
   No, Bella can not give Ms. Smith's information to Rosie due to HIPPA regulation.

3. Mr. Green had before-and-after pictures taken as he was going through bariatric surgery and weight loss. He requests that these pictures be given to his new provider. What is the typical process to transfer pictures to another agency?
   EHR transfer picture to another agency

4. Mr. Thomas is a 39-year-old dependent adult. During the rooming process, the medical assistant suspects that Mr. Thomas is a victim of neglect. What should the medical assistant do?

If medical assistant suspect victim neglect immediately report supervisor.

INTERNET ACTIVITIES

1. Using the internet, research your state's disease reporting public health statutes. Create a poster presentation, PowerPoint presentation, or paper summarizing the reporting process for each category of diseases (e.g., urgent public health concern, less urgent, and HIV and AIDS). List three diseases for the urgent and less urgent categories.

2. Using the internet, review the Child Welfare Information Gateway website (www.childwelfare.gov) for content related to your state. You can also use government websites from your state. Create a poster presentation, PowerPoint presentation, or paper summarizing child protection in your state. Focus on related statutes, the reporting process, and who mandatory reporters are.

3. Using the internet, research prevention of elder abuse, neglect, and exploitation. Focus on resources in your state. Briefly summarize your findings and cite the websites used.

Procedure 4.1 Protecting a Patient's Privacy

Name _____ **Date** _____ **Score** _____

Tasks: Apply HIPAA rules, and protect a patient's privacy. Demonstrate sensitivity to a patient and his rights.

Scenario: Ken Thomas (date of birth [DOB] 10/25/61) saw Jean Burke N.P. (nurse practitioner) this past week. He was diagnosed with acute leukemia after several tests. You work with N.P. Burke and were involved with arranging Ken's tests. Today, Ken's adult child, Alex Thomas, calls you. Alex wants to know what is going on with Ken. You look at Ken's health record and see that Alex is not on the disclosure authorization form or a medical records release form. Per the facility's policy, for information to be given to a patient's family, a disclosure authorization form must be completed.

Later, Ken calls and asks why you didn't update Alex on his condition. He sounds upset while he is talking with you.

Equipment and Supplies:
- Patient record
- Disclosure authorization form (electronic or paper) (See Figure 4.2)

Standard: Complete the procedure and all critical steps in _____ minutes with a minimum score of 85% within two attempts (*or as indicated by the instructor*).

Scoring: Divide the points earned by the total possible points. Failure to perform a critical step, indicated by an asterisk (*), results in grade no higher than an 84% (*or as indicated by the instructor*).

Time: Began_____ Ended_____ Total minutes: _____

Steps:	Point Value	Attempt 1	Attempt 2
1. Using the scenario, role-play the situation with a peer. You are the medical assistant and just realized that Alex is not on the release form. a. Be professional and respectful as you apply HIPAA to the situation. *(Refer to the Checklist for Affective Behaviors - Respect.)*	15*		
2. Inform Alex that his name is not on a disclosure authorization form. Discuss the purpose of the disclosure authorization form.	15		
3. Explain to Alex how you would be able to give him information. Encourage Alex to talk with his father about the situation.	10*		
4. (Your peer should now be Ken.) When Ken calls, be professional and respectful as you hear his complaints. Keep your voice even and do not raise the volume.	10		
5. Inform Ken that you understand his frustration. Explain why you could not give information to Alex. a. Show sensitivity to his feelings and his rights. *(Refer to the Checklist for Affective Behaviors - Sensitivity.)*	15*		
6. Discuss with Ken how you could prepare the disclosure authorization form. Make plans for how Ken would sign the form.	15		
7. Document the phone call with Alex and Ken. Describe the facts and the plan to complete the release form.	20*		
Total Points	100		

Checklist for Affective Behaviors

Affective Behavior	*Directions:* Check behaviors observed during the role-play.					
Respect	**Negative, Unprofessional Behaviors**	**Attempt**		**Positive, Professional Behaviors**	**Attempt**	
		1	**2**		**1**	**2**
	Rude, unkind			Courteous		
	Disrespectful, impolite			Polite		
	Unwelcoming			Welcoming		
	Brief, abrupt			Took time with patient		
	Unconcerned with person's dignity			Maintained person's dignity		
	Negative nonverbal behaviors			Positive nonverbal behaviors		
	Other:			Other:		
Sensitivity	Distracted; not focused on the other person			Focused full attention on the other person		
	Judgmental attitude; not accepting attitude			Nonjudgmental, accepting attitude		
	Failed to clarify what the person verbally or nonverbally communicated			Used summarizing or paraphrasing to clarify what the person verbally or nonverbally communicated		
	Failed to acknowledge what the person communicated			Acknowledged what the person communicated		
	Rude, discourteous			Pleasant and courteous		
	Disregards the person's dignity and rights			Maintains the person's dignity and rights		
	Other:			Other:		

Grading for Affective Behaviors		**Point Value**	**Attempt 1**	**Attempt 2**
Does not meet Expectation	• Response was disrespectful and/or insensitive. • Student demonstrated more than 2 negative, unprofessional behaviors during the interaction.	**0**		
Needs Improvement	• Response was disrespectful and/or insensitive. • Student demonstrated 1 or 2 negative, unprofessional behaviors during the interaction.	**0**		
Meets Expectation	• Response was respectful and sensitive; no negative, unprofessional behaviors observed. • More practice is needed for behavior to appear natural and for student to appear comfortable and at ease.	**15**		

Occasionally Exceeds Expectation	• Response was respectful and sensitive; no negative, unprofessional behaviors observed. • At times student appeared comfortable and at ease; but more practice is needed for behavior to become natural and consistent with a professional medical assistant.	15		
Always Exceeds Expectation	• Response was respectful and sensitive; no negative, unprofessional behaviors observed. • Student's behaviors appeared natural and comfortable. Behaviors are consistent with a professional medical assistant.	15		

Documentation

Comments

CAAHEP Competencies	Steps
X.P.2.a. Apply HIPAA rules in regard to: privacy	1-3, 6
X.A.1. Demonstrate sensitivity to patient rights	5
ABHES Competencies	**Steps**
4. Medical Law and Ethics b. Institute federal and state guidelines when: 1) Releasing medical records or information	Entire procedure
4.f. Comply with federal, state, and local health laws and regulations as they relate to healthcare settings	1-3, 6
4.h. Demonstrate compliance with HIPAA guidelines, the ADA Amendments Act, and the Health Information Technology for Economic and Clinical Health (HITECH) Act	1-3, 6

Procedure 4.2 Completing a Release of Record Form for a Release of Information

Name _____ Date _____ Score _____

Tasks: Apply HIPAA rules, and complete a release of record form for a release of information.

Scenario: Aaron Jackson was seen at Walden Hospital for a high fever. You need to help Aaron's mother complete a record release form so his record from the emergency department visit can be sent to the clinic. She needs to request all records from the visit on the first of this month. The clinic information is on the form. The release will expire in 1 month.

Aaron's information	Walden Hospital's information
DOB: 10/17/2011 **SSN:** 164-72-4618 **Address:** 555 McArthur Avenue, Anytown, AL 12345-1234 **Phone:** (123) 814-7844 **Mother:** Patricia Jackson	**Address:** Walden Hospital 123 Healing Way Anywhere, AL 12345-1234 **Phone:** (123) 814-4563 **Fax:** (123) 814-6544

Equipment and Supplies:
- Records release form (electronic or paper) (See Work Product 4.1)
- Patient record

Standard: Complete the procedure and all critical steps in _____ minutes with a minimum score of 85% within two attempts (*or as indicated by the instructor*).

Scoring: Divide the points earned by the total possible points. Failure to perform a critical step, indicated by an asterisk (*), results in grade no higher than an 84% (*or as indicated by the instructor*).

Time: Began_____ Ended_____ Total minutes: _____

Steps:	Point Value	Attempt 1	Attempt 2
1. Using the medical record release form, insert the patient information (Work Product 4.1). Add the patient's name, DOB, and social security number (SSN). Include the current address and phone number that is found in the patient record. If an electronic form is used, select the correct patient and the fields will auto-populate.	10*		
2. Complete the parts of the form that specify who authorizes the release and who is to release the information.	15*		
3. Check the box(es) of the information that needs to be released. If required, write in what other records need to be released.	15*		
4. Add the date of the visit. Add the name and contact information for the facility where the records need to be sent.	15*		
5. Indicate how the released information will be used.	15		
6. Indicate when the authorization should expire. Proofread the form for accuracy. If using an electronic form, save the form to the patient's record. Print the form so the mother can sign.	10		

7.	During a role-play with the patient's mother, explain what the provider is requesting. Ensure she can understand and read English. Have the mother read the form.	**10**		
8.	Ask the mother if she has any questions. Answer any questions and then explain where she needs to sign if she agrees with the documentation.	**10**		
	Total Points	**100**		

Comments

CAAHEP Competencies	Step(s)
X.P.2.b. Apply HIPAA rules in regard to: release of information	Entire procedure
ABHES Competencies	**Step(s)**
4. Medical Law and Ethics b. Institute federal and state guidelines when: 1) Releasing medical records or information	Entire procedure
4. f. Comply with federal, state, and local health laws and regulations as they relate to healthcare settings	Entire procedure
4.h. Demonstrate compliance with HIPAA guidelines, the ADA Amendments Act, and the Health Information Technology for Economic and Clinical Health (HITECH) Act	Entire procedure

Work Product 4.1 Records Release Form

Name _____ Date _____ Score _____

WALDEN-MARTIN
FAMILY MEDICAL CLINIC
1234 ANYSTREET | ANYTOWN, ANYSTATE 12345
PHONE 123-123-1234 | FAX 123-123-5678

Medical Records Release

Patient Name: _____ Date of Birth: _____

SSN: _____ Phone: _____

Address:

I, _____ authorize _____

to disclose/release the following information (check all applicable):

☐ All Records   ☐ Abstract/Summary

☐ Laboratory/pathology records   ☐ Pharmacy/prescription records

☐ X-ray/radiology records   ☐ Other

☐ Billing records

Note: *If these records contain any information from previous providers or information about HIV/AIDS status, cancer diagnosis, drug alcohol abuse, or sexually transmitted disease, you are hereby authorizing disclosure of this information. A copy of this signed authorization must be given to the individual.*

These records are for services provided on the following date(s):_____

Please send the records listed above to (use additional sheets if necessary):

Name: _____ Phone: _____

Address: Fax: _____

The information may be used/disclosed for each of the following purposes:

☐ At patient's request   ☐ For employment purposes

☐ For patient's health care   ☐ Other

☐ For payment/insurance

This authorization shall expire no later than: _____ or upon the following event _____ , and may not be valid for greater than one year from the date of signature for medical records.

I understand that after the custodian of records discloses my health information, it may no longer be protected by federal privacy laws. I understand that this authorization is voluntary and I may refuse to sign this authorization which will not affect my ability to obtain treatment; receive payment; or eligibility for benefits unless allowed by law. By signing below I represent and warrant that I have authority to sign this document and authorize the use or disclosure of protected health information and that there are no claims or orders that would prohibit, limit, or otherwise restrict my ability to authorize the use or disclosure of this protected health information.

_____   _____

Patient signature
(or patient's personal representative)   **Date**

_____   _____

Printed name of patient representative   **Representative's authority to sign for patient**
                                                           (i.e. parent, guardian, power of attorney, executor)

Procedure 4.3 Perform Disease Reporting

Name _____ Date _____ Score _____

Tasks: Research the state's disease reporting public health statutes and complete the disease reporting paperwork based on public health statutes. Document the activity in the patient's health record.

Scenario: Jean Burke N.P. received the test results for Ken Thomas. He tested positive for gonorrhea. She wants you to file the report with the public health department. Here is the information from his health record and the clinic. For any missing information, follow the instructor's directions or make it up if no directions were provided.

Patient Information	Provider and Lab Information	Health Record Information
Ken Thomas 398 Larkin Avenue Anytown, AL 12345-1234 Anycounty k.thomas@anytown.mail Phone: (123) 784-1118 DOB: 10/25/61 Race: Multiple races Ethnicity: Unknown Marital status: Single Living with Sandy Brown, who was not treated	Provider: Jean Burke, N.P. Walden-Martin Family Medical Clinic 1234 Anystreet Anytown, AL 12345-1234 Phone: (123) 123-1234 Fax: (123) 123-5678 Lab: Walden-Martin Family Medical Clinic Lab	Diagnosis: Gonorrhea Symptoms: Started 5 days ago, greenish discharge from penis, burning with urination Test: Urine specimen was collected yesterday; gonorrhea nucleic acid amplification test NAAT test done yesterday, results are positive Treatment: Patient treated today with ceftriaxone 250 mg intramuscular (IM) single dose and azithromycin 1 g orally single dose

Equipment and Supplies:
- Computer with internet access and printer
- Patient record (see table with information)
- Black pen

Standard: Complete the procedure and all critical steps in _____ minutes with a minimum score of 85% within two attempts (*or as indicated by the instructor*).

Scoring: Divide the points earned by the total possible points. Failure to perform a critical step, indicated by an asterisk (*), results in grade no higher than an 84% (*or as indicated by the instructor*).

Time: Began _____ Ended _____ Total minutes: _____

Steps:	Point Value	Attempt 1	Attempt 2
1. Using the internet, search for the disease reporting procedure in your state's public health department or similar facility. Read the procedure.	10		
2. Identify which form is required based on the patient's diagnosis. Print the form.	10		

3. Use a black pen to complete the form. Neatly complete the patient's demographic information section using the information from the health record.	**25**		
4. Complete the diagnosis, symptoms, testing, and treatment information.	**25**		
5. Complete the rest of the form. Review the form for accuracy. Make any changes required before submitting the form to the instructor.	**20**		
6. Document in the patient's health record that the disease reporting paperwork was completed and submitted	**10**		
Total Points	**100**		

Documentation

Comments

CAAHEP Competencies	Step(s)
X.P.5. Perform compliance reporting based on public health statutes	Entire procedure
ABHES Competencies	**Step(s)**
4. Medical Law and Ethics f. Comply with federal, state, and local health laws and regulations as they relate to healthcare settings	Entire procedure
4.b.2) Entering orders in and utilizing electronic health records	6

Procedure 4.4   Report Illegal Activity

Name _____   Date _____   Score _____

Task: Report an illegal activity in the healthcare setting following proper protocol.

Scenario: Today, you witnessed a coworker, Sally Brown, taking medical samples from the supply cabinet. You see her sticking them in her purse. She sees you and states, "This was the same medication I had to pay $200 for the last time I was sick. I don't see why we need to pay for medications when we have samples that we give free to patients. We should be able to use them too." You know the facility's professional policy prohibits taking medical samples from the sample cabinet for personal reasons.

Facility's Compliance Reporting Protocol:
Walden-Martin Family Medical Clinic's Compliance Program has a phone number and email address for employees to report suspected violations, suspected illegal activity, fraud, abuse, theft, and workplace safety concerns. Concerns can be left on the voicemail or emailed without fear of retribution or retaliation. Please include as many details as possible, including date(s), names, and the situation.

Any employee who seeks retribution or retaliation against another employee for reporting an offense needs to be aware of criminal penalties for such actions.

Equipment and Supplies:
- Computer with email and internet access or phone
- Instructor's email address or voicemail phone number
- Pen and paper
- Facility's compliance reporting protocol (See box)

Standard: Complete the procedure and all critical steps with a minimum score of 85% within two attempts (*or as indicated by the instructor*).

Scoring: Divide the points earned by the total possible points. Failure to perform a critical step, indicated by an asterisk (*), results in grade no higher than an 84% (*or as indicated by the instructor*).

Steps:	Point Value	Attempt 1	Attempt 2
1. Read the facility's corporate compliance reporting protocol.	10		
2. Using the paper and pen, write down the facts of what you witnessed.	10		
3. Using the paper and pen, compose the message you want to email or leave on the voicemail for the compliance office.	30		
4. Proofread the message and make any changes required. Make sure to include the date, names of people involved, and the details of the situation.	20		
5. Using your email or phone, send a message to the corporate compliance office. Use the email address or phone number provided by your instructor.	30		
Total Points	100		

Comments

CAAHEP Competencies	**Step(s)**
X.P.6. Report an illegal activity in the healthcare setting following proper protocol	Entire procedure
ABHES Competencies	**Step(s)**
4. Medical Law and Ethics f. Comply with federal, state, and local health laws and regulations as they relate to healthcare settings	Entire procedure

Procedure 4.5 Complete Incident Report

Name _____ Date _____ Score _____

Task: Complete an incident report form for a medication error.

Scenario: Johnny Parker (DOB 06/15/10) saw Jean Burke N.P. for a well-child visit. Johnny is off schedule with his hepatitis B vaccine series and today he is to get his last hepatitis B booster. You (a medical assistant) prepare the medication and give the injection in his right deltoid muscle. Later in the day, you realize that hepatitis B was out of stock for 1 week. You must have given a hepatitis A booster to Johnny. You realized that you failed to read the label three times during the preparation of the medication. You reported the mistake to Jean Burke N.P. and your supervisor. Your supervisor called Lisa Parker, Johnny's mother. They will come back next week for the hepatitis B vaccine. You need to complete the incident report.

Equipment and Supplies:
- Incident Report form (Work Product 4.2) and black pen or computer with an internet and SimChart for the Medical Office (SCMO)

Standard: Complete the procedure and all critical steps in _____ minutes with a minimum score of 85% within two attempts (*or as indicated by the instructor*).

Scoring: Divide the points earned by the total possible points. Failure to perform a critical step, indicated by an asterisk (*), results in grade no higher than an 84% (*or as indicated by the instructor*).

Time: Began_____ Ended_____ Total minutes: _____

Steps:	Point Value	Attempt 1	Attempt 2
1. SCMO method: Access SCMO and enter the Simulation Playground. If a popup window appears, select "Return to previous session with saved patient information" and click Start. On the Calendar screen, click on the Form Repository icon. Click on Office Forms on the left Info Panel and select Incident Report. For both methods: Accurately complete the information from the date down to the reason for the patient's visit.	20		
2. For both methods: Specify the incident description, immediate action and outcome, and contributing factors, and fill in the prevention boxes. Provide as much detail as possible. Be honest and concise with your facts.	20		
3. For both methods: Complete the reported by, position, and contact phone number sections. Your information should be in these fields. Make up a contact phone number.	20		
4. For both methods: Complete the other persons involved, position, and contact phone number sections. Jean Burke's information should be in these fields. Make up her contact phone number.	20		
5. For both methods: Review the form for accuracy. Make any changes required before submitting the form to the instructor. (For the SCMO method: Save or print the form based on your instructor's directions.)	20		
Total Points	100		

Comments

CAAHEP Competencies	Step(s)
X.P.7. Complete an incident report related to an error in patient care	Entire procedure
ABHES Competencies	**Step(s)**
4. Medical Law and Ethics e. Perform risk management procedures	Entire procedure

Work Product 4.2 Incident Report Form

Name _____ Date _____ Score _____

WALDEN-MARTIN
FAMILY MEDICAL CLINIC
1234 ANYSTREET | ANYTOWN, ANYSTATE 12345
PHONE 123-123-1234 | FAX 123-123-5678

Incident Report

Date: _____ **Time:** _____

Incident Type: ☐ Staff ☐ Patient ☐ Visitor ☐ Equipment/Property

Witness: ☐ Staff ☐ Patient ☐ Visitor

Department: _____ **Exact Location:** _____

Medical Team: _____

Patient Reason for Visit: _____ **Medication Incident:** ☐ Yes ☐ No

Incident Description:

Immediate Actions and Outcome:

Contributing Factors:

Prevention:

Next of kin / guardian notified / patient? ☐ Yes ☐ No ☐ N/A   **Medical staff notified?** ☐ Yes ☐ No ☐ N/A

Reported By: _____ **Position:** _____

Contact Phone Number: _____

Other Persons Involved: _____ **Position:** _____

Contact Phone Number: _____

Medical Report (Document patient's assessment and list investigations and treatments):

_____

Provider: _____ **Designation:** _____

Provider Signature: _____ **Date/Time:** _____

Healthcare Ethics

CAAHEP Competencies	Assessment
V.C.17.c. Discuss the theories of: Kübler-Ross	Skills and Concepts – C. 18 a-e; Certification Preparation – 6
X.C.7.e. Define: Uniform Anatomical Gift Act	Skills and Concepts – C. 26
X.C.7.f. Define: living will/advanced directives	Vocabulary Review – D. 3, 5; Certification Preparation – 7
X.C.7.g. Define: medical durable power of attorney	Vocabulary Review – D. 4
X.C.7.h. Define: Patient Self Determination Act (PSDA)	Skills and Concepts – C. 20
XI.C.1.a. Define: ethics	Vocabulary Review – D. 1; Certification Preparation – 1
XI.C.1.b. Define: morals	Vocabulary Review – D. 2; Certification Preparation – 2
XI.C.2. Differentiate between personal and professional ethics	Skills and Concepts – A. 3; Certification Preparation – 3
XI.C.3. Identify the effect of personal morals on professional performance	Skills and Concepts – A. 2
XI.P.1. Develop a plan for separation of personal and professional ethics	Procedure 5.1
XI.P.2. Demonstrate appropriate response(s) to ethical issues	Procedure 5.2
XI.A.1. Recognize the impact personal ethics and morals have on the delivery of healthcare	Procedure 5.1, 5.2

ABHES Competencies	Assessment
4. Medical Law and Ethics g. Display compliance with the Code of Ethics of the profession	Skills and Concepts – A. 6 Procedure 5.1, 5.2

VOCABULARY REVIEW

Using the word pool on the right, find the correct word to match the definition. Write the word on the line after the definition.

Group A

1. Codes of conduct stated by an employer or professional association _____

2. Basic units of heredity _____

3. Rod-shaped structures found in the cell's nucleus; they contain genetic information _____

4. A set of rules about good and bad behavior

   _____

5. An individual's code of conduct _____

6. The freedom to determine one's own actions and decisions

   _____

7. People who study the ethical effect of biomedical advances

   _____

8. To treat patients fairly and give them care that is due and appropriate _____

9. To do good _____

10. To do no harm _____

Word Pool
- autonomy
- chromosomes
- beneficence
- code of ethics
- justice
- genes
- nonmaleficence
- professional ethics
- personal ethics
- bioethicists

Group B

1. The inability to get pregnant after 1 year of unprotected intercourse _____

2. Nonreproductive cells; they do not include sperm and egg cells

   _____

3. Cells can make copies of themselves _____

4. Sperm and egg cells _____

5. Cells can develop into specialized cells _____

6. The process of creating a genetically identical biological entity

   _____

7. The entire genetic makeup of an organism

   _____

8. A branch of medicine involved with using patients' genomic information as part of their clinical care _____

9. A branch of pharmacology that studies the genetic factors that influences a person's response to a medication

   _____

10. The manipulation of genetic material in cells to change hereditary traits or produce a specific result _____

Word Pool
- genomic medicine
- differentiate
- self-renew
- genome
- cloning
- genetic engineering
- somatic cells
- germline cells
- pharmacogenomics
- infertility

Group C

1. A competent adult can appoint a person to make healthcare decisions in the event he or she is unable to do so

   _____

2. Withholding a life-saving treatment (e.g., feeding tube) and letting the person die _____

3. A branch of knowledge, learning, or instruction; for instance, medicine, nursing, social work, and physical therapy

   _____

4. Incorporating the most current and valid research results into the practice of healthcare, thus providing the best patient care

   _____

5. Latin for "father of the country" _____

6. Involves removing egg cells from a female's ovaries, fertilizing them with sperm outside of the body, and then implanting the fertilized egg in the uterus _____

7. To help relieve the symptoms of a serious illness

   _____

8. A type of palliative care for people who have about 6 months or less to live _____

9. Bringing to an end _____

10. The act of killing a person who is suffering from an incurable disease _____

11. To preserve by freezing at low temperatures

    _____

12. A physician who has graduated from medical school and is finishing specialized clinical training _____

13. An immature ovum _____

14. A person who acts on behalf of another person or takes the place of another person _____

15. A group composed of members from a variety of disciplines that analyzes ethical issues _____

16. Any procedure where nonhuman cells, tissues, or organs are implanted or infused into a person _____

Word Pool
- cessation
- evidence-based practices
- in-vitro fertilization
- *parens patriae*
- healthcare proxy
- discipline
- xenotransplantation
- resident
- hospice
- euthanasia
- cryopreservation
- oocyte
- ethics committees
- passive euthanasia
- palliative
- surrogate

Group D
Define each word or phrase.

1. Ethics: _____

   _____

2. Morals: _____

   _____

3. Advance directives: _____

   _____

4. Medical durable power of attorney:_____

   _____

5. Living will:_____

   _____

ABBREVIATIONS
Write out what each of the following abbreviations stands for.

1. AMA _____
2. CEJA _____
3. AAMA _____
4. GMOs _____
5. FDA _____
6. ART _____
7. IUI _____
8. STI _____
9. NHI _____
10. PSDA _____
11. DNR _____
12. CPR _____
13. POLST _____
14. UDDA _____
15. UAGA _____
16. NOTA _____
17. OPTN _____

SKILLS AND CONCEPTS

Answer the following questions. Write your answer on the line or in the space provided.

A. Personal and Professional Ethics

1. Describe morals and their impact on a person's life._____

   _____

   _____

2. Identify the effect of personal morals on professional performance. _____

   _____

   _____

3. Describe the difference between personal and professional ethics. _____

   _____

   _____

4. What are codes of ethics and who publishes them? _____

   _____

   _____

5. What is the CEJA and what does it do?_____

   _____

   _____

6. Summarize the Medical Assisting Code of Ethics. _____

   _____

   _____

7. How can a medical assistant approach a situation if it involves his or her biases? _____

   _____

   _____

8. When looking for employment, why is it important to consider one's biases before applying for certain jobs?

   _____

   _____

B. Principles of Healthcare Ethics

1. List the four ethical principles. _____

_____

2. How can a medical assistant follow the ethical principle of autonomy when caring for patients?

_____

_____

3. How can a medical assistant follow the ethical principle of nonmaleficence when caring for patients?

_____

_____

4. How can a medical assistant follow the ethical principle of beneficence when caring for patients?

_____

_____

5. How can a medical assistant follow the ethical principle of justice when caring for patients?

_____

_____

C. Ethical Issues

1. Describe the positions of advocates and opponents of human cloning. _____

_____

_____

2. What is the Human Genome Project and what resulted from the project? _____

_____

_____

3. _____ can identify issues with a person's chromosomes, genes, or proteins.

4. List seven types of genetic testing. _____

_____

_____

5. When using pharmacogenomics, what is an advantage to a patient? _____

_____

6. What are the two main categories of stem cells? _____

_____

7. What is gene therapy? _____

_____

8. _____ technique can remove, add, or alter sections of the gene.

9. Describe the difference between genome editing of somatic cells and germline cells. _____

_____

_____

10. What is an ethical issue that may arise with assistive reproductive technology?_____

_____

_____

11. Describe CEJA's opinion on assistive reproductive technology._____

_____

_____

12. Discuss the CEJA's opinion on gamete donation. _____

_____

_____

13. What power does the *parens patriae* doctrine gives the courts? _____

_____

_____

14. Discuss the CEJA's opinion on parental refusal of treatment._____

_____

_____

15. Describe the difference between open and closed adoptions. _____

_____

_____

16. What are the Safe Haven Infant Protection laws and what is the main goal of these laws? _____

_____

_____

17. Describe CEJA's opinion on confidential healthcare for minors. _____

_____

_____

18. Describe the following stages of grief and dying of Elisabeth Kübler-Ross' theory.

   a.   Denial: _____

   _____

   b.   Anger: _____

   _____

   c.   Bargaining: _____

   _____

   d.   Depression: _____

   _____

   e.   Acceptance:_____

   _____

19. Where can hospice care be provided? _____

   _____

20. Describe the importance of the Patient Self-Determination Act (PSDA)._____

   _____

21. What does the CEJA encourage providers to do regarding advance directives? _____

   _____

22. Besides addressing different types of advance directions, list five other topics found on advance directive forms.

   _____

   _____

   _____

   _____

23. Describe importance of the Uniform Determination of Death Act. _____

   _____

   _____

24. What is CEJA's opinion on physician-assisted suicide and euthanasia? _____

   _____

   _____

25. What should a person do if he or she wants to be a potential organ donor at death?_____

   _____

   _____

26. Describe the Uniform Anatomical Gift Act. _____

_____

_____

27. The _____ established the Organ Procurement and Transplant Network (OPTN).

CERTIFICATION PREPARATION
Circle the correct answer.

1. Which term means "rules of conduct that differentiate between acceptable and unacceptable behavior"?
    a. Ethics
    b. Justice
    c. Morals
    d. Code of ethics

2. Which term means "internal principles that distinguish between right and wrong"?
    a. Ethics
    b. Morals
    c. Justice
    d. Nonmaleficence

3. _____ are codes of conduct stated by an employer or professional association.
    a. Personal ethics
    b. Morals
    c. Professional ethics
    d. Code of ethics

4. Which means "to do no harm"?
    a. Autonomy
    b. Justice
    c. Nonmaleficence
    d. Beneficence

5. What is the process of creating a genetically identical biological entity?
    a. Genetic engineering
    b. Cloning
    c. Genetic testing
    d. Pharmacogenetics

6. Which Kübler-Ross stage of grief and dying involves the person refusing to accept the fact?
    a. Anger
    b. Depression
    c. Bargaining
    d. Denial

7. Which advance directive provides instructions about life-sustaining medical treatment to be administered or withheld when the patient has a terminal condition?
    a. Medical durable power of attorney
    b. Healthcare proxy
    c. Living will
    d. Organ donation

8. Which advance directive allows a competent adult to appoint a person (called a *proxy* or *agent*) to make healthcare decisions in the event he or she is unable to do so?
    a. Medical durable power of attorney
    b. Healthcare proxy
    c. Living will
    d. Organ donation

9. Which is the type of euthanasia where the patient consents to the action?
    a. Active
    b. Passive
    c. Voluntary
    d. Involuntary

10. Which act established a national registry for organ matching and also made it a criminal act to exchange organs for transplant for something of value?
    a. Patient Self-Determination Act
    b. Uniform Anatomical Gift Act
    c. Uniform Determination of Death Act
    d. National Organ Transplant Act

WORKPLACE APPLICATIONS

1. Mrs. Johnson called Walden-Martin Family Medical Clinic and Daniela answered the phone. Mrs. Johnson requested an appointment. She stated that she has experienced sleep changes, difficulty concentrating, sadness, and appetite changes since her husband died. Based on what you have read in this chapter, what might be occurring with Mrs. Johnson?

   She was in grieving stages that why she have that all symptoms.

2. Jean is graduating from a medical assistant program. During her practicum, she heard about the dangers of narcotic medications. She does not believe that patients should receive narcotic medications. Jean is an advocate of alternative medications and feels there are reasonable alternatives to narcotic medications. How should Jean approach finding a job, given her bias?

   She had to mention this in her resume or she need to manage this bias.

3. Jan, a certified medical assistant, was discussing advance directives with a patient. The patient asked Jan to explain the importance of advance directives. How would you explain the importance of advance directives?

   An advance directives lets your health care team and loved ones know what kind of health care you want, or who you want to make decisions for you where you can't.

INTERNET ACTIVITIES

1. Using the internet, research your state's advance directive forms. Create a poster presentation, PowerPoint presentation, or paper summarizing the topic areas on the advance directive forms. Cite your resource(s).

2. Using the internet, research your state's Safe Haven laws for children. If your state does not have these laws, select a state that does. Create a poster presentation, PowerPoint presentation, or paper summarizing the Safe Haven laws. Focus on related statutes, maximum age of the child, and locations where the child can be brought. Cite your resource(s).

3. Using the internet, research an ethical issue. Create a poster presentation, PowerPoint presentation, or paper summarizing your findings. In your project, summarize the ethical issue and provide the advocates' and opponents' views of the issue.

Procedure 5.1 Developing an Ethics Separation Plan

Name _____ **Date** _____ **Score** _____

Task: To develop a plan for separation of personal and professional ethics.

Scenario: You are working at WMFM Clinic. Your provider sees many children, including teens. New state laws allow for confidential healthcare for minors. The agency has now adopted policies and procedures to allow providers to see teens 16 years or older without parental consent. The teens can be seen for sexually transmitted infections (STIs) and reproductive issues (including birth control). All health records related to these visits are confidential, meaning parents cannot be told about their child's visit.

Your personal belief is that parents should always be allowed to know what is occurring with their children. They are responsible for the child until age 18 and they pay the bills. You also believe that children (younger than 18) are too young to be in an intimate relationship. This type of activity should only be for adults in a committed relationship. You don't believe in birth control.

Equipment and Supplies:
- Paper and pen
- Medical Assisting Code of Ethics (see box in the textbook)

Standard: Complete the procedure and all critical steps with a minimum score of 85% within two attempts (*or as indicated by the instructor*).

Scoring: Divide the points earned by the total possible points. Failure to perform a critical step, indicated by an asterisk (*), results in grade no higher than an 84% (*or as indicated by the instructor*).

Steps/Criteria:	Point Value	Attempt 1	Attempt 2
1. Read the Medical Assisting Code of Ethics. Write down key themes or phrases.	15		
2. Using the scenario, write down the professional ethics involved in the situation.	15		
3. Using the scenario, write down the personal ethics involved in the situation.	15		
4. Compare the lists. Identify the personal ethics that conflict with the Code of Ethics and the professional ethics of the agency.	15		
5. For each area of conflict, create a plan on how you will separate your personal and professional ethics. Remember as a professional, you need to follow the professional ethics of the agency and the profession. Address how will you handle the situation and what your options would be if you were in the situation.	20*		
6. Describe how the personal ethics and morals in this scenario would impact patient care and the delivery of healthcare. • Describe how a medical assistant's personal ethics and morals could impact how that person provides care. • Describe how patient care may be altered or not up to the standard of care required. • Describe how a medical assistant could respond in a professional manner and maintain the standard of care and personal integrity.	20*		
Total Points	**100**		

Comments

CAAHEP Competencies	Steps
XI.P.1. Develop a plan for separation of personal and professional ethics	5
XI.A.1. Recognize the impact personal ethics and morals have on the delivery of healthcare	6
ABHES Competencies	**Steps**
4. Medical Law and Ethics g. Display compliance with the Code of Ethics of the profession	5

Procedure 5.2 Demonstrate Appropriate Response to Ethical Issues

Name _____ Date _____ Score _____

Tasks: Identify ethical issues and demonstrate appropriate and professional responses. Recognize the impact personal ethics and morals have on the delivery of healthcare.

Scenario 1: You are working at WMFM Clinic. You are responsible for collecting payments from patients. Mr. Smythe, who is visually impaired, paid for his visit in cash. He gives you $500 for a $402 bill. You make change and give him a receipt. At the end of the day, you notice that you have $60 more than what you should have and some of the bills were mixed up in the cashbox. You realize you gave Mr. Smythe the incorrect amount of money.

Scenario 2: You are setting up a laceration repair tray for Dr. Martin to use. As you are preparing the sterile equipment, one of the instruments gets contaminated. You know Dr. Martin urgently needs the tray. You realize the contamination can cause an infection.

Equipment and Supplies:
• Paper and pen

Standard: Complete the procedure and all critical steps in _____ minutes with a minimum score of 85% within two attempts (*or as indicated by the instructor*).

Scoring: Divide the points earned by the total possible points. Failure to perform a critical step, indicated by an asterisk (*), results in grade no higher than an 84% (*or as indicated by the instructor*).

Time: Began_____ Ended_____ Total minutes: _____

Steps:	Point Value	Attempt 1	Attempt 2
1. Read both scenarios. Identify and write down the ethical issues involved.	20		
2. With a peer, role-play Scenario 1. Your peer should be the supervisor in this scenario. Demonstrate a professional and appropriate ethical response to this situation. a. Explain the situation to the supervisor. b. Describe how you felt the error occurred and who received the incorrect change. c. Explain how you would like to handle the situation and correct the error.	30		
3. With a peer, role-play Scenario 2. Your peer should be the provider in this scenario. During the role-play, demonstrate a professional and appropriate ethical response to this situation.	30		
4. In a written response, discuss the potential implications for the patient's health related to not reporting or correcting the error.	20		
Total Points	**100**		

• Ethical issue(s) identified in Scenario 1:

- Ethical issue(s) identified in Scenario 2:

- Discuss the potential implication to the patient's health related to not reporting or correcting the error.

Comments

CAAHEP Competencies	Step(s)
XI.P.2. Demonstrate appropriate response(s) to ethical issues	1-3
XI.A.1. Recognize the impact personal ethics and morals have on the delivery of healthcare	4
ABHES Competencies	**Step(s)**
4. Medical Law and Ethics g. Display compliance with the Code of Ethics of the profession	Entire procedure

Group D

1. The computer process of changing encrypted text to readable or plain text after a user enters a secret key or password _____

2. A person or business that provides a service to a covered entity that involves access to PHI _____

3. Each employee with network access must log in using a unique password _____

4. Devices attached to the monitor that allow visualization of the screen contents only if the user is directly in front of the screen _____

5. Program or hardware that acts as a barrier between the network and the internet _____

6. Something designed to be used at or near where the patient is seen; point-of-care tools and apps are resources for the provider to use when working directly with the patient _____

7. A wireless mobile workstation _____

8. The use of electronic software to communicate with pharmacies and send prescribing information _____

9. A healthcare facility, healthcare provider, pharmacy, health (insurance) plan, or claims clearinghouse that transmits protected health information electronically _____

10. The interval of time during which something, such as hardware or software, is not functioning _____

11. Refers to remote clinical and nonclinical services, such as provider training, meetings, and continuing education _____

Word Pool
- point-of-care
- telehealth
- computer on wheels
- e-prescribing
- business associate
- firewall
- downtime
- covered entity
- privacy filters
- authentication
- decryption

ABBREVIATIONS

Write out what each of the following abbreviations stands for.

1. EHR _____

2. PC _____

3. OCR _____

4. GB _____

5. ISP _____

6. DSL _____

7. IT _____

8. EMR _____

9. HIPAA _____

10. ePHI _____

11. CPU _____

12. ROM _____

13. RAM _____

14. MB _____

15. HITECH _____

16. COW _____

17. CPOE _____

18. RPM _____

19. mHealth _____

20. HHR _____

SKILLS AND CONCEPTS

Answer the following questions. Write your answer on the line or in the space provided.

A. Computers in Ambulatory Care

1. List the three types of personal computers. _____

   _____

2. The PC and peripheral devices are _____.

3. List five input devices. _____

   _____

4. Describe the difference among the function, control, and special-purpose keys on keyboards.

   _____

   _____

   _____

   _____

5. List three ways to move the pointer (cursor) on the screen. _____

   _____

6. What hardware and software are used for telemedicine? _____

   _____

   _____

7. What is a patient portal? _____

   _____

8. Scanners convert images to digital text using a process called _____.

9. List four types of scanners. _____

_____

10. List three output devices. _____

_____

11. Images are created on monitors using _____; the _____ the number, the sharper the image.

12. Describe the advantages of inkjet and laser printers. _____

_____

_____

13. The _____ is the "brains" of the computer and it sits on the _____.

14. Describe the three types of primary memory. _____

_____

_____

_____

15. When saving data to the computer, the data are saved on the _____ drive.

16. Describe cloud storage. _____

_____

_____

17. A(n) _____ is usually considered a character, such as a number, letter, or symbol.

18. Put these data storage capacities in order from smallest to largest: MB, GB, TB, KB_____

_____

19. What two things are required for a healthcare facility's computer network to access the internet?

_____

B. Maintaining Computer Hardware

1. Describe three ways to prevent computer problems. _____

_____

_____

_____

2. Describe how to clean the hardware's casing. _____

_____

_____

3. Describe infection control procedures for computer hardware. _____

_____

_____

_____

_____

C. Computer Workstation Ergonomics

1. _____ is the field of study that involves reducing strain and injuries by improving the workstation design.

2. Describe principles of ergonomics as they apply to a workstation.

   a. Describe principles related to the backrest. _____

   _____

   _____

   b. Describe principles related to the seat and the armrest. _____

   _____

   _____

   c. Describe the position of the torso, neck, and feet when sitting. _____

   _____

   _____

   d. Describe the location of the monitor and document holder._____

   _____

   _____

   e. Describe the location of the keyboard, work surface, and mouse._____

   _____

   _____

   f. Describe when headsets should be used._____

   _____

3. If a person is sitting or standing at a computer for a long period of time, what should the person do every 30 minutes?

_____

D. Software Used in Ambulatory Care

1. Describe the difference between system software and application software. _____

_____

_____

2. Give examples for each of the following application software.

   a. Anti-malware software: _____

   b. Word processing software: _____

   c. Spreadsheet software: _____

   d. Database software: _____

3. Describe the difference among practice management software, electronic medical records, and electronic health records.

   a. Practice management software (PMS): _____

   _____

   b. Electronic medical records (EMR): _____

   _____

   c. Electronic health record (EHR): _____

   _____

4. Describe the difference between interface and interoperability. _____

_____

5. List the useful features of practice management software. _____

_____

_____

_____

E. Computer Network Privacy and Security

1. Describe the Security Rule's administrative safeguards and list four safeguards. _____

_____

_____

2.   Describe the Security Rule's physical safeguards and list four safeguards. _____

_____

_____

3.   Describe three physical safeguards that are part of workstation security. _____

_____

_____

4.   Describe the Security Rule's technical safeguards and list seven safeguards. _____

_____

_____

5.   Describe the data backup process. _____

_____

_____

6.   What is the importance of frequently backing up the network data? _____

_____

_____

F. Continual Technology Advances in Healthcare

1.   Explain e-prescribing. _____

_____

2.   What is computerized provider/physician order entry (CPOE) and who is allowed to use CPOE?

_____

_____

CERTIFICATION PREPARATION

Circle the correct answer.

1.   What is one kilobyte equivalent to?
   a.   1024 bytes
   b.   1024 MB
   c.   1024 GB
   d.   1024 TB

2.   Which software protects computers against viruses?
   a.   Database software
   b.   Presentation software
   c.   Anti-malware software
   d.   Spreadsheet software

3.   What is a physical safeguard that is used over monitors to prevent others from seeing the information?
   a.   Firewalls
   b.   Screen savers
   c.   Authentication
   d.   Privacy filters

4. Which is a type of software that allows the user to enter demographic information, schedule appointments, maintain lists of insurance payers, perform billing tasks, and generate reports?
   a. Electronic health record (EHR)
   b. Electronic medical records (EMR)
   c. Practice management
   d. Microsoft Word and Excel

5. What is an electronic version of a patient's paper record?
   a. Electronic health record (EHR)
   b. Electronic medical records (EMR)
   c. Practice management
   d. A and B

6. What are records of computer activity used to monitor users' actions within software, including additions, deletions, and viewing of electronic records?
   a. Automatic log-off
   b. Authentication
   c. Firewalls
   d. Audit trails

7. What is a program or hardware device that acts as a barrier or filter between the network and the internet?
   a. Firewalls
   b. Screen savers
   c. Authentication
   d. Privacy filters

8. What means potential threats to the computer system security are identified, the likelihood of such occurrence is determined, and additional safeguards are implemented?
   a. Firewalls
   b. Security risk analysis
   c. Authentication
   d. Privacy filters

9. What makes a strong password?
   a. Use a person's name
   b. Use eight or more characters
   c. Use a random combination of upper- and lowercase letters, numbers, and symbols
   d. B and C

10. Which is the computer memory used for loading and running programs?
    a. ROM
    b. RAM
    c. Cache
    d. Hard drive

WORKPLACE APPLICATIONS

1. As part of her role, Christiana is learning about security measures to keep the network secure and confidential. Identify the security measures described.

   a. After a period of inactivity, the workstation logs off. _automatic log-off_

   b. Used to encode or change the information into nonreadable or encrypted data. _encryption software_

   c. Multiple incorrect log-in attempts are flagged, and many times the account is locked. Prevents hackers from cracking passwords.
      monitoring of log-in activity

   d. Each employee is assigned a unique name or number for identifying and tracking user identity.
      unique user identification

2. Christiana is evaluating the scanners in the reception area and the health information management department, which handles scanning documents into the electronic health records. Discuss types of scanners that might be used in both of these areas.

    In the reception area:- An Id card scanner would be used to scan insurance cards, driver license, etc. In the health department:- A sheetfed scanner or a flatbed scanner

3. Christiana would like to have a computer with internet access available for patients to use in the reception area. What are things that she will need to consider?

    The computer could be a dumb terminal where the patients would have access to the internet.

INTERNET ACTIVITIES

1. Review the content of one of the patient education websites listed in the chapter. Create a poster presentation, a PowerPoint presentation, or write a paper summarizing your research.

2. Select a disease. Find two reputable patient education websites that provide information on the disease, diagnostic tests, and treatments. One of your websites must be different than those listed in the chapter. Create a poster presentation, a PowerPoint presentation, or write a paper summarizing your research and include the websites used.

3. You need to purchase a printer for your department. Research a business-size laser printer and an inkjet printer. Create a poster presentation, a PowerPoint presentation, or write a paper summarizing your research and include the websites used. Include the following points for each printer:
    a. Name and model number of the printer
    b. Cost of the printer
    c. Cost of a new printer cartridge
    d. Speed of the printer
    e. Additional features of the printer that would be useful in a business setting

Procedure 6.1 Prepare a Workstation

Name _____ Date _____ Score _____

Tasks: Perform infection control procedures and create an ergonomically friendly workstation.

Equipment and Supplies:
- Nonabrasive disinfectant (hospital grade) wipes or specially made wipes for computer hardware or as indicated by the keyboard manufacturer
- Gloves (if required for using wipes)
- User guide for keyboard or facility's infection control procedure for computer hardware
- Desktop computer with adjustable monitor
- Office chair with an adjustable seat, armrest, and backrest
- Footrest (if needed)
- Foam wrist rest
- Document holder (optional)
- Hand sanitizer (optional)

Standard: Complete the procedure and all critical steps in _____ minutes with a minimum score of 85% within two attempts (*or as indicated by the instructor*).

Scoring: Divide the points earned by the total possible points. Failure to perform a critical step, indicated by an asterisk (*), results in grade no higher than an 84% (*or as indicated by the instructor*).

Time: Began_____ Ended_____ Total minutes: _____

Steps:	Point Value	Attempt 1	Attempt 2
1. While sitting in the chair, adjust the backrest so it supports the upper body and the lumbar support area fits to the small of the back. Adjust the seat pan height so the feet are flat on the floor or footrest. Adjust the armrest to support the forearms with the shoulders in a relaxed position.	20		
2. Adjust the monitor so it is directly in front of the person and the top of the monitor is at or just below the eye level. If using a document holder, position it so it is at the same distance and height as the monitor.	20		
3. Place the keyboard at a height and an angle to allow the wrists to be in a neutral position. Position the mouse so it is at elbow level for typing. Support the wrists with a foam wrist rest.	20		
4. While sitting with your torso and neck vertically and in line, identify if everything is positioned correctly and comfortably. Make any adjustments as needed.	10		
5. Using the keyboard user guide or the facilities infection control procedure for computer hardware, determine the product to use to disinfect the keyboard. Don gloves if needed. Using a disinfectant wipe, clean the surface using friction for 5 seconds in each area. Discard gloves if worn.	20*		
6. Wash hands or use hand sanitizer before using the keyboard.	10*		
Total Points	100		

Comments

ABHES Competencies	Step(s)
8. Clinical Procedures a. Practice standard precautions and perform disinfection/ sterilization techniques	5

Procedure 6.2   Identify a Reliable Patient Education Website

Name _____ Date _____ Score _____

Tasks: Research a disease or condition and evaluate a patient education website.

Equipment and Supplies:
- Computer with internet access, word processing software, and printer

Standard: Complete the procedure and all critical steps in _____ minutes with a minimum score of 85% within two attempts (*or as indicated by the instructor*).

Scoring: Divide the points earned by the total possible points. Failure to perform a critical step, indicated by an asterisk (*), results in grade no higher than an 84% (*or as indicated by the instructor*).

Time: Began_____ Ended_____ Total minutes: _____

Steps:	Point Value	Attempt 1	Attempt 2
1. Select a disease or condition. Using the internet, find a website with information about the disease or condition. Do not use a website listed in the textbook.	10*		
2. Identify the mission or purpose of the website, who supports or runs the website, and and whether there is advertising present on the page. If advertising is present, is the advertising mixed in with the content or text?	20		
3. Identify if the information is current or less than 3 years old.	10		
4. Identify the author(s) and the person's background. Does a panel of healthcare experts review the content?	20		
5. Identify if a person needs to enter personal information to view pages of the website. If so, what does the website's host do with the personal information?	20		
6. Compose a one-page paper on your findings. Use double line spacing and a 12-point font size. Include the website you used. Discuss if the website is reliable and if the content is updated. Proofread and spell-check your document prior to printing it.	20		
Total Points	100		

Comments

ABHES Competencies	Step(s)
7. Administrative Procedure h. Perform basic computer skills	Entire procedure

4. What is the correct format and location for the date? _____

_____

_____

5. What is the purpose of the reference line in a professional letter? _____

_____

6. How would you compose a greeting for a professional letter to John White? _____

_____

_____

7. Where is the closing located and what are typical professional closings? _____

_____

_____

8. What are two ways a reference notation would be keyed if Jean Moore were typing a letter for Dr. Sam Mast?

_____

_____

9. Where is the reference notation placed? _____

_____

10. Describe how to add a copy notation to a letter. _____

_____

11. Name three items that should be on a continuation page. _____

_____

12. Describe the difference between closed and open punctuation in a letter. _____

_____

_____

13. Describe a full block letter format. _____

_____

_____

14. Describe the similarities and differences between the modified block letter format and the semi-block letter format.

_____

_____

_____

15. What are letter templates? _____

_____

16. Business letters should be enclosed in standard _____ envelopes, which measure _____.

17. Letters and memos use the _____ orientation.

18. List the four headings used in memoranda and include the correct punctuation._____

_____

_____

_____

19. Explain why medical assistants need to know how to compose a professional email. _____

_____

_____

20. The following questions relate to composing professional emails.

a. What type of greeting should be used and give an example? _____

_____

b. Refrain from using all capital letters. How may the reader interpret this? _____

_____

c. Can texting abbreviations and emoticons (emojis) be used? _____

_____

d. How should you end your email?_____

_____

e. When emailing a patient, what should occur with a copy of the sent email? _____

_____

21. What type of information is usually on the cover sheet for a fax? _____

_____

_____

C. Mail

1. Describe how an automated mail processing machine reads the address on an envelope. _____

_____

_____

2. Describe five tips to follow when addressing mail._____

   _____

   _____

   _____

   _____

3. List four things that affect the postage rate of mail. _____

   _____

4. When the healthcare facility uses Certified Mail with Return Receipt, what information does the facility get?

   _____

5. Termination letters are sent by _____*employer*_____.

6. ___*Standard insurance*___ is an optional mail service that protects against loss or damage and the cost is based on the declared value of the item.

7. ___*restricted delivery*___ is an optional mail service that requires the addressee or authorized agent to verify identity when signing for the delivery.

8. _____ is an optional mail service that requires the recipient to pay for the merchandise and shipping when the package is received.

CERTIFICATION PREPARATION
Circle the correct answer.

1. Which is a word or group of words that describes a noun or pronoun?
   a. Adverb
   b. Adjective
   c. Verb
   d. Noun

2. Which needs to be capitalized?
   a. The first letter of the first word in a sentence or question
   b. The first letter of proper nouns
   c. The pronoun "I"
   d. All of the above

3. When should a comma be used?
   a. Before a coordinator (and, but, yet, nor, for, or, so) that links two main clauses
   b. To separate items in a list of three or more things
   c. After certain words (e.g., yes, no) at the start of a sentence
   d. All of the above

4. What type of software allows the user to enter demographic information, schedule appointments, maintain lists of insurance payers, perform billing tasks, and generate reports?
   a. Electronic health record (EHR)
   b. Electronic medical records (EMR)
   c. Practice management
   d. Microsoft Word and Excel

5. What includes the initials of the person who composed the letter?
   a. Enclosure notation
   b. Reference notation
   c. Copy notation
   d. Attachment notation

6. Which type of business letter format has the sender's and inside addresses left-justified and the date, closing, and signature blocks starting at the center point or right-justified?
   a. Semi-block
   b. Memo
   c. Modified block
   d. Full block

7. Which is the most commonly used mail service used for envelopes weighing up to 13 ounces, and provides delivery in 3 days or less?
   a. Priority Mail
   b. Priority Mail Express
   (c.) First-Class Mail
   d. Media Mail

8. Which optional mail service is used to protect expensive items, a mailing receipt is provided, and upon request an electronic verification of delivery or delivery attempt can be sent?
   (a.) Registered Mail
   b. Standard Insurance
   c. Certified Mail
   d. Return Receipt

9. Dr. James Smith composed a letter and Cathy Black keyed the letter. What is the correct format for the notation in the letter?
   a. cb:JS
   b. JS:cb
   (c.) CB:js
   d. js:CB

10. Which is *not* a header in a memo?
    a. TO
    b. FROM
    (c.) DEPARTMENT
    d. SUBJECT

WORKPLACE APPLICATIONS

1. Christiana Zwellen CMA (AAMA) is composing the following letters. Indicate the name that should appear in the signature block.

   a. A letter from her to the office supply company. _Dear Sir or Madam_

   b. A letter to Mrs. White from Dr. James Martin. _Mr. and Mrs. James Martin_

   c. A referral letter about a patient from Dr. James Martin to Dr. Robert Black. _Dear Mr. Robert Black, letter about patient._

2. When Christiana Zwellen is composing a letter for Dr. James Martin, indicate two ways she can create the reference notation.

   Reference initials, the business letter template

3. Christiana needs to fold a letter for a #10 envelope. Describe how this is done. _fold a letter in thirds, bring the bottom third of letter up and form a crease. Then fold the third down and make a crease. The second crease of the letter is inserted into envelope first._

INTERNET ACTIVITIES

1. Research professional email etiquette. Describe five ways you can improve your written communication with patients and professionals.

2. Research the two-letter postal abbreviations for the states. Write each address provided as it should appear on an envelope. Use only approved U.S. Postal Service standard street abbreviations and the two-letter postal abbreviation for states.

    a. Walden-Martin Family Medical Clinic, 1234 Any Street, Anytown, Alabama 14453 _____

    _____

    _____

    b. John Smith, 383 E. Center, Anytown, Nebraska 13333-2232 _____

    _____

    _____

    c. Sally Black, 39291 S. Parkway, Anytown, Wisconsin 54334-6443 _____

    _____

    _____

    d. Jeff Jones, 454 Boulevard, Anytown, Minnesota 49932-1234 _____

    _____

    _____

    e. Sam House, 599 State Highway, Anytown, Illinois 69532-1651 _____

    _____

    _____

3. Use the zip code look-up tool on www.usps.com to find the zip codes for the following cities. Write the zip code on the line to the right of the city.

    a. Chicken, AK _____

    b. Rabbit Hash, KY _____

    c. Oatmeal, TX _____

    d. Turkey, TX _____

    e. Popcorn, IN _____

    f. Toast, NC _____

    g. Corn, OK _____

    h. Cucumber, WV _____

    i. Chili, WI _____

    j. Cream, WI _____

Procedure 7.1 Compose a Professional Business Letter Using the Full Block Letter Format

Name _____ Date _____ Score _____

Task: Compose a professional letter using technology. Use the full block letter format and closed punctuation. Address the envelope and fold the letter.

Scenario: Jean Burke NP (nurse practitioner) has requested that you compose a letter to the parent (Lisa Parker) of Johnny Parker (date of birth [DOB]: 06/15/2010) to let her know that Johnny's throat culture from last Wednesday was negative. If he is not improving or if she has any questions, she should call the office. Lisa Parker's address is 91 Poplar Street, Anytown, AL 12345-1234. You are working at Walden-Martin Family Medical Clinic. The healthcare facility's address is 1234 Anystreet, Anytown, AL 12345. The phone number is 123-123-1234 and the fax number is 123-123-5678.

Equipment and Supplies:
- Patient's health record
- Computer with word processing software and printer
- Paper
- #10 envelope

Standard: Complete the procedure and all critical steps with a minimum score of 85% within two attempts (or as indicated by the instructor).

Scoring: Divide the points earned by the total possible points. Failure to perform a critical step, indicated by an asterisk (*), results in grade no higher than an 84% (or as indicated by the instructor).

Steps:	Point Value	Attempt 1	Attempt 2
1. Obtain the intended recipient's contact information and determine the message you want to convey. Using the computer and word processing software, compose the letter using the full block letter format. Use 1-inch margins on all four sides, portrait orientation, and use single line spacing throughout the letter. Use an easy-to-read font (e.g., Times New Roman or Calibri), in a 10- or 12-point size.	5		
2. Create a letterhead in the header of the document. Include the clinic's name, street address or post office box, city, state, and ZIP code.	10		
3. Key (type) the date starting at the left margin. Have one blank line between the date line and the last line of the letterhead.	10		
4. Key the inside address starting at the left margin and use the correct spelling and punctuation. Leave one to nine blank lines between the date and the inside address, to center the body of the letter on the page.	10*		
5. Key the salutation starting at the left margin and use the correct spelling and punctuation. Leave one blank line between the inside address and the salutation.	10		
6. Use your critical thinking skills to compose a concise, accurate message. Type the message in the body of the letter starting at the left margin. Leave one blank line between the salutation and the first line of the body and then between each paragraph of the body. The message should be clear, concise, and professional. Use proper grammar, punctuation, capitalization, and sentence structure.	10		

7.	Key a proper closing starting at the left margin and use the correct spelling and punctuation. Leave one blank line between the last line of the body and the closing.	10		
8.	Key the signature block starting at the left margin and use the correct spelling and punctuation. Leave four blank lines between the closing and the signature block. If you are preparing the letter for a provider, you must include a reference notation.	10		
9.	Spell-check and proofread the document. Check for the proper tone, grammar, punctuation, capitalization, and sentence structure. Check for proper spacing between the parts of the letter. Make any final corrections. Print the document.	5		
10.	Address the envelope, using either the computer and word processing software or a pen and following the correct format.	10		
11.	When using a #10 envelope, fold the letter by pulling up the bottom end until it reaches just below the inside address or two-thirds of the way up the letter. Crease at the fold. Then, fold the top of the letter down so that it is flush with the bottom fold and crease the paper.	5		
12.	File a copy of the letter in the paper medical record or upload an electronic copy of the letter to the electronic health record (EHR).	5		
	Total Points	100		

Comments

CAAHEP Competencies	Step(s)
V.P.8. Compose professional correspondence utilizing electronic technology	Entire procedure
ABHES Competencies	**Step(s)**
7. Administrative Procedures g. Display professionalism through written and verbal communications	Entire procedure
7.h. Perform basic computer skills	Entire procedure

Procedure 7.2   Compose a Professional Business Letter Using the Modified Block Letter Format

Name _____ Date _____ Score _____

Task: Compose a professional letter using technology. Use the modified block letter format (with the center point option). Address the envelope (if needed) and fold the letter.

Scenario: Julie Walden, MD has requested that you compose a letter to Carl C. Bowden (DOB: 04/05/1954 to let him know that his hepatitis C laboratory test was negative. If he has any questions, he should call the office. His address is 19 Beale Street, Anytown, AL 12345-1234. You are working at Walden-Martin Family Medical Clinic. The healthcare facility's address is 1234 Anystreet, Anytown, AL 12345. The phone number is 123-123-1234 and the fax number is 123-123-5678.

Equipment and Supplies:
- Patient's health record
- Computer with word processing software and printer
- Paper
- #10 envelope or window business envelope

Standard: Complete the procedure and all critical steps with a minimum score of 85% within two attempts (or as indicated by the instructor).

Scoring: Divide the points earned by the total possible points. Failure to perform a critical step, indicated by an asterisk (*), results in grade no higher than an 84% (or as indicated by the instructor).

Steps:	Point Value	Attempt 1	Attempt 2
1. Obtain the intended recipient's contact information and determine the message you want to convey. Using the computer and word processing software, compose the letter using the modified block letter format. Use 1-inch margins on all four sides, portrait orientation, and use single line spacing throughout the letter. Use an easy-to-read font (e.g., Times New Roman or Calibri), in a 10- or 12-point size.	5		
2. Create a letterhead in the header of the document. Include the clinic's name, street address or post office box, city, state, and ZIP code.	10		
3. Key (type) the date starting at the center point of the document. Have one blank line between the date line and the last line of the letterhead.	10		
4. Key the inside address starting at the left margin and use the correct spelling and punctuation. Leave one to nine blank lines between the date and the inside address, to center the body of the letter on the page. If using a window business envelope, adjust the address position to fit the window.	10*		
5. Key the salutation starting at the left margin and use the correct spelling and punctuation. Leave one blank line between the inside address and the salutation.	10		

6.	Use your critical thinking skills to compose a concise, accurate message. Type the message in the body of the letter starting at the left margin. Leave one blank line between the salutation and the first line of the body and then between each paragraph of the body. The message should be clear, concise, and professional. Use proper grammar, punctuation, capitalization, and sentence structure.	**10**		
7.	Key a proper closing starting at the center point of the document. Use the correct spelling and punctuation. Leave one blank line between the last line of the body and the closing.	**10**		
8.	Key the signature block starting at the center point of the document. Use the correct spelling and punctuation. Leave four blank lines between the closing and the signature block. If you are preparing the letter for a provider, you must include a reference notation.	**10**		
9.	Spell-check and proofread the document. Check for the proper tone, grammar, punctuation, capitalization, and sentence structure. Check for proper spacing between the parts of the letter. Make any final corrections. Print the document. If needed, address the envelope, using either the computer and word processing software or a pen and following the correct format.	**10**		
10.	When using a #10 envelope, fold the letter by pulling up the bottom end until it reaches just below the inside address or two-thirds of the way up the letter. Crease at the fold. Then, fold the top of the letter down so that it is flush with the bottom fold and crease the paper. For window business envelopes, have the letter's print side facing up and place the envelope over the top third of the letter. Fold the bottom edge of the paper up to the bottom edge of the envelope and crease at the fold. Then, remove the envelope and flip the letter over and fold the top of the letter down to the prior crease line and crease at the fold. Place the letter in the envelope so that the recipient's address shows through the window.	**10**		
11.	File a copy of the letter in the paper medical record or upload an electronic copy of the letter to the electronic health record (EHR).	**5**		
	Total Points	**100**		

Comments

CAAHEP Competencies	Step(s)
V.P.8. Compose professional correspondence utilizing electronic technology	Entire procedure
ABHES Competencies	**Step(s)**
7. Administrative Procedures g. Display professionalism through written and verbal communications	Entire procedure
7.h. Perform basic computer skills	Entire procedure

Procedure 7.3   Compose a Professional Business Letter Using the Semi-Block Letter Format

Name _____ **Date** _____ **Score** _____

Task: Compose a professional letter using technology. Use the semi-block letter format (with the right justified option). Address the envelope and fold the letter.

Scenario: Julie Walden MD has requested that you compose a letter to Amma Patel to let her know that her thyroid test was normal, but her vitamin D level was low. Dr. Walden would like Amma to take 15 mcg of vitamin D each morning. She can purchase this over the counter. She needs to have her vitamin D rechecked in 6 months. She can call to schedule the blood test closer to that time. If she has any questions, she should call the office. Her address is 1346 Charity Lane, Anytown, AL 12345-1234. You are working at Walden-Martin Family Medical Clinic. The healthcare facility's address is 1234 Anystreet, Anytown, AL 12345. The phone number is 123-123-1234 and the fax number is 123-123-5678.

Equipment and Supplies:
- Patient's health record
- Computer with word processing software and printer
- Paper
- #10 envelope or #6¾ envelope

Standard: Complete the procedure and all critical steps with a minimum score of 85% within two attempts (or as indicated by the instructor).

Scoring: Divide the points earned by the total possible points. Failure to perform a critical step, indicated by an asterisk (*), results in grade no higher than an 84% (or as indicated by the instructor).

Steps:	Point Value	Attempt 1	Attempt 2
1. Obtain the intended recipient's contact information and determine the message you want to convey. Using the computer and word processing software, compose the letter using the semi-block letter format. Use 1-inch margins on all four sides, portrait orientation, and use single line spacing throughout the letter. Use an easy-to-read font (e.g., Times New Roman or Calibri), in a 10- or 12-point size.	5		
2. Create a letterhead in the header of the document. Include the clinic's name, street address or post office box, city, state, and ZIP code.	10		
3. Right justify and key (type) the date. Have one blank line between the date line and the last line of the letterhead.	10		
4. Key the inside address starting at the left margin and use the correct spelling and punctuation. Leave one to nine blank lines between the date and the inside address, to center the body of the letter on the page.	10*		
5. Key the salutation starting at the left margin and use the correct spelling and punctuation. Leave one blank line between the inside address and the salutation.	10		

6.	Use your critical thinking skills to compose a concise, accurate message. Type the message in the body of the letter starting at the left margin. Leave one blank line between the salutation and the first line of the body and then between each paragraph of the body. Each paragraph should be indented five spaces. The message should be clear, concise, and professional. Use proper grammar, punctuation, capitalization, and sentence structure.	10		
7.	Right justify and key a proper closing. Use the correct spelling and punctuation. Leave one blank line between the last line of the body and the closing.	10		
8.	Right justify and key the signature block. Use the correct spelling and punctuation. Leave four blank lines between the closing and the signature block. If you are preparing the letter for a provider, you must include a reference notation.	10		
9.	Spell-check and proofread the document. Check for the proper tone, grammar, punctuation, capitalization, and sentence structure. Check for proper spacing between the parts of the letter. Make any final corrections. Print the document.	5		
10.	Address the envelope, using either the computer and word processing software or a pen and following the correct format.	10		
11.	When using a #10 envelope, fold the letter by pulling up the bottom end until it reaches just below the inside address or two-thirds of the way up the letter. Crease at the fold. Then, fold the top of the letter down so that it is flush with the bottom fold and crease the paper. When using a #6¾ envelope, pull the bottom edge of the letter up until it is ½ inch from the top edge of the document and crease at the fold. Bring the right edge two-thirds of the way across the width of the document and crease the paper. Then bring the left edge to the right edge and crease at the fold. Flip the document so the left edge is on the bottom and insert the letter into the envelope.	5		
12.	File a copy of the letter in the paper medical record or upload an electronic copy of the letter to the electronic health record (EHR).	5		
	Total Points	100		

Comments

CAAHEP Competencies	Step(s)
V.P.8. Compose professional correspondence utilizing electronic technology	Entire procedure
ABHES Competencies	**Step(s)**
7. Administrative Procedures g. Display professionalism through written and verbal communications	Entire procedure
7.h. Perform basic computer skills	Entire procedure

Procedure 7.4   Compose a Memorandum

Name _____   Date _____   Score _____

Task: Compose a professional memorandum.

Scenario: You are asked by the supervisor to compose a memo that can be posted in the department. You are to remind the staff about the department meeting next Tuesday at noon in the conference room. Staff can bring their lunches and beverages will be provided.

Equipment and Supplies:
- Computer with word processing software and printer
- Paper

Standard: Complete the procedure and all critical steps with a minimum score of 85% within two attempts (or as indicated by the instructor).

Scoring: Divide the points earned by the total possible points. Failure to perform a critical step, indicated by an asterisk (*), results in grade no higher than an 84% (or as indicated by the instructor).

Steps:	Point Value	Attempt 1	Attempt 2
1. Determine the message you want to convey. Using the computer and word processing software, compose the memo. Use 1-inch margins on all four sides, portrait orientation, and use single line spacing throughout the memo. Use an easy-to-read font (e.g., Times New Roman or Calibri), in a 10- or 12-point size.	15		
2. Left justify the headers and use boldface and capital letters, followed by a colon. Headers include TO, FROM, DATE, and SUBJECT. Leave one blank line between each header.	15		
3. Key (type) the information following the headers in regular font, using a mix of capital and lowercase letters. Using the tab tool, align the information vertically down the page. Key (type) the date as indicated for professional letters.	15		
4. Add a centered black line between the headers and the body (optional). Leave two to three blank lines between the headers and the body of the memo.	15		
5. Key the message in the body of the memo. Left justify the content in the body and use single line spacing. Use proper grammar and correct spelling and punctuation. With multiple paragraphs, skip a single line between paragraphs.	15		
6. The content of the message in the body of the memo is written clearly, concisely, and accurately. Add special notations as needed.	15		
7. Spell-check and proofread the document. Check for the proper tone, grammar, punctuation, capitalization, and sentence structure. Check for proper spacing between the parts of the memo. Make any final corrections. Print the document.	10		
Total Points	100		

Comments

CAAHEP Competencies	Step(s)
V.P.8. Compose professional correspondence utilizing electronic technology	Entire procedure
ABHES Competencies	**Step(s)**
7. Administrative Procedures g. Display professionalism through written and verbal communications	Entire procedure
7.h. Perform basic computer skills	Entire procedure

Procedure 7.5   Compose a Professional Email

Name _____   Date _____   Score _____

Task: Compose a professional email that conveys the message to the reader clearly, concisely, and accurately.

Scenario: Aaron Jackson (DOB: 10/17/2011) has an appointment at 11 AM next Thursday. Send his guardian an appointment reminder via email. Aaron will be seeing David Kahn, M.D. The guardian should bring in any medications Aaron is currently taking. You are working at Walden-Martin Family Medical Clinic. The healthcare facility's address is: 1234 Anystreet, Anytown, AL 12345. The phone number is 123-123-1234 and the fax number is 123-123-5678. Your instructor will supply you with the guardian's name and email address.

Equipment and Supplies:
- Patient's health record
- Computer with email software

Standard: Complete the procedure and all critical steps with a minimum score of 85% within two attempts (or as indicated by the instructor).

Scoring: Divide the points earned by the total possible points. Failure to perform a critical step, indicated by an asterisk (*), results in grade no higher than an 84% (or as indicated by the instructor).

Steps:	Point Value	Attempt 1	Attempt 2
1. Obtain the intended recipient's contact information and determine the message you want to convey.	5		
2. Using the computer and email software, key (type) in the recipient's email address. If the email has two recipients, use a semicolon (;) after the name of the first recipient. Double-check the email addresses for accuracy.	5*		
3. Key in a subject, keeping it simple but focused on the contents of the email.	10		
4. Key a formal greeting, using correct punctuation.	10		
5. Key the message in the body of the email using proper grammar, punctuation, capitalization, and sentence structure. Avoid abbreviations. The message should be clear, concise, and professional.	20		
6. Finish the email with closing remarks.	10		
7. Key a closing, followed by your name and title on the next line. Include the clinic's name and contact information below your name.	10		
8. Spell-check and proofread the email. Check for proper tone, grammar, punctuation, capitalization, and sentence structure. Check for proper spacing between the parts of the email.	10		
9. Make any final revisions, select any features to apply to the email, and then send it.	10		
10. Print a copy of the email to be filed in the paper medical record or upload an electronic copy of the email to the patient's electronic health record (EHR).	10		
Total Points	100		

Comments

CAAHEP Competencies	Step(s)
V.P.8. Compose professional correspondence utilizing electronic technology	Entire procedure
ABHES Competencies	**Step(s)**
7. Administrative Procedures g. Display professionalism through written and verbal communications	Entire procedure
7.h. Perform basic computer skills	Entire procedure

Procedure 7.6   Complete a Fax Cover Sheet

Name _____ Date _____ Score _____

Task: Complete a fax cover sheet clearly and accurately.

Scenario: Lisa Parker, mother of Johnny Parker (DOB: 06/15/2010) requested his immunization history be sent to Anytown School, attention: Susie Payne. The school's phone number is 123-123-5784 and the fax number will be supplied by your instructor. The release of medical records has been completed and signed by Lisa, Johnny's guardian/mother. Your phone number is the main clinic number listed on the header of the fax cover sheet.

Equipment and Supplies:
- Document to be faxed (optional)
- Fax machine and fax number (optional)
- Pen
- Fax cover sheet (Work Product 7.1, HIPAA-Compliant Fax Cover Sheet)

Standard: Complete the procedure and all critical steps with a minimum score of 85% within two attempts (or as indicated by the instructor).

Scoring: Divide the points earned by the total possible points. Failure to perform a critical step, indicated by an asterisk (*), results in grade no higher than an 84% (or as indicated by the instructor).

Steps:	Point Value	Attempt 1	Attempt 2
1. Using a pen and the fax cover sheet, clearly and accurately write your name, phone number, and the date.	20		
2. Clearly and accurately write the name of the person receiving the fax. Also include the company, fax number, and the phone number.	20		
3. Write the number of pages. The cover sheet must be counted in the total.	20		
4. Complete Re: by indicating the subject of the fax. Be general with the subject and refrain from including anything confidential.	20		
5. Proofread the fax cover sheet. Verify the name, agency, and contact information of the recipient. Verify the document(s) being sent are correct. Organize the documents so the coversheet is on top and fax to the recipient (optional).	20		
Total Points	**100**		

Comments

ABHES Competencies	Step(s)
7. Administrative Procedures g. Display professionalism through written and verbal communications	Entire procedure

Work Product 7.1   HIPAA-Compliant Fax Cover Sheet

To be used with Procedure 7.6.

Name _____   Date _____   Score _____

WALDEN-MARTIN
FAMILY MEDICAL CLINIC
1234 ANYSTREET | ANYTOWN, ANYSTATE 12345
PHONE 123-123-1234 | FAX 123-123-5678

Fax

To: _____   **From:** _____

Company: _____   **Phone:** _____

Fax: _____   **Date:** _____

Phone: _____

Pages: _____

Re: _____

CONFIDENTIAL NOTICE

The material enclosed with this facsimile transmission is confidential and private. The material is the property of the sender and some or all of the information may be protected by the Health Insurance Portability & Accountability Act (HIPAA). This information is intended exclusively for the addressed person or agency indicated above. If you are not the intended individual or entity of this information, you are hereby notified that any use, duplication, circulation, or transmission of the information is strictly prohibited under state and federal law. Please notify the sender immediate using the telephone number indicated above.

Telephone Techniques

CAAHEP	Assessments
V.P.6. Demonstrate professional telephone techniques	Procedure 8.1
V.P.7. Document telephone messages accurately	Procedure 8.2
V.P.11. Report relevant information concisely and accurately	Procedure 8.2

ABHES	Assessments
7. Administrative Procedures g. Display professionalism through written and verbal communications	Procedure 8.1, 8.2

VOCABULARY REVIEW

Using the word pool on the right, find the correct word to match the definition. Write the word on the line after the definition.

Group A

1. A commercial service that answers telephone calls for its clients
   answering service

2. An unexpected, life-threatening situation that requires immediate action _emergency_

3. A business telephone system that allows for more than one telephone line _multiple line telephone system_

4. A feature that states who the caller is and displays the telephone numbers of incoming calls made to a particular line
   caller ID

5. The depth of a tone or sound; a distinctive quality of sound
   pitch

6. A telephone feature that allows calls made to one number to be sent to another specified number _call forwarding_

7. An applied science concerned with designing and arranging things needed to do your job in an efficient and safe way
   ergonomics

8. An individual or company that supplies medical care and services to a patient or the public _~~provider~~ ~~pitch~~ provider_

9. A telephone with a loudspeaker and a microphone; it can be used without having to pick up and hold the handset
   speakerphone

10. A telephone function in which a selected stored number can be dialed by pressing only one key _speed dialing_

11. An electronic system that allows messages from telephone callers to be recorded and stored _voice mail_

12. A two-way communication system with a microphone and loudspeaker at each station; often a feature of business telephones
    intercom

Word Pool
- multiple line telephone system
- ergonomics
- speakerphone
- caller ID
- voice mail
- emergency
- call forwarding
- answering service
- intercom
- provider
- speed dialing
- pitch

CERTIFICATION PREPARATION

Circle the correct answer.

1. Which best describes the primary goal of "screening" telephone calls?
   a. Preventing calls from reaching the provider
   b. Handling calls at the lowest level possible
   c. Selecting which calls should be forwarded to which staff members through an understanding of the purpose of the call
   d. Determining whether the calls are emergencies

2. Active listening involves
   a. giving the same attention to a person on the telephone as would be given to a person face to face.
   b. concentrating on the conversation at hand.
   c. discovering vital information.
   d. all of the above.

3. The medical assistant should be extremely careful when using a speakerphone because
   a. the service is expensive.
   b. it is distracting.
   c. the call can be traced.
   d. confidentiality can be violated.

4. Which term would be considered jargon?
   a. Encephalalgia
   b. Rash
   c. Dizziness
   d. Headache

5. The medical assistant may help an angry caller calm down by
   a. getting angry in return.
   b. speaking in a lower tone of voice.
   c. referring the situation to the office manager immediately.
   d. calling the provider into the situation.

6. If your office is in New York and you need to contact a supplier in Seattle, which New York time would be the earliest that you should call to place an order, assuming that the supplier opens at 8 AM?
   a. 8:00 AM
   b. 9:00 AM
   c. 10:00 AM
   d. 11:00 AM

7. Which types of calls should be limited in the professional setting?
   a. Local
   b. Long distance
   c. Toll free
   d. Personal

8. Enunciation is
   a. the choice of words.
   b. the highness or lowness of sound.
   c. articulation of clear sounds.
   d. a change in pitch.

9. Which is *not* required when a telephone message is taken?
   a. The caller's name and phone number
   b. The time and date
   c. The name of the person to whom the call is directed
   d. The caller's account number

10. When placing callers on hold, how often should you check back to make sure the caller still wants to remain on hold?
    a. No longer than 1 minute
    b. Every 2 minutes
    c. Until time is available to talk
    d. It is not necessary to check back; patients will hold until you return to the call

WORKPLACE APPLICATIONS

1. Mr. Ken Thomas calls to get his prescription for Ambien refilled. His pharmacy is Wolfe Drug, and the drugstore phone number is 214-555-4523. Mr. Thomas is allergic to penicillin. His phone number is 214-555-2377. Mr. Thomas' message was received on July 23 at 10:15 AM.

    a. Who should receive this message? _medical assistant_

    b. Questions to ask the patient: _All the information is there to carry out the request, if approved by the doctor._

    c. What action should be taken after speaking with the patient? _Pull the medical record, if not already done. Place the phone message with the record and give it to the physician._

2. Message retrieved from the answering machine, "This is Sarah at AnyTown Lab with a STAT laboratory report. It is 9:35 AM on November 16. The patient's name is Noemi Rodriguez, date of birth November 4, 1971 and her WBC count is 18,000. Please notify Dr. Walden immediately. The laboratory phone number is 800-555-3333 and my extension is 255. If she has any questions, please have her give me a call. Thanks."

    a. Who should receive this message? _Dr. Walden, primarily and secondly, the medical assistant_

    b. Questions to ask Sarah: _There may be no questions for the lab, but patient will need to be contacted contacted._

    c. What action should be taken? _Follow doctor's orders to handle the situation._

3. Denise has been the receptionist for a moderately large clinic for the past 3 months. She replaced Dorothy, who retired. Denise has been overwhelmed with the calls to the clinic, and the office manager has spoken to her twice about missing calls. Denise insists that she is constantly on the phone answering and transferring calls. She is beginning to lose faith in herself, but as she considers why she is failing at her job, she realizes that two new physicians have joined the practice since Dorothy left, and numerous calls come to the clinic for those two providers. Denise wants to suggest to the office manager that perhaps the time has come for a second receptionist, but she is unsure how to broach the subject. How can Denise begin her conversation with the office manager? What should she not do or say?

She need to discuss regarding the issue with the office manager. She always need to speak the truth.

INTERNET ACTIVITIES

1. Using online resources, locate the following telephone numbers for your city or community.

   a. Nonemergency number for the police department _____

   b. Local social security office _____

   c. American Red Cross office _____

   d. Acute care hospital _____

   e. Meals on Wheels _____

   f. American Cancer Society _____

   g. Local senior center _____

   h. Local food bank _____

   i. Poison control _____

   j. Local child protective services _____

Procedure 8.1   Demonstrate Professional Telephone Techniques

Name _____ Date _____ Score _____

Task: To answer the telephone in a provider's office in a professional manner and respond to a request for action.

Scenario: Charles Johnson, DOB 3/3/1958, an established patient of Dr. Martin, has called to schedule an appointment to have his blood pressure checked. This will be a follow-up appointment that is 15 minutes long. He is requesting that the appointment be on a Friday during his lunchtime between 11:00 and 12:00.

Equipment and Supplies:
- Telephone
- Pen or pencil
- Computer
- Notepad

Standard: Complete the procedure and all critical steps in _____ minutes with a minimum score of 85% within two attempts (*or as indicated by the instructor*).

Scoring: Divide the points earned by the total possible points. Failure to perform a critical step, indicated by an asterisk (*), results in grade no higher than an 84% (*or as indicated by the instructor*).

Time: Began_____ Ended_____ Total minutes: _____

Steps:	Point Value	Attempt 1	Attempt 2
1. Demonstrate telephone techniques by answering the telephone by the third ring.	10		
2. Speak distinctly with a pleasant tone and expression, at a moderate rate, and with sufficient volume for the person to understand every word.	15*		
3. Identify the office and/or provider and yourself.	10		
4. Verify the identity of the caller, and if using an electronic health record, bring the patient's health record to the active screen of the computer.	15*		
5. Screen the call if necessary.	10		
6. Apply active listening skills to assess whether the caller is distressed or agitated and to determine the concern to be addressed.	10*		
7. Determine the needs of the caller and provide the requested information or service if possible. Provide the caller with excellent customer service. Be as helpful as possible. Check the appointment schedule and determine the first Friday that would have an open appointment between 11:00 and 12:00	10		
8. Obtain sufficient patient information to schedule the appointment, including the patient's full name, DOB, insurance information, and preferred contact method. Repeat the date and time of the appointment to ensure that the patient has the correct information.	10		
9. Terminate the call in a pleasant manner and replace the receiver gently, always allowing the caller to hang up first.	10		
Total Points	100		

Comments

CAAHEP Competencies	Step(s)
V.P.6. Demonstrate professional telephone techniques	Entire procedure
ABHES Competencies	**Step(s)**
7. Administrative Procedures g. Display professionalism through written and verbal communications	Entire procedure

Procedure 8.2   Document Telephone Messages and Report Relevant Information Concisely and Accurately

Name _____ Date _____ Score _____

Tasks: To take an accurate telephone message and follow up on the requests made by the caller.

Scenario: Norma Washington, DOB 8/1/1944, an established patient of Dr. Martin, has called to report her blood pressure readings that she has been taking at home. Dr. Martin had made a recent change in her medication and wanted her to monitor her BP at home for 3 days and call in with the results. She has taken her blood pressure in the morning and in the evening for the past 3 days, with the following results:
- Day 1: 144/92 in the AM, 156/94 in the PM
- Day 2: 136/84 in the AM, 142/86 in the PM
- Day 3: 132/80 in the AM, 138/82 in the PM

Equipment and Supplies:
- Telephone
- Computer or message pad
- Pen or pencil
- Health record

Standard: Complete the procedure and all critical steps in _____ minutes with a minimum score of 85% within two attempts (*or as indicated by the instructor*).

Scoring: Divide the points earned by the total possible points. Failure to perform a critical step, indicated by an asterisk (*), results in grade no higher than an 84% (*or as indicated by the instructor*).

Time: Began_____ Ended_____ Total minutes: _____

Steps:	Point Value	Attempt 1	Attempt 2
1. Demonstrate telephone techniques by answering the telephone using the guidelines in Procedure 8.1.	15		
2. Using a message pad or the computer, take the phone message (either on paper or by data entry into the computer) and obtain the following information: • Name of the person to whom the call is directed • Name of the person calling • Caller's telephone number • Reason for the call • Action to be taken • Date and time of the call • Initials of the person taking the call	15*		
3. Apply active listening skills and repeat the information back to the caller after recording the message.	10		
4. End the call and wait for the caller to hang up first.	10		
5. Document the telephone call with all pertinent information in the patient's health record.	10*		
6. Deliver the phone message to the appropriate person.	10		

7.	Follow up on important messages.	**10**		
8.	If using paper messaging, keep old message books for future reference. Carbonless copies allow the facility to keep a permanent record of phone messages. If using an electronic system, the message will be saved to the patient's record automatically.	**10**		
9.	File pertinent phone messages in the patient's health record. Make sure the computer record is closed after the documentation has been done.	**10**		
	Total Points	**100**		

Comments

CAAHEP Competencies	**Step(s)**
V.P.6. Demonstrate professional telephone techniques	1, 3, 4
V.P.7. Document telephone messages accurately	2, 5
ABHES Competencies	**Step(s)**
7. Administrative Procedures g. Display professionalism through written and verbal communications	Entire procedure

Scheduling Appointments and Patient Processing

CAAHEP	Assessments
VI.C.1. Identify different types of appointment scheduling methods	Skills and Concepts – C. 1-6
VI.C.2.a. Identify advantages and disadvantages of the following appointment systems: manual	Skills and Concepts – C. 2
VI.C.2.b. Identify advantages and disadvantages of the following appointment systems: electronic	Skills and Concepts – C. 3
VI.C.3. Identify critical information required for scheduling patient procedures	Skills and Concepts – G. 1
VI.P.1. Manage appointment schedule using established priorities	Procedure 9.1, 9.2, 9.4
VI.P.2. Schedule a patient procedure	Procedure 9.5
VI.A.1. Display sensitivity when managing appointments	Procedure 9.2, 9.4, 9.5
VII.P.3. Obtain accurate patient billing information	Procedure 9.2
V.P.4.a. Coach patients regarding: office policies	Procedure 9.3
ABHES	**Assessments**
7. Administrative Procedures e. Apply scheduling principles	Procedure 9.1, 9.2, 9.4, 9.5

VOCABULARY REVIEW

Using the word pool on the right, find the correct word to match the definition. Write the word on the line after the definition.

Group A

1. Documentation in the medical record to track the patient's condition and progress _____

2. Space of time between events _____

3. An unexpected event that throws a plan into disorder; an interruption that prevents a system or process from continuing as usual or as expected _____

4. Skilled as a result of training or practice _____

5. A rule that controls how something should be done; guidelines or boundaries _____

6. An appointment type used when a patient needs to see the provider after a condition should have been resolved or to monitor an ongoing condition _____

7. The environment where something is created or takes shape; a base on which to build _____

8. Statistical data of a population; in healthcare this includes patient name, address, date of birth, employment, and other details

   _____

9. A type of software that allows the user to enter demographic information, schedule appointments, maintain lists of insurance payers, perform billing tasks, and generate reports

   _____

10. Essential; being an indispensable part of a whole

   _____

Word Pool

- parameters
- demographics
- integral
- intervals
- matrix
- follow-up appointment
- proficiency
- practice management software
- progress notes
- disruption

Group B

1. A means of achieving a particular end, as in a situation requiring urgency or caution _____

2. The process of confirming health insurance coverage for the patient _____

3. A written document describing the healthcare facility's privacy practices _____

4. A system for examining and separating into different groups; in the healthcare facility, it means determining the severity of illness that patients experience and prioritizing appointments based on that severity _____

5. The process of determining if a procedure or service is covered by the insurance plan and what the reimbursement is for that procedure or service _____

6. To sort out and classify the injured; used in the military and in emergency settings to determine the priority of a patient to be treated _____

7. A patient who has been treated previously by the healthcare provider within the past 3 years _____

8. A secure online website that gives patients 24-hour access to personal health information using a username and password _____

9. When a patient fails to keep an appointment without giving advance notice _____

10. The process of determining if a procedure or service is covered by the insurance plan and what the reimbursement is for that procedure or service _____

Word Pool
- Notice of Privacy Practices
- preauthorization
- precertification
- established patients
- screening
- no-show
- expediency
- triage
- patient portal
- verification of eligibility

ABBREVIATIONS
Write out what each of the following abbreviations stands for.

1. ECG _____
2. NPP _____
3. MRI _____
4. CT _____
5. EMT _____
6. EHR _____
7. HIPAA _____
8. CDC _____

SKILLS AND CONCEPTS

Answer the following questions. Write your answer on the line or in the space provided.

Scheduling Appointments

A. Establishing the Appointment Schedule

1. When developing an appointment schedule, _____ and _____ must be considered.

2. _____ information includes the patient's address, insurance information, and email address.

B. Creating the Appointment Matrix

1. Time would be blocked out in the schedule for what four reasons when setting up the appointment matrix?

   a. _____

   b. _____

   c. _____

   d. _____

2. How can the medical assistant handle a provider who habitually spends more than the allotted time with patients?

   _____

   _____

   _____

   _____

3. Using the appointment schedule page that follows, schedule these appointments, blocking out the appropriate amount of time:

   Recheck appointment   15 minutes

   Complete physical examination (PE)   45 minutes

   a. Jana Green; recheck appointment, prefers Wednesdays
   b. Pedro Gomez; complete physical examination, prefers Tuesdays
   c. Truong Tran; recheck, prefers Thursdays after 9:00 AM
   d. Walter Biller; complete physical examination, prefers Mondays as early as possible
   e. Reuven Ahmad; complete physical examination, prefers Fridays

	Monday	Tuesday	Wednesday	Thursday	Friday
8:00					
8:15					
8:30					
8:45					
9:00					
9:15					
9:30					
9:45					
10:00					

C. Methods of Scheduling Appointments

1. Identify the different scheduling methods._____

    _____

    _____

2. Identify the advantages and disadvantages of a manual appointment system. _____

    _____

    _____

    _____

    _____

    _____

3. Identify advantages and disadvantages of an electronic appointment system. _____

    _____

    _____

    _____

    _____

    _____

D. Types of Appointment Scheduling

Briefly describe each type of scheduling and list one advantage and one disadvantage of each.

1. Time-specified (stream) scheduling _____

   _____

   _____

   _____

   _____

   _____

   _____

2. Open office hours _____

   _____

   _____

   _____

   _____

   _____

   _____

3. Wave scheduling _____

   _____

   _____

   _____

   _____

   _____

4. Modified wave scheduling _____

   _____

   _____

   _____

   _____

   _____

   _____

5. Double booking _____

_____

_____

_____

_____

_____

_____

6. Grouping procedures _____

_____

_____

_____

_____

_____

_____

_____

E. Telephone Scheduling

1. When scheduling an appointment over the telephone, what options are available to remind patients of the appointment?

_____

F. Scheduling Appointments for New Patients

1. To determine how much time to allow for an appointment, the medical assistant needs to obtain information about the _____.

2. New patients should be asked to arrive _____ minutes early to complete necessary paperwork.

3. An ideal tool to provide new patients with information is a(n) _____.

G. Scheduling Other Types of Appointments

1. Identify critical information required for scheduling patient procedures. _____

_____

_____

_____

_____

_____

_____

2. Identify the special requests that a provider may have for inpatient surgeries. _____

_____

_____

_____

_____

H. Special Circumstances

1. What is the difference between an emergency appointment and an urgent appointment? _____

_____

_____

_____

_____

2. How does the medical assistant handle a patient who arrives at the clinic to see the provider but does not have an appointment?

_____

_____

_____

_____

I. Increasing Appointment Show Rates
Practice completing appointment reminder cards on the forms provided. Students should be able to fill out the appointment cards with the information provided without difficulty.

1. Tai Yan has an appointment for August 23, 20XX, at 3:00 PM with Dr. Martin.

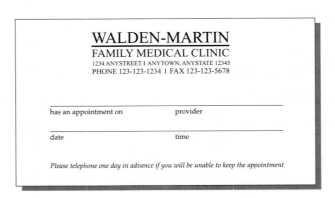

WALDEN-MARTIN
FAMILY MEDICAL CLINIC
1234 ANYSTREET I ANYTOWN, ANYSTATE 12345
PHONE 123-123-1234 I FAX 123-123-5678

_____ has an appointment on _____ provider

_____ date _____ time

Please telephone one day in advance if you will be unable to keep the appointment

2.   Diego Lopez has an appointment for May 1, 20XX, at 9:00 AM with Dr. Walden.

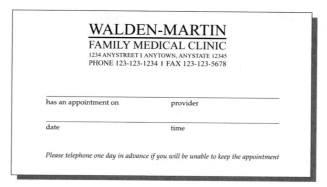

3.   Julia Berkley has an appointment for June 13, 20XX, at 11:45 AM with Dr. Walden.

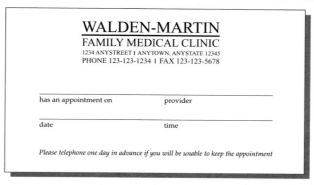

4.   Monique Jones has an appointment for September 12, 20XX, at 2:40 PM with Jean Burke, N.P.

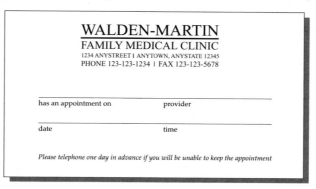

5.   Ken Thomas has an appointment for December 15, 20XX, at 4:30 PM with Dr. Martin.

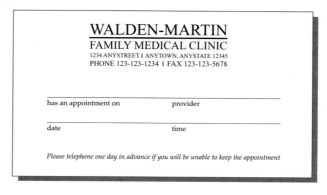

Patient Processing Tasks

1. When screening patients at the reception desk, what patient conditions require immediate action by the medical assistant?

    _____

    _____

2. What action should the medical assistant take when patients have emergent conditions? _____

    _____

    _____

    _____

3. If a medical assistant is unable to greet a patient at the reception desk, what actions can help acknowledge the person?

    _____

    _____

4. List six features of a HIPAA-appropriate sign-in register. _____

    _____

    _____

    _____

    _____

    _____

    _____

5. List three features that would cause a HIPAA violation with sign-in registers. _____

    _____

    _____

    _____

    _____

6. How does a medical assistant take steps to protect other patients in the reception area? _____

    _____

    _____

    _____

    _____

7. What must occur if a patient refuses to sign the NPP form? _____

_____

_____

_____

_____

8. How should a medical assistant review a new patient brochure with a new patient? _____

_____

_____

_____

_____

9. During the check-in process, what three things must the medical assistant do for all patients? _____

_____

_____

_____

_____

10. If the provider is delayed, what should the medical assistants do with the patients who are waiting?

_____

_____

_____

_____

11. How should a medical assistant handle a situation when a patient is angry? _____

_____

_____

_____

_____

12. What occurs during the checkout process?_____

_____

_____

_____

_____

CERTIFICATION PREPARATION

Cirle the correct answer.

1. The medical assistant may help an angry caller to calm down by
   a. getting angry in return.
   b. speaking in a lower tone of voice.
   c. referring the situation to the office manager immediately.
   d. calling the provider into the situation.

2. Why is it necessary to include a note in the patient's chart when the person does not show up for a scheduled appointment?
   a. To bill the patient for the time
   b. To keep count of the number of no-shows for a possible drop in the future
   c. To be prepared for future legal consequences regarding the patient's care
   d. To provide the medical assistant with a reminder to call and reschedule

3. What is the appointment-setting method by which a patient logs onto the internet and views a facility's schedule to set his or her own appointment?
   a. Flexible office hours
   b. Self-scheduling
   c. Grouping procedures
   d. Advance booking

4. An obstetrician who devotes two afternoons a week to seeing pregnant patients is using an appointment scheduling method called
   a. wave scheduling.
   b. advance booking.
   c. grouping procedures.
   d. modified wave scheduling.

5. Which type of scheduling is an attempt to create short-term flexibility within each hour?
   a. Time-specified scheduling
   b. Wave scheduling
   c. Stream scheduling
   d. Modified-wave scheduling

6. All patients want to be kept informed about how long they should expect to wait to see the provider. Any delay longer than _____ minutes should be explained.
   a. 15
   b. 20
   c. 30
   d. No explanation is necessary

7. When screening patients at the reception desk, which patient has an emergent condition and requires immediate care?
   a. Chest pain
   b. Sore throat
   c. Tick bite
   d. Ankle injury

8. When calling a patient from the reception room to escort him to an exam room, how should the medical assistant call the patient?
   a. "James Brown, Dr. Walden is ready for you."
   b. "James Brown with the sore throat"
   c. "James Brown with a birthdate of June 6"
   d. "James Brown"

9. The statistical characteristics of human populations are called
   a. numbers.
   b. perceptions.
   c. demographics.
   d. phonetics.

10. An effective way to deal with patients who are always late for appointments is to
    a. refuse to schedule them after this happens several times.
    b. have them wait until it is convenient for the physician.
    c. advise them that they disrupt the office schedule.
    d. give them the last appointment of the day.

WORKPLACE APPLICATIONS

1. Janie Haynes consistently arrives at the clinic between 15 and 45 minutes late. She always has a "good" excuse, but she could make her appointments on time if she had better time management skills. The office manager has mentioned to Paula, the receptionist, that Janie is to be scheduled at 4:45 PM and if she is late, she will not be seen by the provider. Paula books Janie's next three appointments at that time, and Janie actually arrives early. However, on the fourth appointment, Janie arrives at 5:50 PM, and Paula knows that it is her responsibility to tell Janie that she cannot see the provider. How does Paula handle this task? What are the options for Paula?

_____

_____

_____

_____

_____

2. Jill is the receptionist for Drs. Boles and Bailey, who are psychiatrists. Each week, Sara Ables comes to her appointments but brings her two small children, Joey and Julie, ages 8 and 6 years, respectively. When Sara goes back for her appointment, the children are almost uncontrollable in the reception area. Although there are never more than two patients waiting, the kids are a serious disruption in the clinic. When Jill mentioned the problem to Dr. Boles, he said that Sara really needed the sessions and that Jill should try to work with Sara on this issue. What can Jill do to remedy the situation?

_____

_____

_____

_____

_____

INTERNET ACTIVITIES

1. Using online resources, research group appointments. Create a poster presentation, a PowerPoint presentation, or write a paper summarizing your research. Include the following points in your project:
   a. Description of a group appointment
   b. List the types of conditions that are best suited for group appointments
   c. Explain whose confidentiality is maintained with group appointments
   d. List the benefits for patients and providers when group appointments are used

Procedure 9.1   Establish the Appointment Matrix

Name _____ Date _____ Score _____

Task: To establish the matrix of the appointment schedule.

Scenario: You have been asked to set up the schedule matrix for Dr. Julie Walden, Dr. James Martin, and Dr. Angela Perez. Block off the following times in the appointment schedule:

Dr. Julie Walden:
- Lunch; daily from 11:30 AM to 12:30 PM
- Hospital Rounds; Mondays and Wednesday from 8:00 AM to 9:00 AM

Dr. James Martin:
- Lunch; daily from 12:00 PM to 1:00 PM
- Hospital Rounds; Tuesdays and Thursday from 8:00 AM to 9:00 AM

Dr. Angela Perez:
- Lunch; daily from 12:30 PM to 1:30 PM
- Hospital Rounds; Fridays from 8:00 AM to 9:00 AM

Equipment and Supplies:
- Appointment book or computer with scheduling software
- Office procedure manual (optional)
- Black pen, pencil, and highlighters
- Calendar

Standard: Complete the procedure and all critical steps in _____ minutes with a minimum score of 85% within two attempts (*or as indicated by the instructor*).

Scoring: Divide the points earned by the total possible points. Failure to perform a critical step, indicated by an asterisk (*), results in grade no higher than an 84% (*or as indicated by the instructor*).

Time: Began_____ Ended_____ Total minutes: _____

Steps:	Point Value	Attempt 1	Attempt 2
1. Using the calendar, determine when the office is not open (e.g., holidays, weekends, evenings). If using the appointment book and a black pen, draw an *X* through the times the office is not open. If using the scheduling software, block the times the office is not open.	25*		
2. Identify the times each provider is not available. If using the appointment book, write in the providers' names on each column and then draw an *X* through their unavailable times. If using the scheduling software, select each provider and block the times the provider is unavailable.	25*		
3. Using the office procedure manual or providers' preferences, determine when each provider performs certain types of examinations. In the appointment book, indicate these examinations either by writing the examination time or by highlighting the examination times. Follow the office's procedure on indicating these examination times in the appointment book. When using scheduling software, set up the times for the examinations or use the highlighting feature if available.	25*		

4.	Using the office procedure manual or the list of providers' preferences and availability, identify other times to block on the scheduling matrix. Some providers require catch-up times and these time slots are blocked. Some medical facilities save appointment times for same-day appointments. When saving time blocks for same-day appointments, make sure to use pencil so it can be erased and the patient's information entered on the day of the appointment. For the scheduling software, block those times when patients cannot be booked and indicate the times for the same-day appointments.	25*	
	Total Points	100	

Comments

CAAHEP Competencies	Steps
VI.P.1. Manage appointment schedule using established priorities	Entire procedure
ABHES Competencies	**Steps**
7. Administrative Procedures e. Apply scheduling principles	Entire procedure

Procedure 9.2   Schedule a New Patient

Name _____ Date _____ Score _____

Task: To schedule a new patient for a first office visit and identify the urgency of the visit using established priorities.

Scenario: Patricia Black, a new patient, calls. She just moved to the area and her asthma has flared up over the last 24 hours, but her albuterol inhaler is empty, and she needs a new prescription for it. She states that she is doing okay, but without the albuterol she knows it will get worse within the next few days. According to your screening guidelines, she needs to be seen today and scheduling guidelines indicate she needs a 45-minute appointment.

Equipment and Supplies:
- Appointment book or computer with scheduling software
- Scheduling and screening guidelines
- Pencil

Standard: Complete the procedure and all critical steps in _____ minutes with a minimum score of 85% within two attempts (*or as indicated by the instructor*).

Scoring: Divide the points earned by the total possible points. Failure to perform a critical step, indicated by an asterisk (*), results in grade no higher than an 84% (*or as indicated by the instructor*).

Time: Began_____ Ended_____ Total minutes: _____

Steps:	Point Value	Attempt 1	Attempt 2
1. Obtain the patient's demographic information (e.g., full name, birth date, address, and telephone number). Write this information down or enter it into the scheduling software. Verify the information.	15*		
2. Determine whether the patient was referred by another provider.	10		
3. Determine the patient's chief complaint and when the first symptoms occurred. Utilize the scheduling and screening guidelines as needed. (*Refer to the Checklist for Affective Behaviors*)	15*		
4. Search the appointment book or scheduling software for the first suitable appointment time and an alternate time. Offer the patient a choice of these dates and times. Be open to alternative times if the patient cannot make the initial options you gave. Provide additional appointment options as needed.	10*		
5. Enter the mutually agreeable time into the schedule. Enter the patient's name, telephone number, and add *NP* for new patient.	10		
6. Obtain the patient's insurance information. If new patients are expected to pay at the time of the visit, explain this financial arrangement when the appointment is made.	15*		
7. Provide the patient with directions to the healthcare facility and parking instructions if needed.	10		
8. Before ending the call, ask if the patient has any questions. Reinforce the date and time of the appointment. Politely and professionally end the call, making sure to thank the patient for calling. (*Refer to the Checklist for Affective Behaviors*)	15		
Total Points	**100**		

Checklist for Affective Behaviors

Affective Behavior	Directions: Check behaviors observed during the role-play.					
Respect	**Negative, Unprofessional Behaviors**	**Attempt 1**	**Attempt 2**	**Positive, Professional Behaviors**	**Attempt 1**	**Attempt 2**
	Rude, unkind			Courteous		
	Disrespectful, impolite			Polite		
	Unwelcoming			Welcoming		
	Brief, abrupt			Took time with patient		
	Unconcerned with person's dignity			Maintained person's dignity		
	Negative nonverbal behaviors			Positive nonverbal behaviors		
	Other:			Other:		
Sensitivity	Distracted; not focused on the other person			Focused full attention on the other person		
	Judgmental attitude; not accepting attitude			Nonjudgmental, accepting attitude		
	Failed to clarify what the person verbally or nonverbally communicated			Used summarizing or paraphrasing to clarify what the person verbally or nonverbally communicated		
	Failed to acknowledge what the person communicated			Acknowledged what the person communicated		
	Rude, discourteous			Pleasant and courteous		
	Disregarded the person's dignity and rights			Maintained the person's dignity and rights		
	Other:			Other:		

Grading for Affective Behaviors		Point Value	Attempt 1	Attempt 2
Does not meet Expectation	• Response was disrespectful and/or insensitive. • Student demonstrated more than 2 negative, unprofessional behaviors during the interaction.	0		
Needs Improvement	• Response was disrespectful and/or insensitive. • Student demonstrated 1 or 2 negative, unprofessional behaviors during the interaction.	0		
Meets Expectation	• Response was respectful and sensitive; no negative, unprofessional behaviors observed. • More practice is needed for behavior to appear natural and for student to appear comfortable and at ease.	15		
Occasionally Exceeds Expectation	• Response was respectful and sensitive; no negative, unprofessional behaviors observed. • At times student appeared comfortable and at ease; but more practice is needed for behavior to become natural and consistent with a professional medical assistant.	15		
Always Exceeds Expectation	• Response was respectful and sensitive; no negative, unprofessional behaviors observed. • Student's behaviors appeared natural and comfortable. Behaviors are consistent with a professional medical assistant.	15		

Comments

CAAHEP Competencies	Step(s)
VI.P.1. Manage appointment schedule using established priorities	1-7
VI.A.1. Display sensitivity when managing appointments	3, 8
VII.P.3. Obtain accurate patient billing information	6
ABHES Competencies	**Step(s)**
7. Administrative Procedures e. Apply scheduling principles	1-7

Procedure 9.3   Coach Patients Regarding Office Policies

Name _____ Date _____ Score _____

Tasks: Create a new patient brochure and then role-play ways to coach patients regarding office policies.

Scenario: You work at Walden-Martin Family Medical Clinic. Your supervisor asks you to create a new patient brochure for the clinic. The healthcare facility's information is listed here. After you complete the brochure, you coach the following patients regarding office procedures:
- Mr. Charles Johnson (he has a question regarding the payment policy)
- Ms. Monique Jones (she has a question regarding the medication refill procedure)

Healthcare Facility	Providers
Walden-Martin Family Medical Clinic 1234 Anystreet Anytown, Anystate 12345 Phone: 123-123-1234 Fax: 123-123-5678	Julie Walden, M.D. James Martin, M.D. Angela Perez, M.D. David Kahn, M.D. Jean Burke, N.P.

Equipment and Supplies:
- Computer with word processing software and printer
- Office procedure manual (optional)

Standard: Complete the procedure and all critical steps with a minimum score of 85% within two attempts (*or as indicated by the instructor*).

Scoring: Divide the points earned by the total possible points. Failure to perform a critical step, indicated by an asterisk (*), results in grade no higher than an 84% (*or as indicated by the instructor*).

Steps:	Point Value	Attempt 1	Attempt 2
1. Using word processing software, design an informational brochure for patients that provides information about the healthcare facility and describes practice procedures. At a minimum, the information should include the following: 　a. Description of the healthcare facility (e.g., type of practice, mission statement) 　b. Location or a map of the facility 　c. Contact information (i.e., telephone numbers, emails, and website addresses) 　d. Providers' names and credentials 　e. Services offered 　f. Hours of operation 　g. How appointments can be scheduled 　h. Healthcare facility's policies and procedures (e.g., payment policies, appointment cancellations, medication refills, assistance after hours) 　i. Insurance plans accepted	55		
2. Proofread the brochure. Revise as needed. Print the brochure.	5		
3. Using the scenario for the first patient, give a brief summary of the different parts of the brochure. Use words the patient will understand.	10*		

4.	Ask if the patient has any questions. Actively listen to the patient's concerns. Address those concerns.	**10***		
5.	Using the scenario for the second patient, give a brief summary of the different parts of the brochure. Use words that the patient understands.	**10***		
6.	Ask if the patient has any questions. Actively listen to the patient's concerns. Address those concerns.	**10***		
	Total Points	**100**		

Comments

CAAHEP Competencies	**Step(s)**
V.P.4.a. Coach patients regarding: office policies	3-6

Procedure 9.4   Schedule an Established Patient

Name _____ Date _____ Score _____

Task: To manage the provider's schedule by scheduling appointments for an established patient and handling rescheduling and a no-show appointment.

Scenario: Celia Tapia has just finished seeing Dr. Martin and is checking out at your desk. You see that she needs to schedule a follow-up appointment in 2 weeks. The scheduling guidelines indicate a follow-up appointment is 15 minutes long.

Equipment and Supplies:
- Appointment book or computer with scheduling software
- Scheduling guidelines
- Pencil, red pen
- Reminder card
- Patient's health record

Standard: Complete the procedure and all critical steps in _____ minutes with a minimum score of 85% within two attempts (*or as indicated by the instructor*).

Scoring: Divide the points earned by the total possible points. Failure to perform a critical step, indicated by an asterisk (*), results in grade no higher than an 84% (*or as indicated by the instructor*).

Time: Began_____ Ended_____ Total minutes: _____

Steps:	Point Value	Attempt 1	Attempt 2
1. Obtain the patient's name and information, purpose of the visit, the provider to be seen, and any scheduling preferences. If using the scheduling software, enter the patient's name and date of birth (DOB). Verify the correct patient is selected.	15		
2. Identify the length of the appointment by using the scheduling guidelines.	15*		
3. Search the appointment book or scheduling software for the first suitable appointment time and an alternate time. Offer the patient a choice of these dates and times. Be open to alternative times if the patient cannot make the initial options you gave. Provide additional appointment options as needed.	15		
4. Using a pencil, write the patient's name and phone number in the appointment book and block out the correct amount of time. Add in any other relevant information per the facility's procedures. If using the scheduling software, create the appointment per the facility's guidelines.	15*		
5. Complete the appointment reminder card and ensure the date and time on the card matches the appointment time. Give the card to the patient.	10		

Scenario continues: Later that day, Celica Tapia calls and needs to reschedule her appointment for the next day at the same time.				
6. When a patient calls to reschedule an appointment, follow steps #1 through #4. When the new appointment is made, make sure to erase the old appointment from the appointment log. With the scheduling software, ensure the old appointment time is removed from the schedule. Repeat the appointment date and time to the patient. *(Refer to the Checklist for Affective Behaviors)*	**15**			
Scenario continues: Celia Tapia no-shows for her follow-up appointment.				
7. In the appointment book, using red pen, indicate the patient no-showed. Using the patient's health record, document that the patient failed to show for the follow-up examination with the provider. In an electronic system change the appointment status to no-show and ensure that it is documented in the health record.	**15**			
Total Points	**100**			

Checklist for Affective Behaviors

Affective Behavior	*Directions: Check behaviors observed during the role-play.*					
Respect	**Negative, Unprofessional Behaviors**	**Attempt**		**Positive, Professional Behaviors**	**Attempt**	
		1	**2**		**1**	**2**
	Rude, unkind			Courteous		
	Disrespectful, impolite			Polite		
	Unwelcoming			Welcoming		
	Brief, abrupt			Took time with patient		
	Unconcerned with person's dignity			Maintained person's dignity		
	Negative nonverbal behaviors			Positive nonverbal behaviors		
	Other:			Other:		
Sensitivity	Distracted; not focused on the other person			Focused full attention on the other person		
	Judgmental attitude; not accepting attitude			Nonjudgmental, accepting attitude		
	Failed to clarify what the person verbally or nonverbally communicated			Used summarizing or paraphrasing to clarify what the person verbally or nonverbally communicated		
	Failed to acknowledge what the person communicated			Acknowledged what the person communicated		
	Rude, discourteous			Pleasant and courteous		
	Disregarded the person's dignity and rights			Maintained the person's dignity and rights		
	Other:			Other:		

Grading for Affective Behaviors		Point Value	Attempt 1	Attempt 2
Does not meet Expectation	• Response was disrespectful and/or insensitive. • Student demonstrated more than 2 negative, unprofessional behaviors during the interaction.	0		
Needs Improvement	• Response was disrespectful and/or insensitive. • Student demonstrated 1 or 2 negative, unprofessional behaviors during the interaction.	0		
Meets Expectation	• Response was respectful and sensitive; no negative, unprofessional behaviors observed. • More practice is needed for behavior to appear natural and for student to appear comfortable and at ease.	15		
Occasionally Exceeds Expectation	• Response was respectful and sensitive; no negative, unprofessional behaviors observed. • At times student appeared comfortable and at ease; but more practice is needed for behavior to become natural and consistent with a professional medical assistant.	15		
Always Exceeds Expectation	• Response was respectful and sensitive; no negative, unprofessional behaviors observed. • Student's behaviors appeared natural and comfortable. Behaviors are consistent with a professional medical assistant.	15		

Comments

CAAHEP Competencies	Steps
VI.P.1. Manage appointment schedule using established priorities	All
VI.A.1. Display sensitivity when managing appointments	6
ABHES Competencies	**Steps**
7. Administrative Procedures e. Apply scheduling principles	All

Procedure 9.5   Schedule a Patient Procedure

Name _____ **Date** _____ **Score** _____

Task: To schedule a patient for a procedure within the time frame needed by the provider, confirm with the patient, and issue all required instructions.

Scenario: Monique Jones has just completed seeing Dr. Walden and is checking out at your desk. She gives you an order from the provider that states she needs to have a magnetic resonance image (MRI) of her left ankle within a week. The radiology department in your facility performs MRIs.

Equipment and Supplies:
- Provider's order detailing the procedure required
- Computer with order entry software (optional)
- Name, address, and telephone number of facility where procedure will take place
- Patient's demographic and insurance information
- Patient's health record
- Procedure preparation instructions
- Telephone
- Consent form (if required for procedure)

Standard: Complete the procedure and all critical steps in _____ minutes with a minimum score of 85% within two attempts (*or as indicated by the instructor*).

Scoring: Divide the points earned by the total possible points. Failure to perform a critical step, indicated by an asterisk (*), results in grade no higher than an 84% (*or as indicated by the instructor*).

Time: Began_____ Ended_____ Total minutes: _____

Steps:	Point Value	Attempt 1	Attempt 2
1. Obtain an oral or written order from the provider for the exact procedure to be performed.	15		
2. Gather the patient's demographic and insurance information. If using an electronic health record, verify you have the correct patient. *(Refer to the Checklist for Affective Behaviors)*	15		
3. Determine the patient's availability within the time frame provided by the provider for the procedure.	15		

4.   Contact the diagnostic facility and schedule the patient's procedure. If you are using a computerized provider order entry (CPOE) system and your facility performs the procedure, you also need to enter the order using the CPOE system.
  • Provide the patient's diagnosis and provider's exact order, including the name of procedure and time frame.
  • Establish the date and time for the procedure.
  • Give the patient's name, age, address, telephone number, and insurance information (i.e., insurance policy numbers, precertification information, and addresses for filing claims).
  • Determine any special instructions for the patient or special anesthesia requirements.
  • Notify the facility of any urgency for test results.
	20*		

5.	If a consent form is required for the procedure, ensure the provider has reviewed the form with the patient and the patient has signed the consent form. A copy of the consent form may be required by the diagnostic facility before the procedure. The consent form should be scanned and uploaded into the electronic health record or placed in the paper record.	**15**	
6.	Document the details of the scheduled procedure in the patient's health record. If applicable, create a reminder to check on the procedure results after the appointment date.	**20***	
	Total Points	**100**	

Checklist for Affective Behaviors

Affective Behavior	Directions: Check behaviors observed during the role-play.					
Respectful	**Negative, Unprofessional Behaviors**	**Attempt**		**Positive, Professional Behaviors**	**Attempt**	
		1	**2**		**1**	**2**
	Rude, unkind			Courteous		
	Disrespectful, impolite			Polite		
	Unwelcoming			Welcoming		
	Brief, abrupt			Took time with patient		
	Unconcerned with person's dignity			Maintained person's dignity		
	Negative nonverbal behaviors			Positive nonverbal behaviors		
	Other:			Other:		
Sensitivity	Distracted; not focused on the other person			Focused full attention on the other person		
	Judgmental attitude; not accepting attitude			Nonjudgmental, accepting attitude		
	Failed to clarify what the person verbally or nonverbally communicated			Used summarizing or paraphrasing to clarify what the person verbally or nonverbally communicated		
	Failed to acknowledge what the person communicated			Acknowledged what the person communicated		
	Rude, discourteous			Pleasant and courteous		
	Disregarded the person's dignity and rights			Maintained the person's dignity and rights		
	Other:			Other:		

Grading for Affective Behaviors		Point Value	Attempt 1	Attempt 2
Does not meet Expectation	• Response was disrespectful and/or insensitive. • Student demonstrated more than 2 negative, unprofessional behaviors during the interaction.	0		
Needs Improvement	• Response was disrespectful and/or insensitive. • Student demonstrated 1 or 2 negative, unprofessional behaviors during the interaction.	0		
Meets Expectation	• Response was respectful and sensitive; no negative, unprofessional behaviors observed. • More practice is needed for behavior to appear natural and for student to appear comfortable and at ease.	15		
Occasionally Exceeds Expectation	• Response was respectful and sensitive; no negative, unprofessional behaviors observed. • At times student appeared comfortable and at ease; but more practice is needed for behavior to become natural and consistent with a professional medical assistant.	15		
Always Exceeds Expectation	• Response was respectful and sensitive; no negative, unprofessional behaviors observed. • Student's behaviors appeared natural and comfortable. Behaviors are consistent with a professional medical assistant.	15		

Comments

CAAHEP Competencies	Steps
VI.P.2. Schedule a patient procedure	All
VI.A.1. Display sensitivity when managing appointments	2
ABHES Competencies	**Steps**
7. Administrative Procedures e. Apply scheduling principles	All

Health Records

CAAHEP Competencies	Assessment
VI.C.4. Define types of information contained in the patient's medical record	Vocabulary Review – A. 1, 7 Skills and Concepts – A. 1, 4
VI.C.5.a. Identify methods of organizing the patient's medical record based on: problem-oriented medical record (POMR)	Skills and Concepts – B. 1
VI.C.5.b. Identify methods of organizing the patient's medical record based on: source-oriented medical record (SOMR)	Vocabulary Review – C. 5, 9, 10 Skills and Concepts – B. 2
VI.C.6.a. Identify equipment and supplies needed for medical records in order to: Create	Skills and Concepts – B. 3
VI.C.6.b. Identify equipment and supplies needed for medical records in order to: Maintain	Skills and Concepts – B. 3
VI.C.6.c. Identify equipment and supplies needed for medical records in order to: Store	Skills and Concepts – B. 3
VI.C.7. Describe filing indexing rules	Skills and Concepts – C. 1
VI.C.11. Explain the importance of data back-up	Skills and Concepts – A. 2
VI.C.12. Explain meaningful use as it applies to EMR	Skills and Concepts – A. 3; Workplace Applications – 1; Internet Activities – 1
VI.P.3. Create a patient's medical record	Procedure 10.1, 10.4
VI.P.4. Organize a patient's medical record	Procedure 10.2, 10.4
VI.P.5. File patient medical records	Procedure 10.2, 10.4, 10.5
VI.P.6. Utilize an EMR	Procedure 10.2
VI.P.7. Input patient data utilizing a practice management system	Procedure 10.1, 10.2
X.A.2. Protect the integrity of the medical record	Procedure 10.1, 10.2, 10.3
ABHES Competencies	Assessment
1. General Orientation d. List the general responsibilities and skills of the medical assistant	Skills and Concepts – B.4
4. Medical Law and Ethics a. Follow documentation guidelines	Skills and Concepts – B. 5-9

ABHES Competencies	Assessment
4. Medical Law and Ethics b. Institute federal and state guidelines when: 1) Releasing medical records or information 2) Entering orders in and utilizing electronic health records	Procedure 10.1, 10.2
7. Administrative Procedures a. Gather and process documents	Procedure 10.2, 10.4, 10.5
7. Administrative Procedures b. Navigate electronic health records systems and practice management software	Procedure 10.1, 10.2

VOCABULARY REVIEW

Using the word pool on the right, find the correct word to match the definition. Write the word on the line after the definition.

Group A

1. Data or information obtained from the patient
   _____

2. A process to ensure the reliability of test results
   _____

3. Using as few words as possible to express the message
   _____

4. A computerized record that conforms to nationally recognized standards and contains health-related information about a specific patient _____

5. A temporary diagnosis made before all test results have been received _____

6. The smooth continuation of care from one provider to another that allows the patient to receive the most benefit and no interruption or duplication of care _____

7. Data obtained through physical examination, laboratory and diagnostic testing, and by measurable information
   _____

8. The likely outcome of a disease including chance of recovery
   _____

9. Passed from parents to offspring through the genes
   _____

10. How often something happens _____

Word Pool
- electronic health record (EHR)
- quality control
- prognosis
- continuity of care
- incidence
- subjective information
- objective information
- hereditary
- concise
- provisional diagnosis

Group B

1. The ability to work with other systems _____

2. A method or plan for retaining or keeping health records and for their movement from active to inactive to closed _____

3. Occurring later or after _____

4. A rule that controls how something should be done; guidelines or boundaries _____

5. An interconnection between systems _____

6. A secure online website that gives patients 24-hour access to personal health information using a username and password _____

7. The use of electronic software to communicate with pharmacies and send prescribing information _____

8. The process of entering medication orders or other provider instructions into the EHR _____

9. Meeting the standards and regulations of the practice's established policies and procedures _____

10. Granted or endowed with a particular authority, right, or property; to have a special interest in _____

Word Pool
- subsequent
- patient portal
- vested
- interoperability
- e-prescribing
- compliance
- computerized provider/physician order entry (CPOE)
- parameters
- interface
- retention schedule

Group C

1. The age at which a person is recognized by law to be an adult; it varies by state _____

2. A heading, title, or subtitle under which records are filed _____

3. To say something aloud for another person to write down _____

4. A chronologic file used as a reminder that something must be dealt with on a certain date _____

5. The filing of records, correspondence, or cards by number _____

6. To make a written copy of dictated material _____

7. A sturdy cardboard or plastic file-sized card used to replace a folder temporarily removed from the filing space _____

8. To remove or destroy all traces of; do away with; destroy completely _____

9. The most recent item is on top and oldest item is last _____

10. Any system that arranges names or topics according to the sequence of the letters in the alphabet _____

Word Pool
- age of majority
- reverse chronologic order
- obliteration
- transcription
- dictation
- out guides
- caption
- alphabetic filing
- numeric filing
- tickler file

ABBREVIATIONS
Write out what each of the following abbreviations stands for.

1. AMA _____

2. CPOE _____

3. CPT _____

4. EHRs _____

5. HHS _____

6. HIE _____

7. HIPAA _____

8. HIV _____

9. ICD _____

10. NPP _____

11. ONC _____

12. PCP _____

13. PHI _____

14. PHR _____

15. POR _____

16. SOR _____

17. TPR _____

SKILLS AND CONCEPTS
Answer the following questions. Write your answer on the line or in the space provided.

A. Health Record Basics

1. Describe the following types of information found in a patient's health record.

   Demographics: _____

   _____

   _____

   _____

   _____

   _____

Past health history: _____

_____

_____

_____

_____

_____

Family history:_____

_____

_____

_____

_____

_____

Social history: _____

_____

_____

_____

_____

_____

Chief complaint: _____

_____

_____

_____

_____

_____

Vital signs and anthropometric measurements:_____

_____

_____

_____

_____

_____

Diagnosis:_____

_____

_____

_____

_____

_____

Progress notes:_____

_____

_____

_____

_____

_____

_____

2. Explain the importance of data backup. _____

_____

_____

3. Define *meaningful use.*_____

_____

_____

_____

4. Note whether the following information is usually subjective or objective.

    Patient's address: _____

    Yellowed eyes: _____

    Patient's email address: _____

    Insurance information: _____

    Elevated blood pressure: _____

    Bloated stomach: _____

    Complaint of headache: _____

    Weight of 143 pounds: _____

    Bruises on upper arms: _____

    Patient's phone number: _____

B. Organization and Documentation in a Health Record

1. Identify the categories used for organizing information in a POR system. _____

    _____

    _____

    _____

    _____

    _____

2. Identify the method of organizing information in an SOR system. _____

    _____

    _____

    _____

    _____

    _____

3. Identify equipment and supplies needed to create, maintain, and store health records. _____

    _____

    _____

    _____

    _____

    _____

4. Describe the medical assistant's responsibilities when documenting in the health record including skills and responsibilities.

_____

_____

_____

_____

_____

_____

Correct the following entries as would be done in the health record. Then rewrite the entries correctly. Handwritten corrections are acceptable on these exercises.

5. The correct date of the appointment below was October 12, 20XX.

   10-21-20XX 1330 Patient did not arrive for scheduled appointment. P. Smith, RMA

   _____

   _____

   _____

   _____

6. The patient stated that the chest pain began 2 weeks ago.

   1-31-20XX 10:00 AM Patient complained of chest pain for the past 2 months. No pain noted in arms. No nausea. Desires ECG and blood work to check for heart problems. R. Smithee, CMA (AAMA)

   _____

   _____

   _____

   _____

Document the following exercises.

7. Eric Robertson canceled his surgical follow-up appointment today for the third time. Document this information.

   _____

   _____

   _____

   _____

8. Angela Adams called to report that she was not feeling any better since her office visit on Monday. She wants the doctor to call in a refill for her antibiotics. The chart says that she was to return to the clinic on Thursday if she was not feeling better. Today is Monday, and she says she cannot come into the clinic this week. The physician wants to see her before prescribing any other medication. Document this information.

_____

_____

_____

_____

_____

9. Mary Elizabeth Smith called the physician's office to report redness around an injection site. She was in the office 3 hours ago and received an injection of penicillin. She says she also is itching quite a bit around the site and is having trouble breathing. The doctor has left the office for the day. Office policy states that if the physician is out of the office and a patient presents or calls with an emergency, he or she is to be referred to the ER. Document the action that the medical assistant should take.

_____

_____

_____

_____

_____

C. Indexing and Filing Rules

1. Describe the indexing rules for alphabetic filing. _____

_____

_____

_____

_____

_____

_____

_____

_____

2. Using alphabetic filing, place the names below in correct alphabetic order.

Cassidy Kay Hale	1.	_____
Candace Cassidy LeGrand	2.	_____
Taylor Ann Jackson	3.	_____
Anton Douglas Conn	4.	_____
Mitchel Michael Gibson	5.	_____
Lorienda Gaye Robison	6.	_____
LaNelle Elva Crumley	7.	_____
Allison Gaile Yarbrough	8.	_____
Sarah Kay Haile	9.	_____
Marie Gracelia Stuart	10.	_____
Karry Madge Chapmann	11.	_____
Randi Ann Perez	12.	_____
Cecelia Gayle Raglan	13.	_____
Sarah Sue Ragland	14.	_____
Riley Americus Belk	15.	_____
Starr Ellen Beall	16.	_____
Mitchell Thomas Gibson	17.	_____
George Scott Turner	18.	_____
Winston Roger Murchison	19.	_____
Sara Suzelle Montgomery	20.	_____
Tamika Noelle Frazier	21.	_____
Alisa Jordan Williams	22.	_____
Alisha Dawn Chapman	23.	_____
Bentley James Adams	24.	_____
Montana Skye Kizer	25.	_____
Dakota Marie LaRose	26.	_____
Robbie Sue Metzger	27.	_____
Thomas Charles Bruin	28.	_____
Percival "Butch" Adams	29.	_____
Carlos Perez Santos	30.	_____

3. Why might color-coded files be more efficient than an alphabetic filing system? _____

_____

_____

_____

_____

_____

4. Using terminal filing, place the numbers below in the correct order.

01-64-22	1. _____
72-55-20	2. _____
44-41-20	3. _____
17-41-20	4. _____
56-42-21	5. _____
91-88-21	6. _____
15-24-22	7. _____
82-49-20	8. _____
08-94-21	9. _____
24-42-22	10. _____

D. Miscellaneous

1. Describe the difference between an EMR and a practice management system. _____

_____

_____

_____

_____

_____

2. Describe a manual tickler file._____

_____

_____

_____

_____

3. Correspondence related to the operation of the of the office is considered _____ correspondence.

CERTIFICATION PREPARATION
Circle the correct answer.

1. Information that is obtained by questioning the patient or that is taken from a form is called _____ information.
   a. confidential
   b. subjective
   c. necessary
   d. objective

2. How would you properly index the name "Amanda M. Stiles-Duncan" for filing?
   a. Stilesduncan, Amanda M.
   b. Stiles Duncan, Amanda M.
   c. Duncanstiles, Amanda M.
   d. Duncan, Amanda M. Stiles

3. Who is the legal owner of the information stored in a patient's record?
   a. The patient
   b. The provider or agency where services were provided
   c. The patient's insurance company
   d. Both the patient and the provider

4. Which is *not* objective information?
   a. Progress notes
   b. Family history
   c. Diagnosis
   d. Physical examination and findings

5. Many healthcare facilities now use voice recognition software for transcription. The system can be used to dictate which types of reports?
   a. Progress notes
   b. Letters
   c. Emails
   d. All of the above

6. Perhaps the most essential action for the medical assistant working with a patient and using an electronic record is to
   a. type in every word the patient says.
   b. make sure the patient is not hiding any part of the health history.
   c. make frequent eye contact with patient and smile.
   d. sit in a chair across from the patient so that the person cannot see the screen.

7. Which EHR system backup requires the least amount of hardware?
   a. Online backup system
   b. External hard drives
   c. Full server backup
   d. Thumb drive backup

8. The concise account of the patient's symptoms in his or her own words is the _____.
   a. Objective information
   b. Provisional diagnosis
   c. Chief complaint
   d. Caption

9. To completely remove all traces of an entry in a health record is _____.
   a. interface
   b. obliteration
   c. dictation
   d. compliance

10. The process of electronic data entry of a provider's instructions for the treatment of patients is called _____.
   a. progress notes
   b. computerized physician/provider order entry
   c. direct filing system
   d. continuity of care

WORKPLACE APPLICATIONS

1. Dr. Martin wants to be sure the Walden-Martin Family Medical (WMFM) Clinic is meeting all of the requirements for meaningful use that are specified in the HITECH Act. He has asked Susan to put together a list of what WMFM Clinic should be doing to meet those requirements. What would be on Susan's list?

   _____

   _____

   _____

   _____

2. Susan has been learning about the various EHR systems available. She has also been learning about the need to back up to protect the information stored in the EHR. Susan has asked the office manager at WMFC how the EHR is backed up at their facility. The office manager states that they currently use an external hard drive, but would like to look more closely at other options. She asks Susan to determine what other options are available. Write a brief description of each of the options below:

   a. External hard drive:_____

      _____

   b. Full server backup: _____

      _____

   c. Online backup system: _____

      _____

INTERNET ACTIVITIES

1. Using online resources, research EHR systems. Choose the one you think would be the best option and create a poster presentation, a PowerPoint presentation, or write a paper summarizing your research. Include the following points in your project:
   a. Description of the EHR
   b. Description of the practice management functions
   c. Does it include backup features?
   d. How does it meet the meaningful use requirements?

2. Using online resources, research a voice recognition software. Create a poster presentation, a PowerPoint presentation, or write a paper summarizing your research. Include the following points in your project:
   a. Description voice recognition software
   b. List the uses for voice recognition software
   c. Compare three different products
   d. Determine which one would be the best product

Procedure 10.1 Register a New Patient in the Practice Management Software

Name _____ Date _____ Score _____

Task: Register a new patient in the practice management software, prepare a Notice of Privacy Practices (NPP) form and a Disclosure Authorization form for the new patient, and document this in the electronic health record (EHR).

Scenario: You need to register a new patient. The facility's policies and procedures require that the medical assistant search the EHR database for the patient to prevent duplicate records.

Equipment and Supplies:
- Computer with SimChart for the Medical Office or practice management and EHR software
- Completed patient registration form (Figure 10.1)
- Scanner

Standard: Complete the procedure and all critical steps in _____ minutes with a minimum score of 85% within two attempts (*or as indicated by the instructor*).

Scoring: Divide the points earned by the total possible points. Failure to perform a critical step, indicated by an asterisk (*), results in grade no higher than an 84% (*or as indicated by the instructor*).

Time: Began_____ Ended_____ Total minutes: _____

Steps:	Point Value	Attempt 1	Attempt 2
1. Obtain the new patient's completed registration form. Log into the practice management software.	10		
2. To help ensure the integrity of the practice management and EHR systems, a search for the new patient's name must always be done before registering that patient. Using the patient's last and first names and date of birth, search the database for the patient. To help ensure the integrity of the practice management and EHR systems, a search for the new patient's name must always be done before registering that person. This prevents a double record from being created if the patient had been entered into the database at an earlier time. (*Refer to the Checklist for Affective Behaviors*)	15*		
3. If the database does not contain the patient's name, add a new patient and enter the patient's demographics from the completed registration form.	10*		
4. Correctly spell the patient's name and accurately enter the patient's date of birth. (*Refer to the Checklist for Affective Behaviors*)	15*		
5. Verify that the information entered is correct and that all fields are completed before saving the data.	10		
6. Using the EHR software, prepare and print a copy of the NPP and a Disclosure Authorization form for the new patient. The Disclosure Authorization form should indicate the disclosure will be to the patient's insurance company.	15		
Scenario Update: The patient received both documents and signed the Disclosure Authorization form.			
7. Using the EHR, document that the patient received a copy of the NPP and signed the Disclosure Authorization form. Scan the Disclosure Authorization form and upload it into the EHR.	15*		
8. Log out of the software upon completion of the procedure.	10		
Total Points	**100**		

Checklist for Affective Behaviors

Affective Behavior	*Directions:* Check behaviors observed during the role-play.					
Ethical	Failed to adequately follow the facility's policy			Adequately followed the facility's policy		
	Incorrectly entered patient's information (e.g., misspelled name) during the database search			Correctly entered patient's information (e.g., misspelled name) when searching database		
	Incorrectly entered patient's information (e.g., misspelled name) when registering patient			Correctly entered patient's information (e.g., misspelled name) when registering patient		
	Other:			Other:		

Grading for Affective Behaviors	Point Value	Attempt 1	Attempt 2
Does not meet Expectation • Response was unethical. • Student demonstrated more than 2 negative, unprofessional behaviors during the interaction.	0		
Needs Improvement • Response was unethical • Student demonstrated 1 or 2 negative, unprofessional behaviors during the interaction.	0		
Meets Expectation • Response was ethical; no negative, unprofessional behaviors observed. • More practice is needed for behavior to appear natural and for student to appear comfortable and at ease.	15		
Occasionally Exceeds Expectation • Response was ethical; no negative, unprofessional behaviors observed. • At times student appeared comfortable and at ease; but more practice is needed for behavior to become natural and consistent with a professional medical assistant.	15		
Always Exceeds Expectation • Response was ethical; no negative, unprofessional behaviors observed. • Student's behaviors appeared natural and comfortable. Behaviors are consistent with a professional medical assistant.	15		

CAAHEP Competencies	Steps
VI.P.3. Create a patient's medical record	All
X.A.2. Protect the integrity of the medical record	2, 4
ABHES Competencies	**Steps**
7. Administrative Procedures b. Navigate electronic health records systems and practice management software	All

Figure 10.1   Patient Information Form

Patient Information:
Name: Jonathan S. Scott
Address: 922 Golf Road, Anytown, AK 12345
Date of Birth: 08/01/1990
Email: jscott16@anytown.mail
Sex: M
Home Phone: 123-123-3098
SSN: 987-66-1223
Emergency Contact Name: Callie Scott
Emergency Contact Phone: 123-123-0857

Guarantor Information:
Relationship of Guarantor to Patient: Self
Employer Name: Anytown Bank
Work Phone: 123-567-9012
Primary Provider: David Kahn, MD

Insurance Information:
  Primary Insurance:
    Insurance: Aetna
    Name of Policyholder: Jonathan S. Scott
    SSN of Policyholder: 987-66-1223
    Policy/ID Number: JS8884910
    Group Number: 66574W
    Claims Address: 1234 Insurance Way, Anytown, AL 12345-1234
    Claims Phone Number: 180-012-3222

Procedure 10.2   Upload Documents to the EHR

Name _____ Date _____ Score _____

Task: Scan paper records and upload digital files to the EHR.

Scenario: A new patient brings in a laboratory report and a radiology report that he would like to have added to his EHR. You need to scan in the original documents and upload them to the EHR.

Equipment and Supplies:
- Scanner
- Computer with SimChart for the Medical Office or EHR software
- Patient's laboratory and radiology reports (Figures 10.2 and 10.3)

Standard: Complete the procedure and all critical steps in _____ minutes with a minimum score of 85% within two attempts (*or as indicated by the instructor*).

Scoring: Divide the points earned by the total possible points. Failure to perform a critical step, indicated by an asterisk (*), results in grade no higher than an 84% (*or as indicated by the instructor*).

Time: Began_____ Ended_____ Total minutes: _____

Steps:	Point Value	Attempt 1	Attempt 2
1. Obtain the patient's name and date of birth if not on the reports.	10		
2. Using a scanner that is connected to the computer, scan each document, creating an individual digital image for each.	20		
3. Locate the file of the two scanned images in the computer drive. Open the files to ensure the images are clear.	15*		
4. To help ensure the integrity of the practice management and EHR systems, a search for the new patient's name must always be done. In the EHR, search for the patient, using the patient's last and first name. Verify the patient's date of birth. (*Refer to the Checklist for Affective Behaviors*)	15*		
5. Locate the window to upload diagnostic/laboratory results and add a new result. Enter the date of the test. Select the correct type of result. Browse for the image file of the laboratory file and attach it. Save the information.	15*		
6. Select the option to add a new result and repeat the steps to upload the second report.	10*		
7. To help ensure the integrity of the EHR system, verify that the correct documents were uploaded and specific headers (titles) were given to the document. (*Refer to the Checklist for Affective Behaviors*)	15*		
Total Points	100		

Checklist for Affective Behaviors

Affective Behavior	*Directions: Check behaviors observed during the role-play.*					
Ethical	Failed to adequately follow the facility's policy			Adequately followed the facility's policy		
	Incorrectly entered patient's information (e.g., misspelled name) during the database search			Correctly entered patient's information (e.g., misspelled name) when searching database		
	Incorrectly uploaded a document			Correctly uploaded the document		
	Incorrectly titled the document uploaded			Correctly titled the document uploaded		
	Other:			Other:		

Grading for Affective Behaviors		Point Value	Attempt 1	Attempt 2
Does not meet Expectation	• Response was unethical • Student demonstrated more than 2 negative, unprofessional behaviors during the interaction.	0		
Needs Improvement	• Response was unethical. • Student demonstrated 1 or 2 negative, unprofessional behaviors during the interaction.	0		
Meets Expectation	• Response was ethical; no negative, unprofessional behaviors observed. • More practice is needed for behavior to appear natural and for student to appear comfortable and at ease.	15		
Occasionally Exceeds Expectation	• Response was ethical; no negative, unprofessional behaviors observed. • At times student appeared comfortable and at ease; but more practice is needed for behavior to become natural and consistent with a professional medical assistant.	15		
Always Exceeds Expectation	• Response was ethical; no negative, unprofessional behaviors observed. • Student's behaviors appeared natural and comfortable. Behaviors are consistent with a professional medical assistant.	15		

CAAHEP Competencies	Steps
VI.P.4. Organize a patient's medical record	2-5
VI.P.5. File patient medical records	2-5
X.A.2. Protect the integrity of the medical record	4, 7
ABHES Competencies	**Steps**
7. Administrative Procedures a. Gather and process documents	2-5
7. Administrative Procedures b. Navigate electronic health records systems and practice management software	All

Figure 10.2 Laboratory Report

AnyTown Laboratory

Date Reported:	04/25/20XX	**Date Received:**	04/25/20XX
Patient Name:	Jonathan S. Scott	**DOB:**	08/01/1990
Ordering Provider:	George St. Cyr, MD		
Date Collected:	04/15/20XX	**Time Collected:**	0830
Test Requested:	Lipid Panel	**Fasting?:**	Yes

Test	Result	Flag	Reference Range
Cholesterol, total	210	High	<200 mg/dL
HDL Cholesterol	26	Low	>40 mg/dL
LDL Cholesterol	142	High	<130 mg/dL
Triglycerides	236	High	<150 mg/dL
Total Cholesterol/HDL ratio	5.8	High	<4.5

Figure 10.3   Radiology Report

AnyTown Radiology

Date: 10/31/20XX **Time:** 1430
Patient Name: Jonathan S. Scott **DOB:** 08/01/1990
Exam Type: Chest x-ray 2 views **Ordering Provider:** George St. Cyr, MD

Final Report:
History: Cough and fever
Report: Frontal and lateral views of the chest
Comparison: None

Findings:
Lungs: The lungs are well inflated and clear. There is no evidence of pneumonia or pulmonary edema.
Pleura: There is no pleural effusion or pneumothorax.
Heart and mediastinum: The cardiomediastinal silhouette is normal.
Impression: Clear lungs without evidence of pneumonia.
Recommendation: None.
Provider: Bones, Seymore MD

Procedure 10.3   Protect the Integrity of the Medical Record

Name _____ Date _____ Score _____

Tasks: Protect the integrity of the medical record.

Scenario: You are mentoring a medical assistant student who is in practicum. You notice the student routinely does not sign out of the electronic health record before leaving the desk. The facility's policy is to sign out or lock the computer before leaving it.

Directions: Role-play the scenario with a peer, who plays the student. You, the medical assistant, must explain to the "student" the facility's policy. Also address the hazards of not protecting the medical record. If the student does not change his/her behavior, you will need to address the situation with the department supervisor.

Standard: Complete the procedure and all critical steps in _____ minutes with a minimum score of 85% within two attempts (*or as indicated by the instructor*).

Scoring: Divide the points earned by the total possible points. Failure to perform a critical step, indicated by an asterisk (*), results in grade no higher than an 84% (*or as indicated by the instructor*).

Time: Began_____ Ended_____ Total minutes: _____

Steps:	Point Value	Attempt 1	Attempt 2
1. Professionally and respectfully discuss the situation with the student. *(Refer to the Checklist for Affective Behaviors – Respect.)*	25		
2. Inform the student about the facility's policy and the hazards of not protecting the electronic health record. *(Refer to the Checklist for Affective Behaviors – Ethics.)*	25		
3. Provide the student with strategies to protect the electronic health record. *(Refer to the Checklist for Affective Behaviors – Ethics.)*	25		
4. Inform the student what will occur if he/she does not protect the electronic record. *(Refer to the Checklist for Affective Behaviors – Respect.)*	25		
Total Points	**100**		

Checklist for Affective Behaviors

Affective Behavior	Directions: Check behaviors observed during the role-play.					
Respect	**Negative, Unprofessional Behaviors**	**Attempt**		**Positive, Professional Behaviors**	**Attempt**	
		1	**2**		**1**	**2**
	Rude, discourteous			Pleasant and courteous		
	Disregarded the person's dignity and rights			Maintained the person's dignity and rights		
	Failed to clearly and/or professionally address the situation			Clearly and professionally addressed the situation		
	Brief, abrupt			Took time to explain the situation		
	Used inappropriate terminology and/or language for a professional setting			Used appropriate terminology and/or language for a professional setting		
	Voice level and tone was unprofessional			Kept voice at a professional level and tone		
	Negative nonverbal behaviors			Positive nonverbal behaviors		
	Other:			Other:		
Ethical	Failed to adequately explain facility's policy			Adequately explained the facility's policy		
	Failed to adequately discuss the hazards of not protecting the electronic health record			Adequately explained the legal and ethical results of not protecting the electronic health record. Addressed the consequences to the clinic, employee, and patient		
	Failed to adequately explain how to protect the electronic health record			Adequately explained how to protect the electronic health record (e.g., log off before leaving the station, keep passwords private)		
	Other:			Other:		

Grading for Affective Behaviors		Point Value	Attempt 1	Attempt 2
Does not meet Expectation	• Response was disrespectful and/or unethical. • Student demonstrated more than 2 negative, unprofessional behaviors during the interaction.	**0**		
Needs Improvement	• Response was disrespectful and/or unethical. • Student demonstrated 1 or 2 negative, unprofessional behaviors during the interaction.	**0**		
Meets Expectation	• Response was respectful and ethical; no negative, unprofessional behaviors observed. • More practice is needed for behavior to appear natural and for student to appear comfortable and at ease.	**25**		
Occasionally Exceeds Expectation	• Response was respectful and ethical; no negative, unprofessional behaviors observed. • At times student appeared comfortable and at ease; but more practice is needed for behavior to become natural and consistent with a professional medical assistant.	**25**		
Always Exceeds Expectation	• Response was respectful and ethical; no negative, unprofessional behaviors observed. • Student's behaviors appeared natural and comfortable. Behaviors are consistent with a professional medical assistant.	**25**		

Comments

CAAHEP Competencies	Step(s)
X.A.2. Protect the integrity of the medical record	Entire procedure

Procedure 10.4   Create and Organize a Patient's Paper Health Record

Name _____ Date _____ Score _____

Task: Create a paper health record for a new patient. Organize health record documents in a paper health record.

Equipment and Supplies:
- End tab file folder
- Completed patient registration form (Figure 10.1)
- Divider sheets with different color labels (4)
- Progress note sheet (1)
- Name label
- Color-coding labels (first two letters of last name and first letter of first name)
- Year label
- Allergy label
- Black pen or computer with word processing software to process labels
- Health record documents (i.e., prior records, laboratory reports) (Figures 10.2 and 10.3)
- Hole puncher

Standard: Complete the procedure and all critical steps in _____ minutes with a minimum score of 85% within two attempts (*or as indicated by the instructor*).

Scoring: Divide the points earned by the total possible points. Failure to perform a critical step, indicated by an asterisk (*), results in grade no higher than an 84% (*or as indicated by the instructor*).

Time: Began_____ Ended_____ Total minutes: _____

Steps:	Point Value	Attempt 1	Attempt 2
1. Obtain the patient's first and last name.	5		
2. Neatly write or word process the patient's name on the name label. Left-justify the last name, followed by a comma, the first name, middle initial and a period (e.g., Smith, Mary J.).	10		
3. Adhere the name label to the bottom left side of the record tab. When the record is held by the main fold in your left hand, the writing should be easy to read. (For directional purposes, assume the record main fold is on the left and the tab is at the bottom.)	10		
4. Put the color-coding labels on the bottom right edge of the folder. Start by placing the first letter of the last name at the farthest right edge. Working left, place the second letter of the last name, then the first letter of the first name, and lastly the year label. The year label should be close to the name label.	15*		
5. Place the allergy label on the front of the record. If allergies are known, clearly write the allergy on the label in red ink.	10*		
6. Place the divider labels on the record divider sheets, if they come separately. Ensure the labels on the divider sheets are staggered so they do not overlap. Print the name of the section on the front and back of the label. The print should be easy to read when the record is held by the main fold.	10		

7.	Using the prongs on the left-hand side of the record, secure the registration form.	**10**		
8.	Using the prongs on the right-hand side of the record, secure the index dividers with a progress note sheet under the progress note tab.	**10**		
Scenario Update: The patient authorized his/her prior provider to send health records to your agency. You need to organize these records within the paper health record.				
9.	To help ensure the integrity of the practice management and EHR systems, a search for the new patient's name must always be done. This prevents errors in documentation. Verify the name and the date of birth on the health records and ensure they match the information on the health record. *(Refer to the Checklist for Affective Behaviors)*	**10***		
10.	Open the prongs on the right side of the record and carefully remove the record to the point of where the documents need to be inserted. For the documents being inserted, punch holes in the proper location. Insert the papers into the record and then reassemble the remaining part of the record. Continue to do this until all the documents are filed within the health record.	**10**		
	Total Points	**100**		

Checklist for Affective Behaviors

Affective Behavior	***Directions:*** *Check behaviors observed during the role-play.*					
Ethical	Fails to adequately explain facility's policy.			Adequate explains the facility's policy.		
	Fails to adequately discuss the hazards of not protecting the paper health record.			Adequately explains the legal and ethical results of not protecting the paper health record. Addresses the consequences to the clinic, employee, and patient.		
	Fails to adequately explain how to protect the paper health record.			Adequately explains how to protect the paper health record (e.g., close files when done, turn so that the patient name is not visible)		
	Other:			Other:		

Grading for Affective Behaviors		Point Value	Attempt 1	Attempt 2
Does not meet Expectation	• Response was disrespectful. • Student demonstrated more than 2 negative, unprofessional behaviors during the interaction.	0		
Needs Improvement	• Response was disrespectful. • Student demonstrated 1 or 2 negative, unprofessional behaviors during the interaction.	0		
Meets Expectation	• Response was respectful; no negative, unprofessional behaviors observed. • More practice is needed for behavior to appear natural and for student to appear comfortable and at ease.	15		
Occasionally Exceeds Expectation	• Response was respectful; no negative, unprofessional behaviors observed. • At times student appeared comfortable and at ease; but more practice is needed for behavior to become natural and consistent with a professional medical assistant.	15		
Always Exceeds Expectation	• Response was respectful; no negative, unprofessional behaviors observed. • Student's behaviors appeared natural and comfortable. Behaviors are consistent with a professional medical assistant.	15		

CAAHEP Competencies	Steps
VI.P.4. Organize a patient's medical record	6, 7, 8, 10
VI.P.5. File patient medical records	10
X.A.2. Protect the integrity of the medical record	9
ABHES Competencies	**Steps**
7. Administrative Procedures a. Gather and process documents	10

Procedure 10.5   File Patient Health Records

Name _____ Date _____ Score _____

Task: File patient health records using two different filing systems: the alphabetic system and the numeric system.

Scenario: The agency utilizes the alphabetic system. You need to file health records in the correct location.

Equipment and Supplies:
- Paper health records using the alphabetic filing system
- Paper health records using the numeric filing system
- File box(es) or file cabinet

Standard: Complete the procedure and all critical steps in _____ minutes with a minimum score of 85% within two attempts (*or as indicated by the instructor*).

Scoring: Divide the points earned by the total possible points. Failure to perform a critical step, indicated by an asterisk (*), results in grade no higher than an 84% (*or as indicated by the instructor*).

Time: Began_____ Ended_____ Total minutes: _____

Steps:	Point Value	Attempt 1	Attempt 2
1. Using alphabetic guidelines, place the records to be filed in alphabetic order.	20		
2. Using the file box or file cabinet, locate the correct spot for the first file.	10		
3. Place the health record in the correct location. Continue these filing steps until all the health records are filed.	20*		
4. Using numeric guidelines, place the records to be filed in numeric order.	20		
5. Using the file box or file cabinet, locate the correct spot for the first file.	10		
6. Place the health record in the correct location. Continue these filing steps until all the health records are filed.	20*		
Total Points	100		

CAAHEP Competencies	Steps
VI.P.5. File patient medical records	3, 6
ABHES Competencies	**Steps**
7. Administrative Procedures a. Gather and process documents	All

Daily Operations and Safety

chapter

11

CAAHEP Competencies	Assessment
VI.C.9. Explain the purpose of routine maintenance of administrative and clinical equipment	Skills and Concepts – B. 5; Certification Preparation – 5
VI.C.10. List steps involved in completing an inventory	Skills and Concepts – B. 9
VI.P.8. Perform routine maintenance of administrative or clinical equipment	Procedure 11.2
VI.P.9. Perform an inventory with documentation	Procedure 11.1, 11.3
XII.C.3. Discuss fire safety issues in an ambulatory healthcare environment	Skills and Concepts – C. 15-18; Certification Preparation – 7, 9
XII.C.4. Describe fundamental principles for evacuation of a healthcare setting	Skills and Concepts – C. 12-14; Internet Activities – 3
XII.C.7.a. Identify principles of: body mechanics	Skills and Concepts – C. 1-3; Certification Preparation – 6; Workplace Application – 2
XII.C.8. Identify critical elements of an emergency plan for response to a natural disaster or other emergency	Skills and Concepts – C. 8; Certification Preparation – 8; Internet Activities – 3
XII.P.2.b. Demonstrate proper use of: fire extinguishers	Procedure 11.6
XII.P.3. Use proper body mechanics	Procedure 11.4
XII.P.4. Participate in a mock exposure event with documentation of specific steps	Procedure 11.5
XII.P.5. Evaluate the work environment to identify unsafe working conditions	Procedure 11.4
XII.A.1. Recognize the physical and emotional effects on persons involved in an emergency situation	Procedure 11.5
XII.A.2. Demonstrate self-awareness in responding to an emergency situation	Procedure 11.5
ABHES Competencies	**Assessment**
7. Administrative Procedures f. Maintain inventory of equipment and supplies	Procedure 11.1, 11.3

VOCABULARY REVIEW

Using the word pool on the right, find the correct word to match the definition. Write the word on the line after the definition.

Group A

1. A commercial service that answers telephone calls for its clients

   _____

2. A process to ensure the reliability of test results, often using manufactured samples with known values

   _____

3. The process of replacing the supplies that were used

   _____

4. The ability to start a task and independently complete it

   _____

5. The process of removing all microorganisms

   _____

6. To destroy or render pathogenic organisms inactive; this does not include spores, tuberculosis bacilli, and certain viruses

   _____

7. Documentation in the paper health record that can be used to track the patient's condition and progress

   _____

8. The process of cleaning equipment and instruments with detergent and water to remove debris and reduce the number of microorganisms _____

9. Emergency medications and equipment (e.g., oxygen, intravenous [IV], and airway supplies) stored in a cart and ready for an emergency _____

10. A detailed list of equipment and supplies owned and stored; the process of counting the supplies in stock

    _____

Word Pool
- initiative
- sterilize
- restock
- crash cart
- disinfect
- inventory
- answering service
- progress notes
- sanitize
- quality control

Group B

1. Amount of supplies that need to be ordered
   _____

2. A lack of similarity between what is stated and what is found; for instance, the computer inventory count is different than the physical count _____

3. The point at which low inventory requires the product to be ordered _____

4. A document that accompanies purchased merchandise and shows what is in the box or package _____

5. Unique number assigned by the ordering facility that allows the facility to track or reference the order _____

6. Assistance (i.e., service) that is provided by a healthcare provider and can be billed to the insurance company or patient
   _____

7. To diminish in value (e.g., the value of an item) over a period of time; a concept used for tax purposes _____

8. Refers to how often an item is purchased; this depends on how frequently the item is used and the storage space available for it
   _____

9. Companies that sell supplies, equipment, or services to other companies or individuals _____

10. Billing statements that list the amount owed for goods or services purchased _____

Word Pool
- reorder point
- packing slip
- quantity to reorder
- purchase order number
- buying cycle
- billable service
- vendors
- discrepancy
- depreciate
- invoice

Group C

1. An order placed for an item that is temporarily out of stock and will be sent later _____

2. Money owed by a company to other companies for services and goods; pertains to paying the bills of the facility
   _____

3. To reduce the level or intensity; bring down a person's anger or elevated emotions _____

4. Unforeseen situations that threaten employees and visitors; they can disrupt services provided _____

5. Doors made of fire-resistant materials; close manually or automatically during a fire to prevent the spread of the fire
   _____

6. Involves evacuating everyone from the building to a safe location outside the building _____

7. Evacuation to an interior room with no windows used in case of tornados and other severe storms _____

8. Involves moving one or more people out of immediate danger
   _____

9. Involves evacuating people off of the same floor as the emergency situation _____

10. Involves evacuating people who are located on the floors above and below the situation _____

Word Pool
- accounts payable
- de-escalating
- backordered
- shelter-in-place evacuation
- vertical evacuation
- fire doors
- workplace emergencies
- building evacuation
- horizontal evacuation
- local evacuation

ABBREVIATIONS

Write out what each of the following abbreviations stands for.

1. EHR _____

2. GPOs _____

3. PBGs _____

4. PO _____

5. OSH Act _____

6. OSHA _____

7. ADA _____

8. GAS _____

9. BTL _____

10. BX _____

11. CS _____

12. EA _____

13. PKG _____

14. DDL _____

15. PPD _____

16. PYMT _____

17. QTY _____

SKILLS AND CONCEPTS

Answer the following questions. Write your answer on the line or in the space provided.

A. Opening and Closing the Healthcare Facility

1. Describe three opening tasks for the clinical medical assistant. _____

    _____

    _____

    _____

2. Describe three opening tasks for the administrative medical assistant._____

    _____

    _____

    _____

3. List four closing duties of the clinical medical assistant. _____

_____

_____

_____

_____

4. List four closing duties of the administrative medical assistant._____

_____

_____

_____

B. Equipment and Supplies

1. Describe why the facility should have an inventory list of equipment._____

_____

_____

2. Describe how the practice's accountant can use the equipment inventory list. _____

_____

_____

3. Explain how supervisors can use the equipment inventory list._____

_____

_____

4. List seven items that should be documented for each piece of equipment on the inventory list. _____

_____

_____

_____

5. Explain the purpose of routine maintenance of administrative and clinical equipment. _____

_____

_____

_____

_____

6. Describe three factors that are taken into consideration when deciding to replace a piece of equipment with a newer model.

_____

_____

_____

7. Explain two reasons that a supervisor or provider may opt to lease a piece of equipment versus buying it.

_____

_____

8. List eight items that should be recorded for each supply in inventory. _____

_____

_____

9. List steps involved in completing an inventory. _____

_____

_____

_____

10. Describe the usefulness of purchase order numbers for the vendor and the medical facility. _____

_____

_____

11. On receiving supply deliveries, describe why it is important to check the merchandise as soon as possible.

_____

_____

_____

12. Explain how the packing slip is used when ordered supplies arrive. _____

_____

_____

C. Safety and Security

1. When lifting an object, explain how your feet should be placed. _____

_____

_____

2. Describe the position of your knees and back when lifting. _____

_____

_____

3. List four other principles of body mechanics. _____

_____

_____

_____

4. List four ways to keep safe in the work environment. _____

_____

_____

_____

5. List five high-risk situations inside the facility that can lead to accidents. _____

_____

_____

_____

6. List four ways a medical assistant can help prevent injuries and fires. _____

_____

_____

_____

7. Describe an emergency response plan. _____

_____

_____

_____

8. Identify six critical elements of an emergency plan for response to a natural disaster or other emergency.

_____

_____

_____

9. Floor maps with _____ and _____ should be posted throughout the facility.

10. _____ must be clearly marked and well-lit.

11. Exit routes should be clear of _____ and _____ at all times.

12. List evacuation priorities by locations. Start with the most critical or highest priority to evacuate.

_____

_____

_____

13. List evacuation priorities by people. Start with the most critical or highest priority to evacuate._____

_____

_____

_____

14. Describe the five types of evacuations. _____

_____

_____

_____

_____

15. List five items that should be located throughout the facility per state code for fire response. _____

_____

_____

16. Describe RACE._____

_____

_____

_____

17. Describe PASS or how to use most fire extinguishers. _____

_____

_____

_____

18. What two types of fire extinguishers are used for a paper or wood fire? _____

_____

19. Describe the stages of general adaptation syndrome (GAS)._____

_____

_____

_____

CERTIFICATION PREPARATION

Circle the correct answer.

1. What is an opening task for the administrative medical assistant?
   a. Unlock supply cabinets.
   b. Perform quality-control tests on laboratory equipment.
   c. Update the voicemail message.
   d. Follow up on outstanding patient issues from the prior day.

2. What should be disinfected in the healthcare facility?
   a. Exam table
   b. Writing table
   c. Computer keyboard
   d. All of the above

3. How often do crash carts and other emergency supplies need to be inventoried?
   a. Every week
   b. Every other week
   c. Every month
   d. Every 6 months

4. What is *not* found on a routine maintenance log?
   a. Equipment name, serial number, and location of the machine
   b. Manufacturer's name and date of purchase
   c. Store name where the machine was purchased
   d. Warranty information and service provider information

5. What the purpose of routine maintenance of administrative and clinical equipment?
   a. Prevent injury to the patients
   b. Prevent costly damage to the equipment
   c. Prevent injury to staff members
   d. All of the above

6. What is *not* a principle of proper body mechanics?
   a. When lifting an object, maintain a wide, stable base with your feet.
   b. Get help if the item is too heavy to lift by yourself.
   c. Keep your movements smooth.
   d. When reaching for an object, you can stand on tiptoes.

7. What is the correct way to operate most fire extinguishers?
   a. Pull the pin, squeeze the handle, aim the nozzle, and sweep the nozzle from side to side
   b. Pull the pin, aim the nozzle, sweep the nozzle from side to side, and squeeze the handle
   c. Pull the pin, sweep the nozzle from side to side, squeeze the handle, and aim the nozzle
   d. Pull the pin, aim the nozzle, squeeze the handle, and sweep the nozzle from side to side

8. What is a critical element of an emergency response plan?
   a. Evacuation policy and procedure
   b. Methods to report emergencies
   c. Critical shutdown procedures
   d. All of the above

9. Which is a dry chemical fire extinguisher that is used on fires related to electrical sources?
   a. A
   b. B
   c. C
   d. D

10. Which is *not* a symptom of stress?
    a. Anger
    b. Low blood pressure
    c. Anxiety
    d. Fear

WORKPLACE APPLICATION

1. Catherine is working at the reception desk and the procedure has been to place the cashbox on the receptionist's desk. Patients arrive, make payments, and the cashbox remains on the desk visible to all and in easy access to the public. How might Catherine safeguard the money in the cashbox?

   _____

   _____

2. Maria is lifting heavy boxes. Describe how she should lift and carry heavy boxes. _____

   _____

   _____

   _____

3. Maria sometimes needs to room patients who make her uncomfortable. Describe four ways she could keep safe in these situations.

   _____

   _____

   _____

INTERNET ACTIVITIES

1. Obtain a vaccine name from the instructor and research the storage directions for that medication.

2. Research guidelines for storing vaccines in the refrigerator. Create a poster that provides the key guidelines that must be followed for safe storage.

3. Using the OSHA website (www.osha.gov), research emergency action plans. Create a poster, PowerPoint, or paper summarizing your research. Focus on these areas:
   - The minimum requirements for the emergency action plan
   - Evacuation elements
   - Shelter-in-place requirements and procedures

Procedure 11.1 Perform an Equipment Inventory with Documentation

Name _____ Date _____ Score _____

Tasks: Perform an equipment inventory. Document the inventory on the equipment inventory form.

Equipment and Supplies:
- Pens
- Administrative and/or clinical equipment
- Purchase information (e.g., date, cost, and supplier) and warranty information (e.g., start and end date, warranty coverage)
- Equipment inventory form (Work Product 11.1)

Standard: Complete the procedure and all critical steps with a minimum score of 85% within two attempts (*or as indicated by the instructor*).

Scoring: Divide the points earned by the total possible points. Failure to perform a critical step, indicated by an asterisk (*), results in grade no higher than an 84% (*or as indicated by the instructor*).

Steps:	Point Value	Attempt 1	Attempt 2
1. For each piece of equipment to be inventoried, gather the following information: a. Name of equipment, manufacturer, and serial number b. Location and facility number (if applicable) c. Purchase date, cost, supplier, and warranty information	20		
2. Complete an equipment inventory form (Work Product 11.1) by adding the gathered information for each item inventoried.	60		
3. Review the document created. Make any necessary revisions.	20		
Total Points	**100**		

Comments

CAAHEP Competencies	Step(s)
VI.P.9. Perform an inventory with documentation	Entire procedure
ABHES Competencies	**Step(s)**
7. Administrative Procedures f. Maintain inventory of equipment and supplies	Entire procedure

Work Product 11.1   Equipment Inventory Form

Name _____ **Date** _____ **Score** _____

To be used with Procedure 11.1.

Equipment Name	Manufacturer/ Serial Number	Location/Facility Number	Purchase Date/ Supplier	Cost	Warranty Information

Procedure 11.2   Perform Routine Maintenance of Equipment

Name _____ **Date** _____ **Score** _____

Tasks: Perform routine maintenance of administrative or clinical equipment. Document the maintenance on the log.

Equipment and Supplies:
- Maintenance log(s) (Work Product 11.2)
- Administrative or clinical equipment (e.g., oral thermometers)
- Supplies for routine maintenance (e.g., battery)
- Operation manual if needed
- Pens
- Information regarding the equipment (i.e., name, serial number, location, facility number, manufacturer, purchase date, warranty information, frequency of inspections, and service provider)

Standard: Complete the procedure and all critical steps with a minimum score of 85% within two attempts (*or as indicated by the instructor*).

Scoring: Divide the points earned by the total possible points. Failure to perform a critical step, indicated by an asterisk (*), results in grade no higher than an 84% (*or as indicated by the instructor*).

Steps:	Point Value	Attempt 1	Attempt 2
1. Gather information on the piece of equipment identified for routine maintenance including name, serial number, location, facility number, manufacturer, purchase date, warranty information, frequency of inspections, and service provider.	20		
2. Fill in the equipment details on the log (Work Product 11.2).	20*		
3. To perform the maintenance activities, gather the required supplies. If you are not familiar with the procedure or the required supplies, refer to the operation manual.	10		
4. Perform the maintenance activities as directed in the operation manual. Take any required safety precautions necessary to protect yourself and others.	20*		
5. Clean up the work area.	10		
6. Using a pen, document the date, time, the maintenance activity performed, and include your signature on the log.	20		
Total Points	**100**		

Comments

CAAHEP Competencies	Step(s)
VI.P.8. Perform routine maintenance of administrative or clinical equipment	Entire procedure

Work Product 11.2   Maintenance Logs

Name _____   **Date** _____   **Score** _____

To be used with Procedure 11.2.

Maintenance Log

Equipment: _____   Serial #: _____   Location: _____

Facility #: _____   Manufacturer: _____   Purchased: _____

Warranty Information: _____

Frequency of Inspections: _____

Service Provider: _____

Date	Time	Maintenance Activities	Signature

Maintenance Log

Equipment: _____   Serial #: _____   Location: _____

Facility #: _____   Manufacturer: _____   Purchased: _____

Warranty Information: _____

Frequency of Inspections: _____

Service Provider: _____

Date	Time	Maintenance Activities	Signature

Maintenance Log

Equipment: _____   Serial #: _____   Location: _____

Facility #: _____   Manufacturer: _____   Purchased: _____

Warranty Information: _____

Frequency of Inspections: _____

Service Provider: _____

Date	Time	Maintenance Activities	Signature

Maintenance Log

Equipment: _____   Serial #: _____   Location: _____

Facility #: _____   Manufacturer: _____   Purchased: _____

Warranty Information: _____

Frequency of Inspections: _____

Service Provider: _____

Date	Time	Maintenance Activities	Signature

Procedure 11.3   Perform a Supply Inventory with Documentation While Using Proper Body Mechanics

Name _____ Date _____ Score _____

Tasks: Perform a supply inventory using correct body mechanics. Document the inventory on the supply inventory form.

Equipment and Supplies:
- Pens
- Administrative or clinical supplies to be inventoried
- Purchase information (e.g., item number, cost, and supplier) for supplies in inventory
- Reorder point and quantity to reorder for each item in inventory
- Supply inventory form (Work Product 11.3)

Standard: Complete the procedure and all critical steps with a minimum score of 85% within two attempts (*or as indicated by the instructor*).

Scoring: Divide the points earned by the total possible points. Failure to perform a critical step, indicated by an asterisk (*), results in grade no higher than an 84% (*or as indicated by the instructor*).

Steps:	Point Value	Attempt 1	Attempt 2
1. For the supplies in inventory, gather the following information for each item: • Name, size, quantity (e.g., purchased individually, 100 per box) • Item number, supplier's name, cost • Reorder point and quantity to reorder	5		
2. For each supply item, enter information on the inventory form (Work Product 11.3). Make sure the appropriate entry is in the right location. Note: The "Stock Available" column will be empty for now.	15*		
3. Review the document. Make any necessary revisions.	10		
4. Using the supply inventory list, inventory the supplies in the department. Identify how the supply should be counted (e.g., individually, by the box) and count the number of items in stock.	15		
5. Add the number in the appropriate row under the "Stock Available" header.	10		
6. Compare the reorder point number to the stock available number. If the stock available number is at or below the reorder point, indicate that the item needs to be reordered by checking the appropriate column.	10*		
7. Make sure the supplies are neatly arranged. The older stock should be in front of the newer stock.	5		
8. Repeat steps 5 through 7 until all supplies are inventoried.	10		
9. Use proper body mechanics when lifting and moving supplies by maintaining a wide, stable base with your feet. Your feet should be shoulder-width apart and you should have good footing. Bend at the knees, keeping your back straight. Lift smoothly with the major muscles in your arms and legs. Use the same technique when putting the item down.	10*		

10. Use proper body mechanics when reaching for an object. Clear away barriers and use a step stool if needed. Your feet should face the object. Avoid twisting or turning with a heavy load.	**10***		
Total Points	**100**		

Comments

CAAHEP Competencies	Step(s)
VI.P.9. Perform an inventory with documentation	1-8
XII.P.3. Use proper body mechanics	9, 10
ABHES Competencies	**Step(s)**
7. Administrative Procedures f. Maintain inventory of equipment and supplies	1-8

Work Product 11.3   Supply Inventory Form

Name _____   **Date** _____   **Score** _____

To be used with Procedure 11.3.

Item Name	Size	Quantity	Item Number	Supplier's Name	Reorder Point	Quantity to Reorder	Cost	Stock Available	Order (✓)

Procedure 11.4   Evaluate the Work Environment

Name _____ Date _____ Score _____

Task: Evaluate the work environment to identify unsafe working conditions.

Equipment and Supplies:
- Work environment evaluation form (Work Product 11.4)
- Pen

Standard: Complete the procedure and all critical steps with a minimum score of 85% within two attempts (*or as indicated by the instructor*).

Scoring: Divide the points earned by the total possible points. Failure to perform a critical step, indicated by an asterisk (*), results in grade no higher than an 84% (*or as indicated by the instructor*).

Steps:	Point Value	Attempt 1	Attempt 2
1. Observe the environment for slipping, tripping, or fall risks. Document your findings on the work environment evaluation form (Work Product 11.4).	20		
2. Observe the environment for safety and security issues. Document your findings.	20		
3. Observe the environment for fire risks and electrical issues. Document your findings.	20		
4. Observe the environment for fire containment and evacuation strategies. Document your findings.	20		
5. Based on your observations, summarize your findings. If risks are present, create a list of issues that need to be addressed. Describe what needs to be done for each risk.	20*		
Total Points	100		

Comments

CAAHEP Competencies	Step(s)
XII.P.5. Evaluate the work environment to identify unsafe working conditions	Entire procedure

Work Product 11.4   Work Environment Evaluation Form

Name _____ **Date** _____ **Score** _____

To be used with Procedure 11.4.

Directions: *Check either in the "Yes" or "No" column for each question. Check "NA" if it is not applicable. Include any issues in the comment column. Summarize your findings for each area, using the space indicated.*

Slipping, tripping, or fall risks	Yes	No	NA	Comments
• Is the lighting appropriate?				
• Are any lights burned out? Are any areas dim?				
• Is the flooring and carpeting ripped or pulled up?				
• If rugs/mats are present, are they folded?				
• Is water on the floor?				
• Is signage present warning of the water?				
• Are items cluttering the hallway, making walking difficult?				
• Are cords, cables, and other items in the walkway?				
• Is trash on the floor?				
• Are heavy items on high shelves?				
• Is a sturdy step stool available?				
Safety and security issues	**Yes**	**No**	**NA**	**Comments**
• Are rooms available that can be locked and used during workplace violence?				
• Is there limited visibility from the hallway into the room?				
• Are there areas in the building with limited visibility?				
• If the building is accessible to the public, are there any safe zones or areas for staff?				
• Are the emergency call lights in the exam rooms and bathrooms functioning?				
• Are the oxygen tanks (if available) checked per the facility's policy?				
Fire risks and electrical issues	**Yes**	**No**	**NA**	**Comments**
• Are electrical cords and plugs free from cracks, fraying, or other damage?				
• Are power strips overloaded?				
• Is electricity being used near a water source?				
• Are flammable chemicals and supplies stored according to manufacturers' guidelines?				
• Are combustibles (e.g., paper, cardboard, cloth, flammable chemicals) away from heat sources?				

Fire containment and evacuation strategies	Yes	No	NA	Comments
• Are building diagrams posted on walls indicating exit routes (two or more), fire alarms, and fire extinguishers?				
• Are exit routes uncluttered?				
• Are exit signs visible and lit?				
• Are fire doors unblocked and able to be closed in an emergency?				
• Are interior rooms available for severe storms?				
• Are smoke detectors located throughout the building?				
• Are fire alarms available?				
• Are fire extinguishers available and checked routinely (per the facility's policy)?				
• Are flammable products (e.g., oxygen tanks, chemicals) stored along the exit routes?				

Based on your observations, summarize your findings.

If risks are present, create a list of issues that need to be addressed. Describe what needs to be done for each risk.

Procedure 11.5 Participate in a Mock Exposure Event

Name _____ Date _____ Score _____

Tasks: Demonstrate self-awareness in an emergency situation. Participate in a mock exposure event and document specific steps taken. Recognize the physical and emotional effects on individuals involved in an emergency situation.

Scenario: You and Beth are in the autoclave room and two chemicals spill, creating toxic fumes. Beth is having trouble breathing. The staff, patients, and visitors present include:

Rooms	Staff and Reception Areas
1—Teen and his mother	Reception Area A—Four people waiting
2—Older woman in a wheelchair	Reception Area B—Five people waiting
3—Mother with three little children	
4—Adult female	**Staff**
5—Empty	Tim—In MA station 3
6—An older couple	Rose—At the insurance desk
7—Adult male	Dave and Patty—At the reception desk
8—Empty	Julie Walden, MD—In provider office 1
Procedure room—Empty	Angela Perez, MD—In room 3
	Jean Burke, NP—In room 7

Directions: Create a paper and address the points in the checklist. Use reliable internet resources to research the physical and emotional effects of stress on the body. Include your findings in the paper as indicated in the checklist. Use 1-inch margins, double spacing, and 12-point font. Length should be at least two pages.

Equipment and Supplies:
- Paper
- Pen
- Floor map (see Figure 11.11 in the textbook)
- Computer with internet access

Standard: Complete the procedure and all critical steps with a minimum score of 85% within two attempts (*or as indicated by the instructor*).

Scoring: Divide the points earned by the total possible points. Failure to perform a critical step, indicated by an asterisk (*), results in grade no higher than an 84% (*or as indicated by the instructor*).

Steps:	Point Value	Attempt 1	Attempt 2
1. Using the scenario, describe how you would handle the emergency exposure situation with Beth. • Identify four steps a medical assistant could take to demonstrate self-awareness while responding to this emergency situation. • Describe exposure control mechanisms or how you might limit the exposure to other people once you remove Beth from the room.	15*		

2.	*Scenario continues: Dr. Walden informed the staff to evacuate from the building. The outdoor safe meeting location is at the back of the parking lot.* Document the steps to handle the exposure event and evacuation from the building. • Describe what each staff member and provider should do to help with the evacuation procedure and notify 911. • Describe the steps (evacuations) in the order that they should occur. • Describe how the staff may ensure all individuals are out of the building.	**15***		
3.	Dr. Walden is in charge during the emergency. Describe what her responsibilities include.	**5**		
4.	Dave took the patient registry. Describe why the patient registry is important.	**5**		
5.	*Scenario continues: Two weeks after the event, Beth confides to you that she is not doing well. She recovered from the exposure, but since the event she has had difficulty sleeping. She is anxious when she goes into the autoclave room. She is having trouble concentrating on her job. She mentioned she has had two nightmares of emergencies occurring in the department in which she gets injured.* • Describe what might be occurring with Beth and the symptoms that relate to it. • Discuss what you might encourage her to do about the situation.	**15***		
6.	Research the physical and emotional effects of stress on the body. Identify four physical effects and four emotional effects of stress on persons involved in an emergency situation. Cite your resources.	**15***		
7.	Describe how the physical and emotional effects of stress would be different for Beth, you, the providers, and the other employees present.	**15**		
8.	Describe how a medical assistant could limit the physical and emotional effects of stress on each person/group: Beth, the providers, the other employees present in the facility, and yourself.	**15**		
	Total Points	**100**		

Comments

CAAHEP Competencies	Step(s)
XII.P.4. Participate in a mock exposure event with documentation of specific steps	1-2
XII.A.1. Recognize the physical and emotional effects on persons involved in an emergency situation	5-8
XII.A.2. Demonstrate self-awareness in responding to an emergency situation	1

Procedure 11.6 Use a Fire Extinguisher

Name _____ Date _____ Score _____

Tasks: Select the correct fire extinguisher and demonstrate its use.

Equipment and Supplies:
- Fire extinguisher

Scenarios:
a. You are working in the medical laboratory and an electrical fire starts. 911 was called.
b. You are working in the clinic and fire starts in a wastebasket. 911 was called.
c. You are working in the medical laboratory and a chemical fire starts (combustible metal fire). 911 was called.

Standard: Complete the procedure and all critical steps with a minimum score of 85% within two attempts (*or as indicated by the instructor*).

Scoring: Divide the points earned by the total possible points. Failure to perform a critical step, indicated by an asterisk (*), results in grade no higher than an 84% (*or as indicated by the instructor*).

Steps:	Point Value	Attempt 1	Attempt 2
1. Using the scenario, identify the type of fire extinguisher required to put out the fire.	20		
2. Hold the extinguisher by the handle with the hose or nozzle pointing away from you. Pull out the pin that is located below the trigger.	20		
3. Stand about 10 feet from the fire. Aim the extinguisher hose or nozzle at the base of the fire. Keep the extinguisher in an upright position as you work.	20		
4. Squeeze the trigger slowly and evenly.	20		
5. Sweep from side to side until the fire is out.	20		
Total Points	**100**		

Comments

CAAHEP Competencies	Step(s)
XII.P.2.b. Demonstrate proper use of: fire extinguishers	Entire procedure

Health Insurance Essentials

CAAHEP Competencies	Assessment
VIII.C.1.a. Identify: types of third party plans	Skills and Concepts – B. 1
VIII.C.2. Outline managed care requirements for patient referral	Skills and Concepts – B. 4
VIII.C.3.a. Describe processes for: verification of eligibility for services	Skills and Concepts – D. 2
VIII.C.3.c. Describe processes for: preauthorization	Skills and Concepts – D. 3, 4
ABHES Competencies	**Assessment**
5. Human Relations c. Assist the patient in navigating issues and concerns that may arise (i.e., insurance policy information, medical bills, and physician/provider orders)	Case Scenario 2

VOCABULARY REVIEW

Using the word pool on the right, find the correct word to match the definition. Write the word on the line after the definition.

Group A

1. A set dollar amount that the policyholder must pay before the insurance company starts to pay for services

   _____

2. Poor, needy, impoverished _____

3. The amount paid or to be paid by the policyholder for coverage under the contract, usually in periodic installments

   _____

4. Services provided to help prevent certain illnesses or that lead to an early diagnosis _____

5. When the policyholder pays a certain percentage of the bill and the insurance company pays the rest _____

6. A formal request for payment from an insurance company for services provided _____

7. A written agreement between two parties, in which one party (the insurance company) agrees to pay another party (the patient) if certain specified circumstances occur _____

8. Services that are necessary to improve the patient's current health

   _____

9. A set dollar amount that the policyholder must pay for each office visit _____

10. The person responsible for the payment of the premium

    _____

Word Pool
- policy
- premium
- subscriber
- deductible
- coinsurance
- copayment
- claim
- medically necessary
- preventive care
- indigent

Group B

1. Government insurance plan for dependents of military personnel _____

2. Those covered by Medicare; a designated person who receives funds from an insurance policy _____

3. Government insurance plan for employees who are injured or become ill due to work-related issues _____

4. Low-income Medicare patients who qualify for Medicaid for their secondary insurance _____

5. Government insurance plan for those age 65 or older _____

6. A list of fixed prices for services _____

7. Government insurance plan for surviving spouses and dependent children of veterans who died in the line of duty _____

8. A document sent by the insurance company to the provider and the patient explaining the allowed charge amount, the amount reimbursed for services, and the patient's financial responsibilities _____

9. Government insurance plan for those with low income _____

10. A system used to determine how much providers should be paid for services provided; used by Medicare and many other health insurance companies _____

Word Pool
- Medicare
- Medicaid
- TRICARE
- Civilian Health and Medical Program of the Veterans Administration
- Workers' compensation
- beneficiary
- resource-based relative value scale
- explanation of benefits
- fee schedule
- Qualified Medicare Beneficiaries

Group C

1. In charge of coordinating the patient's care _____

2. When the patient has authorized the insurance company to make the payment directly to the provider _____

3. An approved list of physicians, hospitals, and other providers _____

4. An organization that processes claims and provides administrative services for another organization _____

5. A process required by some insurance carriers in which the provider obtains permission to perform certain procedures or services _____

6. An online marketplace where you can compare and buy individual health insurance plans _____

7. The primary care provider who is in charge of a patient's treatment _____

8. The amount paid for a medical service in a geographic area based on what providers in the area usually charge for the same or similar service _____

9. Insurance plan funded by a large company or organization for their own employees _____

10. An order from a primary care provider for the patient to see a specialist or get certain medical services _____

Word Pool
- self-funded plan
- third-party administrator
- health insurance exchange
- assignment of benefits
- usual, customary, and reasonable
- primary care provider
- referral
- preauthorization
- gatekeeper
- provider network

Group D

1. The maximum that the insurance plan will pay for a procedure or service _____

2. Reviews individual cases to ensure that services are medically necessary _____

3. The provider is paid a set amount for each enrolled person assigned to him or her, per period of time, whether or not that person has received services _____

4. The length of time a patient waits for disability insurance to pay after the date of injury _____

5. Low- to middle-income Americans can compare plans and lower their costs for healthcare coverage _____

6. Providers are contracted with the insurance plan and have agreed to accept the contracted fee schedule as payment in full _____

7. A health problem that was present before new health insurance coverage started _____

8. A service provided by various insurance companies for providers to look up a patient's insurance benefits, eligibility, claims status, and explanation of benefits _____

9. A decision-making process used by managed care organizations to manage healthcare costs; involves case-by-case assessments of the appropriateness of care _____

Word Pool
- capitation
- utilization management
- utilization review committee
- participating provider
- allowable charge
- online insurance web portal
- waiting period
- preexisting condition
- health insurance marketplaces

ABBREVIATIONS
Write out what each of the following abbreviations stands for.

1. ACA _____

2. STI _____

3. CHAMPVA _____

4. ESRD _____

5. CMS _____

6. HHS _____

7. RBRVS _____

8. UCR _____

9. EOB _____

10. QMBs _____

11. CHIP _____

12. TPA _____

13. UCR _____

14. MCO _____

15. PCP _____

16. HMO _____

17. PPO _____

18. EPO _____

19. IPA _____

20. PAR _____

SKILLS AND CONCEPTS

Answer the following questions. Write your answer on the line or in the space provided.

A. Health Insurance Plans

1. Match the following terms and definitions:

   _____ Medicaid

   _____ Medicare

   _____ Medigap

   a. A federally funded health insurance program for those older than 65 years or disabled individuals younger than 65 years

   b. A term sometimes applied to private insurance products that supplement Medicare insurance benefits

   c. A health insurance program that is funded by both the federal and state governments for the medically indigent

2. List two different populations who qualify for Medicare. _____

   _____

3. The RBRVS includes the following three parts:

   a. _____

   b. _____

   c. _____

4. The intermediary and administrator who coordinates patients and providers and processes claims for self-funded plans is called a(n) _____.

5. Prescription drugs are covered by Medicare _____.

6. List four different populations who qualify for Medicaid. _____

   _____

7. Active duty military personnel, family members of active duty personnel, and military retirees and their eligible family members younger than age 65 are covered by _____.

8. The health benefits program run by the Department of Veterans Affairs (VA) that helps eligible beneficiaries pay the cost of specific healthcare services and supplies is the (give acronym) _____.

9. List the services covered by workers' compensation plans._____

_____

_____

_____

_____

10. Private health insurance plans are obtained from two sources. List those sources._____

_____

B. Health Insurance Models

1. Traditional health insurance plans are also referred to as _____ plans.

2. For each of the following managed care plans, describe the deductible, coinsurance, and copayment requirements:

    a. Health maintenance organization (HMO): _____

_____

_____

_____

_____

_____

    b. Preferred provider organization (PPO):_____

_____

_____

_____

_____

    c. Exclusive provider organization (EPO):_____

_____

_____

_____

_____

3. A(n) _____ is a review of individual cases by a committee to make sure services are medically necessary and to study how providers use medical care resources.

4. Describe the managed care requirements for a patient referral. _____

_____

_____

_____

_____

C. Participating Provider Contracts

1. A(n) _____ is a healthcare provider who enters into a contract with a specific insurance company or program and agrees to accept the contracted fee schedule.

2. The _____ is the maximum that third-party payers will pay for a procedure or service.

D. The Medical Assistant's Role

1. One of the medical assistant's responsibilities is verifying eligibility. Describe the processes available for the verification of eligibility for services.

_____

_____

_____

2. Describe how the patient's insurance eligibility is confirmed. _____

_____

_____

_____

3. What items should the medical assistant gather when using the paper method to obtain a precertification for a service or procedure?

_____

_____

_____

4. Describe the processes for precertification using the paper method. What does the medical assistant need to do?

_____

_____

_____

E. Other Types of Insurance

1. Match the types of insurance benefits with their description.

_____ Disability

_____ Liability insurance

_____ Life insurance

_____ Long-term care insurance

a. Provides payment of a specified amount upon the insured's death
b. Covers a continuum of broad-range maintenance and health services to chronically ill, disabled, or mentally disabled individuals
c. A form of insurance that provides income replacement if the patient has a non-work–related injury
d. Often includes benefits for medical expenses related to traumatic injuries and lost wages payable to individuals who are injured in the insured person's home or in an automobile accident

CERTIFICATION PREPARATION

Circle the correct answer.

1. A policy that covers a number of people under a single master contract issued to the employer or to an association with which they are affiliated and that is not self-funded is usually called
   a. a group policy.
   b. an individual policy.
   c. a government plan.
   d. a self-insured plan.

2. The maximum amount of money third-party payers will pay for a specific procedure or service is called the
   a. benefit.
   b. allowed amount.
   c. allowable service.
   d. incurred amount.

3. A provider who enters into a contract with an insurance company and agrees to certain rules and regulations is called a _____ provider.
   a. paying
   b. physician
   c. participating
   d. none of the above

4. A review of individual cases by a committee to make sure that services are medically necessary and to study how providers use medical care resources is called a(n)
   a. credentialing committee review.
   b. peer review committee evaluation.
   c. utilization review.
   d. audit committee review.

5. Which type of HMO model consists of physicians with separately owned practices who formally organize into a group but continue to practice in their own offices?
   a. Staff model
   b. Independent practice association
   c. Group model
   d. None of the above

6. Which individuals would not normally be eligible for Medicare?
   a. A 66-year-old retired woman
   b. A blind teenager
   c. A 23-year-old recipient of Temporary Assistance for Needy Families (TANF)
   d. A person on dialysis

7. Which expenses would be paid by Medicare Part B?
   a. Inpatient hospital charges
   b. Hospice services
   c. Home healthcare charges
   d. Physician's office visits

8. A type of insurance that protects workers from loss of wages after an industrial accident that happened on the job is called
   a. an individual policy.
   b. workers' compensation.
   c. unemployment insurance.
   d. disability insurance.

9. A payment method in which providers are paid for each individual enrolled in a plan, regardless of whether the person sees the provider that month, is called a _____ plan.
   a. capitation
   b. self-insured
   c. managed care
   d. fee-for-service

10. What should the medical assistant always verify prior to the patient's appointment?
    a. Eligibility
    b. Benefits and exclusions
    c. Effective date of insurance
    d. All of the above

WORKPLACE APPLICATIONS

1. After reading the following paragraph, fill the blanks in the statements.

   The medical assistant's tasks related to health insurance processing are initiated when the patient encounters the provider by appointment, as a walk-in, or in the emergency department or hospital. To complete insurance billing and coding properly, the medical assistant must perform the following tasks:

   a. Obtain information from the patient and/or the guarantor, including _____ and _____ data.

   b. Verify the patient's _____ for insurance payment with the insurance carrier or carriers, as well as insurance _____, exclusions, and whether _____ is required to refer patients to specialists or to perform certain services or procedures such as surgery or diagnostic tests.

   c. Obtain _____ for referral of the patient to a specialist or for special services or procedures that require advance permission.

2. Julia Berkley has just gotten a new insurance policy and is struggling with all of the terminology she is seeing in her policy. She would like you to explain just what *premium, deductible, coinsurance,* and *copayment* really mean.

   _____

   _____

   _____

   _____

INTERNET ACTIVITIES

1. Using online resources, research TRICARE and CHAMPVA. Create a poster presentation, a PowerPoint presentation, or write a paper summarizing your research. Include the following points in your project:
   a. Describe both TRICARE and CHAMPVA
   b. List who is eligible for TRICARE and who is eligible for CHAMPVA
   c. Explain what is involved when a provider participates in TRICARE

2. Using online resources, research Preferred Provider Organizations (PPO). Create a poster presentation, a PowerPoint presentation, or write a paper summarizing your research. Include the following points in your project:
   a. Description what a PPO is
   b. List the ranges for deductibles and coinsurance amounts found
   c. Explain how a PPO is different from an HMO
   d. Describe why a patient might want to have a PPO policy instead of traditional insurance

Diagnostic Coding Essentials

chapter
13

CAAHEP Competencies	Assessments
IX.C.2. Describe how to use the most current diagnostic coding classification system	Skills and Concepts – B. 1
IX.C.5. Define medical necessity as it applies to procedural and diagnostic coding	Skills and Concepts – A. 1
IX.P.2. Perform diagnostic coding	Procedure 13.1

ABHES Competencies	Assessments
1. General Orientation d. List the general responsibilities and skills of the medical assistant	Procedure 13.1

VOCABULARY REVIEW

Using the word pool on the right, find the correct word to match the definition. Write the word on the line after the definition.

Group A

1. The relative frequency of deaths in a specific population
   _____

2. Information about a patient's diagnosis or diagnoses that has been taken from the medical documentation _____

3. Any meeting between a patient and a healthcare provider
   _____

4. Radiology, pathology, and laboratory reports
   _____

5. The study of the causes or origin of diseases
   _____

6. The branch of medicine dealing with the incidence, distribution, and control of disease in a population _____

7. Determining the cause of a condition, illness, disease, injury, or congenital defect _____

8. Accepted healthcare services that are appropriate for the evaluation and treatment of a disease, condition, illness, or injury and are consistent with the applicable standard of care

   _____

9. Software that will apply diagnostic or procedure codes to medical conditions or procedures _____

10. To make repayment for an expense or a loss incurred
    _____

Word Pool
- diagnosis
- reimbursement
- mortality
- epidemiology
- encounter
- encoder
- diagnostic statement
- ancillary diagnostic services
- medically necessary
- etiology

Group B

1. A mental disorder in which the individual experiences a progressive loss of memory, personality alterations, confusion, loss of touch with reality, and stupor _____

2. Patient's chief complaint or statements about why the patient is seeking medical care _____

3. Developing slowly and lasting for a long time, generally 3 or more months _____

4. Suggest that it should not be used _____

5. An abnormal condition resulting from a previous disease _____

6. A document used to capture the services/procedures and diagnoses for a patient visit _____

7. The quality or state of being specific _____

8. A statement in the patient's own words that describes the reason for the visit _____

9. Abbreviations, punctuation, symbols, instructional notations, and related entities _____

10. Collecting important information from the health record _____

Word Pool
- chronic
- specificity
- conventions
- sequela
- dementia
- abstract
- encounter form
- chief complaint
- contraindicate
- subjective findings

Group C

1. Progressive loss of transparency of the lens of the eye _____

2. The signs and symptoms of a disease _____

3. The period from the last month of pregnancy to 5 months postpartum _____

4. Imminently threatening _____

5. First 6 weeks after delivery _____

6. The study of body tissues _____

7. Any measurable indicators found during the physical examination _____

8. Pregnancy _____

9. Advanced hypothyroidism in adulthood _____

Word Pool
- objective findings
- manifestation
- cataract
- myxedema
- impending
- histologic
- antepartum
- postpartum
- peripartum

ABBREVIATIONS

Write out what each of the following abbreviations stands for.

1. ICD-10-CM _____

2. CMS _____

3. WHO _____

4. EHR _____

5. HPI _____

6. H&P _____

7. CC _____

8. HIV _____

9. AIDS _____

10. DM _____

SKILLS AND CONCEPTS
Answer the following questions. Write your answer on the line or in the space provided.

A. What Is Diagnostic Coding?

1. Define *medically necessary* and explain how it applies to diagnostic coding. Give an example. _____

_____

_____

_____

_____

B. Getting to Know the ICD-10-CM

1. Fill in the blanks in the following statements with terms from the word bank to describe how to use the most current diagnostic coding classification system.

Word Bank:

code	coding guidelines	character
convention	diagnostic	diagnostic statements
essential modifier	exclusion	ICD-10-CM
main term	Tabular List	

a. Abstract the correct diagnosis from the _____ found in the patient health record.

b. Use the _____ to look up the diagnosis in the Alphabetic Index.

c. Review the _____ under the main term.

d. Choose the correct code based on the _____ statement.

e. Look up the code from the Alphabetic Index in the _____.

f. Check for any _____, _____, inclusion notes, _____ notes, or additional _____ symbol.

g. Assign the final _____ diagnosis code.

2. ICD-10-CM codes can have up to _____ characters. A(n) _____ "x" is used to fill in for positions that don't have characters.

3. What are the seventh characters used for encounter types and what do they indicate? _____

_____

_____

_____

4. Four basic forms of punctuation are used in the Tabular Index. List them and what they are used for.

5. Match the following terms.

_____ Main terms

_____ Nonessential modifiers

_____ Subterms

_____ Essential modifiers

a. These terms are indented under the main term; they change the description of the diagnosis in bold type
b. Appear in bold
c. Are found after the main term and are enclosed in parentheses
d. Indented under the essential modifier

6. Review the following diagnostic statements and determine the main term and essential modifier in the Alphabetic Index.

a. Morgan Smith had an acute myocardial infarction, commonly referred to as a *heart attack*.

Main Term: _____   Essential Modifier: _____

b. Georgia Summers went into anaphylactic shock after drinking milk.

Main Term: _____   Essential Modifier: _____

c. Roger Costen has benign essential hypertension.

Main Term: _____   Essential Modifier: _____

d. Raul Castro has been diagnosed with iron-deficiency anemia.

Main Term: _____   Essential Modifier: _____

e. Stephanie Thompson has a urinary tract infection.

Main Term: _____   Essential Modifier: _____

f. Mabel Johnson has rheumatoid arthritis.

Main Term: _____   Essential Modifier: _____

g. Amanda Smith was diagnosed with multiple sclerosis.

Main Term: _____   Essential Modifier: _____

h. Hudson Madison suffered a ruptured abdominal aneurysm.

Main Term: _____   Essential Modifier: _____

i. Don Julius died last week from congestive heart failure.

Main Term: _____   Essential Modifier: _____

j. Betty White has allergic gastroenteritis.

Main Term: _____   Essential Modifier: _____

C. Preparing for Diagnostic Coding

1. The SOAP notes system of documentation divides the information into what four areas?

a. _____

b. _____

c. _____

d. _____

2. To prepare for medical coding, the coder must analyze the patient's health record and _____ the diagnostic statement.

3. Information pertinent to code selection can be abstracted from a variety of medical documents. List the documents where the diagnostic statement may be found.

_____

_____

_____

_____

_____

4. The _____ is the provider's health history evaluation and physical assessment of the patient.

5. The _____ is a statement in the patient's own words that describes why the person is seeking medical attention.

6. The _____ is used for extracting procedure and diagnostic information for patients who underwent surgery.

D. Steps in ICD-10-CM Coding

1. Code the following diagnoses to the highest level of specificity using either the ICD-10-CM coding manual or the TruCode encoder.

    a. Kayla Swift was diagnosed with infectious mononucleosis. _____

    b. Gerald Weaver has osteoarthritis in his right shoulder region. _____

    c. Jeffrey Rush has a personal history of alcoholism. _____

    d. Barry White's alcoholism has caused cirrhosis of the liver without ascites. _____

    e. Frank Emmett had atherosclerosis of the extremities with gangrene. _____

    f. Ginger Chan experienced dermatitis from using facial cosmetics. _____

    g. The Lewises' first child was born with Down syndrome. _____

    h. Lee Anna has experienced painful menstruation during her last three cycles. _____

    i. Gary Stevens was diagnosed with cardiomegaly. _____

    j. Jerry Stein developed Kaposi's sarcoma in his lymph nodes during the final stages of AIDS. _____

    k. Terri Holden attempted suicide for the second time using a handful of lithium. _____

    l. Susan French was stung by a jellyfish while swimming off the coast of Mexico. _____

    m. Riley Brown has acute myocarditis. _____

    n. Ordell Thompson has acute esophagitis. _____

    o. Korney Ralphy was diagnosed with systemic lupus erythematosus. _____

    p. Marcia Radson had a skin condition known as *bullous pemphigoid*, in which blisters form in patches all over her skin. _____

    q. Osteomalacia caused by malnutrition made it impossible for Robbie Hernandez to walk. _____

    r. Henry Casper has oral leukoplakia, which may have been caused by smoking a pipe. _____

    s. Patricia Kielty has had uterine endometriosis for several years and may require a hysterectomy in the future. _____

    t. Robert Bauer dislocated his right shoulder while playing baseball; it was a closed anterior dislocation. _____

CERTIFICATION PREPARATION

Circle the correct answer.

1. Which term defines a malignant neoplasm as the absence of invasion of surrounding tissues?
    a. Primary
    b. Secondary
    c. In situ
    d. Benign

2. Which code will be used for a patient with a history of myocardial infarction with no symptoms but diagnosed by means of an electrocardiogram?
    a. I21
    b. I25.2
    c. I21.3
    d. None of the above

3. Which term applies to the period from the last month of pregnancy to 5 months after giving birth?
    a. Antepartum
    b. Childbirth
    c. Postpartum
    d. Peripartum

4. The abbreviation that is the equivalent of "unspecified" is _____.
    a. NEC
    b. NOS
    c. NOW
    d. NCL

5. If the provider has documented "rule out" in the diagnostic statement, the medical assistant must code what?
    a. Whatever phrase follows "rule out"
    b. Lab results
    c. Signs/symptoms
    d. None of the above

6. A diagnosis is
    a. a third party's opinion of a patient's illness.
    b. determining the cause of a patient's illness.
    c. the process of finding a patient's past medical history.
    d. both b and c.

7. Currently in the United States, the book used for coding diagnoses in physicians' offices is the
    a. Diagnostic Guide for Medicare and Medicaid Services.
    b. Diagnostic Codes for Third-Party Payers.
    c. International Classification of Disease, 10th Edition, Clinical Modifications.
    d. AMA Manual of Essential Diagnostic Codes, Volume 1.

8. Morbidity is the presence of illness or disease, whereas mortality is
    a. the determination of the nature of a disease.
    b. the deaths that occur from a disease.
    c. classification of a disease.
    d. All of the above.

9. In ICD-10, codes longer than three characters always have a decimal point between the
    a. fourth and fifth characters.
    b. fifth and sixth characters.
    c. third and fourth characters.
    d. sixth and seventh characters.

10. In the ICD-10-CM coding system, a lowercase "x" is used
    a. as a placeholder character within a code.
    b. to denote an obsolete code.
    c. as a cross-reference guide.
    d. to indicate the external causes of morbidity.

WORKPLACE APPLICATIONS

1. Dr. Martin has diagnosed Maude Crawford in the past with congestive heart failure and diabetes mellitus type 2 (insulin-dependent, long-term). She comes to the clinic today complaining of chest pain and has a fever of 101.8° F. Code all of these conditions. In which order should these codes be sequenced?

   a. _____

   b. _____

   c. _____

   d. _____

   e. _____

2. Dr. Perez has documented the following for Reuven Ahmad:

   CC: Shortness of breath, chest pain, nausea, and excessive sweating
   DX: 1. probable myocardial infarction, 2. rule out gastroesophageal reflux disease

   What are the correct diagnosis codes for this patient?

   Note to instructors: Remind students that codes may change with updated versions of ICD.

INTERNET ACTIVITIES

1. Using online resources, research diagnostic code encoders. Create a poster presentation, a PowerPoint presentation, or write a paper summarizing your research. Include the following points in your project:
   a. Describe the purpose of an encoder.
   b. List three reasons why a healthcare organization would want to use an encoder for diagnostic coding.
   c. Explain how using an encoder is different than using the ICD-10-CM coding manuals.

2. Using online resources, research the history and development of ICD. Create a poster presentation, a PowerPoint presentation, or write a paper summarizing your research. Include the following points in your project:
   a. Describe the ICD system.
   b. Explain how and why it was originally developed.
   c. List five reasons why ICD-10-CM was developed.

Procedure 13.1 Perform Coding Using the Current ICD-10-CM Manual or Encoder

Name _____ Date _____ Score _____

Task: To perform accurate diagnosis coding using the ICD-10-CM manual or encoder.

Scenario: The encounter form and progress notes both show that the diagnosis for this patient encounter is acute colitis. Locate the most accurate ICD-10-CM code for this diagnostic statement.

Equipment and Supplies:
- ICD-10-CM manual (current year) *or*
- Encoder software such as TruCode

Standard: Complete the procedure and all critical steps in _____ minutes with a minimum score of 85% within two attempts (*or as indicated by the instructor*).

Scoring: Divide the points earned by the total possible points. Failure to perform a critical step, indicated by an asterisk (*), results in grade no higher than an 84% (*or as indicated by the instructor*).

Time: Began_____ Ended_____ Total minutes: _____

Steps:	Point Value	Attempt 1	Attempt 2
Alphabetic Index			
1. Determine and locate the main terms from the diagnostic statement in the Alphabetic Index.	**10**		
2. Locate the essential modifiers listed under the main term in the Alphabetic Index.	**10**		
3. Review the conventions, punctuation, and notes in the Alphabetic Index.	**10**		
4. Choose a tentative code, codes, or code range from the Alphabetic Index that matches the diagnostic statement as closely as possible.	**15***		
Tabular List			
5. Look up the codes chosen from the Alphabetic Index in the Tabular List.	**10**		
6. Review notes, conventions, and the Official Coding Guidelines associated with the code and code description in the Tabular List. a. Review conventions and punctuation. b. Review instructional notations: • *Includes* and *excludes* notes • *Code first, code also,* and *code additional* notes • *and, or,* and *with* statements	**10**		
7. Verify the accuracy of the tentative code in the Tabular List. a. Make sure all elements of the diagnostic statement are included in the codes selected. b. Make sure the code description does not include anything not documented in the diagnostic statement.	**10**		
8. Extend the codes to their highest level of specificity (up to the 7th character, if required). If a 7th character is required, and no codes are present for the 4th, 5th, or 6th characters, it is appropriate to use the dummy placeholder X for these positions.	**10**		

9.	Assign the code (or codes) selected from the Tabular List as the appropriate code for the patient's condition by documenting it in the patient's health record.	**15***		
	Total Points	**100**		
Alternate - Using the TruCode Encoder Software				
1.	Type in the main term from the diagnostic statement in the search box.	**20**		
2.	The software will provide a list of main terms that could be related to the diagnosis typed in the search box. The coder chooses the main term that best represents the diagnostic statement.	**20**		
3.	Based on the main term chosen, a list of essential modifiers is presented. The coder must review the diagnostic statement to ensure that all documented modifying terms are identified. If the provider does not document a modifying term, the coder should not assume that a modifying term was implied.	**20**		
4.	To determine the most accurate code, follow these coding guidelines.	**20**		
5.	Once all the menus of essential modifiers have been presented, choose the most accurate and specific code based on the diagnostic statement.	**20***		
	Total Points	**100**		

CAAHEP Competencies	**Steps**
IX.P.2. Perform diagnostic coding	Entire procedure

Procedural Coding Essentials

CAAHEP	Assessments
IX.C.1. Describe how to use the most current procedural coding system	Skills and Concepts – G. 1
IX.C.3. Describe how to use the most current HCPCS level II coding system	Skills and Concepts – K. 1
IX.C.4.a. Discuss the effects of: upcoding	Skills and Concepts – E. 3
IX.C.4.b. Discuss the effects of: downcoding	Skills and Concepts – E. 4
IX.C.5. Define medical necessity as it applies to procedural and diagnostic coding	Skills and Concepts – E. 5
IX.P.1. Perform procedural coding	Procedure 14.1, 14.2
IX.A.1. Utilize tactful communication skills with medical providers to ensure accurate code selection	Procedure 14.3

VOCABULARY REVIEW

Using the word pool on the right, find the correct word to match the definition. Write the word on the line after the definition.

Group A

1. An online journal, supported by the AMA, that addresses subjects such as appealing insurance denials, validating coding to auditors, training staff members, and answering day-to-day coding questions _____

2. The use of a lower-level procedure code than is justified _____

3. Pertaining to, involving, or affecting two or both sides _____

4. The regular collection of data to assess whether the correct processes are being performed and desired results are being achieved _____

5. Additional medical documentation required to confirm the need for the use of unlisted, unusual, or newly adopted medical procedures code _____

6. Two-digit numeric codes that report or indicate specific criteria, specific condition, or special circumstance _____

7. The quality or state of being specific _____

8. The use of a higher-level procedure code than is supported in the documentation or medical necessity _____

9. In medical terms, a medical diagnosis or procedure named for the person who discovered it _____

10. The surgical removal of dead, damaged, or infected tissue to improve the function of healthy tissue _____

Word Pool
- performance measurement
- eponym
- specificity
- CPT Assistant
- débridement
- special report
- upcoding
- downcoding
- modifiers
- bilaterally

Group B

1. Concentrates on the chief complaint; it looks at the symptoms, severity, and duration of the problem _____

2. A list of questions related to each organ system designed to uncover potential disease processes _____

3. Includes chief complaint, extended history of present illness, problem-pertinent system review including a review of a limited number of additional systems and pertinent past, family, and/or social histories directly related to the patient's problems

   _____

4. The process of collecting pertinent medical information needed to assign the correct code _____

5. A statement in the patient's own words that describes the reason for the visit _____

6. The relative incidence of disease _____

7. Includes chief complaint, extended history of present illness, ROS that is directly related to the problem or problems identified in the history of the present illness, review of all additional body systems, in addition to complete past, family, and social histories

   _____

8. Special symbols used to provide additional information about specific codes _____

9. Includes symptoms, severity, and duration of the chief complaint, and a review of systems that relate to the chief complaint

   _____

10. Relates to the number of deaths from a given disease

   _____

Word Pool
- conventions
- abstract
- chief complaint
- review of systems
- problem-focused history
- expanded problem-focused history
- detailed history
- comprehensive history
- morbidity
- mortality

Group C

1. An extended examination is performed on the affected body area and related body areas or organ systems _____

2. Determine the amount of drug present _____

3. Limited to the affected body area or single system mentioned in the chief complaint _____

4. Each step of the procedure is listed separately _____

5. Medical services and procedures performed for the patient before, during, and after a surgical procedure _____

6. A complete multisystem examination is performed or a complete examination of a single organ system _____

7. Based on the type of drug found _____

8. In addition to the limited body area or system, related body areas or organ systems are examined _____

9. Includes services related to prepping the patient for the procedure, performing the procedure, and suturing to complete the procedure _____

10. A nursing healthcare professional who is certified to administer anesthesia _____

Word Pool
- problem-focused examination
- expanded problem-focused examination
- detailed examination
- comprehensive examination
- Certified Registered Nurse Anesthetist
- global services
- bundled code
- unbundled code
- qualitative
- quantitative

ABBREVIATIONS
Write out what each of the following abbreviations stands for.

1. CPT _____

2. HCPCS _____

3. AMA _____

4. EHR _____

5. H&P _____

6. E/M _____

7. POS _____

8. NP _____

9. EP _____

10. ROS _____

11. CRNA _____

12. NCCI _____

13. MRI _____

14. TURP _____

15. ASA _____

16. RVG _____

SKILLS AND CONCEPTS

Answer the following questions. Write your answer on the line or in the space provided.

A. Introduction to the CPT Manual

1. The CPT was developed and is maintained by the _____.

2. The CPT manual is updated every year on _____.

B. Code Categories in the CPT Manual

1. The CPT code is a five-digit code also known as a(n) _____ code.

2. Category II codes are primarily used for _____ and are optional.

3. Category _____ codes are for new experimental procedures or emerging technology.

C. Organization of the CPT Manual

1. The CPT coding manual organizes codes into the Alphabetic Index and the _____.

2. The six sections of the CPT manual include:

    a. _____

    b. _____

    c. _____

    d. _____

    e. _____

    f. _____

D. Unlisted Procedure or Service Code

1. When using an unlisted procedure code, a(n) _____ must be sent with the insurance claim.

E. General CPT Coding Guidelines

1. _____ are found at the beginning of each of the six sections of the CPT coding manual, and the medical assistant refers to them often when coding procedures.

2. Code additions that explain circumstances that alter a provided service or provide additional clarification or detail are called _____.

3. Define *upcoding* and discuss the effects. _____

_____

4. Define *downcoding* and discuss the effects. _____

_____

_____

5. Define *medical necessity* as it applies to procedural coding. _____

_____

_____

F. Documentation for CPT Coding

1. List the sources used for procedural coding. _____

_____

_____

G. Steps for Efficient CPT Coding

1. Describe how to use the most current procedural coding system. _____

_____

H. Using the Alphabetic Index

1. Describe the four primary classifications of main and modifying terms. _____

_____

2. Explain the difference between "see" and "see also". _____

_____

I. Using the Tabular List

1. Provide the full description for CPT code 47563
   47562   Laparoscopy, surgical; cholecystectomy
   47363   cholecystectomy with cholangiography

_____

_____

_____

J. CPT Coding Guidelines

1. _____ codes provide information on the healthcare facility where services were rendered.

2. Codes in which the components of a procedure are separated and reported separately are called _____ codes.

K. Common HCPCS Coding Guidelines

1. Describe how to use the most current HCPCS level II coding system. _____

   _____

   _____

   _____

   _____

   _____

   _____

   _____

CODING EXERCISES

Code the following procedures with modifiers if appropriate.

CPT Coding

1. Dr. Smith visits Eula Fairbanks, a patient with dementia, in the nursing home for less than 30 minutes and performs an expanded problem-focused examination with MDM of low complexity.

   _____

2. Jessica Lundy, a newborn, was admitted to the pediatric critical care unit after her birth, where Dr. Williams provided her initial care.

   _____

3. Dr. Partridge participated in a complex, lengthy telephone call lasting 30 minutes, regarding a patient who was scheduled for multiple surgeries.

   _____

4. When Terri Anderson was involved in a major car accident, the emergency department physician took a comprehensive history, performed a comprehensive examination, and then made highly complex decisions.

   _____

5. Tim Taylor is a new patient with a small cyst on his back. Dr. Young took a problem-focused history, performed a problem-focused examination, and then made straightforward medical decisions.

   _____

6. Jim Angelo, an established patient, saw the physician for a minor cut on the back of his hand. The physician spent approximately 10 minutes with Jim.

   _____

7. Because Lucille Westerman had multiple health problems, she was admitted for observation after a fainting spell. Dr. Adams took a comprehensive history and performed a comprehensive examination, then made medical decisions of high complexity regarding her care.

   _____

8. Dr. Wray saw Tammy Luttrell in the office as a new patient. He took a detailed history and performed a detailed examination, and then made medical decisions of low complexity.

   _____

9. Dr. Tompkins visited a new patient at her home and spent about 20 minutes diagnosing and treating her for the flu. A problem-focused history and examination with straightforward MDM was performed.

   _____

10. Vera Carpenter was admitted to the hospital for diabetes mellitus, congestive heart failure, and an infection of unknown origin. Dr. Antonetti performed a consultation by doing a detailed history and examination, and MDM of low complexity that took about an hour, including the time spent writing orders in her medical record.

    _____

11. Sylvia Julius, an established patient, saw Dr. Bridges for her allergies. The physician took a problem-focused history, performed a problem-focused examination, and made straightforward decisions regarding her care.

    _____

12. Anesthesia for vaginal delivery

    _____

13. Anesthesia was provided for a brain-dead patient whose organs were being harvested for donation.

    _____

14. Laparoscopic biopsy of the left ovary

    _____

15. Treatment of a clavicular fracture without manipulation

    _____

16. Removal of nasal polyp, right nostril

    _____

17. Tonsillectomy and adenoidectomy, younger than 12

   _____

18. Left ectopic pregnancy

   _____

19. Closed treatment of a coccygeal fracture

   _____

20. A radiologic examination of mastoids, two views

   _____

21. A chest x-ray examination, four views

   _____

22. Magnetic resonance imaging (MRI) of spinal canal

   _____

23. Computed tomography (CT) scan of abdomen with contrast medium

   _____

24. Outpatient kidney imaging with vascular flow

   _____

25. Creatine phosphokinase (CPK) total lab test

   _____

26. Electrolyte panel

   _____

27. Adrenocorticotropic hormone (ACTH) stimulation panel

   _____

28. Obstetric panel

   _____

29. Total protein urine test

   _____

30. Blood alcohol level

   _____

31. Acute hepatitis panel

   _____

32. Urine pregnancy test

   _____

33. Polio vaccine, intramuscular route

   _____

34. Human papillomavirus (HPV) vaccine, nine types, three-dose schedule, intramuscular route

   _____

35. Psychotherapy for crisis; first 60 minutes

   _____

HCPCS Coding

1. Standard wheelchair

   _____

2. Gradient compression stocking below-knee, 40-50 mm Hg each

   _____

3. Above-knee, short prosthesis, no knee joint (stubbies), with articulated ankle/foot, dynamically aligned, right leg

   _____

4. Disposable contact lens, per lens, one set

   _____

5. Ambulance waiting time, 1 hour

   _____

CERTIFICATION PREPARATION
Circle the correct answer.

1. The CPT coding manual is updated annually on
   a. January 1.
   b. December 1.
   c. October 1.
   d. June 1.

2. To find the most accurate code, coders use which progression?
   a. Categories, subcategories, sections, subsections
   b. Sections, subsections, categories, subcategories
   c. Sections, categories, subsections, subcategories
   d. Subsections, subcategories, sections, categories

3. The evaluation and management CPT codes are used for insurance reimbursement in the following healthcare settings *except*
   a. medical office.
   b. weight loss clinic.
   c. nursing home.
   d. hospital.

4. Which codes can be used to help measure performance and outcomes?
   a. Category I codes
   b. Category II codes
   c. Category III codes
   d. Both a and b

5. Which section uses the code range between 70000 and 79999?
   a. Anesthesia section
   b. Surgery section
   c. Radiology section
   d. Medicine section

6. When searching the alphabetic index, "humerus" is an example of a(n)
   a. procedure or service.
   b. organ or anatomic site.
   c. condition, illness, or injury.
   d. eponym, synonym, abbreviation, or acronym.

7. Which level of history includes a review of the systems that relate to the chief complaint?
   a. Problem-focused history
   b. Expanded problem-focused history
   c. Detailed history
   d. Comprehensive history

8. Which HCPCS codes range from A4000 to A8999?
   a. Ambulance transport
   b. Medical supplies
   c. Surgical supplies
   d. Both b and c

9. Which modifier indicates a professional component and is used when a separate technician performs the service but the provider reviews the report and makes a diagnosis?
   a. -50
   b. -62
   c. -26
   d. -RT, -LT

10. Which code is assigned to an urgent care facility as the place of service?
    a. 01
    b. 13
    c. 20
    d. 23

WORKPLACE APPLICATIONS

Identify all procedures that need to be coded for billing purposes in the following situations. Using the most current CPT manual or an encoder such as TruCode, determine the correct CPT codes.

1. Monique Jones is a new patient who saw Dr. Walden to report feeling tired all the time. She stated that she was exhausted even after a full 8 hours of sleep at night. Monique said that she did not have much of an appetite and that she had been eating mostly salads and chicken with a bowl of fruit as snacks. She is not overweight, and her blood pressure and other vital signs were normal. Dr. Walden decided to perform a complete blood count, an electrolyte panel, and a lipid panel. She also ordered a urinalysis, an iron-binding capacity, and a vitamin B12 test. The provider asked the patient if she had noticed any blood in her urine or stool, and she denied blood in the urine but did mention she had several episodes of diarrhea. Dr. Walden added an occult blood test and a stool culture to check for pathogens. The physician placed Monique on multivitamin therapy and told her to return in 1 week to discuss her laboratory test results. She spent approximately 30 minutes with Monique, taking a detailed history and performing a detailed examination, making low-complexity medical decisions. Monique scheduled her appointment for the following week and left the clinic.

2. **Diagnosis:** Left cheek laceration
   Procedure: Repair left cheek laceration

   After the patient was prepped with local anesthetic to the left cheek area, the cheek was dressed and draped with Betadine. The 1.7 cm chin laceration of the skin was closed with three interrupted 6-0 silk sutures. Gentamicin ointment was applied to the lacerations and a dressing was placed on the left cheek. The patient tolerated the procedure well.

What is the appropriate CPT code for this procedure? _____

Can a modifier be used for this procedure? _____ If so, what would be the most appropriate? _____

Because anesthesia was used, can an appropriate anesthesia CPT code be used? _____

3. **Diagnosis:** Abdominal pain
   Procedure: Esophagogastroduodenoscopy with biopsy

   The patient was premedicated and brought to the endoscopy suite where his throat was anesthetized with Cetacaine spray. He then was placed in the left lateral position and given 2 mg Versed, IV. An Olympus gastroscope was advanced into the esophagus, which was well visualized with no significant spasms. Subsequently the scope was advanced into the distal esophagus, which was essentially normal. Then the scope was advanced into the stomach, which showed evidence of erythema and gastritis. The pylorus was intubated and the duodenal bulb visualized. The duodenal bulb showed severe erythema suggestive of duodenitis. Biopsies of both the duodenum and the stomach were obtained. The scope was withdrawn. The patient tolerated the procedure well.

   In the Alphabetic Index, which main term should be used to look up the correct CPT code? _____

   What is the appropriate CPT code for this procedure? _____

   CPT code 43236 is a similar code with submucosal injection. Can this be used if the physician usually performs it, but forgot to document? _____

INTERNET ACTIVITIES

1. Using online resources, research job postings on the internet that relate to medical billing and coding. Review job qualifications and requirements to qualify for these positions. Create a poster presentation, a PowerPoint presentation, or write a paper summarizing your research. Include the following points in your project:
   a. List the qualifications and requirements for a position in the medical billing and coding field.
   b. Explain how a graduate from your program would meet the requirements.
   c. Explain what additional training would be beneficial for someone looking for a position in the medical billing and coding field.

2. Visit http://www.cms.gov/ and use the search words "CPT Coding" to explore the topics related to CPT and HCPCS coding. Create a poster presentation, a PowerPoint presentation, or write a paper summarizing your research. Include the following points in your project:
   a. Explain the differences between CPT coding and HCPCS coding.
   b. Explain when each would be used.
   c. Describe two things that you learned about CPT codes.
   d. Describe two things you learned about HCPCS codes.

Procedure 14.1   Perform Procedural Coding: Surgery

Name _____ Date _____ Score _____

Task: To use the steps for CPT procedural coding to find the most accurate and specific CPT surgery code.

Equipment and Supplies:
• CPT coding manual (current year) or TruCode encoder software
• Operative report (Figure 14.1)

Standard: Complete the procedure and all critical steps in _____ minutes with a minimum score of 85% within two attempts (*or as indicated by the instructor*).

Scoring: Divide the points earned by the total possible points. Failure to perform a critical step, indicated by an asterisk (*), results in grade no higher than an 84% (*or as indicated by the instructor*).

Time: Began_____ Ended_____ Total minutes: _____

Steps Using the CPT Coding Manual:	Point Value	Attempt 1	Attempt 2
1. Abstract the procedures and/or services from the procedural statement in the surgical report.	10		
2. Select the most appropriate main term to begin the search in the Alphabetic Index.	10		
3. Once the main term has been located in the Alphabetic Index, review and select the modifying term or terms if required. If the main term cannot be found in the Alphabetic Index, repeat steps 2 and 3 using a different main term, possibly based on the procedural statement.	10		
4. Once the CPT code or code range is identified in the Alphabetic Index, disregard any code or code range containing additional descriptions or modifying terms not found in the health record.	10		
5. Record the code or code ranges that best match the procedural statements in the surgical report.	10		
6. Turn to the Tabular List and find the first code or code range from your search of the Alphabetic Index. Compare the description of the code with the procedural statement in the surgical report. Verify that all or most of the health record documentation matches the code description and that there is no additional information in the code description that is not found in the documentation.	10		
7. Review the coding guidelines and notes for the section, subsection, and code to ensure that there are no contraindications to use of the code. Review the coding conventions and add-on codes, if any.	10		
8. Determine whether a modifier is needed.	10		
9. Determine whether a Special Report is required.	10		
10. Record the CPT code selected in the health record documentation next to the procedure or service performed and in the appropriate block of the insurance claim form.	10*		
Total Points	**100**		

Alternate Method Steps Using the TruCode Software			
1. Abstract the procedures and/or services from the procedural statement in the surgical report.	**20**		
2. Type the main term into the encoder Search box and select the CPT. Then click on Show All Results.	**20**		
3. If the main term cannot be found through the search, repeat steps 2 and 3 using a different main term based on the procedural statement.	**20**		
4. Choose the procedure description that is closest to the procedural statement in the surgical report.	**20***		
5. Record the CPT code that best matches the procedural statements in the surgical report in the patient's health record.	**20**		
Total Points	**100**		

Comments

CAAHEP Competencies	Step(s)
IX.P.1. Perform procedural coding	Entire procedure

Figure 14.1 Operative Report

Name _____ Date _____ Score _____

Operative Report

PATIENT NAME: Sonia Sample
ROOM NUMBER: 222 West
MR NUMBER: 12-34-56

DATE OF PROCEDURE: 04/22/00
PREOPERATIVE DIAGNOSIS: Acute cholecystitis
POSTOPERATIVE DIAGNOSIS: Acute cholecystitis
NAME OF PROCEDURE: 1. Laparoscopic cholecystectomy
                                            2. Intraoperative cystic duct cholangiogram
SURGEON: Claude St. John, M.D.
ASSISTANT: Mark Weiss, D.O.
ANESTHESIOLOGIST: Angela Adams, M.D.
ANESTHESIA: General

DESCRIPTION OF THE OPERATION:
    The patient was placed in the supine position under general anesthesia. The oral gastric tube was placed. The Foley catheter was placed. The patient received appropriate antibiotics. The abdomen was prepped with iodine and draped in the usual fashion. Using a midline subumbilical incision, we entered the subcutaneous fat to find the aponeurosis of the rectus abdominis. Two stay sutures were placed 0.5 cm from the midline bilaterally and we left on these sutures, creating an opening in the linea alba.
    Under direct vision, the catheter was placed. The Hasson cannula was placed in the abdominal cavity and all was normal except an acute necrotizing and probably gangrenous gallbladder. There were multiple omental adhesions. Three other trocars were placed in the right subcostal plane in the midline, midclavicular line, and midaxillary line using a #10, #5, and #5 mm trocar, respectively. The gallbladder was punctured and emptied of clear white bile indicating a hydrops of the gallbladder. It was grasped at its fundus and at Hartmann's pouch retracted cephalad and to the right, respectively. We found the cystic duct and the cystic artery after circumferential dissection and isolated the cystic duct completely.
    When we were sure that this structure was a deep cystic duct, the clip was placed at the most distal aspect to make an opening immediately proximally and we placed a Reddick cholangiocatheter into it via #14 gauge percutaneous catheter. The cholangiogram showed normal arborization of the liver radicals. Normal bifurcation of the common hepatic duct. Normal common hepatic duct. Long large cystic duct. The common bile duct had numerous stones within it. They could not be emptied from the common bile duct. There was good flow into the duodenum.
    The impression was choledocholithiasis. This was corroborated by the radiologist. The decision was made to prepare the patient most probably for endoscopic retrograde cholangiopancreatography postoperatively, and no further intervention of the common bile duct was done in this setting.
    The cholangiocatheter was removed. An attempt was made to milk the bile out, but no stones came out. Three clips were placed on the proximal aspect of the cystic duct and the duct was then cut distally. The artery was isolated and double clipped proximally and single clipped distally and cut in the intervening section. We then peeled the gallbladder off the gallbladder bed with some difficulty because of the intense edema and inflammation. It was then removed from the liver bed completely. Cautery, suctioning and irrigation were used copiously to create a bloodless field. A last check was made and there was no bleeding and no bile leaking. A #15 Jackson-Pratt type drain was placed into Morrison's pouch and brought out through the lateral most port. We then removed, with great difficulty, the gallbladder from the umbilicus. Because of its enormous size and a 3 cm stone within it that was very difficult to macerate, the opening of the umbilicus had to be enlarged.
    As this was done, we removed the gallbladder completely and sent it for pathologic section. Two separate figure-of-eight 0 PDS were used to close the abdominal fascia. The Jackson-Pratt drain was then sutured in place with 2.0 nylon. The skin was closed throughout with subcuticular 3-0 PDS after copious irrigation of the subcutaneous plane. Mastisol and Steri-Strips were placed on the wound. The patient remained stable although she did have bigeminy during surgery and was on a Lidocaine drip. She will be going to the intensive care unit but as she left, she was extubated in the recovery room and was fully alert. She is moving all limbs.
    I will discuss with the gastroenterologist postoperative endoscopic retrograde cholangiopancreatography.
    SPECIMEN: Gallbladder.

_____

Claude St. John, M.D.
CSJ/ld:
D: 04/22/00
T: 04/22/00 9:21 am
CC: Maria Acosta, M.D.

Procedure 14.2   Perform Procedural Coding: Office Visit and Immunizations

Name _____   Date _____   Score _____

Task: To use the steps for CPT Evaluation and Management coding and HCPCS coding to find the most accurate and specific CPT E/M and HCPCS codes using the coding manuals or the TruCode encoder.

Equipment and Supplies:
- CPT coding manual (current year)
- HCPCS coding manual (current year) or TruCode encoder software
- Progress note

Progress Note for Daniel Miller (DOB 03/12/2012): 04/08/20XX Daniel was seen today for a follow-up visit for his recent case of otitis media in the left ear. The ear infection has completely cleared, and he is now able to receive his hepatitis B vaccine. The office visit involved a problem-focused history, problem-focused examination, and medical decision-making of low complexity.

Standard: Complete the procedure and all critical steps in _____ minutes with a minimum score of 85% within two attempts (*or as indicated by the instructor*).

Scoring: Divide the points earned by the total possible points. Failure to perform a critical step, indicated by an asterisk (*), results in grade no higher than an 84% (*or as indicated by the instructor*).

Time: Began_____ Ended_____ Total minutes: _____

Steps Part A: CPT E/M Coding	Point Value	Attempt 1	Attempt 2
1. Determine the place of service from the progress note.	15		
2. Determine the patient's status.	15		
3. Identify the subsection, category, or subcategory of service in the E/M section.	10		
4. Determine the level of service: • Determine the extent of the history obtained. • Determine the extent of the examination performed. • Determine the complexity of medical decision-making. If necessary, compare the medical documentation against examples in Appendix C, Clinical Examples, of the CPT manual.	15		
5. Select the appropriate level of E/M service code, and document it in the patient's health record.	10		
Part B: HCPCS Coding with TruCode Encoder Software			
6. Review the provider documentation.	10		
7. Type the main term into the Search box of the encoder and choose the HCPCS Tabular code set for accurate coding. If no modifying term produces an appropriate code or code range, review the documentation again and choose another main term.	10		
8. Compare the description of the code with the medical documentation. Select the appropriate HCPCS immunization code, and document it in the patient's health record.	15		
Total Points	100		

Comments

CAAHEP Competencies	Step(s)
IX.P.1. Perform procedural coding	Entire procedure

Procedure 14.3   Working with Providers to Ensure Accurate Code Selection

Name _____ Date _____ Score _____

Task: Communicate respectfully and tactfully with medical providers to ensure accurate code selection.

Background: Using tactful communication skills means using good manners as you provide truthful sensitive information to another person, while considering the person's feelings. Tactful communication skills include verbal and nonverbal communication that shows respect, discretion, compassion, honesty, diplomacy, and courtesy. When you use tactful behaviors, you demonstrate professionalism and you preserve relationships by avoiding conflicts and finding common ground.

Many times, the medical coder is the expert on the accurate CPT and ICD code selections. The highest level of specificity must be used when coding so that appropriate reimbursement can occur. It is not uncommon for the medical coder to interact with providers and assist them in understanding the coding process. During these interactions, it is crucial that the medical coder provides the information in a professional, organized, and logical manner. Using tactful communication skills is critical to maintaining a healthy working relationship with the providers.

Scenario: You are a new medical coder for the medical practice. You have been on the job for 6 weeks and have been seeing a trend that charges are being downcoded. The required documentation is present in the health records, but the providers have been selecting less specific codes for the appointment types. Your goal today is to explain to the providers accurate code selection for the appointment types.

Directions: Using the scenario, role-play with two peers, who will play the providers. You need to discuss the importance of selecting the correct code for reimbursement. You need to demonstrate respect during the conversation and utilize tactful communication skills.

Standard: Complete the role-play in _____ minutes with a minimum score of 100% within two attempts (*or as indicated by the instructor*).

Scoring: Divide the points earned by the total possible points. Met competency: 100% (10 points). Not met competency: 0% (0 points).

Time: Began_____ Ended_____ Total minutes: _____

Affective Behavior	Directions: Check behaviors observed during the role-play.					
Respect	**Negative, Unprofessional Behaviors**	**Attempt**		**Positive, Professional Behaviors**	**Attempt**	
		1	**2**		**1**	**2**
	Rude, unkind, disrespectful, and/or impolite			Courteous and polite		
	Brief, abrupt; appeared rushed with the conversation			Took time with providers		
	Unconcerned with person's dignity			Maintained person's dignity		
	Poor eye contact			Proper eye contact		
	Negative nonverbal behaviors			Positive nonverbal behaviors		
	Other:			Other:		

Tactful	Improper and/or inappropriate			Proper and appropriate		
	Spoke and/or acted in a manner that was offensive to others; lacked compassion and/or courtesy			Spoke and acted without offending others; showed compassion and courtesy		
	Failed to be sensitive to others when explaining the situation			Explained the situation in a clear and diplomatic way		
	Failed to explain the downcoding issue and/or the importance of proper coding			Explained the issues with downcoding and the importance of accurate coding for reimbursement		
	Failed to offer a solution for the situation			Offered a solution for the situation		
	Failed to answer questions; or answers were inappropriate and/or inaccurate			Answered questions appropriately and accurately		
	Other:			Other:		

Grading		Point Value	Attempt 1	Attempt 2
Does not meet Expectation	• Response was disrespectful and/or not tactful. • Student demonstrated more than 2 negative, unprofessional behaviors during the interaction.	0		
Needs Improvement	• Response was disrespectful and/or not tactful. • Student demonstrated 1 or 2 negative, unprofessional behaviors during the interaction.	0		
Meets Expectation	• Response was respectful and tactful; no negative, unprofessional behaviors observed. • More practice is needed for behavior to appear natural and for student to appear comfortable and at ease.	10		
Occasionally Exceeds Expectation	• Response was respectful and tactful; no negative, unprofessional behaviors observed. • At times student appeared comfortable and at ease; but more practice is needed for behavior to become natural and consistent with a professional medical assistant.	10		
Always Exceeds Expectation	• Response was respectful and tactful; no negative, unprofessional behaviors observed. • Student's behaviors appeared natural and comfortable. Behaviors are consistent with a professional medical assistant.	10		

Comments

CAAHEP Competencies	Step(s)
IX.A.1. Utilize tactful communication skills with medical providers to ensure accurate code selection	Entire role-play

Medical Billing and Reimbursement Essentials

CAAHEP Competencies	Assessment
VII.C.5 Identify types of information contained in the patient's billing record	Skills and Concepts – B. 1
VII.C.6. Explain patient financial obligations for services rendered	Skills and Concepts – K. 1- 4
VII.A.1. Demonstrate professionalism when discussing patient's billing record	Procedure 15.2, 15.6
VII.A.2. Display sensitivity when requesting payment for services rendered	Procedure 15.2, 15.6
VII.P.4. Inform a patient of financial obligations for services rendered	Procedure 15.6
VIII.C.1.b. Identify: information required to file a third-party claim	Skills and Concepts – B. 1
VIII.C.1.c. Identify: the steps for filing a third-party claim	Skills and Concepts – F. 2, 3
VIII.C.2 Outline managed care requirements for patient referral	Skills and Concepts – C. 3
VIII.C.3.a. Describe processes for: verification of eligibility for services	Skills and Concepts – A. 3
VIII.C.3.b. Describe processes for: precertification	Skills and Concepts – C. 1, 2
VIII.C.3.c. Describe processes for: preauthorization	Skills and Concepts – C. 1, 2
VIII.C.4. Describe processes for: Define a patient-centered medical home (PCMH)	Skills and Concepts – G. 3
VIII.C.5. Differentiate between fraud and abuse	Skills and Concepts – D. 1
VIII.P.1. Interpret information on an insurance card	Procedure 15.1
VIII.P.2. Verify eligibility for services including documentation	Procedure 15.6
VIII.P.3. Obtain precertification or preauthorization including documentation	Procedure 15.3
VIII.P.4. Complete an insurance claim form	Procedure 15.4
VIII.A.1. Interact professionally with third party representatives	Procedure 15.2

CAAHEP Competencies	Assessment
VIII.A.2. Display tactful behavior when communicating with medical providers regarding third party requirements	Procedure 15.2
VIII.A.3. Show sensitivity when communicating with patients regarding third party requirements	Procedure 15.2
IX.P.3. Utilize medical necessity guidelines	Procedure 15.5
ABHES Competencies	**Assessment**
7. Administrative Procedures c. Perform billing and collection procedures	Procedure 15.1, 15.2, 15.3, 15.5, 15.6
7. Administrative Procedures d. Process insurance claims	Procedure 15.4

VOCABULARY REVIEW

Using the word pool on the right, find the correct word to match the definition. Write the word on the line after the definition.

Group A

1. The standard form used for all government and most commercial insurance companies _____

2. A process completed before claims submission in which claims are examined for accuracy and completeness _____

3. A document sent by the insurance company to the provider and the patient explaining the allowed charge amount, the amount reimbursed for services, and the patient's financial responsibilities _____

4. The process of determining if a procedure or service is covered by the insurance plan and what the reimbursement is for that procedure or service _____

5. The electronic transfer of data between two or more entities _____

6. Meeting the stipulated requirements to participate in the healthcare plan _____

7. When the provider is paid a set amount for each enrolled person assigned to him or her, per period of time, whether or not that person has received services _____

8. A set dollar amount that the patient must pay for each office visit _____

9. A form completed by the patient that authorizes the medical office to release medical records to the insurance company for health insurance reimbursement _____

10. An organization that accepts the claim data from the provider, reformats the data to meet the specifications outlined by the insurance plan, and submits the claim _____

Word Pool
- copayment
- explanation of benefits
- eligibility
- precertification
- CMS-1500 Health Insurance Claim Form
- claims clearinghouse
- release of information
- capitation
- electronic data interchange
- audit

Group B

1. Services or supplies that are used to treat the patient's diagnosis meet the accepted standard of medical practice _____

2. Agrees to accept the terms of the agreement with the insurance company, as well as accept what the plan states as an allowed amount for the services provided _____

3. When the insured and the insurance company share the cost of covered medical services after the deductible has been met _____

4. Knowingly and willfully attempting to execute a scheme to take from any healthcare benefit program _____

5. The person legally responsible for the entire bill _____

6. A set dollar amount that the policyholder is responsible for each year before the insurance company begins to reimburse the healthcare provider _____

7. To settle or determine judicially _____

8. Unintended action that directly or indirectly results in an overpayment to the healthcare provider _____

9. Software that finds common billing errors before the claim is sent to the insurance company _____

10. A number assigned by the Centers for Medicare and Medicaid Services (CMS) that classifies the healthcare provider by license and medical specialties _____

Word Pool
- adjudicate
- National Provider Identifier
- participating provider
- fraud
- abuse
- claim scrubber
- medical necessity
- deductible
- coinsurance
- guarantor

ABBREVIATIONS

Write out what each of the following abbreviations stands for.

1. EOB _____
2. CHAMPVA _____
3. CMPs _____
4. CPT _____
5. EIN _____
6. EMG _____
7. EPSDT _____
8. FECA _____
9. H&P _____
10. HCPCS _____
11. MCO _____
12. NPI _____

13. NUCC _____

14. PAR _____

15. PCMH _____

16. PCP _____

17. POS _____

18. RA _____

19. SSN _____

SKILLS AND CONCEPTS

Answer the following questions. Write your answer on the line or in the space provided.

A. Medical Billing Process

1. List four types of information collected when a patient calls to schedule an appointment.

   a. _____

   b. _____

   c. _____

   d. _____

2. At the time of the appointment, what two things are copied or scanned into the computer? _____

   _____

3. Describe how the patient's insurance eligibility is confirmed. _____

   _____

   _____

   _____

   _____

4. Referring to the information on the ID card, answer the following questions.

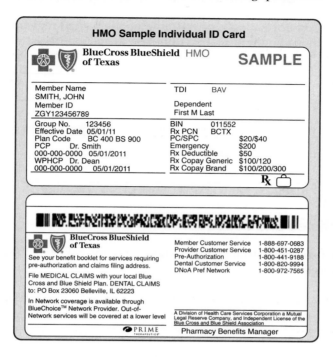

a. What is the member's name? _____

b. What is the member's ID number? _____

c. What is the group number? _____

d. Who is the member's primary care provider (PCP)? _____

e. What is the effective date of the plan? _____

f. What is the deductible for prescriptions (Rx)? _____

g. What is the copay for primary care (PC)? _____

h. What number should the patient call if he has a concern? _____

i. What number should you call if you need to get a preauthorization? _____

j. What number should a healthcare professional working with Dr. Smith call if there is a question about the coverage?

_____

B. Types of Information Found in the Patient's Billing Record

1. The patient's billing record information is often found on the patient registration form. Using Figure 15.1 in the textbook, list the billing information found on the patient registration form.

    _____

    _____

    _____

    _____

    _____

C. Managed Care Policies and Procedures

1. What items should the medical assistant gather when using the paper method to obtain a precertification for a service or procedure?

    _____

    _____

    _____

    _____

    _____

2. Describe the processes for precertification using the paper method. What does the medical assistant need to do?

    _____

    _____

    _____

    _____

    _____

3. Describe the managed care requirements for a patient referral. _____

    _____

    _____

    _____

    _____

    _____

D. Submitting Claims to Third-Party Payers

1. In your own words, identify the steps for filing a third-party claim. _____

_____

_____

_____

_____

_____

_____

_____

E. Generating Electronic Claims

1. Describe the electronic claim form. _____

_____

_____

_____

_____

2. Describe two ways electronic claims can be submitted. _____

_____

_____

_____

_____

3. Describe direct billing. _____

_____

_____

_____

_____

_____

_____

_____

4. Explain the role of a claims clearinghouse. _____

_____

_____

_____

_____

F. Completing the CMS-1500 Health Insurance Claim Form

1. The medical assistant obtained precertification for a procedure. After the procedure was completed, what are six items needed to complete the CMS-1500 Health Insurance Claim Form?

    a. _____

    b. _____

    c. _____

    d. _____

    e. _____

    f. _____

2. Name the three sections of the claim form.

    a. _____

    b. _____

    c. _____

3. Identify information required to file a third-party claim.

    a. What information must be included in Section 1 of the claim form? _____

    _____

    b. Name 13 pieces of information required in Section 2.

        1. _____

        2. _____

        3. _____

        4. _____

        5. _____

        6. _____

        7. _____

        8. _____

9. _____

10. _____

11. _____

12. _____

13. _____

c.   Name 19 pieces of information required in Section 3.

1. _____

2. _____

3. _____

4. _____

5. _____

6. _____

7. _____

8. _____

9. _____

10. _____

11. _____

12. _____

13. _____

14. _____

15. _____

16. _____

17. _____

18. _____

19. _____

G. Accurate Coding to Prevent Fraud and Abuse

1. Differentiate between fraud and abuse. _____

    _____

    _____

    _____

    _____

    _____

    _____

    _____

2. What are the possible consequences of coding fraud and abuse? _____

    _____

    _____

    _____

    _____

3. In your own words, define *patient-centered medical home* (PCMH). _____

    _____

    _____

    _____

    _____

    _____

    _____

    _____

H. Preventing Rejection of a Claim

1. What is the purpose of "claim scrubbers"? _____

    _____

    _____

    _____

I. Checking the Status of a Claim

1. Insurance companies will typically take _____ days to process insurance claims electronically.

2. What information is needed to verify the claim status with insurance company?_____

_____

_____

_____

_____

J. Explanation of Benefits

01/20/20XX

XYZ Insurance Company Explanation of Benefits

Walden-Martin Family Medical Clinic
1234 Anystreet
Anytown, AK 12345-1234

Patient Name	Treatment Dates	CPT Code	Charge Amount	Reason Code	Covered Amount	Deductible Amount	Co-Pay Amount	Paid At	Payment Amount
Yan, Tai	01/06/20XX	99205	132.28	03	125.00	0.00	0.00	80%	100.00
	01/06/20XX	82947	15.00		15.00	0.00	0.00	80%	12.00
	01/06/20XX	86580	11.34		11.34	0.00	0.00	80%	9.07
	Totals		158.62		151.34				121.07
Gomez, Pedro	01/07/20XX	99212	28.55		28.55	0.00	0.00	80%	22.84
	Totals		28.55		28.55				22.84
Green, Jana	01/04/20XX	99203	70.92	03	69.23	0.00	0.00	80%	55.38
	01/04/20XX	71020	40.97	03	34.95	0.00	0.00	80%	27.96
	Totals		111.89		104.18				83.34

Reason Code: 03 Allowed amount per insurance contract

Check No: 56390 $227.25

Using the explanation above answer the following questions:

1. For Tai Yan's office visit, 99205, there is a difference between the Charge Amount and Covered Amount. Based on the reason code supplied what will be done with the difference?

_____

_____

_____

_____

2.   How much is Tai Yan responsible for? _____

_____

3.   How much will be written off for Jana Green? _____

_____

4.   How much is Jana Green responsible for? _____

_____

5.   What is the covered amount services provided to Pedro Gomez? _____

_____

K. The Patient's Financial Responsibility

Calculating Coinsurance and Deductible
Use the following information as you answer the following questions.

```
Patient: Zach Green
Deductible: $750
Coinsurance: 80/20
Patient out-of-pocket expense maximum: $2000
```

1.   During Zach's first visit of the year, he incurred a $500 bill. Who pays this bill?_____

_____

_____

2.   During Zach's second visit of the year, he incurred a $450 bill. Describe how much is paid by Zach and the insurance carrier.

_____

_____

3.   Zach had surgery, which was his third claim of the year. He had a bill of $5000. Considering the prior visits, what is Zach's portion of this bill and what is the responsibility of the insurance carrier?

_____

_____

_____

_____

4.   How much is Zach responsible for so far this year considering his first three visits? _____

_____

_____

CERTIFICATION PREPARATION

Circle the correct answer.

1. To examine claims for accuracy and completeness before they are submitted is to _____ the claims.
   a. correct
   b. audit
   c. revise
   d. reject

2. Block 1 of the CMS-1500 form contains what information?
   a. Patient's name
   b. Insured's name
   c. Type of insurance coverage
   d. Carrier address

3. The patient's name is found in block
   a. 1.
   b. 2.
   c. 3.
   d. 4.

4. CPT codes are found in what block?
   a. 24a
   b. 24b
   c. 24d
   d. 24e

5. Claims with incorrect, missing, or insufficient data are called
   a. clean.
   b. dingy.
   c. incomplete.
   d. dirty.

6. Which is a common reason why insurance claims are rejected?
   a. When a procedure listed is not an insurance benefit
   b. Medical necessity
   c. Preauthorization not obtained
   d. All of the above

7. Which is a fixed amount per visit that is typically paid at the time of medical services?
   a. Copayment
   b. Deductible
   c. Coinsurance
   d. Both a and b

8. Patients sign a(n) _____ of benefits form so that the physician will receive payment for services directly.
   a. release
   b. assignment
   c. turning
   d. sending

9. Claims submitted to a _____ are forwarded to individual insurance carriers.
   a. direct biller
   b. third-party administrator
   c. clearinghouse
   d. post office

10. Electronic data interchange is
    a. transferring data back and forth between two or more entities.
    b. sending information to one insurance carrier.
    c. sending information to one clearinghouse for processing.
    d. None of the above

WORKPLACE APPLICATIONS

1. Sally is the only medical biller in her healthcare agency. One of the two providers orders and performs tests and procedures before getting the needed preauthorizations from the patients' insurance carriers. As a result, the insurance carriers are not covering the claims and the clinic has had to write off thousands of dollars. Discuss how Sally should deal with the situation.

   a. How might she display tactful behavior when communicating with the provider about the third-party requirements?

   _____

   _____

   _____

b. How would you deal with this situation if you were Sally?

_____

_____

_____

2. Christi Brown is meeting with you regarding the bill she received in the mail. When she called to make the appointment, she voiced her confusion about the bill, stating she thought her insurance covered everything. You check her record and see that she met her deductible and now needs to pay 20% of the billed amount. She owes $170. Explain what a deductible and coinsurance are.

_____

_____

_____

INTERNET ACTIVITIES

1. Using online resources, research your insurance carrier or an insurance carrier popular in your area. Research the appeal process for denied claims. Create a poster presentation, a PowerPoint presentation, or write a paper summarizing your research. Include the following points in your project:
    a. Who can start the appeal process?
    b. What steps are involved in the appeal process?
    c. What is the time frame for getting a response to the appeal?

2. Visit http://www.nucc.org and research the resources available on this website. Create a poster presentation, a PowerPoint presentation, or write a paper summarizing your research. Include the following points in your project:
    a. What resources are available for a medical biller on this website?
    b. List three that you think would be most helpful to a medical assistant who does medical billing.
    c. What information is available about the CMS-1500 claim form?
    d. Describe two things you learned from this website.

3. Using online resources, research the most common errors that occur when submitting claims. Create a poster presentation, a PowerPoint presentation, or write a paper summarizing your research. Include the following points in your project:
    a. What are the most common errors?
    b. How can these errors be prevented?
    c. What can a medical assistant do to prevent those errors?

Procedure 15.1   Interpret Information on an Insurance Card

Name _____ **Date** _____ **Score** _____

Task: To identify essential information on the health insurance identification (ID) card to confirm copayment obligations and obtain accurate health insurance information for claims submission.

Equipment and Supplies:
- Patient's health insurance ID, both sides (Figure 15.1)

Standard: Complete the procedure and all critical steps in _____ minutes with a minimum score of 85% within two attempts (*or as indicated by the instructor*).

Scoring: Divide the points earned by the total possible points. Failure to perform a critical step, indicated by an asterisk (*), results in grade no higher than an 84% (*or as indicated by the instructor*).

Time: Began_____ Ended_____ Total minutes: _____

Steps:	Point Value	Attempt 1	Attempt 2
1. Review the patient's health insurance ID card and identify the insured on the health insurance ID card. If the patient is different than the insured, then obtain the relationship with the insured and the insured's date of birth and gender.	20*		
2. Identify the insurance plan.	20		
3. Identify the insured's identification number and group number.	20		
4. Identify the patient's copayment, which is due before the appointment. Collect the correct amount.	20		
5. On the back of the health insurance ID card, ensure that a customer service phone number and medical claims address is present.	20		
Total Points	100		

Comments

CAAHEP Competencies	Step(s)
VIII.P.1. Interpret information on an insurance card	Entire procedure
ABHES Competencies	**Step(s)**
7. Administrative Procedures c. Perform billing and collection procedures	Entire procedure

Figure 15.1   Patient's Health Insurance ID Card

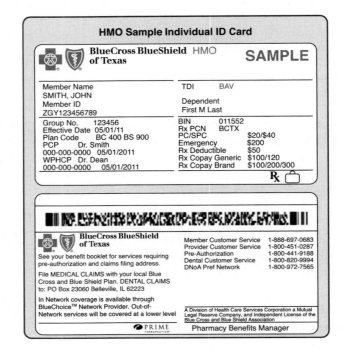

Procedure 15.2 Show Sensitivity when Communicating with Patients Regarding Third-Party Requirements

Name _____ Date _____ Score _____

Tasks: Communicate in an assertive, professional manner with a third-party representative. Demonstrate sensitivity through verbal and nonverbal communication when discussing third-party requirements with a patient. Display tactful behavior when communicating with a provider regarding third-party requirements.

Equipment and Supplies:
- Copy of patient's health insurance ID card
- Prescription for new medication

Scenario: Ken Thomas saw Jean Burke N.P. for his asthma today. He was prescribed a fluticasone inhaler 220 mcg and a refill on his albuterol inhaler. When Ken stops at the checkout desk to make a follow-up appointment, he looks concerned. You inquire how you can help him and he states that he is wondering if his new insurance will pick up the fluticasone inhaler. He further explains that he has used it in the past with great results, but he recently switched insurance plans and he is finding it doesn't have the same coverage as his old plan.

- *Role-play #1: You call the insurance company and discuss the coverage with the insurance carrier's representative. The representative tells you that the fluticasone inhaler is not covered for his condition. The representative gave you names of two other inhalers that would be covered.*
  When you ask if the drug would be covered through the exceptions process, the representative indicated that the provider must send a letter indicating the drug is appropriate for the patient's condition because all other drugs covered by the plan have not been effective or those drugs have side effects that may be harmful to the patient or the patient is allergic to the other drugs.
- *Role-play #2: You must explain to Ken, who is upset with his insurance coverage, that he would have to cover the $250 inhaler.*
- *Role-play #3: Ken explains he does not have $250 for the inhaler. He asks what else he should do. You mention the exception process and Ken requests the provider to send a letter. You need to role-play notifying the provider of the third-party requirements.*

Directions: Role-play the scenarios with a peer. The peer will play the part of the insurance representative, the patient, and the provider. You need to be professional and assertive with the insurance representative. When working with the patient, you need to show sensitivity. When communicating with the provider, you need to be professional and tactful.

Standard: Complete the procedure and all critical steps in _____ minutes with a minimum score of 85% within two attempts (*or as indicated by the instructor*).

Scoring: Divide the points earned by the total possible points. Failure to perform a critical step, indicated by an asterisk (*), results in grade no higher than an 84% (*or as indicated by the instructor*).

Time: Began_____ Ended_____ Total minutes: _____

Steps:	Point Value	Attempt 1	Attempt 2
1. Obtain a copy of the patient's health insurance ID card and the prescription for the new medication.	10		
2. Review the insurance card for coverage information and the phone number for providers.	20		

Scenario: Role-play #1 with a peer. The peer will be the insurance representative. 3. Contact the insurance company and clearly state the patient's information, the patient's question, and the new medication. Write down information provided by the representative.	**10***		
4. Demonstrate professionalism through verbal communication skills, by stating a respectful, assertive, clear, organized message while pronouncing medical terminology and medications correctly. *(Refer to the Checklist for Affective Behaviors - Respect)*	**10***		
Scenario: Role-play #2 with a peer. The peer will be the patient. 5. Explain to the patient the message from the insurance representative using language that can be understood by the patient. *(Refer to the Checklist for Affective Behaviors - Respect and Sensitivity)*	**10***		
6. Demonstrate sensitivity to the patient by paying attention to and responding appropriately to the patient's nonverbal body language and verbal message. *(Refer to the Checklist for Affective Behaviors - Respect and Sensitivity)*	**10***		
7. Demonstrate sensitivity to the patient by showing empathy and clarifying that you understand what the patient is stating. Give the patient your full attention during the conversation and reserve judgment. *(Refer to the Checklist for Affective Behaviors - Respect and Sensitivity)*	**10***		
8. Demonstrate sensitivity to the patient by using a pleasant, courteous tone of voice. Use body language to communicate respect (e.g., eye contact if culturally appropriate, keep arms uncrossed and relaxed). *(Refer to the Checklist for Affective Behaviors - Respect and Sensitivity)*	**10***		
Scenario: Role-play #3 with a peer. The peer will be the provider. 9. Demonstrate tactful behavior when explaining the third-party requirements to the provider. *(Refer to the Checklist for Affective Behaviors - Tactful)*	**10***		
Total Points	**100**		

Affective Behavior	***Directions:*** *Check behaviors observed during the role-play.*					
Respect	**Negative, Unprofessional Behaviors**	**Attempt**		**Positive, Professional Behaviors**	**Attempt**	
		1	**2**		**1**	**2**
	Rude, unkind			Courteous		
	Disrespectful, impolite			Polite		
	Unwelcoming			Welcoming		
	Brief, abrupt			Took time with patient		
	Unconcerned with person's dignity			Maintained person's dignity		
	Negative nonverbal behaviors			Positive nonverbal behaviors		
	Other:			Other:		

Sensitivity	Distracted; not focused on the other person			Focused full attention on the other person		
	Judgmental attitude; not accepting attitude			Nonjudgmental, accepting attitude		
	Failed to clarify what the person verbally or nonverbally communicated			Used summarizing or paraphrasing to clarify what the person verbally or nonverbally communicated		
	Failed to acknowledge what the person communicated			Acknowledged what the person communicated		
	Rude, discourteous			Pleasant and courteous		
	Disregarded the person's dignity and rights			Maintained the person's dignity and rights		
	Other:			Other:		
Tactful	Improper and/or inappropriate			Proper and appropriate		
	Spoke and/or acted in a manner that was offensive to others; lacked compassion and/or courtesy			Spoke and acted without offending others; showed compassion and courtesy		
	Failed to be sensitive to others when explaining the situation			Explained the situation in a clear and diplomatic way		
	Failed to answer questions; or answers were inappropriate and/or inaccurate			Answered questions appropriately and accurately		
	Other:			Other:		

Grading for Affective Behaviors		**Point Value**	**Attempt 1**	**Attempt 2**
Does not meet Expectation	• Response was insensitive and/or disrespectful. • Student demonstrated more than 2 negative, unprofessional behaviors during the interaction.	0		
Needs Improvement	• Response was insensitive and/or disrespectful. • Student demonstrated 1 or 2 negative, unprofessional behaviors during the interaction.	0		
Meets Expectation	• Response was sensitive and respectful; no negative, unprofessional behaviors observed. • More practice is needed for behavior to appear natural and for student to appear comfortable and at ease.	10		
Occasionally Exceeds Expectation	• Response was sensitive and respectful; no negative, unprofessional behaviors observed. • At times student appeared comfortable and at ease; but more practice is needed for behavior to become natural and consistent with a professional medical assistant.	10		

Always Exceeds Expectation	• Response was sensitive and respectful; no negative, unprofessional behaviors observed. • Student's behaviors appeared natural and comfortable. Behaviors are consistent with a professional medical assistant.	10		

Comments

CAAHEP Competencies	**Step(s)**
VII.P.4 Inform a patient of financial obligations for services rendered	5
VII.A.1. Interact professionally with third party representatives	3-4
VII.A.2 Display sensitivity when requesting payment for services rendered	7
VIII.A.2. Display tactful behavior when communicating with medical providers regarding third party requirements	9
VIII.A.3. Show sensitivity when communicating with patients regarding third party requirements	5-8
ABHES Competencies	**Step(s)**
7. Administrative Procedures c. Perform billing and collection procedures	Entire procedure

Procedure 15.3   Perform Precertification with Documentation

Name _____ Date _____ Score _____

Task: To obtain precertification from a patient's insurance carrier for requested services or procedures.

Equipment and Supplies:
- Paper method: Patient's health record, Prior Authorization (Precertification) Request form, copy of patient's health insurance ID card, a pen
- Electronic method: Electronic health record system such as SimChart for the Medical Office (SCMO)

Scenario: You are working with Dr. Julie Walden at Walden-Martin Family Medical Clinic. Erma Willis (DOB 12/09/19XX) was seen for excessive snoring and Dr. Walden ordered a sleep study. You need to complete a prior authorization/certification form for the sleep study, which will be conducted by Dr. Jim Sandman. You checked and there is a signed release of information form.

Insurance Information Aetna 1234 Insurance Way Anytown, AL 112345-1234 Member ID Number: EW8884910 Group Number: 66574W	**Clinic and Provider Information** Walden-Martin Family Medical Clinic 1234 Anystreet Anytown, AL 12345 Provider: Julie Walden, MD Fax: 123-123-5678 Phone: 123-123-1234 Provider Contact Name: (your name)
Service Information Place: Walden-Martin Family Medicine Clinic Service Requested: Sleep study Starting Service Date: 1 week from today Ending Service Date: 1 week from today Service Frequency: once ICD-10-CM code: R06.83 CPT code: 95807 Not related to an injury or workers' compensation	

Standard: Complete the procedure and all critical steps in _____ minutes with a minimum score of 85% within two attempts (*or as indicated by the instructor*).

Scoring: Divide the points earned by the total possible points. Failure to perform a critical step, indicated by an asterisk (*), results in grade no higher than an 84% (*or as indicated by the instructor*).

Time: Began _____ Ended _____ Total minutes: _____

Steps:	Point Value	Attempt 1	Attempt 2
1. For the paper method, gather the health record, precertification/prior authorization request form, copy of the health insurance ID card, and a pen. For the electronic method, access the Simulation Playground in SCMO.	20		
2. Using the health record, determine the service or procedure that requires precertification/preauthorization.	20*		

3.	For the paper method, complete the Precertification/Prior Authorization Request form. For the electronic method, click on the Form Repository icon in SCMO. Select Prior Authorization Request from the left INFO PANEL. Use the Patient Search button at the bottom to find the patient. Complete the remaining fields of the form.	**20**		
4.	Proofread the completed form and make any revisions needed.	**20**		
5.	Paper method: File the document in the health record after it is faxed to the insurance carrier. Electronic method: Print and fax or electronically send the form to the insurance company and save the form to the patient's record.	**20**		
	Total Points	**100**		

Comments

CAAHEP Competencies	Step(s)
VIII.P.2 Verify eligibility for services including documentation	Entire procedure
VIII.P.3. Obtain precertification or preauthorization including documentation	Entire procedure
ABHES Competencies	**Step(s)**
7. Administrative Procedures c. Perform billing and collection procedures	Entire procedure

Procedure 15.4   Complete an Insurance Claim Form

Name _____ Date _____ Score _____

Task: To accurately complete a CMS-1500 Health Insurance Claim Form.

Equipment and Supplies:
- Patient's health record
- Copy of patient's insurance ID card or cards
- Patient registration/intake form
- Encounter form
- Insurance claims processing guidelines (Table 15.2)
- Blank CMS-1500 Health Insurance Claim Form (Work Product 15.1)

Background: Almost all medical billing is done electronically through practice management billing software. The paper CMS-1500 Health Insurance Claim Form is provided only to help students practice and develop their medical billing skills.

Directions: Complete each block (as appropriate) of the CMS-1500 (see Table 15.2 for block descriptions).

Scenario: Mr. Walter Biller had an appointment with Dr. Walden on November 16, 20XX. He came in for an influenza vaccine, and while he was there, he wanted Dr. Walden to look at his ear because he was having problems hearing. His right ear canal was impacted with cerumen, which was irrigated and the cerumen was removed during the visit.

Patient Demographics	Clinic and Provider Information	
Walter B. Biller (patient and insured) 87 Willoughby Lane Anytown, AL 12345-1234 Phone: 123-237-3748 DOB: 01/04/1970 SSN: 285-77-7796 HIPAA form on file: Yes – March 19, 20XX Signature on file: Yes – March 19, 20XX	Walden-Martin Family Medical Clinic 1234 Anystreet Anytown, AL 12345 123-123-1234 POS – 04 Independent clinic Established patient of Julie Walden, MD Federal Tax ID# 651249831 NPI# 1467253823	
Insurance Information Account Number: 16611 Aetna Policy/ID Number: CH8327753 Group Number: 33347H		
Diagnosis:	**ICD-10-CM code**	
Impacted cerumen, right ear	H61.21	
Service	**CPT Code**	**Fee**
Est. minimal OV	99211	$24.00
Cerumen removal	69210	$46.00
Vaccine – Flu, 3 Y+	90658	$24.00
Preventive - Flu Administration	G0008	$7.00

Standard: Complete the procedure and all critical steps in _____ minutes with a minimum score of 85% within two attempts (*or as indicated by the instructor*).

Scoring: Divide the points earned by the total possible points. Failure to perform a critical step, indicated by an asterisk (*), results in grade no higher than an 84% (*or as indicated by the instructor*).

Time: Began_____ Ended_____ Total minutes: _____

Steps:	Point Value	Attempt 1	Attempt 2
1. Gather the documents required to complete the claim form.	**10**		
2. Complete the claim form using a pen. Use capital letters. Do not use punctuation (commas or dollar signs) unless indicated in the insurance manual or guidelines. Use a hyphen to hyphenate last names.	**10**		
3. Using the patient's health insurance ID card, determine the type of insurance, and the insurance ID number. Enter this information into block 1 and 1a.	**10**		
4. Using the ID card, the encounter form, and the registration/intake form, determine the patient's information and insured individual's information. Accurately complete blocks 2, 3, 5, 6, 9, and 10 a-c by entering in the patient's information. Complete 4, 7, and 11, a-d with the insured's information.	**10**		
5. Complete blocks 12 and 13 by entering "signature on file" and the date.	**10**		
6. Accurately enter the physician or supplier information by completing blocks 14 through 23. Use the eight (8)–digit format (MM/DD/YYYY) when needed.	**10**		
7. Using the encounter form, complete the appropriate blocks from 24A through 24H. **Note:** • Block 24A: Enter the dates of service, both From and To. For ambulatory services, enter the same date in the FROM and TO fields. Enter a date for each procedure, service, or supply in eight (8)–digit format (MM/DD/YYYY). • Block 24F: Enter the charge for the listed service or procedure. *Do not use commas when reporting dollar amounts.* The cents column is the small column to the right. • Block 24G: Enter the number of days or units. This block is usually used for multiple visits, units of supplies, anesthesia units or minutes, or oxygen volume. If only one service is performed, enter 1.0	**10**		
8. Complete blocks 24I through 27 by entering information on the provider's or healthcare facility where the service was provided and the patient's account number. Check the correct box to indicate acceptance of assignment of benefits.	**10**		
9. Complete blocks 28 through 29 by entering the total charges, total amount paid, and the total amount due. Complete blocks 31 through 33a by entering in the provider's and facility's information.	**10**		
10. Review the claim for accuracy and completeness before submitting. Correct any errors or missing information.	**10***		
Total Points	**100**		

Comments

CAAHEP Competencies	Step(s)
VIII.P.4. Complete an insurance claim form	Entire procedure
ABHES Competencies	**Step(s)**
7. Administrative Procedures d. Process insurance claims	Entire procedure

Work Product 15.1   CMS-1500 Health Insurance Claim Form

HEALTH INSURANCE CLAIM FORM

APPROVED BY NATIONAL UNIFORM CLAIM COMMITTEE (NUCC) 02/12

CARRIER

| | PICA | | | | | | | | PICA | | |

1. MEDICARE   MEDICAID   TRICARE   CHAMPVA   GROUP HEALTH PLAN   FECA BLK LUNG   OTHER
☐ (Medicare#) ☐ (Medicaid#) ☐ (ID#/DoD#) ☐ (Member ID#) ☐ (ID#) ☐ (ID#) ☐ (ID#)

1a. INSURED'S I.D. NUMBER   (For Program in Item 1)

2. PATIENT'S NAME (Last Name, First Name, Middle Initial)

3. PATIENT'S BIRTH DATE   MM   DD   YY   SEX   M ☐   F ☐

4. INSURED'S NAME (Last Name, First Name, Middle Initial)

5. PATIENT'S ADDRESS (No., Street)

6. PATIENT RELATIONSHIP TO INSURED   Self ☐   Spouse ☐   Child ☐   Other ☐

7. INSURED'S ADDRESS (No., Street)

CITY   STATE

8. RESERVED FOR NUCC USE

CITY   STATE

ZIP CODE   TELEPHONE (Include Area Code)   (   )

ZIP CODE   TELEPHONE (Include Area Code)   (   )

9. OTHER INSURED'S NAME (Last Name, First Name, Middle Initial)

10. IS PATIENT'S CONDITION RELATED TO:

11. INSURED'S POLICY GROUP OR FECA NUMBER

a. OTHER INSURED'S POLICY OR GROUP NUMBER

a. EMPLOYMENT? (Current or Previous)   ☐ YES   ☐ NO

a. INSURED'S DATE OF BIRTH   MM   DD   YY   SEX   M ☐   F ☐

b. RESERVED FOR NUCC USE

b. AUTO ACCIDENT?   ☐ YES   ☐ NO   PLACE (State)

b. OTHER CLAIM ID (Designated by NUCC)

c. RESERVED FOR NUCC USE

c. OTHER ACCIDENT?   ☐ YES   ☐ NO

c. INSURANCE PLAN NAME OR PROGRAM NAME

d. INSURANCE PLAN NAME OR PROGRAM NAME

10d. CLAIM CODES (Designated by NUCC)

d. IS THERE ANOTHER HEALTH BENEFIT PLAN?   ☐ YES   ☐ NO   *If yes*, complete items 9, 9a, and 9d.

PATIENT AND INSURED INFORMATION

READ BACK OF FORM BEFORE COMPLETING & SIGNING THIS FORM.

12. PATIENT'S OR AUTHORIZED PERSON'S SIGNATURE I authorize the release of any medical or other information necessary to process this claim. I also request payment of government benefits either to myself or to the party who accepts assignment below.

SIGNED _____   DATE _____

13. INSURED'S OR AUTHORIZED PERSON'S SIGNATURE I authorize payment of medical benefits to the undersigned physician or supplier for services described below.

SIGNED _____

14. DATE OF CURRENT ILLNESS, INJURY, or PREGNANCY (LMP)   MM   DD   YY   QUAL.

15. OTHER DATE   QUAL.   MM   DD   YY

16. DATES PATIENT UNABLE TO WORK IN CURRENT OCCUPATION   FROM MM DD YY   TO MM DD YY

17. NAME OF REFERRING PROVIDER OR OTHER SOURCE   17a.   17b. NPI

18. HOSPITALIZATION DATES RELATED TO CURRENT SERVICES   FROM MM DD YY   TO MM DD YY

19. ADDITIONAL CLAIM INFORMATION (Designated by NUCC)

20. OUTSIDE LAB?   ☐ YES   ☐ NO $ CHARGES

21. DIAGNOSIS OR NATURE OF ILLNESS OR INJURY Relate A-L to service line below (24E)   ICD Ind. |
A. |____   B. |____   C. |____   D. |____
E. |____   F. |____   G. |____   H. |____
I. |____   J. |____   K. |____   L. |____

22. RESUBMISSION CODE   ORIGINAL REF. NO.

23. PRIOR AUTHORIZATION NUMBER

24. A. DATE(S) OF SERVICE						B. PLACE OF SERVICE	C. EMG	D. PROCEDURES, SERVICES, OR SUPPLIES (Explain Unusual Circumstances)		E. DIAGNOSIS POINTER	F. $ CHARGES	G. DAYS OR UNITS	H. EPSDT Family Plan	I. ID. QUAL.	J. RENDERING PROVIDER ID. #
From			To					CPT/HCPCS	MODIFIER						
MM	DD	YY	MM	DD	YY										
1														NPI	
2														NPI	
3														NPI	
4														NPI	
5														NPI	
6														NPI	

25. FEDERAL TAX I.D. NUMBER   SSN ☐ EIN ☐

26. PATIENT'S ACCOUNT NO.

27. ACCEPT ASSIGNMENT? (For govt. claims, see back)   ☐ YES   ☐ NO

28. TOTAL CHARGE $

29. AMOUNT PAID $

30. Rsvd for NUCC Use

31. SIGNATURE OF PHYSICIAN OR SUPPLIER INCLUDING DEGREES OR CREDENTIALS (I certify that the statements on the reverse apply to this bill and are made a part thereof.)

SIGNED _____   DATE _____

32. SERVICE FACILITY LOCATION INFORMATION

a. NPI   b.

33. BILLING PROVIDER INFO & PH # (   )

a. NPI   b.

PHYSICIAN OR SUPPLIER INFORMATION

NUCC Instruction Manual available at: www.nucc.org   ***PLEASE PRINT OR TYPE***   APPROVED OMB-0938-1197 FORM 1500 (02-12)

Procedure 15.5   Utilize Medical Necessity Guidelines: Respond to a "Medical Necessity Denied" Claim

Name _____ Date _____ Score _____

Task: To resolve the insurance company's denial of a claim for medical necessity by completing an accurate claim.

Equipment and Supplies:
- Paper method: Patient's health record, copy of patient's insurance ID card or cards, patient registration form, encounter form, blank CMS-1500 Health Insurance Claim Form (Work Product 15-2), and a pen
- Electronic method: SimChart for the Medical Office
- Insurance denial letter or scenario (see below)

Scenario: You are working at Walden-Martin Family Medical Clinic, 1234 Anystreet, Anytown, AL 12345 (phone: 123-123-1234). You receive a letter indicating that Medicare has denied the following claim for not being medically necessary:

Patient: Norma B. Washington	DOB: 08/07/1944	Policy/ID Number: 847744144A
Date of Service: 06/13/20XX	ICD: G43.101 (Migraine)	CPT: J3420 (B-12 injection)
Provider: Julie Walden MD		

You did some research and the information above was the only information sent to Medicare for that encounter. The following information was the correct information for the encounter:

Patient: Norma B. Washington	DOB: 08/01/1944	Date of Service: 06/15/20XX
ICD: G43.101 (Migraine)	CPT: J1885 (Toradol 15 mg—$15.50) and 90772 (Injection, Ther/Proph/Diag—$25.00)	
ICD: D51.0 (Vitamin B_{12} deficiency anemia) CPT: J3420 (B_{12} injection—$24.00) and 90772 (Injection, Ther/Proph/Diag—$25.00)		
To be billed to: Medicare, 1234 Insurance Road, Anytown, AL 12345-1234		

Standard: Complete the procedure and all critical steps in _____ minutes with a minimum score of 85% within two attempts (*or as indicated by the instructor*).

Scoring: Divide the points earned by the total possible points. Failure to perform a critical step, indicated by an asterisk (*), results in grade no higher than an 84% (*or as indicated by the instructor*).

Time: Began_____ Ended_____ Total minutes: _____

Steps:	Point Value	Attempt 1	Attempt 2
1. Review the insurance denial letter (scenario) carefully. Compare the patient's information from the denial letter to the health record, claim, and encounter form. Look for errors in the patient's name and date of birth.	20*		
2. Compare the insurance denial letter (scenario) to the health record, claim, and encounter form. Look for errors in the date of service, the diagnosis, and the procedure codes. The procedure must be medically necessary for the diagnosis indicated.	20*		

3.	Complete a claim (either CMS-1500 or an electronic claim using SimChart) by entering in the information about the carrier, patient, and insured.	**20**		
4.	Enter the information regarding the physician, procedures, and diagnosis. Make sure to include all of the information from the encounter.	**20**		
5.	Proofread the claim form for accuracy before submitting the claim.	**20**		
	Total Points	**100**		

Comments

CAAHEP Competencies	Step(s)
IX.P.3. Utilize medical necessity guidelines	Entire procedure
ABHES Competencies	**Step(s)**
7. Administrative Procedures c. Perform billing and collection procedures	Entire procedure

Work Product 15.2 CMS-1500 Health Insurance Claim Form

HEALTH INSURANCE CLAIM FORM

APPROVED BY NATIONAL UNIFORM CLAIM COMMITTEE (NUCC) 02/12

CARRIER

| | | PICA | | | | | | | | PICA | | |

1. MEDICARE ☐ (Medicare#) MEDICAID ☐ (Medicaid#) TRICARE ☐ (ID#/DoD#) CHAMPVA ☐ (Member ID#) GROUP HEALTH PLAN ☐ (ID#) FECA BLK LUNG ☐ (ID#) OTHER ☐ (ID#)

1a. INSURED'S I.D. NUMBER (For Program in Item 1)

2. PATIENT'S NAME (Last Name, First Name, Middle Initial)

3. PATIENT'S BIRTH DATE MM DD YY   SEX M ☐ F ☐

4. INSURED'S NAME (Last Name, First Name, Middle Initial)

5. PATIENT'S ADDRESS (No., Street)

6. PATIENT RELATIONSHIP TO INSURED
Self ☐ Spouse ☐ Child ☐ Other ☐

7. INSURED'S ADDRESS (No., Street)

CITY   STATE

8. RESERVED FOR NUCC USE

CITY   STATE

ZIP CODE   TELEPHONE (Include Area Code) (   )

ZIP CODE   TELEPHONE (Include Area Code) (   )

9. OTHER INSURED'S NAME (Last Name, First Name, Middle Initial)

10. IS PATIENT'S CONDITION RELATED TO:

11. INSURED'S POLICY GROUP OR FECA NUMBER

a. OTHER INSURED'S POLICY OR GROUP NUMBER

a. EMPLOYMENT? (Current or Previous) YES ☐ NO ☐

a. INSURED'S DATE OF BIRTH MM DD YY   SEX M ☐ F ☐

b. RESERVED FOR NUCC USE

b. AUTO ACCIDENT? YES ☐ NO ☐ PLACE (State) ____

b. OTHER CLAIM ID (Designated by NUCC)

c. RESERVED FOR NUCC USE

c. OTHER ACCIDENT? YES ☐ NO ☐

c. INSURANCE PLAN NAME OR PROGRAM NAME

d. INSURANCE PLAN NAME OR PROGRAM NAME

10d. CLAIM CODES (Designated by NUCC)

d. IS THERE ANOTHER HEALTH BENEFIT PLAN? YES ☐ NO ☐ *If yes*, complete items 9, 9a, and 9d.

READ BACK OF FORM BEFORE COMPLETING & SIGNING THIS FORM.

12. PATIENT'S OR AUTHORIZED PERSON'S SIGNATURE I authorize the release of any medical or other information necessary to process this claim. I also request payment of government benefits either to myself or to the party who accepts assignment below.

SIGNED _____ DATE _____

13. INSURED'S OR AUTHORIZED PERSON'S SIGNATURE I authorize payment of medical benefits to the undersigned physician or supplier for services described below.

SIGNED _____

14. DATE OF CURRENT ILLNESS, INJURY, or PREGNANCY (LMP) MM DD YY QUAL.

15. OTHER DATE QUAL. MM DD YY

16. DATES PATIENT UNABLE TO WORK IN CURRENT OCCUPATION FROM MM DD YY TO MM DD YY

17. NAME OF REFERRING PROVIDER OR OTHER SOURCE

17a. ____ 17b. NPI ____

18. HOSPITALIZATION DATES RELATED TO CURRENT SERVICES FROM MM DD YY TO MM DD YY

19. ADDITIONAL CLAIM INFORMATION (Designated by NUCC)

20. OUTSIDE LAB? YES ☐ NO ☐ $ CHARGES

21. DIAGNOSIS OR NATURE OF ILLNESS OR INJURY Relate A-L to service line below (24E) ICD Ind. ____

A. ____ B. ____ C. ____ D. ____
E. ____ F. ____ G. ____ H. ____
I. ____ J. ____ K. ____ L. ____

22. RESUBMISSION CODE ____ ORIGINAL REF. NO. ____

23. PRIOR AUTHORIZATION NUMBER

24. A. DATE(S) OF SERVICE						B. PLACE OF SERVICE	C. EMG	D. PROCEDURES, SERVICES, OR SUPPLIES (Explain Unusual Circumstances) CPT/HCPCS MODIFIER	E. DIAGNOSIS POINTER	F. $ CHARGES	G. DAYS OR UNITS	H. EPSDT Family Plan	I. ID. QUAL.	J. RENDERING PROVIDER ID. #
From MM	DD	YY	To MM	DD	YY									
1													NPI	
2													NPI	
3													NPI	
4													NPI	
5													NPI	
6													NPI	

25. FEDERAL TAX I.D. NUMBER SSN ☐ EIN ☐

26. PATIENT'S ACCOUNT NO.

27. ACCEPT ASSIGNMENT? (For govt. claims, see back) YES ☐ NO ☐

28. TOTAL CHARGE $

29. AMOUNT PAID $

30. Rsvd for NUCC Use

31. SIGNATURE OF PHYSICIAN OR SUPPLIER INCLUDING DEGREES OR CREDENTIALS (I certify that the statements on the reverse apply to this bill and are made a part thereof.)

SIGNED _____ DATE _____

32. SERVICE FACILITY LOCATION INFORMATION

a. NPI   b.

33. BILLING PROVIDER INFO & PH # (   )

a. NPI   b.

PHYSICIAN OR SUPPLIER INFORMATION

PATIENT AND INSURED INFORMATION

NUCC Instruction Manual available at: www.nucc.org   **PLEASE PRINT OR TYPE**   APPROVED OMB-0938-1197 FORM 1500 (02-12)

Procedure 15.6 Inform a Patient of Financial Obligations for Services Rendered

Name _____ Date _____ Score _____

Tasks: Inform patient of his/her financial obligation and to demonstrate professionalism and sensitivity when discussing the patient's billing record.

Equipment and Supplies:
- Facility's payment policy
- Copy of patient's insurance card (or see information in the scenario)
- Patient's account record (or see information in the scenario)

Obtaining Payments – WMFM Clinic Policy

• For patients with copayments, all copayments must be collected before the patient leaves the clinic.
• For patients with balances overdue:
  • Patients must pay 20% of the balance before an appointment can be scheduled.
  • Or patients can establish a 6- or 12-month interest-free payment plan, making the first payment before the next visit can be scheduled.
• Payments can be made using VISA, Mastercard, personal check (no starter checks accepted), or cash. Payments can also be made online.

Scenario #1: Mr. Walter Biller arrives for his appointment. You need to check his eligibility for services and also if he has a copayment for today's visit. His insurance information: account number: 16611; Aetna, Policy/ID Number: CH8327753; and Group Number: 33347H

Scenario #2: Christi Brown is meeting with you regarding the bill she received in the mail. She called to make the appointment and she voiced her confusion about the bill. She stated that she thought her insurance covered everything. You check her record and see that she met her deductible and now needs to pay 20% of the billed amount. She owes $170.

Directions: Role-play the scenarios with a peer. The peer will be the insurance representative in Scenario #1, and then the patient in Scenario #2. You will be the medical assistant. You need to be professional and sensitive when working with patients regarding payments. You also need to follow the clinic's policy.

Standard: Complete the procedure and all critical steps in _____ minutes with a minimum score of 85% within two attempts (*or as indicated by the instructor*).

Scoring: Divide the points earned by the total possible points. Failure to perform a critical step, indicated by an asterisk (*), results in grade no higher than an 84% (*or as indicated by the instructor*).

Time: Began_____ Ended_____ Total minutes: _____

Steps:	Point Value	Attempt 1	Attempt 2
Scenario #1: Role-play with a peer who will be the insurance representative. 1. Contact the patient's insurance company and verify the patient's eligibility for services. Provide the representative with the patient's information. Find out if the patient has a copayment for today's visit. Document the information obtained.	20*		

Scenario #1 update: You need to provide the patient with the information that he owes a copayment for today's visit. 2. Inform the patient of his financial obligation of the copayment.	**10***		
Scenario update: He states he does not have the cash with him. 3. Inform the patient of the clinic policy regarding copayments and how the payment can be made.	**10**		
4. Demonstrate sensitivity and professionalism when discussing the payment. *(Refer to the Checklist for Affective Behaviors - Respect and Sensitivity)*	**15***		
Scenario #2: Role-play with a peer who will be the patient. 5. Determine the amount the patient owes by reviewing the patient's account record. Inform the patient the amount owed for services rendered.	**15***		
Scenario update: Patient stated she does not have the money to pay the entire bill today. 6. Inform the patient of the clinic policy regarding overdue accounts and scheduling appointments. Provide the patient with options for the overdue amount based on the clinic policy.	**15**		
7. Demonstrate sensitivity and professionalism when discussing the payment and the situation. *(Refer to the Checklist for Affective Behaviors - Respect and Sensitivity)*	**15***		
Total Points	**100**		

Affective Behavior	***Directions:*** *Check behaviors observed during the role-play.*					
	Negative, Unprofessional Behaviors	**Attempt**		**Positive, Professional Behaviors**	**Attempt**	
Respect		**1**	**2**		**1**	**2**
	Rude, unkind			Courteous, professional; assertive as required		
	Disrespectful, impolite			Polite, patient		
	Negative verbal communication (e.g., harsh words, disrespectful comments)			Professional verbal communication (e.g., respectful and understanding communication)		
	Brief, abrupt			Took time with person		
	Unconcerned with person's dignity			Maintained person's dignity		
	Negative nonverbal behaviors			Positive nonverbal behaviors		
	Other:			Other:		

Sensitivity	Distracted; not focused on the other person			Focused full attention on the other person		
	Judgmental attitude; not accepting attitude			Nonjudgmental, accepting attitude		
	Failed to clarify what the person verbally or nonverbally communicated			Used summarizing or paraphrasing to clarify what the person verbally or nonverbally communicated		
	Failed to acknowledge what the person communicated			Acknowledged what the person communicated		
	Rude, discourteous			Pleasant and courteous		
	Disregarded the person's dignity and rights			Maintained the person's dignity and rights		
	Other:			Other:		

Grading for Affective Behaviors		Point Value	Attempt 1	Attempt 2
Does not meet Expectation	• Response was insensitive and/or disrespectful. • Student demonstrated more than 2 negative, unprofessional behaviors during the interaction.	0		
Needs Improvement	• Response was insensitive and/or disrespectful. • Student demonstrated 1 or 2 negative, unprofessional behaviors during the interaction.	0		
Meets Expectation	• Response was sensitive and respectful; no negative, unprofessional behaviors observed. • More practice is needed for behavior to appear natural and for student to appear comfortable and at ease.	15		
Occasionally Exceeds Expectation	• Response was sensitive and respectful; no negative, unprofessional behaviors observed. • At times student appeared comfortable and at ease; but more practice is needed for behavior to become natural and consistent with a professional medical assistant.	15		
Always Exceeds Expectation	• Response was sensitive and respectful; no negative, unprofessional behaviors observed. • Student's behaviors appeared natural and comfortable. Behaviors are consistent with a professional medical assistant.	15		

Comments

CAAHEP Competencies	Step(s)
VII.A.1. Demonstrate professionalism when discussing patient's billing record	4, 7
VII.A.2. Display sensitivity when requesting payment for services rendered	4, 7
VIII.P.2. Verify eligibility for services including documentation	1
VII.P.4. Inform a patient of financial obligations for services rendered	2, 5
ABHES Competencies	**Step(s)**
7. Administrative Procedures c. Perform billing and collection procedures	Entire procedure

Patient Accounts and Practice Management

chapter

16

CAAHEP Competencies	Assessment
II.C.1. Demonstrate knowledge of basic math computations	Skills and Concepts – D. 13
VII.C.1.a. Define the following bookkeeping terms: charges	Skills and Concepts – B. 2.4
VII.C.1.b. Define the following bookkeeping terms: payments	Skills and Concepts – B. 2.5
VII.C.1.c. Define the following bookkeeping terms: accounts receivable	Skills and Concepts – B. 2.2
VII.C.1.d. Define the following bookkeeping terms: accounts payable	Skills and Concepts – B. 2.1
VII.C.1.e. Define the following bookkeeping terms: adjustments	Skills and Concepts – B. 2.3
VII.C.2. Describe banking procedures as related to the ambulatory care setting	Skills and Concepts – D. 1-5
VII.C.3.a. Identify precautions for accepting the following types of payments: cash	Skills and Concepts – D. 7
VII.C.3.b. Identify precautions for accepting the following types of payments: check	Skills and Concepts – D. 6
VII.C.3.c. Identify precautions for accepting the following types of payments: credit card	Skills and Concepts – D. 8
VII.C.3.d. Identify precautions for accepting the following types of payments: debit card	Skills and Concepts – D. 8
VII.C.4.a. Describe types of adjustments made to patient accounts including: non-sufficient funds (NSF) check	Skills and Concepts – C. 6
VII.C.4.b. Describe types of adjustments made to patient accounts including: collection agency transaction	Skills and Concepts – C. 4
VII.C.4.c. Describe types of adjustments made to patient accounts including: credit balance	Skills and Concepts – C. 5
VII.C.4.d. Describe types of adjustments made to patient accounts including: third party	Skills and Concepts – C. 3

CAAHEP Competencies	Assessment
VII.C.5. Identify types of information contained in the patient's billing record	Skills and Concepts – C. 7
VII.C.6. Explain patient financial obligations for services rendered	Workplace Applications – 1
VII.P.1.a. Perform accounts receivable procedures to patient accounts including posting: charges	Procedure 16.1
VII.P.1.b. Perform accounts receivable procedures to patient accounts including posting: payments	Procedure 16.1, 16.3
VII.P.1.c. Perform accounts receivable procedures to patient accounts including posting: adjustments	Procedure 16.3
VII.P.2. Prepare a bank deposit	Procedure 16.4
VII.P.3. Obtain accurate patient billing information	Procedure 16.2
VII.P.4. Inform a patient of financial obligations for services rendered	Procedure 16.2
VII.A.1. Demonstrate professionalism when discussing patient's billing record	Procedure 16.2
VII.A.2. Display sensitivity when requesting payment for services rendered	Procedure 16.2
ABHES Competencies	**Assessment**
1. General Orientation d. List the general responsibilities and skills of the medical assistant	Skills and Concepts – D.
7. Administrative Procedures c. Perform billing and collection procedures	Procedures 16.1, 16.2, 16.3, 16.4

VOCABULARY REVIEW

Using the word pool on the right, find the correct word to match the definition. Write the word on the line after the definition.

Group A

1. The person legally responsible for the entire bill
_____

2. A document sent by the insurance company to the provider and the patient explaining the allowed charge amount, the amount reimbursed for services, and the patient's financial responsibilities
_____

3. The process of recording financial transactions
_____

4. A manual bookkeeping system that uses a day sheet to record all financial transactions for the date of service and maintains patient account balances by using physical ledger cards
_____

5. Poor, needy, impoverished _____

6. To come into or acquire _____

7. A list of fixed fees for services _____

8. A minor who has been granted emancipation by the court; the minor can assume the rights and responsibilities of adulthood
_____

9. The amount of money the healthcare facility has in the bank that can be withdrawn as cash _____

10. A running balance of all financial transactions for a specific patient
_____

Word Pool
- bookkeeping
- incurred
- cash on hand
- patient account
- guarantor
- pegboard system
- fee schedule
- explanation of benefits
- emancipated minor
- indigent

Group B

1. Something of value that cannot be touched physically
_____

2. Hostile and aggressive _____

3. A special court established to handle small claims or debts, without the services of lawyers _____

4. A chronologic file used as a reminder that something must be dealt with on a certain date _____

5. All property available for the payment of debts
_____

6. An oath or swear word _____

7. An individual or party who brings the suit to court
_____

8. Debt that is not guaranteed by something of value; credit card debt is the most common type _____

9. An individual assigned to make financial decisions about the estate of a deceased patient _____

10. The coordinator of financial resources assigned by the court during a bankruptcy case _____

Word Pool
- belligerent
- expletive
- tickler file
- intangible
- executor
- assets
- unsecured debt
- trustee
- small claims court
- plaintiff

Group C

1. Money the bank pays the account holder on the amount in their account for using the money in the account _____

2. Global technology that includes imbedded microchips that store and protect cardholder data; also called *chip and PIN* and *chip and signature* _____

3. Money in a bank account that is not assigned to pay for any office expenses _____

4. An imitation intended to be passed off fraudulently or deceptively as genuine; forgery _____

5. A fixed compensation periodically paid to a person for regular work _____

6. The central bank of the United States _____

7. The misuse of a healthcare facility's funds for personal gain _____

8. An individual or business against whom a lawsuit is filed _____

9. To bring into agreement _____

10. A document guaranteeing payment of a specific amount of money to the payer named on the document _____

Word Pool
- defendant
- interest
- Federal Reserve Bank
- discretionary income
- negotiable instrument
- counterfeit
- EMV chip technology
- embezzlement
- reconciliation
- salaried

ABBREVIATIONS

Write out what each of the following abbreviations stands for.

1. EOB _____
2. A/R _____
3. A/P _____
4. TILA _____
5. FTC _____
6. PIN _____
7. POS _____
8. EFT _____

SKILLS AND CONCEPTS

Answer the following questions. Write your answer on the line or in the space provided.

A. Managing Funds in the Healthcare Facility

1. What items should appear on the financial records of any business at all times? _____

_____

_____

_____

_____

B. Bookkeeping in the Healthcare Facility

1. Examine the fee schedule and answer the following questions.

FEE SCHEDULE

BLACKBURN PRIMARY CARE ASSOCIATES, PC
1990 Turquiose Drive
Blackburn, WI 54937
608-459-8857

Federal Tax ID Number: 00-0000000

BCBS Group Number: 14982
Medicare Group Number: 14982

OFFICE VISIT, NEW PATIENT

Focused, 99201	$45.00
Expanded, 99202	$55.00
Intermediate, 99203	$60.00
Extended, 99204	$95.00
Comprehensive, 99205	$195.00
Consultation, 99245	$250.00

OFFICE VISIT, ESTABLISHED PATIENT

Minimal, 99211	$40.00
Focused, 99212	$48.00
Intermediate, 99213	$55.00
Extended, 99214	$65.00
Comprehensive, 99215	$195.00

OFFICE PROCEDURES

ECG, 12 lead, 93000	$55.00
Stress ECG, Treadmill, 93015	$295.00
Sigmoidoscopy, Flex; 45330	$145.00
Spirometry, 94010	$50.00
Cerumen Removal, 69210	$40.00
Collection & Handling	
Lab Specimen, 99000	$9.00
Venipuncture, 35415	$9.00
Urinalysis, 81000	$20.00
Urinalysis, 81002 (Dip Only)	$12.00
Influenza Injection, 90724	$20.00
Pneumococcal Injection, 90732	$20.00
Oral Polio, 90712	$15.00
DTaP, 90700	$20.00
Tetanus Toxoid, 90703	$15.00
MMR, 90707	$25.00
HIB, 90737	$20.00
Hepatitis B, newborn to age 11 years, 90744	$60.00
Hepatitis B, 11-19 years, 90745	$60.00
Hepatitis B, 20 years and above 90746	$60.00
Intramuscular Injection, 90788	
Penicillin	$30.00
Cephtriaxone	$25.00
Solu-Medrol	$23.00
Vitamin B-12	$13.00
Subcutaneous Injection, 90782	
Epinephrine	$18.00
Susphrine	$25.00
Insulin, U-100	$15.00

COMMON DIAGNOSTIC CODES

Acute coronary thrombosis without myocardial infarction I24.0
Other forms of acute ischemic heart disease I24.8
Chronic ischemic heart disease I25.9
Essential hypertension (arterial)(benign) (essential)(malignant)(primary)(systemic) I10
Hypertensive heart disease with heart failure I11.0
Unspecified asthma, uncomplicated J45.909
Asthma with COPD J44.9
Other asthma J45.998
Unspecified asthma with status asthmaticus J45.902
Postural kyphosis M40.00
Osteoporosis M81.0
Acute otitis media H66.0
Chronic otittis media H66.3

---

a. What is the charge for a consultation? _____

b. What is the charge for CPT code 99203? _____

c. What is the most expensive procedure on the list? _____

d. Which injection is more expensive, insulin or vitamin B_{12}? _____

2. Match the following terms with the correct definition:

<table>
<tr><td align="center">**Terms**</td><td align="center">**Definitions**</td></tr>
</table>

1. Accounts payable _____

2. Accounts receivable _____

3. Adjustments _____

4. Charges _____

5. Payments _____

a. Money that is expected but has not yet been received
b. Fees applied to the patient account when services are rendered
c. The management of debt incurred and not yet paid
d. Money given to the provider in exchange for services
e. Credits posted to the patient account when the provider's fee exceeds the amount allowed stated on the EOB

C. Accounts Receivable

1. What are the pitfalls of fee adjustments? _____

_____

_____

_____

_____

_____

2. Briefly explain how "skips" can be traced. _____

_____

_____

_____

_____

_____

_____

3. When a provider's fee exceeds the allowed amount stated on the explanation of benefits from the insurance company, a(n) _____ is posted to the patient account record for that difference.

4. When a patient account is turned over to a collection agency, what adjustment is posted to the account?

_____

_____

5. When a patient has a credit balance on his or her account, what adjustment is posted to the account?

_____

_____

_____

_____

6. Describe the adjustments that are made to the patient's account when an NSF check is received by the healthcare facility.

_____

_____

_____

_____

7. What information should be included on the patient ledger? _____

_____

_____

_____

_____

_____

D. Accounts Payable

1. In the ambulatory care setting, what is the checking account used for? _____

_____

_____

2. In the ambulatory care setting, what is a savings account used for? _____

_____

_____

3. You are a medical assistant in a small practice and have been told that you now have the responsibility for paying the bills by writing out and signing the checks. What is the first action you need to take before writing out the first check?

_____

_____

4. Name six activities that can be done with basic online banking services.

a. _____

b. _____

c. _____

d. _____

e. _____

f. _____

5. List the four requirements for a check to be negotiable.

   a. _____

   b. _____

   c. _____

   d. _____

6. Describe five precautions for accepting checks in the healthcare facility.

   a. _____

   b. _____

   c. _____

   d. _____

   e. _____

7. Describe four precautions to take if a patient is paying with cash.

   a. _____

   b. _____

   c. _____

   d. _____

8. Describe precautions to take when a patient pays with a debit card or a credit card._____

   _____

   _____

   _____

   _____

   _____

   _____

9. Describe the banking procedures as related to the ambulatory care setting and include the medical assistant's role with each procedure.

   a. Making bank deposits: _____

   _____

   _____

   _____

b. Preparing a bank deposit:_____

_____

_____

_____

c. Endorsing checks: _____

_____

_____

_____

d. Writing checks:_____

_____

_____

_____

10. Describe three ways to do a mobile deposit of a check.

a. _____

b. _____

c. _____

11. Describe each type of endorsement.

a. Blank endorsement:_____

_____

_____

_____

b. Restrictive endorsement: _____

_____

_____

_____

c. Special endorsement: _____

_____

_____

_____

12. List three reasons a stop-payment would be done.

    a. _____

    b. _____

    c. _____

13. When preparing the bank deposit, you have the following in cash:
    (3) $50 bills
    (22) $20 bills
    (20) $10 bills
    (46) $5 bills
    (68) $1 bills

    What is the total for currency that you would record on the deposit slip? _____

E. Employee Payroll

1. If an employee is paid with a(n) _____, their _____ paycheck will always be the same dollar amount.

2. Each employee must complete a W-4 form. What information is indicated on that form? _____

    _____

    _____

    _____

    _____

CERTIFICATION PREPARATION

Circle the correct answer.

1. Which agreement for payment plans is not subject to Truth in Lending Act and does not require a signed Truth in Lending statement?
   a. Specific agreement for less than four installments and finance charge
   b. Specific agreement with more than four installments and finance charge
   c. Credit card or loan specifically for health-care treatment
   d. All of the above

2. What should be considered when using a collection agency?
   a. Net back
   b. Fee percentage
   c. Fee charged by the collection agency
   d. Both a and b

3. Accounts _____ are debts incurred but not yet paid.
   a. receivable
   b. delinquent
   c. payable
   d. bookkeeping

4. The recording of business and accounting transactions is called _____.
   a. receivables
   b. payables
   c. accounting
   d. bookkeeping

5. Which does *not* conform to the general rules for telephone collections?
   a. Call only between 8 AM and 9 PM.
   b. Assume a positive attitude.
   c. Leave a message at work revealing the nature of the call.
   d. Keep the conversation brief and to the point.

6. When should checks from patients and other sources be deposited?
   a. At the same time bills are paid
   b. The same day that they are received
   c. When the bank statement is reconciled each month
   d. At the end of the week

7. Which is *not* one of the four types of endorsements?
   a. Blank
   b. Quality
   c. Restrictive
   d. Special

8. A check drawn on the bank's own account and signed by an authorized bank official is called a _____.
   a. bank draft
   b. voucher check
   c. cashier's check
   d. certified check

9. The country is divided into how many Federal Reserve districts?
   a. 8
   b. 10
   c. 12
   d. 14

10. Which endorsement includes words specifying the person to whom the endorser makes the check payable?
    a. Blank endorsement
    b. Restrictive endorsement
    c. Qualified endorsement
    d. Special endorsement

WORKPLACE APPLICATIONS

1. Mr. Sanchez comes to the desk to check out after seeing the provider. When Laura tells him that his bill is $95, he complains that he only saw the provider for 10 minutes. The fee is in accordance with evaluation and management guidelines. Explain the fees to Mr. Sanchez.

_____

_____

_____

2. In Laura's new role at Walden-Martin Family Medical Clinic, she will be writing checks to take care of the accounts payable for the clinic. A practicum student has just started at the clinic and will be working with Laura for the next several days. How should Laura describe this aspect of her job?

_____

_____

_____

_____

INTERNET ACTIVITIES

1. Using online resources, research the role of an accountant. Create a poster presentation, a PowerPoint presentation, or write a paper summarizing your research. Include the following points in your project:
    a. Why most healthcare providers employ one to handle financials for the office
    b. What an accountant does for the provider
    c. How a medical assistant helps the accountant do his or her job

2. Using online resources, research mobile deposit technology. Create a poster presentation, a PowerPoint presentation, or write a paper summarizing your research. Include the following points in your project:
    a. Describe three different mobile deposit technologies available for healthcare facilities.
    b. Describe which technology would work best for a small provider's office, large provider's office, and physical therapy rehabilitation facility.

Procedure 16.1   Post Charges and Payments to Patient Accounts

Name _____ Date _____ Score _____

Task: To enter charges into the patient account record manually and electronically.

Equipment and Supplies:
- Patient account ledger card (Work Product 16.1)
- SimChart for the Medical Office software
- Encounter form/superbill
- Provider's fee schedule

Scenario: Ken Thomas is a returning patient of Dr. Martin. He makes his $50 copayment at the time of the office visit.

Standard: Complete the procedure and all critical steps in _____ minutes with a minimum score of 85% within two attempts (*or as indicated by the instructor*).

Scoring: Divide the points earned by the total possible points. Failure to perform a critical step, indicated by an asterisk (*), results in grade no higher than an 84% (*or as indicated by the instructor*).

Time: Began_____ Ended_____ Total minutes: _____

Steps for Posting Charges Manually:	Point Value	Attempt 1	Attempt 2
1. For new patients, create the patient account by entering the following information on a patient account ledger card: • Patient's full name, address, and at least two contact phone numbers • Date of birth • Health insurance information, including the subscriber number, group number, and effective date • Subscriber's name and date of birth (if the subscriber is not the patient) For returning patients, review the account record to see whether a balance is due. If there is a balance, bring this to the patient's attention when he or she comes for the appointment. Respectfully explain that the provider would appreciate a payment on the previous balance before he or she can care for the patient.	50		
2. After seeing the patient, the provider completes the encounter form, which includes all procedures and the associated fee schedule. Using the completed encounter form (see Figure 16.1 in textbook), enter the charges manually on the ledger card for the patient's account record. Total all the charges on the encounter form for the services rendered. Then subtract the copayment made from the total charges. The previous balance, if any, is added to this new total. Use the following worksheet to calculate the new balance. The new balance due amount should be presented to the patient before he or she leaves the healthcare facility. 	Total Charges	$
Amount paid (copayment)	$
+ Previous balance (if any)	$
= New Balance Due	$		50*		
Total Points	**100**		

Steps for Posting Charges in SimChart for the Medical Office			
1. After logging into SimChart, locate the established patient by clicking on Find Patient, enter the patient's name, verify DOB, and click on the radio button. This will bring you to the Clinical Care tab. If there is no encounter shown, create an encounter by clicking on Office Visit under Info Panel on the left, select a visit type, and click on Save. Once an encounter has been created, return to the Patient Dashboard and click on the Superbill link on the right (or click on the Coding and Billing tab).	20		
2. From the Superbill area, in the Encounters Not Coded section, click on the encounter (in blue). On page 1, enter the diagnosis in the Diagnosis field and document the services provided (additional services are found on pages 2-3 of the Superbill).	20		
3. Complete the information needed on page 4 of the Superbill and submit.	20*		
4. Click on Ledger on the left and search for your patient. Once your patient has been located, click on the arrow across from the name in the ledger.	20		
5. Enter the payment received. The balance will be auto-calculated for you.	20		
Total Points	100		

Comments

CAAHEP Competencies	Step(s)
VII.P.1.a. Perform accounts receivable procedures to patient accounts including posting: charges	Manual: 2 SimChart: 2
VII.P.1.b. Perform accounts receivable procedures to patient accounts including posting: payments	Manual: 2 SimChart: 5
ABHES Competencies	**Step(s)**
7. Administrative Procedures c. Perform billing and collection procedures	Entire procedure

Work Product 16.1 Ledger

Ledger:

Blue Cross Blue Shield				
ID # KT4496785				
Group # 55124T				
Subscriber: Ken Thomas	Ken Thomas			
	398 Larkin Avenue			
DOB: 10/25/1961	Anytown, Anystate 12345-1234			

Date	Service Description	Charges	Payments	Adjustments	Balance

Procedure 16.2   Inform a Patient of Financial Obligations for Services Rendered

Name _____ Date _____ Score _____

Tasks: Inform a patient of his/her financial obligation and demonstrate professionalism and sensitivity when discussing the patient's billing record.

Equipment and Supplies:
- Facility's payment policy
- Copy of patient's insurance card (or see information in the scenario)
- Patient's account record (or see information in the scenario)

Obtaining Payments – WMFM Clinic Policy

- For patients with copayments, all copayments must be collected before the patient leaves the clinic.
- For patients with balances overdue:
  - Patients must pay 20% of the balance before an appointment can be scheduled.
  - Or patients can establish a 6- or 12-month interest-free payment plan, making the first payment before the next visit can be scheduled.
- Payments can be made using VISA, Mastercard, personal check (no starter checks accepted), or cash. Payments can also be made online.

Scenario #1: Mr. Walter Biller arrives for his appointment. You need to check his eligibility for services and also if he has a copayment for today's visit. His insurance information: account number: 16611; Aetna, Policy/ID Number: CH8327753; and Group Number: 33347H

Scenario #2: Christi Brown is meeting with you regarding the bill she received in the mail. She called to make the appointment and she voiced her confusion about the bill. She stated that she thought her insurance covered everything. You check her record and see that she met her deductible and now needs to pay 20% of the billed amount. She owes $170.

Directions: Role-play the scenarios with a peer. The peer will be the insurance representative in Scenario #1, and then the patient in Scenario #2. You will be the medical assistant. You need to be professional and sensitive when working with patients regarding payments. You also need to follow the clinic's policy.

Standard: Complete the procedure and all critical steps in _____ minutes with a minimum score of 85% within two attempts (*or as indicated by the instructor*).

Scoring: Divide the points earned by the total possible points. Failure to perform a critical step, indicated by an asterisk (*), results in grade no higher than an 84% (*or as indicated by the instructor*).

Time: Began_____ Ended_____ Total minutes: _____

Steps:	Point Value	Attempt 1	Attempt 2
Scenario #1: Role-play with a peer who will be the insurance representative. 1. Contact the patient's insurance company and verify the patient's eligibility for services. Provide the representative with the patient's information. Find out if the patient has a copayment for today's visit. Document the information obtained.	20*		
Scenario #1 update: You need to provide the patient with the information that he owes a copayment for today's visit. 2. Inform the patient of his financial obligation of the copayment.	10*		
Scenario update: He states he does not have the cash with him. 3. Inform the patient of the clinic policy regarding copayments and how the payment can be made.	10		
4. Demonstrate sensitivity and professionalism when discussing the payment. *(Refer to the Checklist for Affective Behaviors - Respect and Sensitivity)*	15*		
Scenario #2: Role-play with a peer who will be the patient. 5. Determine the amount the patient owes by reviewing the patient's account record. Inform the patient the amount owed for services rendered.	15*		
Scenario update: Patient states she does not have the money to pay the entire bill today. 6. Inform the patient of the clinic policy regarding overdue accounts and scheduling appointments. Provide the patient with options for the overdue amount based on the clinic policy.	15		
7. Demonstrate sensitivity and professionalism when discussing the payment and the situation. *(Refer to the Checklist for Affective Behaviors - Respect and Sensitivity)*	15*		
Total Points	**100**		

Affective Behavior	Directions: Check behaviors observed during the role-play.					
Respect	**Negative, Unprofessional Behaviors**	**Attempt**		**Positive, Professional Behaviors**	**Attempt**	
		1	**2**		**1**	**2**
	Rude, unkind			Courteous, professional; assertive as required		
	Disrespectful, impolite			Polite, patient		
	Negative verbal communication (e.g., harsh words, disrespectful comments)			Professional verbal communication (e.g., respectful and understanding communication)		
	Brief, abrupt			Took time with person		
	Unconcerned with person's dignity			Maintained person's dignity		
	Negative nonverbal behaviors			Positive nonverbal behaviors		
	Other:			Other:		
Sensitivity	Distracted; not focused on the other person			Focused full attention on the other person		
	Judgmental attitude; not accepting attitude			Nonjudgmental, accepting attitude		
	Failed to clarify what the person verbally or nonverbally communicated			Used summarizing or paraphrasing to clarify what the person verbally or nonverbally communicated		
	Failed to acknowledge what the person communicated			Acknowledged what the person communicated		
	Rude, discourteous			Pleasant and courteous		
	Disregarded the person's dignity and rights			Maintained the person's dignity and rights		
	Other:			Other:		

Grading for Affective Behaviors		Point Value	Attempt 1	Attempt 2
Does not meet Expectation	• Response was insensitive and/or disrespectful. • Student demonstrated more than 2 negative, unprofessional behaviors during the interaction.	0		
Needs Improvement	• Response was insensitive and/or disrespectful. • Student demonstrated 1 or 2 negative, unprofessional behaviors during the interaction.	0		
Meets Expectation	• Response was sensitive and respectful; no negative, unprofessional behaviors observed. • More practice is needed for behavior to appear natural and for student to appear comfortable and at ease.	15		
Occasionally Exceeds Expectation	• Response was sensitive and respectful; no negative, unprofessional behaviors observed. • At times student appeared comfortable and at ease; but more practice is needed for behavior to become natural and consistent with a professional medical assistant.	15		
Always Exceeds Expectation	• Response was sensitive and respectful; no negative, unprofessional behaviors observed. • Student's behaviors appeared natural and comfortable. Behaviors are consistent with a professional medical assistant.	15		

Comments

CAAHEP Competencies	Step(s)
VII.P.3. Obtain accurate patient billing information	#1
VII.P.4. Inform a patient of financial obligations for services rendered	#2, 5
VII.A.1. Demonstrate professionalism when discussing patient's billing record	#4, 7
VII.A.2. Display sensitivity when requesting payment for services rendered	#4, 7
ABHES Competencies	**Step(s)**
7. Administrative Procedures c. Perform billing and collection procedures	Entire procedure

Procedure 16.3 Post Payments and Adjustments to Patient Account

Name _____ Date _____ Score _____

Task: To demonstrate sensitivity through verbal and nonverbal communication when discussing third-party requirements with patients.

Equipment and Supplies:
*   Patient account ledger card or SimChart for the Medical Office software

Scenario: Monique Jones (06/23/1985) was seen 6 months ago for a wellness visit and lab work. Her insurance had lapsed, and she is completely responsible for the bill. She did not make any payments and resisted all attempts at collection of the balance of $172.00. Her account was turned over to the collection agency and they were able to collect the balance in full. The collection agency retains 50% of what they collect as payment. Post the collection agency payment and adjustment to her account.

Standard: Complete the procedure and all critical steps in _____ minutes with a minimum score of 85% within two attempts (*or as indicated by the instructor*).

Scoring: Divide the points earned by the total possible points. Failure to perform a critical step, indicated by an asterisk (*), results in grade no higher than an 84% (*or as indicated by the instructor*).

Time: Began_____ Ended_____ Total minutes: _____

Steps:	Point Value	Attempt 1	Attempt 2
1. Look up the ledger card for the patient account (or the patient ledger in SimChart). Confirm that you have the correct patient account.	30		
2. Post an adjustment to reverse the adjustment done when the account was turned over to the collection agency.	30		
3. Post the payment and adjustment that reflects the actual dollar amount received from the collection agency and the amount that was retained as payment.	40*		
Total Points	100		

Comments

CAAHEP Competencies	Step(s)
VII.P.1.b. Perform accounts receivable procedures to patient accounts including posting: payments	3
VII.P.1.c. Perform accounts receivable procedures to patient accounts including posting: adjustments	2, 3
ABHES Competencies	**Step(s)**
7. Administrative Procedures c. Perform billing and collection procedures	Entire procedure

Procedure 16.4   Prepare a Bank Deposit

Name _____ Date _____ Score _____

Task: Prepare a bank deposit for currency and checks.

Equipment and Supplies:
- Checks and currency for deposit (see scenario)
- Check for endorsement
- Calculator
- Paper method: bank deposit slip (Work Product 16.2)
- Electronic method: SimChart for the Medical Office (SCMO)

Scenario: The following checks need to be deposited:
- #3456 for $89
- #6954 for $136
- #9854-10 for $1366.65
- #8546 for $653.36
- #9865 for $890.22.

The following currency needs to be deposited:
- (19) $20 bills
- (10) $10 bills
- (46) $5 bills
- (73) $1 bills

The healthcare facility's name is Walden-Martin Family Medical Clinic, account number 123-456-78910, and the bank is Clear Water Bank, Anytown, Anystate.

Standard: Complete the procedure and all critical steps in _____ minutes with a minimum score of 85% within two attempts (*or as indicated by the instructor*).

Scoring: Divide the points earned by the total possible points. Failure to perform a critical step, indicated by an asterisk (*), results in grade no higher than an 84% (*or as indicated by the instructor*).

Time: Began_____ Ended_____ Total minutes: _____

Steps:	Point Value	Attempt 1	Attempt 2
1. Gather the documents to be used. For the electronic method, enter into the Simulation Playground in SCMO. Click on the Form Repository icon. On the INFO PANEL, click on Office Forms and then select Bank Deposit Slip.	10		
2. Add the date on the deposit slip.	10		
3. Using the calculator, calculate the amount of currency to be deposited. Enter the amount in the CURRENCY line, completing the dollar and cent boxes.	15*		
4. Enter the total amount in the TOTAL CASH line.	10		
5. For each check to be deposited, enter the check number, the dollars, and cents. List each check on a separate line.	10		

6.	Calculate the total to be deposited and enter the number in the TOTAL FROM ATTACHED LIST box.	**15***		
7.	Enter the number of items deposited in the TOTAL ITEMS box.	**10**		
8.	Before completing the deposit slip, verify the check amounts listed and recalculate the totals. For the electronic method, click on SAVE.	**10**		
9.	Place a restrictive endorsement on the check(s).	**10**		
	Total Points	**100**		

Comments

CAAHEP Competencies	**Step(s)**
VII.P.2. Prepare a bank deposit	Entire procedure
ABHES Competencies	**Step(s)**
7. Administrative Procedures c. Perform billing and collection procedures	Entire procedure

Work Product 16.2 Bank Deposit Slip

DEPOSIT TICKET

WALDEN-MARTIN FAMLY MEDICAL CLINIC
1234 ANYSTREET
ANYTOWN, ANYSTATE 12345

DEPOSITS MAY NOT BE AVAILABLE FOR
IMMEDIATE WITHDRAWAL

Clear Water Bank
Anytown, Anystate

ACCOUNT NUMBER: 123-456-78910

Endorse & List Checks Separately

DATE _____	Dollars	Cents
CURRENCY		
COIN		
TOTAL CASH		
1.		
2.		
3.		
4.		
5.		
6.		
7.		
8.		
9.		
10.		
11.		
12.		
Less Cash Returned		
Total Items	Total Deposit	

Advanced Roles in Administration

CAAHEP	Assessments
V.C.3 Recognize barriers to communication	Skills and Concepts – D. 4
X.C.7.i. Define: risk management	Skills and Concepts – B. 2
X.C.10a Identify: Health Information Technology for Economic and Clinical Health (HITECH) Act	Skills and Concepts – F. 1

VOCABULARY REVIEW

Using the word pool on the right, find the correct word to match the definition. Write the word on the line after the definition.

1. The environment where something is created or takes shape; a base on which to build _____

2. Obeying, obliging, or yielding _____

3. Sticking together tightly _____

4. Evidence of authority, status, rights, entitlement to privileges _____

5. Contains all documents related to an individual's employment _____

6. To appoint a person as a representative _____

7. A term referring to actions taken by management to keep good employees _____

8. General _____

9. A steady employee whom a new staff member can approach with questions and concerns _____

10. Things that incite or spur to action; rewards or reasons for performing a task _____

11. Slighting; having a negative or degrading tone _____

12. Able to pay all debts _____

Word Pool
- consensus
- credential
- solvent
- matrix
- delegate
- incentive
- cohesive
- disparaging
- mentor
- retention
- human resources file
- compliant

SKILLS AND CONCEPTS

Answer the following questions. Write your answer on the line or in the space provided.

A. Medical Office Management

1. Describe the traits of a successful medical office manager. _____

   _____

   _____

   _____

   _____

   _____

   _____

2. Describe a good relationship between a manager and his or her employees. _____

   _____

   _____

   _____

   _____

   _____

   _____

B. Office Management Responsibilities

1. List five office management responsibilities.

   a. _____

   b. _____

   c. _____

   d. _____

   e. _____

2. Define *risk management*. _____

   _____

   _____

   _____

   _____

C. Office Manager Role

1. List and define in your own words the five Cs of communication. _____

    _____

    _____

    _____

    _____

    _____

2. List four characteristics of a good listener. _____

    _____

    _____

    _____

    _____

    _____

3. Describe the ABC method of time management._____

    _____

    _____

    _____

    _____

    _____

D. Creating a Team Environment

1. What action improves communication in the healthcare workplace? _____

    _____

    _____

    _____

2. Name two positive things that occur when communication improves in the healthcare workplace.

    a. _____

    b. _____

3. Name two actions an office manager can take to improve employee morale. _____

    _____

    _____

4. Describe the following barriers to communication and explain how to overcome them.

    a. Physical separation barrier: _____

    _____

    _____

    _____

    _____

    b. Language barriers: _____

    _____

    _____

    _____

    _____

    c. Status barriers: _____

    _____

    _____

    _____

    _____

    d. Gender difference barriers: _____

    _____

    _____

    _____

    _____

    e. Cultural diversity barriers : _____

    _____

    _____

    _____

    _____

E. Finding the Right Employee for the Job

1. List three effective methods for finding new employees.

    a. _____

    b. _____

    c. _____

2. List five illegal interview questions.

a. _____

b. _____

c. _____

d. _____

e. _____

3. List five legal interview questions.

a. _____

b. _____

c. _____

d. _____

e. _____

4. Discuss topic areas that would be considered illegal and legal during an interview. _____

_____

_____

_____

F. Policies and Procedures

1. Identify three components of the HITECH Act._____

_____

_____

_____

2. List five items that should be included in a personnel policy manual.

a. _____

b. _____

c. _____

d. _____

e. _____

3. Define *sexual harassment*. _____

_____

_____

CERTIFICATION PREPARATION

Circle the correct answer.

1. Which is a quality of an effective leader or office manager?
   a. Has a sense of fairness
   b. Has good communication skills
   c. Uses good judgment
   d. All of the above

2. Something that spurs an individual to action or rewards an individual for performing a task is called
   a. morale.
   b. incentive.
   c. appraisal.
   d. circumvention.

3. Which act protects the employee against unsafe workplaces?
   a. Fair Labor Standards Act
   b. Family and Medical Leave Act
   c. Occupational Safety and Health Act
   d. Age Discrimination Act

4. Some managers assign a person to assist new employees during the initial probationary period; this person is called a
   a. mentor.
   b. supervisor.
   c. coworker.
   d. subordinate.

5. A group of employees who stick together during difficult times could be called
   a. cohesive.
   b. adaptive.
   c. affable.
   d. meticulous.

6. Which subjects cannot be discussed in a job interview?
   a. Religion
   b. Work history
   c. Previous terminations of employment
   d. None of the above

7. The process of inciting a person to some action or behavior is called
   a. reprimand.
   b. motivation.
   c. circumvention.
   d. appraisal.

8. Which is a strong method of improving employee morale and encouraging outstanding performance?
   a. Incentives
   b. Recognition
   c. Fraternizing with subordinates outside work
   d. All of the above

9. Which is critical for good communication and smooth operation of a medical facility?
   a. Scheduling activities that involve the families of employees
   b. Holding regular staff meetings and sending regular emails and memos
   c. Shielding employees from negative information
   d. All of the above

10. Which employee behavior is grounds for immediate dismissal without warning?
    a. Embezzlement
    b. Insubordination
    c. Violation of patient confidentiality
    d. All of the above

WORKPLACE APPLICATIONS

1. Create a job description or job posting for a "dream" job of your choice. Make sure to include the duties, required education, and other details typically found in postings.

   _____

   _____

   _____

   _____

   _____

   _____

2. Create a plan of how to screen applications and résumés for a medical assistant job in a family practice department. Describe the process you would use to evidentially identify the few applicants who should be interviewed.

   _____

   _____

   _____

   _____

   _____

   _____

   _____

   _____

   _____

   _____

   _____

INTERNET ACTIVITIES

1. Using online resources, research team-building exercises designed to promote and build teamwork for a group of employees. Create a poster presentation, a PowerPoint presentation, or write a paper summarizing your research. Include the following points in your project:
   a. Describe three team-building activities.
   b. Why do you think each of these activities will promote and build teamwork?
   c. How would you make sure that these activities are relevant to working in healthcare?

2. Using online resources, research the I-9 form. Create a poster presentation, a PowerPoint presentation, or write a paper summarizing your research. Include the following points in your project:
   a. Describe the purpose of the form.
   b. Summarize the process for completing the I-9 form.
   c. Describe acceptable documentation used to complete the form.

Introduction to Anatomy and Medical Terminology

CAAHEP Competencies

V.C.9. Identify medical terms labeling the word parts	Skills and Concepts – A. 7, 8, 10
I.C.1. Describe structural organization of the human body	Skills and Concepts – B. 1-20
I.C.2. Identify body systems	Skills and Concepts – B. 11-21
I.C.3.a. Describe: body planes	Skills and Concepts – G. 1
I.C.3.b. Describe: directional terms	Skills and Concepts – D. 1-10
I.C.3.c. Describe: quadrants	Skills and Concepts – F. 1-7
I.C.3.d. Describe: body cavities	Skills and Concepts – E. 1-6
V.C.10. Define medical terms and abbreviations related to all body system	Vocabulary Review – A. 1-11, B. 1-12; Abbreviations – 1-46
I.C.7. Describe the normal function of each body system	Skills and Concepts – B. 10-21
I.C.4. List major organs in each body system	Skills and Concepts – B. 10-21, E. 1-6, F. 1-7
I.C.4. List major organs in each body system	Skills and Concepts – B. 10-21, E. 1-6, F. 1-7

ABHES Competencies

3. Medical Terminology	
a. Define and use the entire basic structure of medical terminology and be able to accurately identify the correct context (i.e., root, prefix, suffix, combinations, spelling and definitions)	Skills and Concepts – A. 7, 8, 10
b. Build and dissect medical terminology from roots and suffixes to understand the word element combinations	Skills and Concepts – A. 10
c. Apply medical terminology for each specialty	Vocabulary Review – A. 1-11, B. 1-12; Skills and Concepts – C. 2-15, D. 1-10
d. Define and use medical abbreviations when appropriate and acceptable	Abbreviations – 1-46

VOCABULARY REVIEW

Using the word pool, find the correct word to match the definition. Write the word on the line after the definition.

Group A

1. A rapidly dividing cancer cell that has little to no similarity to normal cells _____

2. Protein substances produced in the blood or tissues in response to a specific antigen that destroy or weaken the antigen; part of the immune system _____

3. A broad dome-shaped muscle used for breathing that separates the thoracic and abdominopelvic cavities

   _____

4. Word parts that appear at the beginning of terms

   _____

5. Process of viewing living tissue that has been removed for the purpose of diagnosis or treatment _____

6. The "subjects" of most terms; they consist of the word root with its respective combining vowel _____

7. Substances that stimulate the production of an antibody when introduced into the body; include toxins, bacteria, viruses, and other foreign substances _____

8. Rod-shaped structures found in the cell's nucleus; they contain genetic information _____

9. Words used in healthcare whose definitions must be memorized without the benefit of word parts _____

10. Describes how malignant tissue looks like the normal tissue it came from; poorly _____ means it does not look like the normal tissue, and well _____ means it looks like the normal tissue

    _____

11. Word parts that appear at the end of terms

    _____

Word Pool

- prefixes
- antigens
- biopsy
- differentiated
- anaplastic
- diaphragm
- combining forms
- suffixes
- antibodies
- nondecodable terms
- chromosomes

Group B

1. A specially trained doctor who diagnoses and treats cancer _____

2. A cell division process by which two daughter cells are formed from one parent cell; each daughter has a complete copy of parent's chromosomes _____

3. Located between cells _____

4. Wavelike motion _____

5. A disease-causing organism _____

6. Structures inside of the cell that have specific functions to maintain the cell _____

7. An examination using a scope with a camera attached to a long, thin tube that can be inserted into the body _____

8. A physician specially trained in the nature and cause of disease _____

9. Contraction of the muscles causing the narrowing of the inside tube of the vessel _____

10. Substances created by microorganisms, plants, or animals and poisonous to humans _____

11. Study of disease _____

12. The internal environment of the body that is compatible with life; a steady state that is created by all the body systems working together to provide a consistent and unvarying internal environment _____

Word Pool
- endoscopy
- pathogen
- homeostasis
- vasoconstriction
- mitosis
- pathology
- toxins
- intercellular
- peristalsis
- oncologist
- organelle
- pathologist

ABBREVIATIONS
Write out what each of the following abbreviations stands for.

1. CARD _____
2. AAMA _____
3. AAMT _____
4. AMA _____
5. ER _____
6. DNA _____
7. IM _____
8. CABG _____
9. TURP _____
10. AP _____
11. PA _____

12. RUQ _____

13. LUQ _____

14. RLQ _____

15. LLQ _____

16. CT _____

17. CAT _____

18. CO_2 _____

19. O_2 _____

20. TNM _____

21. MRI _____

22. PET _____

23. US _____

24. PKU _____

25. RNA _____

26. CRP _____

27. RBC _____

28. WBC _____

29. Hgb _____

30. Hct _____

31. CMP _____

32. ESR _____

33. FSH _____

34. HbA1c or A1c _____

35. PTT _____

36. PT _____

37. INR _____

38. TSH _____

39. C&S _____

40. FIT _____

41. gFOBT _____

42. FOBT _____

43. O&P_____

44. UA_____

45. ERCP_____

46. EGD_____

SKILLS AND CONCEPTS
Answer the following questions. Write your answer on the line or in the space provided.

A. Types of Medical Terms

1. Define *decodable terms* in your own words. _____

_____

_____

2. Define the term *combining vowel*. List the vowels. _____

_____

3. Define *nondecodable terms* in your own words. _____

_____

4. Define the following nondecodable terms.

   a. Acute _____

   _____

   b. Chronic _____

   _____

   c. Sign _____

   _____

   d. Symptom_____

   _____

5. Define the following symbols.

   a. ♂ _____

   b. ♀ _____

   c. ↑ _____

   d. ↓ _____

   e. + _____

   f. − _____

6. Define the acronym CARD.

C _____

A _____

R _____

D _____

7. Using Table 18.1 in the textbook, write the definition of the following combining forms.

  a. ot/o _____

  b. cardi/o _____

  c. nephr/o _____

  d. hepat/o _____

  e. ophthalm/o _____

  f. neur/o _____

8. Using Table 18.2 in the textbook, write the definition of the following suffixes.

  a. -logy _____

  b. -plasty _____

  c. -algia _____

  d. -itis _____

  e. -tomy _____

  f. -scope _____

9. With only a few exceptions, how many spelling rules apply to decodable medical terms? _____

  _____

  _____

10. Using Tables 18.1 through 18.10 in your textbook, decode and define the following terms. Label the word parts as prefix, combining form, or suffix.

  a. ophthalmology _____

  _____

  b. otoplasty _____

  _____

  c. gastralgia _____

  _____

d. cardiomegaly _____

   _____

e. osteomalacia _____

   _____

f. cephalic _____

   _____

g. gastroptosis _____

   _____

h. spirometer _____

   _____

i. splenectomy _____

   _____

j. pericardium _____

   _____

11. For each of the following words, write the plural form using the rules discussed in your textbook under the heading Singular/Plural Rules.

   a. esophagus _____

   b. larynx _____

   c. fornix _____

   d. pleura _____

   e. diagnosis _____

   f. myocardium _____

   g. cardiomyopathy _____

   h. hepatitis _____

ANATOMY REVIEW

B. Structural Organization of the Body

1. The _____ is the basic unit of life.

2. _____ is the process where one cell splits into two identical daughter cells.

3. At what stage of mitosis is the genetic information replicated? _____

4. List the four phases of mitosis. _____

_____

_____

5. _____ is the jelly-like substance that surrounds the organelles and fills the cell.

6. What causes the rough appearance of the rough endoplasmic reticulum? _____

_____

_____

7. _____ is a group of similar cells from the same source that together carry out a specific function.

8. List the four types of tissues and give two examples of each.

    a. epithelial _____

_____

_____

    b. connective _____

_____

_____

    c. muscle _____

_____

_____

    d. nervous _____

_____

_____

9. _____ is a structure composed of two or more types of tissue.

10. A(n) _____ is composed of several organs and their related structures.

11. Which body system contains veins, arteries, and blood? _____

12. Which body system is involved with the breakdown, digestion, and absorption of nutrients? _____

13. Which body system includes the pituitary and the thyroid glands? _____

14. Receiving and processing information and controlling body structures to maintain homeostasis are roles of which body system? _____

15. Which body system is involved with heat production, support, protection, and movement? _____

16. Which body system provides immunity and maintains fluid balance? _____

17. Protection and temperature regulation are some roles of the _____ system; hair and nails are also structures in this system.

18. Which body system is involved with producing children and hormones? _____

19. Delivering oxygen to cells and ridding the body of carbon dioxide are two major roles of which body system? _____

20. Which body system is involved with gathering information from vision, hearing, balance, smell, and taste? _____

21. Eliminating nitrogenous waste from the body and maintaining fluid and electrolytes are important roles for which body system? _____

22. Put the following in order from the simplest to the most complex: organism, organs, cells, body systems, tissue

_____

C. Surface Anatomy Terminology

1. Describe the anatomical position. _____

    _____

    _____

2. *Cervical* refers to the: _____

3. *Frontal* pertains to the: _____

4. *Ocular* refers to the: _____

5. *Axillary* refers to the: _____

6. *Coxal* pertains to the: _____

7. *Sternal* pertains to the: _____

8. *Antecubital* pertains to the: _____

9. *Carpal* refers to the: _____

10. *Femoral* pertains to the: _____

11. *Patellar* pertains to the: _____

12. *Pedal* pertains to the: _____

13. *Acromial* refers to the: _____

14. *Lumbar* pertains to the: _____

15. *Plantar* pertains to the: _____

D. Positional and Directional Terminology

1. *Deep* or *internal* refers to: _____

2. *Anterior* or *ventral* pertains to the:_____

3. *Inferior* or *caudad* pertains to: _____

4. Opposite of *anterior* and refers to the back:_____

5. Pertains to the midline: _____

6. *Contralateral* refers to the:_____

7. *Distal* refers to:_____

8. Pertains to carrying toward a structure: _____

9. Pertains to near the origin: _____

10. Using the directional and positional terms listed in this chapter, write four sentences that use a term in reference to the body. Use four different terms. Example: The fingers are distal to the elbows.

    _____

    _____

    _____

    _____

E. Body Cavities

1. Name the two cavities that make up the dorsal body cavity. _____

    _____

2. Name the two cavities that make up the ventral body cavity._____

    _____

3. Describe the cranial cavity. _____

    _____

    _____

4. Describe the spinal cavity._____

    _____

    _____

5. Describe the thoracic cavity. _____

    _____

    _____

6. Discuss the two cavities that make up the abdominopelvic cavity. _____

_____

_____

F. Abdominopelvic Quadrants and Regions

1. Describe the imaginary lines for the abdominopelvic quadrants._____

_____

2. List three organs found in the right upper quadrant. _____

_____

3. List three organs found in the left upper quadrant. _____

_____

4. List three organs found in the left lower quadrant._____

_____

5. List three organs found in the right lower quadrant. _____

_____

6. Describe the advantage of using the abdominal regions compared to the abdominopelvic quadrants.

_____

_____

7. Using the grid below, create a table showing the locations of the nine abdominal regions. In each box, indicate the region and one organ found in that region.

Right hypochondriac region	Epigastric region	Left hypochondriac region
Right lumbar region	**Umbilical region**	**Left lumbar region**
Right iliac region	**Hypogastric region**	**Left iliac region**

G. Body Planes

1. Using your own words, describe the following planes.

   a. Midsagittal or median plane _____

   _____

   b. Coronal or frontal plane _____

   _____

   c. Transverse or horizontal plane _____

   _____

H. Acid-Base Balance

1. What is the pH of an acidic solution? _____

2. What is the pH of a basic or alkaline solution? _____

3. For the body to maintain homeostasis, what pH range must be maintained in the blood? _____

   _____

4. What three things must work together to maintain the acid-base range in the body? _____

   _____

I. Pathology Basics

1. Describe the difference between the following terms.

   a. Prevalence and incidence _____

   _____

   b. Morbidity and mortality_____

   _____

   c. Acute and chronic _____

   _____

   d. Signs and symptoms _____

   _____

2. List five predisposing factors for disease._____

   _____

3. Describe the difference between noncommunicable diseases and communicable diseases. _____

   _____

4. Describe the characteristics of a benign tumor. _____
_____

5. Describe the characteristics of a malignant tumor. _____
_____
_____

6. Describe grade and stage. _____
_____
_____

CERTIFICATION PREPARATION
Circle the correct answer.

1. What does –*ptosis* mean?
   a. Abnormal condition of softening
   b. Abnormal condition of hardening
   c. Prolapse, drooping, sagging
   d. Enlargement

2. What is the prefix that means between?
   a. inter-
   b. intra-
   c. peri-
   d. pre-

3. What is the prefix that means above, upon?
   a. endo-
   b. hypo-
   c. sub-
   d. epi-

4. What two prefixes mean within?
   a. endo-, intra-
   b. epi-, inter-
   c. ante-, per-
   d. peri-, trans-

5. What is the structural organization of the body from the simplest to the most complex?
   a. Organism, body system, tissues, organs, and cells
   b. Cells, organs, tissues, and body systems
   c. Cells, tissues, organs, body systems, and organism
   d. Cells, tissues, body systems, organs, and organism

6. Which body system produces hormones that circulate in the blood to target tissues that stimulate a particular action?
   a. Cardiovascular
   b. Endocrine
   c. Blood
   d. Integumentary

7. Which body system includes joints, tendons, ligaments, and cartilage?
   a. Integumentary
   b. Nervous
   c. Reproductive
   d. Musculoskeletal

8. Which plane divides the body into the front and back portions?
   a. Frontal plane
   b. Median plane
   c. Midsagittal plane
   d. Transverse plane

9. _____ pertains to the middle and _____ pertains to the side.
   a. Anterior; posterior
   b. Superior; inferior
   c. Ipsilateral; contralateral
   d. Medial; lateral

10. Which cavity is part of the ventral body cavity and contains the heart and lungs?
    a. Spinal cavity
    b. Thoracic cavity
    c. Abdominopelvic cavity
    d. Cranial cavity

WORKPLACE APPLICATIONS

1. Harry is a new student who thinks he might want to become a physician's assistant. He likes to practice decoding terms. What does the combining form mean in each of the following terms?

   a. Cystocele means herniation of the _____ .

   b. Ophthalmology is the study of the _____ .

   c. Otalgia is pain in the _____ .

   d. Osteoma is a tumor in a(n) _____ .

   e. Hepatitis is inflammation of the _____ .

2. Daniela was discussing directional terms with a peer in her class. She was explaining the importance of using directional terms in healthcare. Describe why directional terms are useful when documenting healthcare information.

   _____

   _____

   _____

3. Describe the organizational structure of the body. _____

   _____

   _____

   _____

   _____

INTERNET ACTIVITIES

1. Select one of the causes of disease (e.g., genetics, infectious pathogen). Using online resources, find four diseases that are initiated by that specific cause of disease. Research each disease and the cause of the disease. Create a paper, poster presentation, PowerPoint presentation, or infographic based on your research.

2. Using online resources, research grading and staging of cancers. Create a short paper or PowerPoint describing the difference between grading and staging.

3. Research the difference between acid and base. Write a half-page summary on the importance of the acid-base balance of the body.

4. Research and create a list of the most prevalent forms of cancer for males and females in the United States.

Infection Control

CAAHEP Competencies	Assessment
III.C.1. List major types of infectious agents	Skills and Concepts – B. 3
III.C.2.a. Describe the infection cycle including: the infectious agent	Skills and Concepts – B. 1, 2
III.C.2.b. Describe the infection cycle including: reservoir	Skills and Concepts – B. 1, 2
III.C.2.c. Describe the infection cycle including: susceptible host	Skills and Concepts – B. 1, 2
III.C.2.d. Describe the infection cycle including: means of transmission	Skills and Concepts – B. 1, 2
III.C.2.e. Describe the infection cycle including: portals of entry	Skills and Concepts – B. 1, 2
III.C.2.f. Describe the infection cycle including: portals of exit	Skills and Concepts – B. 1, 2
III.C.3.a. Define the following as practiced within an ambulatory care setting: medical asepsis	Skills and Concepts – G. 1
III.C.3.b. Define the following as practiced within an ambulatory care setting: surgical asepsis	Skills and Concepts – G. 1
III.C.4. Identify methods of controlling the growth of microorganisms	Skills and Concepts – B. 4
III.C.5. Define the principles of standard precautions	Skills and Concepts – E. 1
III.C.6.a. Define personal protective equipment (PPE) for: all body fluids, secretions and excretions	Skills and Concepts – F. 2
III.C.6.b. Define personal protective equipment (PPE) for: blood	Skills and Concepts – F. 2
III.C.6.c. Define personal protective equipment (PPE) for: non-intact skin	Skills and Concepts – F. 2
III.C.6.d. Define personal protective equipment (PPE) for: mucous membranes	Skills and Concepts – F. 2
III.C.7. Identify Center for Disease Control (CDC) regulations that impact healthcare practices	Skills and Concepts – E. 2; Internet Activities – 1
III.P.1. Participate in bloodborne pathogen training	Procedure 19.1

CAAHEP Competencies	Assessment
III.P.2. Select appropriate barrier/personal protective equipment	Procedure 19.3
III.P.3. Perform handwashing	Procedure 19.2

ABHES Competencies	Assessment
8.a. Practice standard precautions and perform disinfection/sterilization techniques	Procedure 19.1, 19.2, 19.3

VOCABULARY REVIEW

Using the word pool on the right, find the correct word to match the definition. Write the word on the line after the definition.

Group A

1. Substances that inhibit the growth of microorganisms on living tissue; they are used to cleanse the skin, wounds, and so on

   _____

2. A thick-walled, dormant form of bacteria that is very resistant to disinfection measures _____

3. Passed from parents to offspring through the genes

   _____

4. Capable of producing disease _____

5. A disease where the body produces antibodies that attack its own tissues, leading to the deterioration of tissue

   _____

6. Diseases spread from person to person either by direct or indirect contact _____

7. To take, as food, into the body _____

8. An illness resulting from the deterioration of tissues and organs

   _____

9. Free from all microorganisms, pathogenic and nonpathogenic

   _____

10. A protein formed when a cell is exposed to a virus; the protein blocks viral action on the cell and protects against viral invasion

    _____

Word Pool
- sterile
- hereditary
- autoimmune
- degenerative
- communicable
- pathogenic
- ingested
- antiseptics
- interferon
- spore

Group B

1. Protein substances produced in the blood or tissues in response to a specific antigen that destroys or weakens the antigen

   _____

2. The presence of pus-forming organisms in the blood

   _____

3. To pass or spread disease _____

4. Animals or insects (e.g., ticks) that transmit a pathogen

   _____

5. To void waste from the bowels through the anus; have a bowel movement _____

6. An infection caused by a yeast, *Candida albicans*, that typically affects the vaginal mucosa and skin _____

7. Not animate; lifeless _____

8. Any fungal skin disease that results in scaling, itching, and inflammation; examples are ringworm, athlete's foot

   _____

9. Agents that destroy pathogenic organisms

   _____

10. To breathe in _____

Word Pool
- candidiasis
- tinea
- vectors
- transmission
- inanimate
- inhalation
- germicides
- defecation
- antibodies
- pyemia

Group C

1. The partial or complete disappearance of the clinical and subjective characteristics of a chronic or malignant disease

   _____

2. Not permitting penetration _____

3. To take into the body by any route other than the digestive tract

   _____

4. Infections that are acquired in a healthcare setting

   _____

5. Any chemical agent used on nonliving objects to destroy or inhibit the growth of harmful organisms; not effective against bacterial spores _____

6. Condition of general bodily weakness or discomfort

   _____

7. Those procedures that do not penetrate human tissue

   _____

8. The recurrence of the symptoms of a disease after apparent recovery _____

9. A set of infection control practices used to prevent transmission of diseases that can be acquired by contact with blood, body fluids, nonintact skin, and mucous membranes _____

10. Extreme tiredness _____

Word Pool
- fatigue
- malaise
- relapse
- remission
- Standard Precautions
- parenteral
- disinfectant
- impervious
- noninvasive procedures
- nosocomial infections

Amandeep Kaur

ABBREVIATIONS

Write out what each of the following abbreviations stands for.

1. OSHA _Occupational Safety and Health Administration_
2. DNA _Deoxyribonucleic Acid_
3. RNA _Ribonucleic Acid_
4. AIDS _Acquired Immune Deficiency Syndrome_
5. HIV _Human Immunodeficiency Virus_
6. CDC _Centers for Disease Control and Prevention_
7. WBC _White Blood Cell_
8. HSV _Herpes Simplex Virus_
9. HBV _Hepatitis B Virus_
10. OPIM _Other Potentially Infectious Material_
11. PPE _Personal Protective Equipment_
12. EPA _Eicosapentaenoic Acid_

SKILLS AND CONCEPTS

Answer the following questions. Write your answer on the line or in the space provided.

A. Disease

1. A(n) _hereditary_ disease is one that is passed from one generation to another.

2. A(n) _autoimmune_ disease is one in which a person's antibodies attack his or her own tissues.

3. A(n) _degenerative_ disease results from a deterioration of the tissues and/or organs.

4. A(n) _communicable_ disease is one that is spread from person to person.

Amandeep Kaur

B. Chain of Infection

1. Label the chain of infection diagram with the following terms. Place the correct number in the chain of infection next to the corresponding letters that follow.

    Infectious agent ___A___

    Reservoir host ___B___

    Portal of exit ___E___

    Mode of transmission ___D___

    Portal of entry ___C___

    Susceptible host ___F___

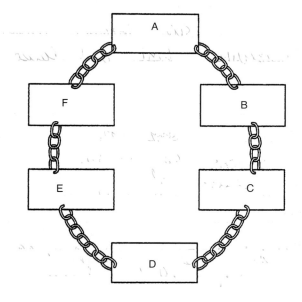

2. In your own words, describe each of the links you listed above. Give an example for each link.

    a. Infectious agent _living and non-living pathogens such as bacteria, viruses, protozoa, parasite, helminths, and prison which cause disease._

    b. Reservoir host _Spices that is infected by a parasite, and which serves as a source of infection for humans._

    c. Portal of exit _the path by which a pathogen leaves its host._

Mandeep Kaur

d. Mode of transmission _It refers as how an infectious agent can be transformed from a reservoir to host._

e. Portals of entry _site through which microorganism enter the susceptible host and cause disease._

f. Susceptible host _Organism that will feel the effects of the infectious disease that has traveled through chain of infection._

3. Describe the characteristics of the five groups of pathogenic microorganisms.

a. _Bacteria :- Tiny, simple cells that produce disease in a variety of ways. Pathogenic bacteria secrete toxin substances that can damage human tissue, act as parasites inside human cells._

b. _Virus :- Viral particles insert their own DNA or RNA into a host cell and then use the host cell to help reproduce more viral particles._

c. _Protoza :- Unicellular parasites that can replicate and multiply rapidly once inside the host._

d. _Fungi :- They are unicellular and multicellular; include organisms as mushrooms, molds and yeasts. Many forms are pathogenic and can cause disease._

e. _Helminths :- They are multicellular includs. tapeworms, roundworms, and flatworms._

Amardeep Kaur

4. Describe the infection cycle and summarize three methods that you can use to break the chain of infection in a medical facility.

Certain factors are required for infectious disease to spread.

Three methods are :-

1) Constant hand washing

2) Proper use of antiseptics.

3) Disinfection and sterilization techniques.

5. The human body has several natural protective mechanisms to defend itself from infections. Summarize them here.

- Intact skin serves as a natural barrier to disease.
- Mucous membranes protect underlying tissues and trapped foreign substances.
- Trapped substances can be expelled by sneezing and coughing.

- The natural pH of many of the body's organ discourage the growth of microbes.

C. Inflammatory Response

1. Describe the impact of the inflammatory response on the body's ability to defend itself against infection.

_____

_____

_____

_____

_____

_____

_____

_____

D. Types of Infection

1. Describe the stages of an acute infection. _____

   _____

   _____

   _____

   _____

   _____

   _____

2. In your own words, describe a latent infection and give two examples. _____

   _____

   _____

   _____

   _____

   _____

   _____

   _____

   _____

3. In your own words, define *opportunistic infections*. _____

   _____

   _____

   _____

   _____

   _____

   _____

   _____

E. Occupational Safety and Health Administration Standards for the Healthcare Setting

1. Explain the principle of Standard Precautions and list the five major areas included in the Occupational Safety and Health Administration (OSHA) compliance guidelines.

   _____

   _____

   _____

   _____

   _____

   _____

   a. _____

   b. _____

   c. _____

   d. _____

   e. _____

2. List five body fluids that have been identified as potentially infectious by the Centers for Disease Control and Prevention (CDC).

   a. _____

   b. _____

   c. _____

   d. _____

   e. _____

3. Summarize safety techniques that can be used when applying OSHA compliance guidelines to accidental blood exposure, other body fluid exposure, and needlesticks.

   _____

   _____

   _____

   _____

   _____

   _____

   _____

4. Identify four safety rules that should be followed in the ambulatory care setting to comply with the OSHA environmental protection guidelines.

   a. _____

   b. _____

   c. _____

   d. _____

F. Aseptic Techniques: Preventing Disease Transmission

1. Place a check mark beside the procedures that require the use of disposable gloves.

   a. _____ Assisting with a vaginal examination

   b. _____ Performing a routine urinalysis

   c. _____ Measuring a patient's temperature, pulse, and respirations

   d. _____ Performing a patient interview

   e. _____ Drawing blood from a 6-year-old child

2. Identify the variety of personal protective equipment (PPE) that can be used when caring for a patient with a suspected infectious disease, including protection from body fluids, secretions, excretions, blood, nonintact skin, and mucous membranes.

   _____

   _____

   _____

   _____

   _____

   _____

G. Role of the Medical Assistant in Asepsis

1. Match the following terms with the correct definition.

_____ Disinfection

_____ Medical asepsis

_____ Surgical asepsis

_____ Sanitization

_____ Sterilization

a. Removal of disease-causing organisms or destruction of the organisms
b. Destruction of all microorganisms
c. Destruction of all organisms
d. A cleansing process that reduces the number of microorganisms to a safe level
e. The process of killing pathogenic organisms or rendering them inactive

CERTIFICATION PREPARATION

Circle the correct answer.

1. What are the two important factors in performing an effective hand wash?
   a. Friction and running warm water
   b. Antibacterial soap and hot water
   c. Length of time spent and type of soap
   d. Position of the hands and temperature of the water

2. The process used to wash and remove blood and tissue from medical instruments is called
   a. asepsis.
   b. disinfection.
   c. sanitization.
   d. sterilization.

3. The method that completely destroys microorganisms is
   a. disinfection.
   b. sterilization.
   c. sanitization.
   d. boiling.

4. Based on the chain of infection, what would be the most effective method of controlling the spread of conjunctivitis in a day care center?
   a. Conjunctivitis is not contagious.
   b. Close the day care center until all children are symptom-free.
   c. Sanitize hands thoroughly after each contact with a symptomatic child.
   d. Immediately send the child home to prevent the spread of the disease.

5. Inflammation mediators that are released at the site of cellular damage perform which function?
   a. Increase blood flow to the site
   b. Increase the permeability of blood vessel walls
   c. Cause more RBCs to be attracted to the site of injury
   d. Both a and b

6. Relapse and remission are seen frequently in what types of infections?
   a. Chronic infections
   b. Latent infections
   c. Infections with rapid onset
   d. Infections that cause fever

7. Viral infections
   a. are treated effectively with antibiotics.
   b. include malaria and gonorrhea.
   c. are treated with a focus on palliative care.
   d. may form spores.

8. The immune system response called *humoral immunity* is
   a. cellular immune reactions.
   b. production of antibodies in response to a foreign substance in the body.
   c. the inflammatory process.
   d. natural protection against disease.

9. Rosa is responsible for training a new employee in medical aseptic handwashing. Which should Rosa emphasize?
   a. Using hot running water
   b. Carefully washing around all rings
   c. Using an adequate amount of soap and rubbing in a circular motion around all fingers
   d. Carefully drying the hands with a sterile disposable drape

10. The key to reducing the prevalence of antibiotic resistance is to
    a. prescribe antibiotics for all cases of the flu.
    b. order antibiotics for a minimum of 2 days.
    c. use an antibiotic that is specific to the pathogen.
    d. all of the above.

WORKPLACE APPLICATIONS

1. Rosa is explaining the signs and symptoms of inflammation to a patient. List the four classic symptoms.

   a. _____

   b. _____

   c. _____

   d. _____

2. A patient asks Rosa why the provider did not prescribe an antibiotic for her viral illness. What should Rosa say to the patient? Include in your discussion the provider's concerns about antibiotic resistance.

   _____

   _____

   _____

   _____

3. While performing venipuncture, Rosa has an accidental needlestick. Describe postexposure actions and follow-up procedures.

   _____

   _____

   _____

   _____

INTERNET ACTIVITIES

1. Visit www.osha.gov. Review the OSHA Bloodborne Pathogens Standards. Create a poster presentation, a PowerPoint presentation, or write a paper summarizing your research. Include the following points in your project:
   a. What can you do in your workplace to prevent accidental exposure to blood-borne pathogens?
   b. What types of equipment can be used to prevent accidental exposure to blood-borne pathogens?

2. Visit the Infection Control area of the CDC site at www.cdc.gov/ncidod/dhqp/index.html. Investigate the material on healthcare-associated infections. Create a poster presentation, a PowerPoint presentation, or write a paper summarizing your research. Include the following points in your project:
   a. Define *healthcare-associated infection*.
   b. What are the most common healthcare-associated infections?
   c. How can a medical assistant prevent healthcare-associated infections?

Procedure 19.1   Remove Contaminated Gloves and Discard Biohazardous Material

Name _____ Date _____ Score _____

Task: To minimize exposure to pathogens by aseptically removing and discarding contaminated gloves.

Equipment and Supplies:
- Disposable gloves
- Biohazard waste container with labeled red biohazard bag

Standard: Complete the procedure and all critical steps in _____ minutes with a minimum score of 85% within two attempts (*or as indicated by the instructor*).

Scoring: Divide the points earned by the total possible points. Failure to perform a critical step, indicated by an asterisk (*), results in grade no higher than an 84% (*or as indicated by the instructor*).

Time: Began_____ Ended_____ Total minutes: _____

Steps:	Point Value	Attempt 1	Attempt 2
1. With the dominant hand, grasp the glove of the opposite hand near the palm and begin removing the first glove. The arms should be held away from the body with the hands pointed down.	15		
2. Pull the glove inside out. After removal, ball it into the palm of the remaining gloved hand.	15		
3. Insert two fingers of the ungloved hand between the edge of the cuff of the other contaminated glove and the hand.	15		
4. Push the glove down the hand, inside out, over the contaminated glove being held, leaving the contaminated side of both gloves on the inside.	15		
5. Properly dispose of the inside-out, contaminated gloves in a biohazard waste container.	20*		
6. Perform a medical aseptic hand wash as described in Procedure 19.2 or sanitize the hands with an alcohol-based sanitizer.	20		
Total Points	100		

Comments

CAAHEP Competencies	Step(s)
III.P.1. Participate in bloodborne pathogen training	Entire procedure
ABHES Competencies	**Step(s)**
8.a. Practice standard precautions and perform disinfection/sterilization techniques	Entire procedure

Procedure 19.2   Perform Hand Hygiene

Name _____   Date _____   Score _____

Task: To minimize the number of pathogens on the hands, thus reducing the risk of transmission of pathogens.

Equipment and Supplies:
- Sink with warm running water
- Liquid soap in a dispenser (bar soap is not acceptable)
- Disposable nail brush or orange stick
- Paper towels in a dispenser
- Water-based lotion
- Covered waste container with foot pedal
- Alcohol-based hand sanitizer

Standard: Complete the procedure and all critical steps in _____ minutes with a minimum score of 85% within two attempts (*or as indicated by the instructor*).

Scoring: Divide the points earned by the total possible points. Failure to perform a critical step, indicated by an asterisk (*), results in grade no higher than an 84% (*or as indicated by the instructor*).

Time: Began_____ Ended_____ Total minutes: _____

Steps:	Point Value	Attempt 1	Attempt 2
1. Remove all jewelry except your wristwatch, if it can be pulled up above your wrist, and a plain wedding ring.	10		
2. Turn on the faucet and regulate the water temperature to lukewarm.	5		
3. Wet your hands, apply soap, and lather using a circular motion with friction while holding your fingertips downward. Rub well between your fingers. If this is the first hand wash of the day, use a nail brush or an orange stick and clean under every fingernail. Inspect your nails thoroughly.	10*		
4. Rinse well, holding your hands so that the water flows from your wrists downward to your fingertips.	10		
5. If this is the first hand wash of the day or if your hands are obviously contaminated, wet your hands again and repeat the scrubbing procedure using a vigorous, circular motion over the wrists and hands for at least 1-2 minutes.	10		
6. Rinse your hands a second time, keeping the fingers lower than your wrists.	10		
7. Dry your hands with paper towels. Do not touch the paper towel dispenser as you are obtaining towels.	10		
8. If the faucet is not foot-operated, turn it off with a dry paper towel.	10		
9. After you finish drying your hands and turning off the faucet, place used towels into a covered waste container.	10		
10. If needed, apply a water-based antibacterial hand lotion to prevent chapped or dry skin.	10		
11. Repeat the procedure as indicated throughout the day.	5		
Total Points	100		

Comments

CAAHEP Competencies	Step(s)
III.P.3. Perform handwashing	Entire procedure
ABHES Competencies	**Step(s)**
8.a. Practice standard precautions and perform disinfection/sterilization techniques	Entire procedure

Procedure 19.3   Sanitizing Soiled Instruments

Name _Amardeep Kaur_   **Date** _____   **Score** _____

Task: Remove all contaminated matter from instruments in preparation for disinfection or sterilization while following Standard Precautions and wearing appropriate personal protective equipment (PPE).

Equipment and Supplies:
- Sink with cold and hot running water
- Sanitizing agent or low-sudsing soap with enzymatic action
- Decontaminated utility gloves that show no signs of deterioration
- Chin-length face shield or goggles and face mask if contamination with blood-borne pathogens is possible
- Impermeable gown
- Disposable brush
- Disposable paper towels
- Instruments for sanitization
- Disinfectant cleaner prepared according to manufacturer's directions
- Covered waste container with foot pedal
- Biohazard waste container with labeled red biohazard bag

Standard: Complete the procedure and all critical steps in _____ minutes with a minimum score of 85% within two attempts (*or as indicated by the instructor*).

Scoring: Divide the points earned by the total possible points. Failure to perform a critical step, indicated by an asterisk (*), results in grade no higher than an 84% (*or as indicated by the instructor*).

Time: Began_____ Ended_____ Total minutes: _____

Steps:	Point Value	Attempt 1	Attempt 2
1. Put on an impermeable gown and face shield or goggles and mask if potential for splashing of infectious material exists.	10		
2. Put on utility gloves.	5		
3. Separate the sharp instruments from other instruments to be sanitized.	10		
4. Rinse the instruments under cold running water.	5		
5. Open hinged instruments and scrub all grooves, crevices, and serrations with a disposable brush.	10*		
6. Rinse well with hot water.	5		
7. Towel-dry all instruments thoroughly and dispose of contaminated towels and disposable brush in a biohazard waste container. Do not touch the paper towel dispenser as you are obtaining towels.	10		
8. Remove the utility gloves and wash your hands according to Procedure 19.2.	10		
9. Towel-dry your hands and put on gloves. Decontaminate the utility gloves and work surfaces using disinfectant cleaner.	10		
10. Dispose of the contaminated towels in a covered waste container.	5		
11. Place sanitized instruments in a designated area for disinfection or sterilization.	10		

12. Remove the gloves according to Procedure 19.1. Dispose of the gloves in a biohazard waste container. Sanitize hands.	**10**		
Total Points	**100**		

Comments   *Body Temperature, Pulse, Respiration*

CAAHEP Competencies	Step(s)
III.P.2. Select appropriate barrier/personal protective equipment	Entire procedure
ABHES Competencies	**Step(s)**
8.a. Practice standard precautions and perform disinfection/sterilization techniques	Entire procedure

Vital Signs

CAAHEP Competencies	Assessment
I.P.1.a. Measure and record: blood pressure	Procedure 20.8
I.P.1.b. Measure and record: temperature	Procedure 20.1, 20.2, 20.3, 20.4, 20.5
I.P.1.c. Measure and record: pulse	Procedure 20.6, 20.7
I.P.1.d. Measure and record: respirations	Procedure 20.7
I.P.1.i. Measure and record: pulse oximetry	Procedure 20.9
I.P.1.e. Measure and record: height	Procedure 20.10
I.P.1.f. Measure and record: weight	Procedure 20.10
II.C.1. Demonstrate knowledge of basic math computations	Skills and Concepts – B. 10 Skills and Concepts – E. 3 Skills and Concepts – H. 1

ABHES Competencies	Assessment
8. Clinical Procedures b. Obtain vital signs, obtain patient history, and formulate chief complaint	Procedure 20.1 through 20.10

VOCABULARY REVIEW

Using the word pool on the right, find the correct word to match the definition. Write the word on the line after the definition.

Group A

1. A waxy secretion in the ear canal; commonly called *ear wax* ___cerumen___

2. To shift back and forth ___fluctuate___

3. Voice box ___larynx___

4. The internal environment of the body that is compatible with life; a steady state that is created by all the body systems working together to provide a consistent and unvarying internal environment ___homeostasis___

5. A term that refers to an area outside of or away from an organ or structure ___peripheral___

6. Pertaining to an elevated body temperature ___febrile___

7. A condition of general bodily weakness or discomfort, often marking the onset of a disease ___malaise___

8. Inflammation or infection of the external auditory canal; commonly called *swimmer's ear* ___otitis externa___

9. A febrile condition or fever ___pyrexia___

10. Fluctuations that occur during each day ___diurnal variation___

Word Pool
- homeostasis
- diurnal variation
- febrile
- pyrexia
- fluctuate
- malaise
- otitis externa
- cerumen
- peripheral
- larynx

Group B

1. A slow heartbeat; a pulse below 60 beats per minute ___bradycardia___

2. To close, shut, or stop up ___occlude___

3. A term used to describe a pulse that feels full because of increased power of cardiac contraction or as a result of increased blood volume ___bounding___

4. An irregular heartbeat that originates in the sinoatrial node (pacemaker) ___sinus arrhythmia___

5. To listen with a stethoscope ___auscultated___

6. A rapid but regular heart rate; one that exceeds 100 beats per minute ___tachycardia___

7. Difficult and/or painful breathing ___dyspnea___

8. A condition in which the radial pulse is less than the apical pulse; it may indicate a peripheral vascular abnormality ___pulse deficit___

9. A term describing a pulse that is thin and feeble ___thready___

10. A pulse in which beats occasionally are skipped ___intermittent pulse___

Word Pool
- bradycardia
- tachycardia
- pulse deficit
- intermittent pulse
- sinus arrhythmia
- bounding
- thready
- occlude
- auscultated
- dyspnea

Group C

1. Abnormally rapid breathing ___tachypnea___
2. Abnormally slow breathing ___bradypnea___
3. Whistling sound made during breathing
   ___wheezing___
4. Excessively deep breathing ___hyperpnea___
5. An abnormal lung sound heard on auscultation, characterized by discontinuous bubbling noises ___rales___
6. A progressive, irreversible lung condition that results in diminished lung capacity ___COPD___
7. Condition of difficult breathing unless in an upright position ___orthopnea___
8. Abnormal, periodic cessation of breathing
   ___apnea___
9. Rapid, shallow breathing ___hyperventilation___
10. Deep, rapid breathing followed by a period of apnea
    ___Cheyne – Stokes respiration___

Word Pool
- chronic obstructive pulmonary disease (COPD)
- bradypnea
- apnea
- tachypnea
- hyperpnea
- hyperventilation
- orthopnea
- wheezing
- Cheyne-Stokes respiration
- rales

Group D

1. Elevated blood pressure of unknown cause that develops for no apparent reason; sometimes called *primary hypertension*
   ___essential hypertension___
2. Heavy snoring ___stertorous___
3. A temporary fall in blood pressure when a person rapidly changes from a recumbent position to a standing position
   ___orthostatic (postural)___
4. To determine or check readings with those of a standard
   ___calibrated___
5. Abnormal rumbling sound heard on auscultation, caused by airways blocked by secretions or muscle contractions
   ___rhonchi___
6. A condition in which extra lymph fluid builds up in tissues and causes swelling ___lymphedema___
7. The difference between the systolic and diastolic blood pressures
   ___pulse pressure___
8. Middle layer and the thickest layer of the heart; composed of cardiac muscles ___myocardium___
9. Of unknown cause ___idiopathic___
10. Thickening, decreased elasticity, and calcification of arterial walls
    ___arteriosclerosis___
11. Fainting; a brief lapse in consciousness ___syncope___
12. Dizziness; abnormal sensation of movement when there is none
    ___vertigo___
13. Blood pressure that is below normal (systolic pressure below 90 mm Hg and diastolic pressure below 50 mm Hg)
    ___hypotension___

Word Pool
- rhonchi
- stertorous
- vertigo
- pulse pressure
- arteriosclerosis
- myocardium
- essential hypertension
- idiopathic
- hypotension
- orthostatic (postural) hypotension
- syncope
- calibrated
- lymphedema

ABBREVIATIONS

Write out what each of the following abbreviations stands for.

1. BMI _Body Mass Index_
2. TPR _Temperature, Pulse, Respiration_
3. BP _Blood Pressure_
4. SpO$_2$ _____
5. PAP _Papanicolaou Test_
6. CPR _Cardiopulmonary Resuscitation_
7. COPD _Chronic Obstructive Pulmonary Disease_
8. CHF _Congestive Heart Failure_
9. CNS _Central Nervous System_

SKILLS AND CONCEPTS

Answer the following questions. Write your answer on the line or in the space provided.

A. Factors that May Influence Vital Signs

1. Vital signs can be influenced by _____ and _____ factors.

2. A medical assistant should be aware of _____ that could indicate discomfort or pain.

B. Temperature

1. A(n) _continuous_ fever rises and falls only slightly during a 24-hour period. It remains above the patient's average normal range.

2. A(n) _intermittent_ fever comes and goes, or it spikes and then returns to the average range.

3. A(n) _remittent_ fever fluctuates greatly (more than 3°F) but does not return to the average range.

4. _Axillary_ temperatures are approximately 1°F lower than accurate oral readings.

5. _Tympanic_ thermometers are an accurate means of taking temperatures in adults and older children because of the closeness to the hypothalamus.

6. _Temporal_ temperatures are an easy, noninvasive, and accurate alternative to taking rectal temperatures in infants.

7. Medication to reduce a fever is called a(n) _antipyretic_.

8. Tympanic thermometers should not be used if the patient has _otitis externa_ or _cerumen_.

9. Temperatures considered febrile include the following:

   a. Aural (ear) temperatures higher than _100.4_ °F (38°C)

   b. Oral temperatures higher than _99.5_ °F (37.8°C)

   c. Axillary temperatures higher than _98.6_ °F (37.2°C)

10. Use the following formulas to convert the temperatures in the chart from one system to the other. Round answers to the nearest tenth.

    Fahrenheit to Celsius: Celsius to Fahrenheit:
    °C = (°F − 32) / 1.8   °F = (°C × 1.8) + 32

    98.6°F = _____ °C

    39.5°C = _____ °F

    97.6°F = _____ °C

    99.4°F = _____ °C

    40°C = _____ °F

    36°C = _____ °F

    38.5°C = _____ °F

    41°C = _____ °F

    102°F = _____ °C

    37.5°C = _____ °F

11. List and describe four factors that may affect body temperature.

    a. _____

    _____

    _____

    b. _____

    _____

    _____

    c. _____

    _____

    _____

    d. _____

    _____

    _____

C. Types of Thermometers and Their Uses

1. When taking an oral temperature, what should the medical assistant ask the patient? _Have you had anything hot or cold, smoked or chewed gum?_

2. A(n) _blue_ probe is used to take an oral temperature and a(n) _red_ probe is used to take a rectal temperature.

3. Explain how to expose the tympanic membrane before taking an aural temperature in children younger than 3 years and those older than 3 years.
   To expose the tympanic membrane in children younger than age 3, gently pull the earlobe down and back; for patients older than age 3, gently pull the pinna (top the ear) up and back.

4. Explain the procedure for taking a temperature using a temporal artery thermometer. _Place the probe in the center of forehead, Depress the button on the scanner and gently stroke the probe across the forehead toward hairline, keep the probe flat on patient's skin, The highest measurement is recorded._

D. Pulse

1. List eight pulse sites and label their correct locations on the figure.

   a. _Temporal pulse_
   b. _carotid pulse_
   c. _Apical pulse_
   d. _Brachial pulse_
   e. _radial pulse_
   f. _femoral pulse_
   g. _popliteal pulse_
   h. _dorsalis pedis pulse_

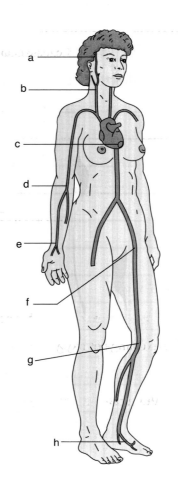

2. What three characteristics should the medical assistant note while measuring a pulse?

   a. Rate

   b. Rhythm

   c. Volume

3. A patient with a significant difference between the apical and brachial pulse counts has a(n) irregular heartbeat.

4. A patient who is anxious or in pain may have an increase in the pulse rate, which is called hyperventilation.

5. The brachial pulse, which is palpated before the blood pressure is taken, is located in the bend of the elbow.

6. Sinus Arrythmia is when the heart rate varies with respirations.

7. The Apical pulse is the most accurate method of taking the pulse of infants and of patients with an arrhythmia.

8. Describe the three-point scale for recording pulse volume. Three-Point scale for measuring pressure. 1) Full, bounding pulse: Pulsation is very strong and doesnot disppear with moderate. 2) Normal pulse: Pulsation is easily felt but disappears with moderate pressure. 3) weak, thready pulse: Pulsation is not easily felt and disappears with slightly pressure.

9. Why might the medical assistant opt to take an adult patient's apical pulse rather than radial? Reason is that you noted irregularities in the heart rate when palpating the radial pulse. Therefore, you should listen to an apical pulse for a full minute to make sure you are accurately counting the no. of beats per min.

10. Explain where to place the stethoscope head when taking an apical pulse. Place the stethoscope at the junction of the fifth intercostal space and the midclavicular line on the left side of the patient's chest.

E. Respiration

1. One full respiration includes both inspiration and expiration.

2. The exchange of oxygen and carbon dioxide in the lungs is called restoration.

3. Carlos counts eight respirations for 30 seconds. The rate is 16 respirations per minute.

4. Breathing rates are controlled by the respiratory center, which is located in the medulla oblongata of the brain.

5. List the three characteristics of respirations.

   a. _Rate_

   b. _Rhythm_

   c. _Depth_

F. Blood Pressure

1. Blood pressure reflects the pressure of the blood against the walls of the _arteries_.

2. Blood pressure is recorded as a fraction; the _Systolic_ reading is the numerator (top number), and the _Diastolic_ reading is the denominator (bottom number).

3. When you subtract the diastolic pressure from the systolic pressure, you get the _Blood Pressure_.

4. _Systole_ is the contraction of the heart.

5. _Diastole_ reflects the relaxation of the heart.

6. Differentiate between essential and secondary hypertension. _____

   _____

   _____

   _____

   _____

7. List and describe the five Korotkoff sounds.

   a. _____

   _____

   b. _____

   _____

   c. _____

   _____

   d. _____

   _____

   e. _____

   _____

8. Discuss the importance of using a correct blood pressure cuff size when monitoring patient blood pressures.

_____

_____

_____

_____

9. Describe how to apply a blood pressure cuff. Why is it important that the edge of the cuff is above the antecubital space?

_____

_____

_____

_____

_____

_____

10. Describe four physiologic factors that can affect an individual's blood pressure.

    a. _____

    b. _____

    c. _____

    d. _____

11. Explain the effects of patient body position on blood pressure. Describe the ideal body position for taking the most accurate blood pressure.

_____

_____

_____

_____

_____

_____

12. Explain four common causes of errors in blood pressure readings. _____

_____

_____

_____

G. Pulse Oximetry

1. List conditions for which a pulse oximetry may be used to assess a patient's oxygenation status.

   _____

   _____

2. A normal pulse oximetry reading would be _____ or higher.

H. Anthropometric Measurements

1. Use the formulas below to convert the following weights from one system to the other.

To Convert Kilograms to Pounds
1 kg = 2.2 lb
Multiply the number of kilograms by 2.2.

To Convert Pounds to Kilograms
1 lb = 0.45 kg
Multiply the number of pounds by 0.45, or divide the number of pounds by 2.2 kg.

145 lb =   _____ kg

54 kg =   _____ lb

60 kg =   _____ lb

112 lb =   _____ kg

50 lb =   _____ kg

CERTIFICATION PREPARATION

Circle the correct answer.

1. How long should the pulse be counted for the most accurate results?
   a. 15 seconds
   b. 30 seconds
   c. 45 seconds
   d. 1 minute

2. What would be considered a normal pulse for an average-sized 37-year-old patient in good health?
   a. 45 beats per minute
   b. 52 beats per minute
   c. 66 beats per minute
   d. 110 beats per minute

3. Which pulse is palpated on the wrist?
   a. Apical
   b. Brachial
   c. Carotid
   d. Radial

4. If a patient is diagnosed with secondary hypertension, this means that the
   a. patient has the most severe form of hypertension.
   b. hypertension is associated with another disease.
   c. patient has the most common form of hypertension.
   d. condition has worsened from essential hypertension.

5. As a blood pressure cuff is deflated, the first tapping sound is the _____ pressure.
   a. mean arterial
   b. systolic
   c. diastolic
   d. pulse

6. The diastolic BP is heard during which Korotkoff phase?
   a. I
   b. II
   c. IV
   d. V

7. How can you help patients feel comfortable about having their weight measured in the office?
   a. Place the scale in a private area of the office.
   b. Reassure them that their weight is at a healthy level.
   c. Have them remain in their shoes and outer clothing.
   d. Allow them to weigh themselves at home and bring in the results.

8. In a healthy adult at rest, the ratio of respirations to pulse beats is typically
   a. 1:3.
   b. 1:4.
   c. 1:5.
   d. 1:8.

9. Mr. Garcia weighs 250 pounds. You are expected to record this weight in kilograms. It is equal to _____ kg.
   a. 113.6
   b. 550.0
   c. 56.8
   d. 226.0

10. Which respiration characteristic frequently occurs in patients with congestive heart failure and COPD?
    a. Orthopnea
    b. Wheezing
    c. Hyperventilation
    d. Hyperpnea

WORKPLACE APPLICATIONS

1. Mrs. Parker stops at the clinic on her way home from work. She does not have an appointment to see the provider but asks if Carlos can take her blood pressure because she hasn't been "feeling herself" the last few days.

   a. Carlos is not sure whether he should use a normal adult-size blood pressure cuff or a large adult cuff. How would he be able to tell if he needs the large adult cuff? Why is this important?

   _____

   _____

   _____

   _____

   b. Carlos has obtained a blood pressure reading of 150/94 mm Hg in the left arm and 160/98 mm Hg in the right arm. Should Carlos wait for a few minutes and then take the pressures again? Why or why not? Concerned about the readings, Carlos decides the patient should see the provider. What type of questions might Carlos want to ask Mrs. Parker?

   _____

   _____

   _____

   _____

2. Sarah, an 18-month-old patient, is being seen today for a possible ear infection. The best method of taking her temperature is _____. Her mother is concerned because Sarah's temperature has been fluctuating between normal and high levels for 2 days; this is called a(n) _____ fever. Carlos should take Sarah's pulse using the _____ method. Sarah's mother has a digital thermometer at home.

   a. What would be the best method she could use to take the baby's temperature and why? _____

   _____

   _____

   _____

   b. What patient education should Carlos give Sarah's mother about taking axillary temperatures accurately?

   _____

   _____

   _____

3. Carlos is responsible for training a new medical assistant in the Occupational Safety and Health Administration (OSHA) guidelines for preventing disease transmission when taking vital signs. What important factors should Carlos include?

   _____

   _____

   _____

INTERNET ACTIVITIES

1. Visit www.heart.org/HBP. Review the links found on this page. Create a poster presentation, a PowerPoint presentation, or write a paper summarizing your research. Include the following points in your project:
   a. What are the blood pressure categories? List the name of the category as well as the systolic and diastolic numbers.
   b. Why is high blood pressure considered the "silent killer"?
   c. How can high blood pressure harm your health?
   d. List tools and resources available for patients.

2. Investigate the patient education materials available at the American Lung Association site (www.lung.org/lung-disease/copd) for individuals with COPD. Create a poster presentation, a PowerPoint presentation, or write a paper summarizing your research. Include the following points in your project:
   a. Describe COPD, including symptoms, causes, risk factors, and examples.
   b. How is COPD diagnosed and treated?
   c. What assistance is available for those patients living with COPD?

Procedure 20.1 Obtain an Oral Temperature Using a Digital Thermometer

Name _____ Date _____ Score _____

Task: To accurately obtain and record a patient's oral temperature using a digital thermometer.

Equipment and Supplies:
- Patient's record
- Digital thermometer and probe covers
- Biohazard waste container

Standard: Complete the procedure and all critical steps in _____ minutes with a minimum score of 85% within two attempts (*or as indicated by the instructor*).

Scoring: Divide the points earned by the total possible points. Failure to perform a critical step, indicated by an asterisk (*), results in grade no higher than an 84% (*or as indicated by the instructor*).

Time: Began_____ Ended_____ Total minutes: _____

Steps:	Point Value	Attempt 1	Attempt 2
1. Wash hands or use hand sanitizer.	15*		
2. Assemble the needed equipment and supplies.	10		
3. Greet the patient. Identify yourself. Verify the patient's identity with full name and date of birth. Explain the procedure to be performed in a manner that is understood by the patient. Answer any questions the patient may have on the procedure. Make sure the patient has not eaten, consumed any hot or cold fluids, smoked, or exercised during the 15 minutes before the temperature is measured.	10		
4. Prepare the probe for use as described in the directions. Make sure probe covers are always used.	10		
5. Place the probe under the patient's tongue and instruct the patient to close the mouth tightly without biting down on the thermometer. Help the patient by holding the probe end, or the patient can hold the probe end if that is more comfortable.	15*		
6. When a beep is heard, remove the probe from the patient's mouth and immediately eject the probe cover into an appropriate biohazard waste container.	10		
7. Note the reading on the display screen of the thermometer.	10		
8. Wash hands or use hand sanitizer and disinfect the equipment as indicated.	10		
9. Document the reading in the patient's health record.	10*		
Total Points	100		

Documentation

Comments

CAAHEP Competencies	Step(s)
I.P.1.b. Measure and record: temperature	Entire procedure
ABHES Competencies	**Step(s)**
8.b. Obtain vital signs, obtain patient history, and formulate chief complaint	Entire procedure

Procedure 20.2 Obtain an Axillary Temperature Using a Digital Thermometer

Name _____ Date _____ Score _____

Task: To accurately determine and record a patient's axillary temperature using a digital thermometer.

Equipment and Supplies:
- Patient's record
- Digital thermometer and probe cover
- Supply of tissues
- Patient gown as needed
- Biohazard waste container

Standard: Complete the procedure and all critical steps in _____ minutes with a minimum score of 85% within two attempts (*or as indicated by the instructor*).

Scoring: Divide the points earned by the total possible points. Failure to perform a critical step, indicated by an asterisk (*), results in grade no higher than an 84% (*or as indicated by the instructor*).

Time: Began_____ Ended_____ Total minutes: _____

Steps:	Point Value	Attempt 1	Attempt 2
1. Wash hands or use hand sanitizer.	10*		
2. Gather the needed equipment and supplies.	5		
3. Greet the patient. Identify yourself. Verify the patient's identity with full name and date of birth. Explain the procedure to be performed in a manner that is understood by the patient. Answer any questions the patient may have on the procedure.	10		
4. Prepare the thermometer in the same manner as for oral use.	5		
5. Expose the axillary region. If necessary, provide the patient with a gown for privacy.	5		
6. Pat the patient's axillary area dry with tissues if needed.	5		
7. Place the probe tip into the center of the armpit. Making sure the thermometer is touching only skin, not clothing.	10*		
8. Instruct the patient to hold the arm snugly across the chest or abdomen until the thermometer beeps.	10		
9. Remove the thermometer, note the digital reading, and dispose of the cover in the biohazard waste container.	10		
10. Disinfect the thermometer if indicated.	10		
11. Wash hands or use hand sanitizer.	10*		
12. Document the reading in the patient's health record.	10*		
Total Points	100		

Documentation

Comments

CAAHEP Competencies	Step(s)
I.P.1.b. Measure and record: temperature	Entire procedure
ABHES Competencies	**Step(s)**
8.b. Obtain vital signs, obtain patient history, and formulate chief complaint	Entire procedure

Procedure 20.3   Obtain a Rectal Temperature of an Infant Using a Digital Thermometer

Name _____ Date _____ Score _____

Task: To accurately determine and record a patient's rectal temperature using a digital thermometer.

Equipment and Supplies:
- Patient's record
- Digital thermometer and probe covers
- Gloves
- Water-soluble lubricant (KY Jelly)
- Biohazard waste container

Standard: Complete the procedure and all critical steps in _____ minutes with a minimum score of 85% within two attempts (*or as indicated by the instructor*).

Scoring: Divide the points earned by the total possible points. Failure to perform a critical step, indicated by an asterisk (*), results in grade no higher than an 84% (*or as indicated by the instructor*).

Time: Began_____ Ended_____ Total minutes: _____

Steps:	Point Value	Attempt 1	Attempt 2
1. Wash hands or use hand sanitizer.	10*		
2. Assemble the needed equipment and supplies. Make sure that the red probe is used.	5		
3. Greet the patient. Identify yourself. Verify the patient's identity with full name and date of birth. Explain the procedure to be performed in a manner that is understood by the patient. Answer any questions the patient may have on the procedure.	10		
4. Have the parent or caregiver undress the infant.	5		
5. Put on gloves.	5		
6. Prepare the probe for use as described in the directions. Make sure probe covers are always used. Lubricate first two inches of probe.	5		
7. Gently insert the thermometer probe 1/2 inch for infants, 5/8 inch for children, 1 inch for adults. Remain with the patient at all times and hold the thermometer in place until a beep is heard.	10*		
8. Remove the probe and immediately eject the probe cover into an appropriate biohazard waste container.	10		
9. Note the reading on the display screen of the thermometer.	10		
10. Remove soiled gloves and discard into an appropriate biohazard waste container.	10		
11. Wash hands or use hand sanitizer and disinfect the equipment as indicated.	10*		
12. Document the reading in the patient's health record.	10*		
Total Points	100		

Documentation

Comments

CAAHEP Competencies	Step(s)
I.P.1.b. Measure and record: temperature	Entire procedure
ABHES Competencies	**Step(s)**
8.b. Obtain vital signs, obtain patient history, and formulate chief complaint	Entire procedure

Procedure 20.4 Obtain a Temperature Using a Tympanic Thermometer

Name _____ Date _____ Score _____

Task: To accurately determine and record a patient's temperature using a tympanic thermometer.

Equipment and Supplies:
- Patient's record
- Alcohol wipes (optional)
- Tympanic thermometer and probe covers

Standard: Complete the procedure and all critical steps in _____ minutes with a minimum score of 85% within two attempts (*or as indicated by the instructor*).

Scoring: Divide the points earned by the total possible points. Failure to perform a critical step, indicated by an asterisk (*), results in grade no higher than an 84% (*or as indicated by the instructor*).

Time: Began_____ Ended_____ Total minutes: _____

Steps:	Point Value	Attempt 1	Attempt 2
1. Wash hands or use hand sanitizer.	15*		
2. Gather the necessary equipment and supplies.	10		
3. Greet the patient. Identify yourself. Verify the patient's identity with full name and date of birth. Explain the procedure to be performed in a manner that is understood by the patient. Answer any questions the patient may have on the procedure.	10		
4. Clean the probe with an alcohol wipe if indicated. Place a disposable cover on the probe.	10		
5. Insert the probe into the ear canal far enough to seal the opening. Do not apply pressure. For children younger than age 3, gently pull the earlobe down and back; for patients older than age 3, gently pull the top of the ear (pinna) up and back.	15*		
6. Press the button on the probe as directed. The temperature will appear on the display screen in 1-2 seconds.	10		
7. Remove the probe, note the reading, and discard the probe cover into a biohazard waste container without touching it.	10		
8. Wash hands or use hand sanitizer and disinfect the equipment if indicated.	10*		
9. Document the reading in the patient's health record.	10*		
Total Points	100		

Documentation

Comments

CAAHEP Competencies	Step(s)
I.P.1.b. Measure and record: temperature	Entire procedure
ABHES Competencies	**Step(s)**
8.b. Obtain vital signs, obtain patient history, and formulate chief complaint	Entire procedure

Procedure 20.5   Obtain a Temperature Using a Temporal Artery Thermometer

Name _____ Date _____ Score _____

Task: To accurately determine and record a patient's temperature using a temporal artery thermometer.

Equipment and Supplies:
- Patient's record
- Professional temporal artery thermometer with probe covers
- Alcohol wipes
- Waste container

Standard: Complete the procedure and all critical steps in _____ minutes with a minimum score of 85% within two attempts (*or as indicated by the instructor*).

Scoring: Divide the points earned by the total possible points. Failure to perform a critical step, indicated by an asterisk (*), results in grade no higher than an 84% (*or as indicated by the instructor*).

Time: Began_____ Ended_____ Total minutes: _____

Steps:	Point Value	Attempt 1	Attempt 2
1. Wash hands or use hand sanitizer.	10*		
2. Gather the necessary equipment and supplies.	5		
3. Greet the patient. Identify yourself. Verify the patient's identity with full name and date of birth. Explain the procedure to be performed in a manner that is understood by the patient. Answer any questions the patient may have on the procedure.	5		
4. Remove the protective cap on the probe. Depending on the facility's infection control procedures, disposable covers can be used on the scanner, or it can be cleaned by lightly wiping the surface with an alcohol wipe.	10		
5. Push the patient's hair up off the forehead to expose the site. Gently place the probe on the patient's forehead, halfway between the edge of the eyebrows and the hairline, at the center of the face (just above the nose).	10*		
6. Depress and hold the SCAN button and lightly glide the probe sideways across the patient's forehead to the hairline just above the ear. As you move the sensor across the forehead, you will hear a beep, and a red light will flash.	10		
7. Keeping the button depressed, lift the thermometer, and place the probe behind the ear lobe. The thermometer may continue to beep, indicating that the temperature is rising.	10		
8. When scanning is complete, release the button and lift the probe. Note the temperature recorded on the digital display. The scanner automatically turns off 15-30 seconds after release of the button.	10		
9. If a probe cover was used, eject it directly into a biohazard waste container. Disinfect the thermometer if indicated and replace the protective cap.	10		
10. Wash hands or use hand sanitizer.	10*		
11. Document the reading in the patient's health record.	10*		
Total Points	100		

Documentation

Comments

CAAHEP Competencies	Step(s)
I.P.1.b. Measure and record: temperature	Entire procedure
ABHES Competencies	**Step(s)**
8.b. Obtain vital signs, obtain patient history, and formulate chief complaint	Entire procedure

Procedure 20.6 Obtain an Apical Pulse

Name _____ **Date** _____ **Score** _____

Task: To accurately determine and record the patient's apical heart rate.

Equipment and Supplies:
- Patient's record
- Watch with a second hand
- Patient gown as needed
- Stethoscope
- Alcohol wipes

Standard: Complete the procedure and all critical steps in _____ minutes with a minimum score of 85% within two attempts (*or as indicated by the instructor*).

Scoring: Divide the points earned by the total possible points. Failure to perform a critical step, indicated by an asterisk (*), results in grade no higher than an 84% (*or as indicated by the instructor*).

Time: Began_____ Ended_____ Total minutes: _____

Steps:	Point Value	Attempt 1	Attempt 2
1. Wash hands or use hand sanitizer and clean the stethoscope earpieces and diaphragm with alcohol wipes.	10*		
2. Greet the patient. Identify yourself. Verify the patient's identity with full name and date of birth. Explain the procedure to be performed in a manner that is understood by the patient. Answer any questions the patient may have on the procedure.	10		
3. If necessary, assist the patient in disrobing from the waist up and provide the patient with a gown that opens in the front.	5		
4. Assist the patient into the sitting or supine position.	5		
5. Hold the stethoscope's diaphragm against the palm of your hand for a few seconds.	10		
6. Place the stethoscope at the left midclavicular line at the fifth intercostal space over the apex of the heart. Do not touch the bell end of the stethoscope.	10*		
7. Listen carefully for the heartbeat. Count the pulse for 1 full minute. Note any irregularities in rhythm and volume.	10*		
8. Help the patient sit up and dress.	10		
9. Disinfect the stethoscope with an alcohol wipe.	10		
10. Wash hands or use hand sanitizer.	10*		
11. Document the reading in the patient's health record.	10*		
Total Points	100		

Documentation

Comments

CAAHEP Competencies	Step(s)
I.P.1.c. Measure and record: pulse	Entire procedure
ABHES Competencies	**Step(s)**
8.b. Obtain vital signs, obtain patient history, and formulate chief complaint	Entire procedure

Procedure 20.7 Assess the Patient's Radial Pulse and Respiratory Rate

Name _____ Date _____ Score _____

Task: To accurately determine and document a patient's radial pulse rate, rhythm, and volume; and respiratory rate, rhythm, and depth.

Equipment and Supplies:
- Patient's record
- Watch with a second hand

Standard: Complete the procedure and all critical steps in _____ minutes with a minimum score of 85% within two attempts (*or as indicated by the instructor*).

Scoring: Divide the points earned by the total possible points. Failure to perform a critical step, indicated by an asterisk (*), results in grade no higher than an 84% (*or as indicated by the instructor*).

Time: Began_____ Ended_____ Total minutes: _____

Steps:	Point Value	Attempt 1	Attempt 2
1. Wash hands or use hand sanitizer.	10*		
2. Greet the patient. Identify yourself. Verify the patient's identity with full name and date of birth. Explain the procedure to be performed in a manner that is understood by the patient. Answer any questions the patient may have on the procedure.	10		
3. Place the patient's arm in a relaxed position, palm at or below the level of the heart.	5		
4. Gently grasp the palm side of the patient's wrist with your first two or three fingertips approximately 1 inch below the base of the thumb.	5		
5. Count the beats for 1 full minute using a watch with a second hand.	10*		
6. While counting the beats, also assess the rhythm and volume of the patient's pulse.	10*		
7. While continuing to hold the patient's arm in the same position used to count the radial pulse, observe the rise and fall of the patient's chest. If you have difficulty noticing the patient's breathing, place the arm across the chest to detect movement.	5		
8. Inhalation and exhalation make up one complete breathing cycle or respiration. Count the respirations for 30 seconds and multiply by 2.	10*		
9. While counting the respirations, also assess the rhythm and depth of the patient's respirations.	10*		
10. Release the patient's wrist.	5		
11. Wash hands or use hand sanitizer.	10*		
12. Document the readings in the patient's health record.	10*		
Total Points	100		

Documentation

Comments

CAAHEP Competencies	Step(s)
I.P.1.c. Measure and record: pulse	Entire procedure
I.P.1.d. Measure and record: respirations	Entire procedure
ABHES Competencies	**Step(s)**
8.b. Obtain vital signs, obtain patient history, and formulate chief complaint	Entire procedure

Procedure 20.8 Determine a Patient's Blood Pressure

Name _____ Date _____ Score _____

Task: To perform a blood pressure measurement that is correct in technique, accurate, and comfortable for the patient.

Equipment and Supplies:
- Patient's record
- Sphygmomanometer
- Stethoscope
- Antiseptic wipes/alcohol wipes

Standard: Complete the procedure and all critical steps in _____ minutes with a minimum score of 85% within two attempts (*or as indicated by the instructor*).

Scoring: Divide the points earned by the total possible points. Failure to perform a critical step, indicated by an asterisk (*), results in grade no higher than an 84% (*or as indicated by the instructor*).

Time: Began_____ Ended_____ Total minutes: _____

Steps:	Point Value	Attempt 1	Attempt 2
1. Wash hands or use hand sanitizer.	5*		
2. Assemble the equipment and supplies needed. Clean the earpieces and diaphragm of the stethoscope with alcohol wipes.	5*		
3. Greet the patient. Identify yourself. Verify the patient's identity with full name and date of birth. Explain the procedure to be performed in a manner that is understood by the patient. Answer any questions the patient may have on the procedure.	3		
4. Select the appropriate arm for application of the cuff (no mastectomy on that side, no injury or disease). If the patient has had a bilateral mastectomy, the blood pressure should be taken using a large thigh cuff with the stethoscope over the popliteal artery.	3		
5. Seat the patient in a comfortable position with the legs uncrossed and the arm resting, palm up, at heart level on the arm of a chair or a table next to where the patient is seated.	2		
6. Roll up the sleeve to about 5 inches above the elbow or have the patient remove the arm from the sleeve.	2		
7. Select the correct cuff size.	5*		
8. Palpate the brachial artery at the antecubital space in both arms. If one arm has a stronger pulse, use that arm. If the pulses are equal, select the right arm.	5		
9. Center the cuff bladder over the brachial artery with the connecting tube away from the patient's body and the tube to the bulb close to the body.	5		
10. Place the lower edge of the cuff about 1 inch above the palpable brachial pulse, normally located in the natural crease of the inner elbow, and wrap it snugly and smoothly.	3		
11. Position the gauge of the sphygmomanometer so that it is easily seen.	2		

12.	Palpate the radial pulse, tighten the screw valve on the air pump, and inflate the cuff until the pulse can no longer be felt. Make a note at the point on the gauge where the pulse could no longer be felt. Mentally add 30 mm Hg to the reading. Deflate the cuff and wait 15 seconds.	**5**		
13.	Insert the earpieces of the stethoscope turned forward into the ear canals.	**5**		
14.	Place the stethoscope's diaphragm over the palpated brachial artery for an adult patient or the bell for a pediatric patient. Press firmly enough to obtain a seal but not so tightly that the artery is constricted. Only touch the edges of the stethoscope head.	**5**		
15.	Close the valve and squeeze the bulb to inflate the cuff, rapidly but smoothly, to 30 mm above the palpated systolic level, which was previously determined.	**5**		
16.	Open the valve slightly and deflate the cuff at a constant rate of 2 to 3 mm Hg per heartbeat.	**5**		
17.	Listen throughout the entire deflation; note the point on the gauge at which you hear the first sound (systolic), the last sound (diastolic) and until the sounds have stopped for at least 10 mm Hg.	**5**		
18.	Do not reinflate the cuff once the air has been released. Wait 30-60 seconds to repeat the procedure if needed.	**5**		
19.	Remove the cuff from the patient's arm.	**5**		
20.	Remove the stethoscope from your ears and document the systolic and diastolic readings and the arm used as BP systolic/diastolic.	**5**		
21.	Clean the earpieces and the head of the stethoscope with an alcohol wipe and return both the cuff and the stethoscope to storage.	**5**		
22.	Wash hands or use hand sanitizer.	**5***		
23.	Document the readings in the patient's health record.	**5***		
	Total Points	**100**		

Documentation

Comments

CAAHEP Competencies	Step(s)
I.P.1.a. Measure and record: blood pressure	Entire procedure
ABHES Competencies	**Step(s)**
8.b. Obtain vital signs, obtain patient history, and formulate chief complaint	Entire procedure

Procedure 20.9 Perform Pulse Oximetry

Name _____ Date _____ Score _____

Task: To assess the adequacy of oxygen levels (or oxygen saturation) in the blood using a pulse oximeter.

Equipment and Supplies:
- Patient's health record
- Pulse oximeter and appropriately sized probe

Standard: Complete the procedure and all critical steps in _____ minutes with a minimum score of 85% within two attempts (*or as indicated by the instructor*).

Scoring: Divide the points earned by the total possible points. Failure to perform a critical step, indicated by an asterisk (*), results in grade no higher than an 84% (*or as indicated by the instructor*).

Time: Began_____ Ended_____ Total minutes: _____

Steps:	Point Value	Attempt 1	Attempt 2
1. Wash hands or use hand sanitizer.	15*		
2. Assemble the equipment.	10		
3. Greet the patient. Identify yourself. Verify the patient's identity with full name and date of birth. Explain the procedure to be performed in a manner that is understood by the patient. Answer any questions the patient may have on the procedure.	10		
4. Turn on the monitor and attach the probe to the finger (preferred) or ear lobe so it is flush with the skin.	10		
5. The light-emitting diode (LED) should be placed on top of the nail. If the patient is wearing nail polish or has artificial nails, these may have to be removed to get a strong pulse signal.	15*		
6. Sanitize the patient probe and the external portion of the monitor with an aseptic cleaner.	10*		
7. Wash hands or use hand sanitizer.	15*		
8. Document the oxygen saturation percentage and pulse in patient's health record. Include date, time, and if the patient is receiving supplemental oxygen record the amount in liters.	15*		
Total Points	100		

Documentation

Comments

CAAHEP Competencies	Step(s)
I.P.1.i. Measure and record: pulse oximetry	Entire procedure
ABHES Competencies	**Step(s)**
8.b. Obtain vital signs, obtain patient history, and formulate chief complaint	Entire procedure

Procedure 20.10   Measuring a Patient's Weight and Height

Name _____ Date _____ Score _____

Task: To accurately weigh and measure a patient as part of the physical assessment procedure.

Equipment and Supplies:
- Balance beam scale with a measuring bar
- Paper towel
- Patient record

Standard: Complete the procedure and all critical steps in _____ minutes with a minimum score of 85% within two attempts (*or as indicated by the instructor*).

Scoring: Divide the points earned by the total possible points. Failure to perform a critical step, indicated by an asterisk (*), results in grade no higher than an 84% (*or as indicated by the instructor*).

Time: Began_____ Ended_____ Total minutes: _____

Steps:	Point Value	Attempt 1	Attempt 2
1. Wash hands or use hand sanitizer.	5*		
2. Greet the patient. Identify yourself. Verify the patient's identity with full name and date of birth. Explain the procedure to be performed in a manner that is understood by the patient. Answer any questions the patient may have on the procedure.	5		
3. Have the patient remove his or her shoes. Place a paper towel on the scale platform. Check to see that the balance bar pointer floats in the middle of the balance frame when all weights are at zero.	5		
4. Help the patient onto the scale. Make sure the patient has removed any heavy objects from pockets and is not holding anything such as a jacket or purse.	5		
5. Move the large weight into the groove closest to the patient's estimated weight.	5		
6. While the patient is standing still, slide the small upper weight to the right along the pound markers until the pointer balances in the middle of the balance frame.	10*		
7. Leave the weights in place.	5		
8. Ask the patient to step off the scale and move the height bar to a point above the patient's height. Extend the bar and ask the patient step back on the scale.	5		
9. Adjust the height bar so that it just touches the top of the patient's head.	5		
10. Leave the elevation bar set.	5		
11. Assist the patient off the scale. Make sure all items that were removed for weighing are given back to the patient.	5		
12. Read the weight scale. Add the numbers at the markers of the large and small weights and document the total to the nearest 1/4 lb in the patient's health record.	10*		

13. Read the height. Read the marker at the movable point of the ruler and document the measurement to the nearest 1/4 inch on the patient's health record.	10*		
14. Use the patient's weight and height to determine the BMI if it is not automatically done by the EHR program.	5		
15. Return the weights and the measuring bar to zero.	5		
16. Remove the paper towel and dispose of in the waste container. Wash hands or use hand sanitizer.	5		
17. Document the results in the patient's health record.	5		
Total Points	100		

Documentation

Comments

CAAHEP Competencies	Step(s)
I.P.1.e. Measure and record: height	9-17
I.P.1.f. Measure and record: weight	3-8
ABHES Competencies	**Step(s)**
8.b. Obtain vital signs, obtain patient history, and formulate chief complaint	Entire procedure

Physical Examination

CAAHEP Competencies	Assessment
I.P.9. Assist provider with a patient exam	Procedures 21.3 through 21.10
V.C.16. Differentiate between subjective and objective information	Skills and Concepts – D. 2
V.P.3. Use medical terminology correctly and pronounced accurately to communicate information to providers and patients	Procedure 21.1
V.P.1.a. Use feedback techniques to obtain patient information including: reflection	Procedure 21.1
V.P.1.b. Use feedback techniques to obtain patient information including: restatement	Procedure 21.1
V.P.1.c. Use feedback techniques to obtain patient information including: clarification	Procedure 21.1
V.P.2. Respond to nonverbal communication	Procedure 21.2
V.P.11. Report relevant information concisely and accurately	Procedure 21.1
V.A.1.a. Demonstrate: empathy	Procedure 21.1
V.A.1.b. Demonstrate: active listening	Procedure 21.1
V.A.1.c. Demonstrate: nonverbal communication	Procedure 21.1
V.A.2. Demonstrate the principles of self-boundaries	Procedure 21.1
V.C.11. Define the principles of self-boundaries	Skills and Concepts – B. 3
VI.C.12. Explain meaningful use as it applies to EMR	Skills and Concepts – A. 4
X.P.3. Document patient care accurately in the medical record	Procedure 21.1
XII.C.7.a. Identify principles of: body mechanics	Skills and Concepts – G. 1, 2
XII.P.3. Use proper body mechanics	Procedure 21.3

Anardeep Kaur

ABHES Competencies	Assessment
4. Medical Law and Ethics a. Follow documentation guidelines	Procedure 21.1
4. Medical Law and Ethics f. Comply with federal, state, and local health laws and regulations as they relate to healthcare settings 3) Comply with meaningful use regulations	Skills and Concepts – A. 4
8.b. Obtain vital signs, obtain patient history, and formulate chief complaint	Procedure 21.1, 21.2
8.c. Assist provider with general/physical examination	Procedure 21.3 through 21.10

VOCABULARY REVIEW

Using the word pool on the right, find the correct word to match the definition. Write the word on the line after the definition.

Group A

1. Arranged in the order of time ___chronologic___
2. Considering the patient as a whole; includes the physical, emotional, social, economic, and spiritual needs of the person ___holistic___
3. Statistical data of a population; in healthcare, this includes the patient's name, address, date of birth, employment, and other details ___demographic___
4. Allows the listener to get additional information ___clarification___
5. A secure online website that gives patients 24-hour access to personal health information using a username and password ___patient portal___
6. A procedure in which a fiber-optic scope is used to examine the large intestine ___colonoscopy___
7. Describes the signs and symptoms from the time of onset ___history of present illness___
8. A statement in the patient's own words that describes the reason for the visit ___chief complaint___
9. Occurring in or affecting members of a family more than would be expected by chance ___familial___
10. To establish an orderly relationship or connection ___correlates___

Word Pool
- chief complaint
- holistic
- patient portal
- correlates
- demographic
- history of present illness
- chronologic
- familial
- clarification
- colonoscopy

Amandeep Kaur

Group B

1. Subjective complaints reported by the patient, such as pain or nausea ___symptoms___
2. A record or recording of electrical impulses of the heart produced by an electrocardiograph ___electrocardiogram___
3. A problem with the function of the nerves outside the spinal cord ___peripheral neuropathy___
4. A relationship of harmony and accord between the patient and the healthcare professional ___rapport___
5. Pertaining to the area between the vaginal opening and the rectum ___perineal___
6. Using good judgment; being discreet, sensible ___judicious___
7. A physical injury or wound caused by external force or violence ___trauma___
8. Agreement; the state that occurs when the verbal expression of the message matches the sender's nonverbal body language ___congruence___
9. To listen with a stethoscope ___auscultate___
10. Objective findings determined by a clinician such as a fever, hypertension, or rash ___signs___

Word Pool
- congruence
- rapport
- judicious
- symptoms
- signs
- electrocardiogram
- auscultate
- peripheral neuropathy
- trauma
- perineal

Group C

1. An abnormal sound heard during auscultation of the heart that may or may not have a pathologic origin ___murmur___
2. Referring to normal skin tension; the resistance of the skin to being grasped between the fingers and released ___turgor___
3. Movement or exercise of a body part by means of an externally applied force ___manipulation___
4. Not noticeable or prominent ___inconspicuous___
5. An abnormal sound or murmur heard on auscultation of an organ, vessel, or gland ___bruit___
6. The manner or style of walking ___gait___
7. The process of stretching out; increasing the angle of a joint ___extension___
8. Similarity in size, form, and arrangement of parts on opposite sides of the body ___symmetry___
9. The process of decreasing the angle of a joint ___flexion___
10. The use of touch during the physical examination to assess the size, consistency, and location of certain body parts ___palpation___

Word Pool
- palpation
- manipulation
- gait
- symmetry
- murmur
- bruit
- flexion
- extension
- inconspicuous
- turgor

Amandeep Kaur

Group D

1. The white part of the eye that forms the orbit
   _____sclera_____

2. Abnormal enlargement of the distal phalanges (fingers and toes) associated with cyanotic heart disease or advanced chronic pulmonary disease _____clubbing_____

3. Thinning and eventual destruction of the alveoli
   _____emphysema_____

4. Small lumps, lesions, or swellings that are felt when the skin is palpated _____nodules_____

5. Inspection of a cavity or organ by passing light through its walls
   _____transillumination_____

Word Pool
- clubbing
- nodules
- sclera
- transillumination
- emphysema

ABBREVIATIONS

Write out what each of the following abbreviations stands for.

1. MRI _____

2. EHR _____

3. HIPAA _____

4. CC _____

5. VS _____

6. HPI _____

7. PH _____

8. PMH _____

9. UCD _____

10. UCHD _____

11. OTC _____

12. FH _____

13. SH _____

14. SR _____

15. ROS _____

16. ECG _____

17. EKG _____

18. ROM _____

19. CVA _____

20. EOM _____

21. BSE _____

22. TSE _____

23. GI_____

SKILLS AND CONCEPTS
Answer the following questions. Write your answer on the line or in the space provided.

A. Medical History

1. What is the difference between a differential diagnosis and a clinical diagnosis?_____

_____

_____

_____

_____

2. Explain the patient factors that should be considered when a patient is treated holistically. _____

_____

_____

_____

_____

3. List and describe the six components of the medical history.

    a. _____

    _____

    b. _____

    _____

    c. _____

    _____

    d. _____

    _____

    e. _____

    _____

    f. _____

    _____

4. What components of the social history meet the requirements of *meaningful use*?_____

_____

B. Understanding and Communicating with the Patient

1. Define the three processes of active listening.

   a. _____

   _____

   b. _____

   _____

   c. _____

   _____

2. Label the following questions as either open-ended or closed.

   a. How have you been feeling? _____

   b. Do you have a headache? _____

   c. Have you ever broken a bone? _____

   d. What brings you to the provider? _____

   e. Are you feeling better? _____

   f. Do you have high blood pressure? _____

   g. Tell me about your back pain. _____

   h. When did the nausea start? _____

   i. Did your mother have a history of cancer? _____

   j. Do you smoke?_____

3. Define the principles of self-boundaries. How do they relate to the field of medical assisting? _____

_____

_____

_____

_____

_____

_____

C. Interviewing the Patient

1. Identify the defense mechanism displayed by the following patients.

   a. A patient who refuses to believe she has breast cancer _____

   _____

   _____

   b. A 5-year-old child who starts to suck his thumb again when he is ill_____

   _____

   _____

   c. A patient who accuses you of being disrespectful when he has acted that way himself _____

   _____

   _____

   d. A patient who explains that she missed her appointment because she was so busy, and she really didn't need to follow up on the biopsy results anyway

   _____

   _____

D. Assessing the Patient

1. Describe the difference between a patient's signs of a disease and his or her possible symptoms._____

   _____

   _____

   _____

2. Label the following as "subjective" (symptom) or "objective" (sign).

   a. Pain _____

   b. Nausea_____

   c. Dizziness_____

   d. Elevated blood pressure _____

   e. Labored respirations_____

   f. Headache _____

   g. Temperature of the skin _____

   h. Back pain_____

   i. Color of the skin_____

   j. Abdominal pain _____

Amardeep Kaur

E. Documentation

1. Complete the following table.

Abbreviation	Definition
Abd	abdomen
a.c	before eating
ASHD	Anteriosclerotic Heart Disease
bid	Twice a day
BUN	blood urea nitrogen
CAD	Coronary Artery Disease
CHF	Congestive Heart Failure
DM	Diabetes Mellitus
FUO	fever of unknown origin
hs	at bedtime
NKA	no known allergies
R/O	rule out
SOB	Shortness Of Breath
STI	Sexually Transmitted Infection
URI	upper respiratory infection

F. Physical Examination

1. Identify three responsibilities of the medical assistant in room preparation. _____

   * Expiration dates must be checked on all packages and discard expired materials
   * Room should be private, well lit, and comfortable temp.
   * Drapes, gowns, and other supplies are arranged before the patient enters.

   _____

   _____

Amardeep Kaur

2. Explain three responsibilities of the medical assistant in patient preparation. _____

   ✶ measure and record patients ht, wt, BMI, VS

   ✶ Assist the patient into and out examination positions as needed.

   ✶ Document patient data in the medical record, completing all forms required.

3. Detail three responsibilities of the medical assistant in assisting the provider. _____

   ✶ Hand him/her instruments and equipment as requested and provide supplies as needed.

   ✶ position and drape the patient during the different phases of the exam.

   ✶ Assist in collecting and properly labeling specimens such as urine, pap smear, and throat cultures.

4. Describe the following methods of assessment.

   a. Inspection The examiner use observation to detect significant physical features or objective data.

   b. Palpation The examiner uses the sense of touch. A part of the body is felt with the hand to determine its condition or the condition of an underlying organ.

   c. Percussion Involves tapping or straining the body, usually with the fingers or small hammer to elicit sounds or vibratory sensations.

   d. Auscultation The physician use a stethoscope, to listen to sound arising from the body.

Amandeep Kaur

e.   Mensuration   _process of measuring_

_____

_____

_____

f.   Manipulation   _Passive movement of a joint to determine the range of extension or flexion of a part of the body._

_____

G. Principles of Body Mechanics

1.   Summarize the major guidelines for proper body mechanics. _____

_____

_____

_____

_____

_____

2.   Outline the principles of safe lifting techniques. _____

_____

_____

_____

_____

H. Transferring a Patient

1.   Explain what must be done when transferring a patient from a chair to the examination table.

_____

_____

_____

2.   A _____ should be used when transferring patients to prevent injury to yourself and safeguard patients from falling.

I. Assisting with the Physical Examination

1. Identify the instruments needed for the physical examination that are shown in the following figures and describe their purpose.

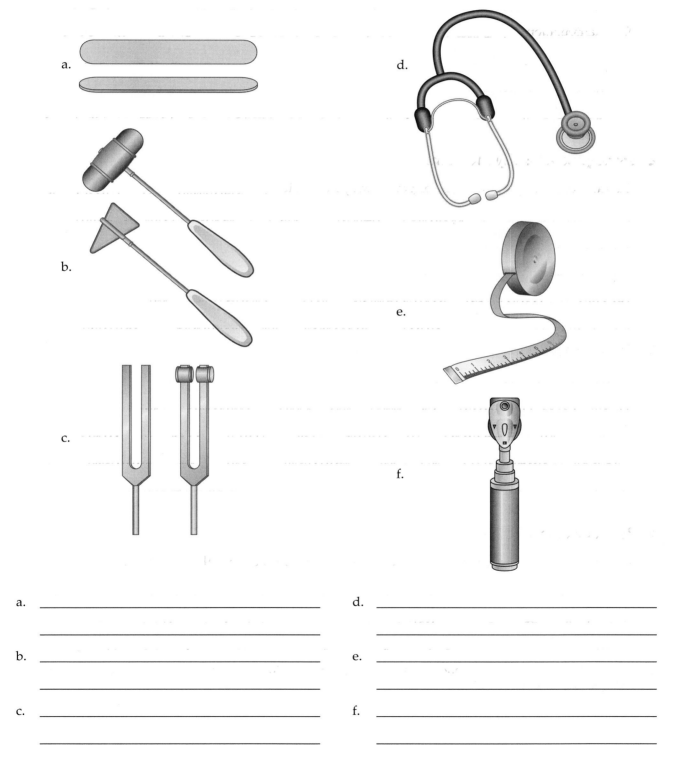

a. _____

   _____

b. _____

   _____

c. _____

   _____

d. _____

   _____

e. _____

   _____

f. _____

   _____

2.   Label the positions for examination shown in the following figures and give an example of a physical examination that is appropriate for each.

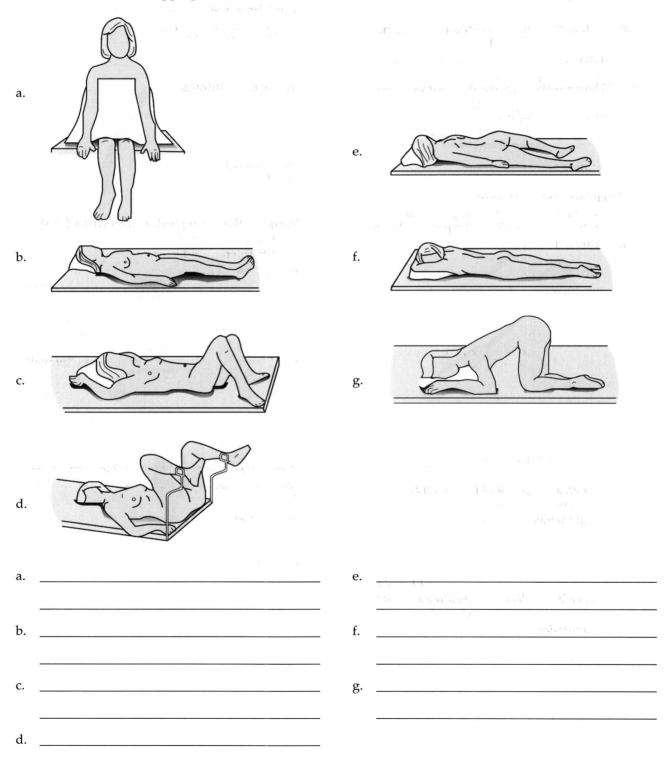

a. _____

b. _____

c. _____

d. _____
_____

e. _____
_____

f. _____
_____

g. _____
_____

CERTIFICATION PREPARATION

Circle the correct answer.

1. What does it mean when medical assistants display *empathy* when dealing with patients?
   a. They feel sorry for patients who have serious health problems.
   b. They are able to hear what patients say without judging the content.
   c. The can detach themselves emotionally from the problems of their patients.
   d. They truly like and care about each of their patients.

2. Which factor is likely to have the most influence on the accuracy and completeness of the information obtained from the patient during the medical history?
   a. The comfort of the chairs in the meeting area.
   b. The medical assistant's ability to take complete and detailed notes.
   c. The privacy of the area in which the interview takes place.
   d. The efficiency of the medical assistant in conducting the interview.

3. Which is an open-ended question?
   a. How old are you?
   b. What brings you to the office today?
   c. Do you smoke?
   d. Does your head hurt?

4. Which is an example of objective data?
   a. Complaints of pain
   b. Social history
   c. Past medical history
   d. Blood pressure recordings

5. During a physical examination, the provider discovers a bruit. What method would she be using to make this discovery?
   a. Auscultation
   b. Palpation
   c. Manipulation
   d. Percussion

6. The provider asks the medical assistant to position a patient on the examination table so that the patient can breathe easier. The most appropriate position is
   a. dorsal recumbent.
   b. lithotomy.
   c. semi-Fowler's.
   d. Trendelenburg.

7. The instrument used to test auditory acuity is the
   a. ophthalmoscope.
   b. otoscope.
   c. tuning fork.
   d. Snellen chart.

8. Where is the tuning fork placed when the Weber test is performed?
   a. On the mastoid process
   b. On the center of the top of the head
   c. One inch from the opening of the ear canal
   d. One foot from the front of the face

9. Which is acceptable when administering the Snellen visual acuity test?
   a. Placing the chart permanently on the wall at the eye level of the average adult
   b. Instructing the patient to close the eye not being tested
   c. Having the patient sit during the test
   d. Allowing the patient to squint

10. A near vision screening test, which can be used in the provider's office, can screen the patient for which vision problem?
    a. Myopia
    b. Presbyopia
    c. Astigmatism
    d. Presbycusis

WORKPLACE APPLICATIONS

In the following scenarios, what types of interview barriers are indicated? Explain how these statements are problematic and may interfere with the patient interview.

1. Mrs. Miller is expressing her concern about a changing mole in her left axillary region. Chris, the medical assistant obtaining her health history, makes the statement, "Mrs. Miller, the dysplastic nevus found in the left axillary region looks as if it could be malignant. You haven't been using sunscreen, have you?"

    _____

    _____

    _____

    _____

2. Mr. Sunsari is being seen today for a suspicious mass in his left lung. The physician has recommended a biopsy of the mass; however, Mr. Sunsari prefers to postpone the procedure. He asks Chris what he should do about scheduling the procedure. Chris states, "I would do it right away."

    _____

    _____

    _____

    _____

3. Carmen Largosi is a diabetic patient who is very concerned about her blood glucose levels. Her mother had diabetes and had to have her left leg amputated. When Carmen expresses her fears, Chris responds with, "I wouldn't worry about that. The doctor is very good with diabetic patients."

    _____

    _____

    _____

    _____

4. Mrs. Xu Nyguen will not establish eye contact with you during the patient interview. Do you think this means Mrs. Nyguen is not telling the truth?

    _____

    _____

    _____

    _____

5. Carl Worth, a 78-year-old patient, is hard of hearing and does not appear to be paying attention when you ask questions for the patient history. His daughter is in the examination room with him, so would it be better to gather patient information from her? Why or why not?

_____

_____

_____

_____

6. Theo Lang is being seen today for a surgical follow-up visit. He asks that his partner, David, accompany him into the examination room. What should you do?

_____

_____

_____

_____

INTERNET ACTIVITIES

1. Using online resources, research a culture other than your own in your area. Research the healthcare and communication practices. Create a poster presentation, a PowerPoint presentation, or write a paper summarizing your research. Include the following points in your project:
   a. How does this culture feel about eye contact?
   b. How does this culture view personal space?
   c. Are there any beliefs that would impact how care is provided in the healthcare setting?

2. Using online resources, research the use of chaperones in the healthcare setting. Create a poster presentation, a PowerPoint presentation, or write a paper summarizing your research. Include the following points in your project:
   a. What are the patient's rights when it comes to having a chaperone in the examination room?
   b. What are the responsibilities of the chaperone?
   c. What should the healthcare facility have in place when using chaperones?

Procedure 21.1   Obtain and Document Patient Information

Name _____ Date _____ Score _____

Task: To use restatement, reflection, and clarification to obtain patient information and document patient care accurately.

Equipment and Supplies:
- History form (Work Product 21.1) or EHR system with the patient history window opened
- If using a paper form—a red pen for recording the patient's allergies, and a black pen to meet legal documentation guidelines
- Quiet, private area

Directions: Complete this procedure with another student playing the role of the patient. To make the experience more realistic, choose a student about whom you know very little. To maintain the student's privacy, he or she does not have to share any confidential information.

Standard: Complete the procedure and all critical steps in _____ minutes with a minimum score of 85% within two attempts (*or as indicated by the instructor*).

Scoring: Divide the points earned by the total possible points. Failure to perform a critical step, indicated by an asterisk (*), results in grade no higher than an 84% (*or as indicated by the instructor*).

Time: Began_____ Ended_____ Total minutes: _____

Steps:	Point Value	Attempt 1	Attempt 2
1. Greet the patient. Identify yourself. Verify the patient's identity with full name and date of birth. Explain your role.	5		
2. Take the patient to a quiet, private area for the interview and explain why the information is needed.	5		
3. Complete the history form by using therapeutic communication techniques, including restatement, reflection, and clarification. Use active listening. Make sure all medical terminology is adequately explained. *(Refer to the Checklist for Affective Behaviors - Active Listening)*	10*		
4. Use appropriate nonverbal communication. Speak in a pleasant, distinct manner, remembering to maintain eye contact with your patient. *(Refer to the Checklist for Affective Behaviors - Nonverbal Communication)*	10*		
5. Demonstrate empathy and remain sensitive to the diverse needs of your patient throughout the interview process. *(Refer to the Checklist for Affective Behaviors - Empathy)*	10*		
6. Record the following statistical information: • Patient's full name, including middle initial • Address, including apartment number and ZIP code • Marital status • Sex (gender) • Age and date of birth • Telephone numbers for home, cell, and work • Insurance information if not already available • Employer's name, address, and telephone number	10		

7. Record the following medical history: • Chief complaint • Present illness • Past medical history • Family history • Social history	**10**			
8. Ask about allergies to drugs and any other substances and record any allergies in red ink on every page of the history form, on the front of the patient record, and on each progress note page; in the EHR, enter allergy information where designated.	**10**			
9. If using a paper form, record all information legibly and neatly and spell words correctly.	**5**			
10. Thank the patient for cooperating and direct him or her back to the reception area.	**5**			
11. Review the record for errors before you pass it to the provider or exit the EHR health history area.	**10**			
12. Protect the integrity of the health record and the confidentiality of patient information. Safeguards mandated by the Health Insurance Portability and Accountability Act (HIPAA) include: • Passwords to secure access to all EHRs • Computer monitor shields to protect patient information if data are left on the screen • Turning monitors away from patient traffic areas to prevent accidental release of information • Securing all medical records	**10**			
Total Points	**100**			

Affective Behavior	***Directions:*** *Check behaviors observed during the role-play.*					
Empathy	**Negative, Unprofessional Behaviors**	**Attempt**		**Positive, Professional Behaviors**	**Attempt**	
		1	**2**		**1**	**2**
	Unsupportive, uninterested, or uncaring			Demonstrated supportive, caring behaviors		
	Did not acknowledge or respond appropriately to the patient's emotional responses; cold, aloof, insensitive, indifferent, or unfeeling			Acknowledged and responded appropriately to the patient's emotional responses; showed sensitivity		
	Failed to reassure patient; did not respond to the patient's concerns			Reassured patient by repeating and responding to the patient's concerns		
	Used language that is hard to understand (e.g., slang, generational terms, medical terminology, too scientific)			Used language that the patient can understand		
	Other:			Other:		

Active Listening	Failed to use therapeutic communication techniques			Asked appropriate open-ended questions; repeated back (paraphrased) and clarifiee important information; responded to patient's emotional responses		
	Did not listen to the patient, interrupted patient			Allowed patient to talk; listened without interrupting		
	Responded with a bias; judgmental and/or condescending to the patient			Responded without bias or judgment; refrained from condescending attitude		
	Failed to address the patient's questions; or answers to patient's questions were inappropriate			Answered the patient's questions appropriately		
	Other:			Other:		
Nonverbal Communication	Spoke in an artificial manner; tone, pitch, and/or volume were unprofessional			Used a natural tone, pitch, and volume when speaking		
	Failed to respond to the patient's nonverbal behaviors			Responded appropriately to patient's nonverbal behaviors		
	Used inappropriate gestures and/or facial expressions			Used appropriate gestures and facial expressions		
	Poor eye contact with patient			Proper eye contact with patient		
	Other:			Other:		

Grading		Point Value	Attempt 1	Attempt 2
Does not meet Expectation	• Response demonstrated lack of active listening, inappropriate nonverbal communication, and/or lacks empathy. • Student demonstrated more than 2 negative, unprofessional behaviors during the interaction.	0		
Needs Improvement	• Response demonstrated lack of active listening, inappropriate nonverbal communication, and/or lacks empathy. • Student demonstrated 1 or 2 negative, unprofessional behaviors during the interaction.	0		

Meets Expectation	• Response demonstrated active listening skills, appropriate nonverbal communication, and empathy; no negative, unprofessional behaviors observed. • More practice is needed for behavior to appear natural and for student to appear comfortable and at ease.	10		
Occasionally Exceeds Expectation	• Response demonstrated active listening skills, appropriate nonverbal communication, and empathy; no negative, unprofessional behaviors observed. • At times student appeared comfortable and at ease; but more practice is needed for behavior to become natural and consistent with a professional medical assistant.	10		
Always Exceeds Expectation	• Response demonstrated active listening skills, appropriate nonverbal communication, and empathy; no negative, unprofessional behaviors observed. • Student's behaviors appeared natural and comfortable. Behaviors are consistent with a professional medical assistant.	10		

Comments

CAAHEP Competencies	Step(s)
V.P.3. Use medical terminology correctly and pronounced accurately to communicate information to providers and patients	3
V.P.1.a. Use feedback techniques to obtain patient information including: reflection	3
V.P.1.b. Use feedback techniques to obtain patient information including: restatement	3
V.P.1.c. Use feedback techniques to obtain patient information including: clarification	3
V.A.1.a. Demonstrate: empathy	3, 4, 5
V.A.1.b. Demonstrate: active listening	3, 4, 5
V.A.1.c. Demonstrate: nonverbal communication	3, 4, 5
V.A.2. Demonstrate the principles of self-boundaries	3, 4, 5
ABHES Competencies	**Step(s)**
8.b. Obtain vital signs, obtain patient history, and formulate chief complaint	7

Work Product 21.1   History Form

Name _____   Date _____   Score _____

MEDICAL RECORD		
NAME	AGE	SEX S / M / D / W
ADDRESS	PHONE	DATE
SPONSOR	ADDRESS	
OCCUPATION	REF BY	ACKN
CHIEF COMPLAINT		
PRESENT ILLNESS		

FAMILY HISTORY

MOTHER		FATHER		SIBLING(S)		
TB	DIAB	MALIG	HT DIS	NEPH	EPILEP	PSYCH

PAST HISTORY — GENERAL HEALTH	GASTROINTESTINAL
CHILDHOOD DISEASES	APPETITE BOWEL HABITS VOMITING
SC FEV RHEUM FEV ASTHMA	INDIGESTION HEMORRHOIDS BLEEDING
OTHER	NAUSEA DIET ITCHING
SOCIAL HISTORY	JAUNDICE PAIN PAIN WITH STOOL
COFFEE TOBACCO ALCOHOL DRUG USE	OTHER
WEIGHT	**URINARY TRACT**
USUAL WEIGHT	NOCTURIA INCONTINENCE INFECTION
RECENT WEIGHT FLUCTUATIONS	PAIN FREQUENCY
HX OF EATING DISORDER	BLEEDING BURNING
REVIEW OF SYSTEMS	**GENITAL TRACT**
E E N T	AGE AT MENST TYPE PERIOD
EYES EARS NOSE THROAT NECK	PAINFUL PERIOD INTERMITTENT BLEEDING
NEUROMUSCULAR	AMENORRHEA DYSMENORRHEA
STRENGTH ANXIETY	VAG DISCH IRRITATION
SLEEP DEPRESSION	BREAST EXAM PROSTATE EXAM
MUSCULAR PAIN PERIPHERAL NEUROPATHY	TESTICULAR EXAM
JOINT PAIN	**L M P**
CARDIOVASCULAR	AGES OF CHILDREN CONTRACEPTION TYPE
HEART DISEASE MI	LMP DATE NO. OF PREGNANCIES
CONGENITAL HEART DEFECTS TIAS	NO. OF LIVE BIRTHS AGES OF CHILDREN
HYPERTENSION STROKE	**OTHER**
EDEMA	_____
LUNGS	_____
PAIN DYSPNEA	**ACCIDENTS**
COUGHING UP BLOOD COUGH	_____
IRREG BREATHING	_____
OPERATIONS	**CURRENT MEDICATIONS AND TREATMENTS**
_____	_____
_____	_____
_____	_____

COMMENTS
_____
_____
_____

Procedure 21.2   Respond to Nonverbal Communication

Name _____   Date _____   Score _____

Task: To observe the patient and respond appropriately to nonverbal communication.

Equipment and Supplies:
• Patient's record

Scenario: Monique Jones is a new patient with the CC of intermittent abdominal pain with alternating diarrhea and constipation. Ms. Jones has experienced this discomfort for several months and appears very frustrated. She is sitting on the end of the exam table with her arms wrapped around her abdomen. She sighs frequently and refuses to maintain eye contact. What is her nonverbal behavior telling you, and how can you establish therapeutic communication with this patient?

Directions: Complete this procedure with another student playing the role of the patient. To make the experience more realistic, choose a student about whom you know very little. To maintain the student's privacy, he or she does not have to share any confidential information.

Standard: Complete the procedure and all critical steps in _____ minutes with a minimum score of 85% within two attempts (*or as indicated by the instructor*).

Scoring: Divide the points earned by the total possible points. Failure to perform a critical step, indicated by an asterisk (*), results in grade no higher than an 84% (*or as indicated by the instructor*).

Time: Began_____ Ended_____ Total minutes: _____

Steps:	Point Value	Attempt 1	Attempt 2
1. Greet the patient. Identify yourself. Verify the patient's identity with full name and date of birth. Explain your role.	20		
2. Ask the patient the purpose of her visit and the onset, duration, and frequency of her symptoms. Pay close attention to her body language to determine whether what she is telling you is congruent with her body language.	20*		
3. Use restatement, reflection, and clarification to gather as much information as possible about the patient's CC. Make sure all medical terminology is adequately explained.	20		
4. Speak in a pleasant, distinct manner, remembering to maintain eye contact with your patient.	20		
5. Continue to observe nonverbal patient behaviors and select the appropriate verbal response to demonstrate your sensitivity to her discomfort, frustration, and anxiety.	20		
Total Points	100		

Comments

CAAHEP Competencies	Step(s)
V.P.2. Respond to nonverbal communication	Entire procedure
ABHES Competencies	**Step(s)**
8. b. Obtain vital signs, obtain patient history, and formulate chief complaint	Entire procedure

Procedure 21.3 Use Proper Body Mechanics

Name _____ Date _____ Score _____

Task: To safely transfer a patient from a wheelchair to an examination table using proper body mechanics.

Equipment and Supplies:
- Patient's record
- Wheelchair
- Examination table with pull-out foot rest
- Gait belt

Standard: Complete the procedure and all critical steps in _____ minutes with a minimum score of 85% within two attempts (*or as indicated by the instructor*).

Scoring: Divide the points earned by the total possible points. Failure to perform a critical step, indicated by an asterisk (*), results in grade no higher than an 84% (*or as indicated by the instructor*).

Time: Began_____ Ended_____ Total minutes: _____

Steps:	Point Value	Attempt 1	Attempt 2
1. Wash hands or use hand sanitizer.	5		
2. Greet the patient. Identify yourself. Verify the patient's identity with full name and date of birth. Explain the procedure to be performed in a manner that is understood by the patient. Determine how much assistance the patient will need to transfer from the wheelchair to the examination table. Do not proceed if you think you will need additional help.	5		
3. Place the wheelchair at a 45-degree angle toward the foot rest at the base of the examination table.	5		
4. Lock the brakes on the wheelchair and move the foot rests of the wheelchair out of the way.	10*		
5. Place the gait belt around the patient's waist over clothing with the buckle in front. Insert the belt through the teeth of the buckle and pull it tight to lock it. The belt should be tight with just enough room to place your fingers under it.	10*		
6. Request that the patient place both feet flat on the floor with the hands on the armrests.	5		
7. Stand directly in front of the patient with your feet apart, back straight, and knees bent.	5		
8. Slide your fingers under the gait belt on opposite sides of the patient's waist.	5		
9. Instruct the patient at the count of three to push off from the armrests while you at the same time grasp the gait belt and, using your leg muscles, straighten your knees so that the patient is in a standing position.	10*		
10. Ask the patient to step up onto the foot rest at the bottom of the exam table and assist the person in pivoting and sitting down on the examination table. Remove the gait belt until the provider has completed the examination.	5		

11. After the examination is complete, place the wheelchair at an angle next to the exam table and lock the wheels. Replace the gait belt. Make sure the patient is positioned at the edge of the table.	**10***		
12. Place yourself directly in front of the patient with your back straight and your knees bent. Slide your fingers under the gait belt on opposite sides of the patient's waist.	**5**		
13. Grasp the gait belt on both sides at the waist. Instruct the patient at the count of three to push off from the examination table and, using your leg muscles, straighten your knees so that the patient is in a standing position on the foot rest.	**10***		
14. Maintaining your hold on the gait belt, ask the patient to step down. Pivot the person so that she can slowly sit in the wheelchair; at the same time, bend your knees but keep your back straight.	**5**		
15. Remove the gait belt. Replace the wheelchair foot rests and unlock the brakes on the wheelchair.	**5**		
Total Points	**100**		

Comments

CAAHEP Competencies	**Step(s)**
I.P.9. Assist provider with a patient exam	Entire procedure
XII.P.3. Use proper body mechanics	Entire procedure
ABHES Competencies	**Step(s)**
8.c. Assist provider with general/physical examination	Entire procedure

Procedure 21.4 Fowler's and Semi-Fowler's Positions

Name _____ Date _____ Score _____

Task: To position and drape the patient for examinations of the head, neck, and chest, or patients who have difficulty breathing when lying flat.

Equipment and Supplies:
- Patient's record
- Examination table
- Table paper
- Patient gown
- Drape
- Disinfectant wipes
- Gloves

Standard: Complete the procedure and all critical steps in _____ minutes with a minimum score of 85% within two attempts (*or as indicated by the instructor*).

Scoring: Divide the points earned by the total possible points. Failure to perform a critical step, indicated by an asterisk (*), results in grade no higher than an 84% (*or as indicated by the instructor*).

Time: Began_____ Ended_____ Total minutes: _____

Steps:	Point Value	Attempt 1	Attempt 2
1. Wash hands or use hand sanitizer.	10		
2. Greet the patient. Identify yourself. Verify the patient's identity with full name and date of birth. Explain the procedure to be performed in a manner that is understood by the patient. Answer any questions the patient may have on the procedure.	10		
3. Give the patient a gown. Explain what clothing must be removed for the particular examination being done and whether the gown should open in the front or the back. Provide assistance as needed. Give the patient privacy while changing. Knock on the examination room door before re-entering to make sure the patient has completed undressing and gowning.	10		
4. For Fowler's position, elevate the head of the bed 90 degrees. If the patient feels more comfortable, she can sit at the end of the table. Extend the foot rest as needed for patient comfort. The patient may be more comfortable in semi-Fowler's position. In this modification of Fowler's position, the head of the table is elevated 45 degrees.	15*		
5. Drape the patient according to the type of examination and the required patient exposure.	10		
6. After the examination has been completed, assist the patient as needed to get off the table and get dressed.	10		
7. Put on gloves and use disinfectant wipes to clean the exam table and all potentially contaminated surfaces. Dispose of used gloves and examination table paper according to facility policies. Pull clean paper over the table.	15		
8. Wash hands or use hand sanitizer.	10		

9. Follow up with the provider's orders regarding scheduling of diagnostic studies, collection of specimens, and/or scheduling of future appointments.	**10**			
Total Points	**100**			

Comments

CAAHEP Competencies	Step(s)
I.P.9. Assist provider with a patient exam	Entire procedure
ABHES Competencies	**Step(s)**
8.c. Assist provider with general/physical examination	Entire procedure

Procedure 21.5 Supine (Horizontal Recumbent) and Dorsal Recumbent Positions

Name _____ Date _____ Score _____

Task: To position and drape the patient for examinations of the abdomen, heart, and breasts in the horizontal recumbent (supine) position, and exams of the rectal, vaginal, and perineal areas in the dorsal recumbent position.

Equipment and Supplies:
- Patient's record
- Examination table
- Table paper
- Patient gown
- Drape
- Disinfectant wipes
- Gloves

Standard: Complete the procedure and all critical steps in _____ minutes with a minimum score of 85% within two attempts (*or as indicated by the instructor*).

Scoring: Divide the points earned by the total possible points. Failure to perform a critical step, indicated by an asterisk (*), results in grade no higher than an 84% (*or as indicated by the instructor*).

Time: Began_____ Ended_____ Total minutes: _____

Steps:	Point Value	Attempt 1	Attempt 2
1. Wash hands or use hand sanitizer.	10		
2. Greet the patient. Identify yourself. Verify the patient's identity with full name and date of birth. Explain the procedure to be performed in a manner that is understood by the patient. Answer any questions the patient may have on the procedure.	10		
3. Give the patient a gown. Explain the clothing that must be removed for the particular examination being done and whether the gown should open in the front or in the back. Provide assistance as needed. For the horizontal recumbent position, the gown should be open in the front. Give the patient privacy while changing. Knock on the examination room door before re-entering to make sure the patient has completed undressing and gowning.	10		
4. Do not place the patient in the necessary positions until the provider is ready for that part of the examination.	10		
5. Pull out the table extension that supports the patient's legs. For the horizontal recumbent (supine) position, help the patient lie flat on the table with the face upward. For the dorsal recumbent position, have the patient lie flat on the back and flex the knees so the feet are flat on the table. If needed, help the patient move down toward the foot of the table for the examination.	10*		
6. Drape the patient from nipple line to feet in the supine position, and diagonally with the point of the drape between the feet for the dorsal recumbent position.	10		
7. After the examination has been completed, assist the patient as needed to get off the table and get dressed.	10		

8. Put on gloves and use disinfectant wipes to clean the exam table and all potentially contaminated surfaces. Dispose of used gloves and examination table paper according to facility policies. Pull clean paper over the table.	**10**		
9. Wash hands or use hand sanitizer.	**10**		
10. Follow up with the provider's orders regarding scheduling of diagnostic studies, collection of specimens, and/or scheduling of future appointments.	**10**		
Total Points	**100**		

Comments

CAAHEP Competencies	Step(s)
I.P.9. Assist provider with a patient exam	Entire procedure
ABHES Competencies	**Step(s)**
8.c. Assist provider with general/physical examination	Entire procedure

Procedure 21.6   Lithotomy Position

Name _____ Date _____ Score _____

Task: To position and drape the patient primarily for vaginal and pelvic examinations and Pap tests.

Equipment and Supplies:
- Patient's record
- Examination table
- Table paper
- Patient gown
- Drape
- Disinfectant wipes
- Gloves

Standard: Complete the procedure and all critical steps in _____ minutes with a minimum score of 85% within two attempts (*or as indicated by the instructor*).

Scoring: Divide the points earned by the total possible points. Failure to perform a critical step, indicated by an asterisk (*), results in grade no higher than an 84% (*or as indicated by the instructor*).

Time: Began_____ Ended_____ Total minutes: _____

Steps:	Point Value	Attempt 1	Attempt 2
1. Wash hands or use hand sanitizer.	5		
2. Greet the patient. Identify yourself. Verify the patient's identity with full name and date of birth. Explain the procedure to be performed in a manner that is understood by the patient. Answer any questions the patient may have on the procedure.	5		
3. Give the patient a gown. Instruct the patient to undress from the waist down with the gown open in the back. If the provider also will be doing a breast examination, the patient should undress completely and put on the gown so that it opens in the front. Provide assistance as needed. Give the patient privacy while changing. Knock on the examination room door before re-entering to make sure the patient has completed undressing and gowning.	10		
4. Do not place the patient in the lithotomy position until the provider is ready for that part of the examination.	10		
5. Pull out the table extension that supports the patient's legs and help the patient lie face upward on the table. Pull out the stirrups, adjust their extension length for the patient's comfort, and lock them in place.	10*		
6. Reinsert the table extension and have the patient move toward the foot of the table with her buttocks on the bottom table edge. Gently place the patient's legs in the stirrups, checking for comfort. Some offices may stock cloth or paper stirrup covers to protect the patient and make the position more comfortable. The patient's arms can be placed alongside the body or across the chest.	10*		
7. Drape the patient diagonally, with the point of the drape between the feet. The drape should be large enough to cover the patient from the nipple line to the ankles and wide enough so the patient's thighs are not exposed.	10		

8.	After the examination has been completed, assist the patient as needed to get off the table and get dressed.	**10**		
9.	Put on gloves and use disinfectant wipes to clean the exam table and all potentially contaminated surfaces. Dispose of used gloves and examination table paper according to facility policies. Pull clean paper over the table.	**10**		
10.	Wash hands or use hand sanitizer.	**10**		
11.	Follow up with the provider's orders regarding scheduling of diagnostic studies, collection of specimens, and/or scheduling of future appointments.	**10**		
	Total Points	**100**		

Comments

CAAHEP Competencies	**Step(s)**
I.P.9. Assist provider with a patient exam	Entire procedure
ABHES Competencies	**Step(s)**
8.c. Assist provider with general/physical examination	Entire procedure

Procedure 21.7   Sims' Position

Name _____ Date _____ Score _____

Task: To position and drape the patient for examination of the rectum, instillation of rectal medication, perineal examination, and some pelvic examinations.

Equipment and Supplies:
- Patient's record
- Examination table
- Patient gown
- Table paper
- Drape
- Disinfectant wipes
- Gloves

Standard: Complete the procedure and all critical steps in _____ minutes with a minimum score of 85% within two attempts (*or as indicated by the instructor*).

Scoring: Divide the points earned by the total possible points. Failure to perform a critical step, indicated by an asterisk (*), results in grade no higher than an 84% (*or as indicated by the instructor*).

Time: Began_____ Ended_____ Total minutes: _____

Steps:	Point Value	Attempt 1	Attempt 2
1. Wash hands or use hand sanitizer.	10		
2. Greet the patient. Identify yourself. Verify the patient's identity with full name and date of birth. Explain the procedure to be performed in a manner that is understood by the patient. Answer any questions the patient may have on the procedure.	10		
3. Give the patient a gown and explain what clothing must be removed for the particular examination being done. Tell the patient that the gown should open in the back. Provide assistance as needed. Give the patient privacy while changing. Knock on the examination room door before re-entering to make sure the patient has completed undressing and gowning.	10		
4. Do not place the patient in the Sims' position until the provider is ready for that part of the examination.	10		
5. Help the patient turn onto the left side; the left arm and shoulder should be drawn back behind the body so that the patient is tilted onto the chest. Flex the right arm upward for support, slightly flex the left leg, and sharply flex the right leg upward. Help the patient move the buttocks to the side edge of the table.	10*		
6. Drape the patient diagonally in a diamond shape, with the point of the diamond dropping below the buttocks. Make sure the drape is large enough to prevent exposure of the patient.	10*		
7. After the examination has been completed, assist the patient as needed to get off the table and get dressed.	10		

8.	Put on gloves and use disinfectant wipes to clean the exam table and all potentially contaminated surfaces. Dispose of used gloves and examination table paper according to facility policies. Pull clean paper over the table.	**10**		
9.	Wash hands or use hand sanitizer.	**10**		
10.	Follow up with the provider's orders regarding scheduling of diagnostic studies, collection of specimens, and/or scheduling of future appointments.	**10**		
	Total Points	**100**		

Comments

CAAHEP Competencies	**Step(s)**
I.P.9. Assist provider with a patient exam	Entire procedure
ABHES Competencies	**Step(s)**
8.c. Assist provider with general/physical examination	Entire procedure

Procedure 21.8   Prone Position

Name _____ **Date** _____ **Score** _____

Task: To position and drape the patient for examination of the back and for certain surgical procedures.

Equipment and Supplies:
- Patient's record
- Examination table
- Patient gown
- Table paper
- Drape
- Disinfectant wipes
- Gloves

Standard: Complete the procedure and all critical steps in _____ minutes with a minimum score of 85% within two attempts (*or as indicated by the instructor*).

Scoring: Divide the points earned by the total possible points. Failure to perform a critical step, indicated by an asterisk (*), results in grade no higher than an 84% (*or as indicated by the instructor*).

Time: Began_____ **Ended**_____ **Total minutes:** _____

Steps:	Point Value	Attempt 1	Attempt 2
1. Wash hands or use hand sanitizer.	5		
2. Greet the patient. Identify yourself. Verify the patient's identity with full name and date of birth. Explain the procedure to be performed in a manner that is understood by the patient. Answer any questions the patient may have on the procedure.	5		
3. Give the patient a gown and explain what clothing must be removed for the particular examination being done. Tell the patient that the gown should open in the back. Provide assistance as needed. Give the patient privacy while changing. Knock on the examination room door before re-entering to make sure the patient has completed undressing and gowning.	10		
4. Do not place the patient in the prone position until the provider is ready for that part of the examination.	10		
5. Pull out the table extension and help the patient lie down on his or her stomach.	15*		
6. Drape the patient over any exposed area that is not included in the examination. For female patients, the drape should be large enough to cover from the breasts to the feet so that the patient is not exposed accidentally if she is asked to roll over.	15		
7. After the examination has been completed, assist the patient as needed to get off the table and get dressed.	10		
8. Put on gloves and use disinfectant wipes to clean the exam table and all potentially contaminated surfaces. Dispose of used gloves and examination table paper according to facility policies. Pull clean paper over the table.	10		
9. Wash hands or use hand sanitizer.	10		

10. Follow up with the provider's orders regarding scheduling of diagnostic studies, collection of specimens, and/or scheduling of future appointments.	10		
Total Points	**100**		

Comments

CAAHEP Competencies	Step(s)
I.P.9. Assist provider with a patient exam	Entire procedure
ABHES Competencies	**Step(s)**
8.c. Assist provider with general/physical examination	Entire procedure

Procedure 21.9   Knee-Chest Position

Name _____ Date _____ Score _____

Task: To position and drape the patient for examinations of the back and rectum and for certain surgical procedures.

Equipment and Supplies:
- Examination table
- Table paper
- Patient gown
- Drape
- Disinfectant wipes
- Gloves

Standard: Complete the procedure and all critical steps in _____ minutes with a minimum score of 85% within two attempts (*or as indicated by the instructor*).

Scoring: Divide the points earned by the total possible points. Failure to perform a critical step, indicated by an asterisk (*), results in grade no higher than an 84% (*or as indicated by the instructor*).

Time: Began_____ Ended_____ Total minutes: _____

Steps:	Point Value	Attempt 1	Attempt 2
1. Wash hands or use hand sanitizer.	5		
2. Greet the patient. Identify yourself. Verify the patient's identity with full name and date of birth. Explain the procedure to be performed in a manner that is understood by the patient. Answer any questions the patient may have on the procedure.	5		
3. Give the patient a gown and explain what clothing must be removed for the particular examination being done. Tell the patient that the gown should open in the back. Provide assistance as needed. Give the patient privacy while changing. Knock on the examination room door before re-entering to make sure the patient has completed undressing and gowning.	10		
4. Do not place the patient in the knee-chest position until the provider is ready for that part of the examination.	10		
5. Pull out the table extension if necessary. Help the patient lie down on his or her back and then turn over into the prone position. Ask the patient to move up onto the knees, spread the knees apart, and lean forward onto the head so that the buttocks are raised. Tell the patient to keep the back straight and turn the face to either side. The patient should rest his or her weight on the chest and shoulders.	10*		
6. If the patient has difficulty maintaining this position, an alternative is to place weight on bent elbows with the head off the table.	10		
7. Drape the patient diagonally so that the point of the drape is on the table between the legs.	10		
8. After the examination has been completed, assist the patient as needed to get off the table and get dressed.	10		

9.	Put on gloves and use disinfectant wipes to clean the exam table and all potentially contaminated surfaces. Dispose of used gloves and examination table paper according to facility policies. Pull clean paper over the table.	**10**		
10.	Wash hands or use hand sanitizer.	**10**		
11.	Follow up with the provider's orders regarding scheduling of diagnostic studies, collection of specimens, and/or scheduling of future appointments.	**10**		
	Total Points	**100**		

Comments

CAAHEP Competencies	Step(s)
I.P.9. Assist provider with a patient exam	Entire procedure
ABHES Competencies	**Step(s)**
8.c. Assist provider with general/physical examination	Entire procedure

Procedure 21.10   Assist Provider with a Patient Exam

Name _____   Date _____   Score _____

Task: To aid the provider in the examination of a patient by preparing the patient and the necessary equipment and ensuring the patient's safety and comfort during the examination.

Equipment and Supplies:
- Patient's record
- Stethoscope
- Gauze
- Ophthalmoscope
- Pen light
- Scale with height measurement bar
- Tuning fork
- Tongue depressor
- Biohazard waste container
- Cotton balls
- Examination light
- Laboratory request forms
- Percussion hammer
- Specimen bottles and laboratory requisitions
- Lubricating gel
- Gloves
- Patient gown
- Sphygmomanometer
- Drapes
- Otoscope with disposable speculum
- Thermometer
- Cotton-tipped applicators
- Tape measure
- Fecal occult blood test supplies
- Disinfectant wipes
- Table paper

Standard: Complete the procedure and all critical steps in _____ minutes with a minimum score of 85% within two attempts (*or as indicated by the instructor*).

Scoring: Divide the points earned by the total possible points. Failure to perform a critical step, indicated by an asterisk (*), results in grade no higher than an 84% (*or as indicated by the instructor*).

Time: Began _____ Ended _____ Total minutes: _____

Steps:	Point Value	Attempt 1	Attempt 2
1. Check the examination room at the beginning of each day and between patients to make sure it is completely stocked with equipment and supplies and that the equipment functions properly.	5		
2. Check expiration dates on all packages and supplies regularly and discard expired materials.	5		
3. Prepare the examination room before and between patients according to acceptable medical rules of asepsis.	5		

4.	Wash hands or use hand sanitizer.	**5**		
5.	Locate the instruments for the procedure. Set them out in order of use within reach of the provider and cover them until the provider enters the examination room.	**10***		
6.	Greet and identify the patient, introduce yourself, and determine whether the patient understands the procedure. If the patient does not, explain what to expect. Refer any unanswered questions to the provider.	**5**		
7.	Review the medical history with the patient and investigate the purpose of the visit. Review current medications and document any changes or prescription refills needed. Document the interview results.	**5**		
8.	Measure and record the patient's vital signs, height, weight, and body mass index (BMI). Instruct the patient on how to collect a urine specimen, if ordered, and hand the patient a properly labeled specimen container. Obtain blood samples for any tests ordered.	**10***		
9.	Hand the patient a gown and drape. Explain what clothes should be removed for the examination and whether the gown should open in the front or the back. Help the patient undress as needed (most patients prefer to undress in privacy). Knock on the door before re-entering the room to protect the patient's privacy.	**5**		
10.	Assist the patient as needed in sitting at the foot of the examination table; place the drape over the patient's lap and legs. If the patient is elderly, confused, or feeling faint or dizzy, do not leave him or her alone.	**5**		
11.	Place the patient's paper health record in the designated area or make sure the computer is ready for the provider to log in and access the patient's electronic health record (EHR). Be careful to safeguard patient confidentiality during this step of the procedure.	**5**		
12.	Assist during the examination by handing the provider instruments as needed and by positioning and draping the patient.	**10**		
13.	When the provider has completed the examination, allow the patient to rest for a moment, then help the patient from the table. Assist with dressing, if necessary. Use proper body mechanics if assistance in transfer is needed.	**5**		
14.	Return to the patient and ask whether he or she has any questions. Give the patient any final instructions, and schedule tests as ordered by the provider and/or the next appointment.	**5**		
15.	Put on gloves and dispose of used supplies and linens in designated biohazard waste containers. Dispose of exam table paper. Use disinfectant wipes to clean the examination table and any other potentially contaminated surface. Disinfect all equipment.	**5**		
16.	Remove the gloves, discard them in the biohazard waste container, and wash hands or use hand sanitizer.	**5**		
17.	Cover the exam table with fresh paper, replace used supplies, and prepare the room for the next patient.	**5**		
	Total Points	**100**		

Comments

CAAHEP Competencies	Step(s)
I.P.9. Assist provider with a patient exam	Entire procedure
ABHES Competencies	**Step(s)**
8.c. Assist provider with general/physical examination	Entire procedure

Patient Coaching

CAAHEP Competencies	Assessment
V.C.6.a. Define coaching a patient as it relates to: health maintenance	Skills and Concepts – A. 4-5; Certification Preparation – 2
V.C.6.b. Define coaching a patient as it relates to: disease prevention	Skills and Concepts – A. 2-3
V.C.6.c. Define coaching a patient as it relates to: compliance with treatment plan	Skills and Concepts – A. 6-7
V.C.6.d. Define coaching a patient as it relates to: community resources	Skills and Concepts – A. 9
V.C.6.e. Define coaching a patient as it relates to: adaptations relevant to individual patient needs	Skills and Concepts – A. 8; C. 16
V.C.12. Define patient navigator	Skills and Concepts – H. 3
V.C.13. Describe the role of the medical assistant as a patient navigator	Skills and Concepts – H. 4-5
V.C.17.b. Discuss the theories of: Erikson	Skills and Concepts – C. 17a-h; Workplace Applications – 1a-h; Certification Preparation – 6
V.C.17.c. Discuss the theories of: Kübler-Ross	Skills and Concepts – B. 1a-e, 2, 3a-e; Certification Preparation – 4
V.P.9. Develop a current list of community resources related to patients' healthcare needs	Procedure 22.2
V.P.10. Facilitate referrals to community resources in the role of a patient navigator	Procedure 22.2
V.P.4.c. Coach patients regarding: disease prevention	Procedure 22.1
V.P.5.b. Coach patients appropriately considering: developmental life stage	Procedure 22.1
V.P.5.c. Coach patients appropriately considering: communication barriers	Procedure 22.1
X.P.3. Document patient care accurately in the medical record	Procedure 22.1, 22.2

ABHES Competencies	Assessment
5. Human Relations b. 3) List organizations and support groups that can assist patients and family members of patients experiencing terminal illnesses	Procedure 22.2
5.d. Adapt care to address the developmental stages of life	Procedure 22.1
8.h. Teach self-examination, disease management and health promotion	Procedure 22.1
8.i. Identify community resources and Complementary and Alternative Medicine practices (CAM)	Procedure 22.2
8.j. Make adaptations for patients with special needs (psychological or physical limitations)	Procedure 22.1
8.k. Make adaptations to care for patients across their lifespan	Procedure 22.1

VOCABULARY REVIEW

Using the word pool on the right, find the correct word to match the definition. Write the word on the line after the definition.

1. The act of sticking to something _____
2. The process of gaining new knowledge or skills through instruction, experience, or study _____
3. Patients are taking the right dose at the right times as prescribed by the provider _____
4. "Doing" domain _____
5. Bringing to an end _____
6. Involves mental processes of recall, application, and evaluation _____
7. Provides personalized patient- and family-centered care in a team-based environment _____
8. "Feeling" domain _____
9. The act of following through on a request or demand _____
10. The inability to feel or experience pleasure during a pleasurable activity _____
11. A person who identifies patients' barriers, works closely with the healthcare team and patients, and guides the patients through the healthcare system _____
12. The set of behaviors, ideas, and customs shared by a specific group of people, which distinguishes the members from other people _____
13. Focuses on the interrelationship among the physical, mental, social, and spiritual aspects of the person's life _____

Word Pool
- medication adherence
- compliance
- cessation
- culture
- adherence
- care coordination
- holistic
- learning
- patient navigator
- affective domain
- anhedonia
- cognitive domain
- psychomotor domain

ABBREVIATIONS
Write out what each of the following abbreviations stands for.

1. Td _____

2. HZV _____

3. PCV13 _____

4. Tdap _____

5. PPSV23 _____

6. BSE _____

7. TSE _____

8. UV _____

9. PSA _____

10. DRE _____

11. AAA _____

12. PHQ-9 _____

13. NIH _____

14. CDC _____

15. ADA _____

16. AHA _____

17. HPV _____

18. DEA _____

19. FDA _____

20. gFOBT _____

21. FIT _____

22. MT-sDNA _____

SKILLS AND CONCEPTS
Answer the following questions. Write your answer on the line or in the space provided.

A. Coaching

1. Describe coaching in your own words. _____

_____

_____

2. Define coaching a patient as it relates to disease prevention. _____
_____

3. List two types of disease prevention coaching a medical assistant may provide. _____
_____

4. Define coaching a patient as it relates to health maintenance._____
_____

5. List two types of health maintenance coaching a medical assistant may provide._____
_____

6. Define coaching a patient as it relates to compliance with a treatment plan. _____
_____
_____

7. How can coaching help increase a patient's compliance or adherence to the treatment plan? _____
_____
_____

8. Define coaching a patient as it relates to adaptations (special needs) relevant to individual patient needs.
_____
_____
_____

9. Define coaching a patient as it relates to community resources._____
_____
_____
_____

B. Making Changes for Health

1. Describe the following grief and dying stages by Kübler-Ross.

   a. Denial _____
   _____

   b. Anger_____
   _____

   c. Bargaining_____
   _____

    d. Depression _____

       _____

    e. Acceptance _____

       _____

2. Describe how grieving may impact a patient's compliance with a treatment plan._____

    _____

    _____

3. List adaptive interactions used for each stage of grief and dying.

    a. Denial _____

       _____

    b. Anger_____

       _____

    c. Bargaining_____

       _____

    d. Depression _____

       _____

    e. Acceptance _____

       _____

4. What does the health belief model help to explain? _____

    _____

5. Briefly describe the three parts of the health belief model. _____

    _____

    _____

    _____

    _____

C. Basics of Teaching and Learning

1. Briefly describe the cognitive domain of learning. _____

    _____

    _____

    _____

2. Related to the cognitive domain, list four ways a medical assistant can help patients remember critical information.

   _____

   _____

   _____

3. List three cognitive teaching strategies._____

   _____

4. List two barriers to the cognitive learning domain. _____

   _____

   _____

5. List three strategies a medical assistant could use to adapt to the cognitive learning barriers. _____

   _____

   _____

6. Briefly describe the psychomotor domain of learning._____

   _____

7. Related to the psychomotor domain, list four ways a medical assistant can help patients remember critical information.

   _____

   _____

   _____

8. List two psychomotor teaching strategies. _____

   _____

9. List two barriers to the psychomotor learning domain. _____

   _____

10. List a strategy a medical assistant could use to adapt to the psychomotor learning barriers. _____

    _____

11. Briefly describe the affective domain of learning. _____

    _____

12. Related to the affective domain, list two ways a medical assistant can help patients remember critical information.

    _____

    _____

13. List two affective teaching strategies. _____

_____

14. List three barriers to the affective learning domain. _____

_____

15. List a strategy a medical assistant could use to adapt to the affective learning barriers. _____

_____

16. List two things a medical assistant should consider when adapting coaching to a patient. _____

_____

_____

17. Describe the goals of each of Erikson's psychosocial development stages.

   a. Trust versus mistrust _____

   _____

   b. Autonomy versus shame and doubt_____

   _____

   c. Initiative versus guilt _____

   _____

   d. Industry versus inferiority _____

   _____

   e. Identity versus role confusion _____

   _____

   f. Intimacy versus isolation _____

   _____

   g. Generativity versus stagnation _____

   _____

   h. Ego integrity versus despair _____

   _____

18. Describe three strategies to use when communicating with patients who have impaired vision.

_____

_____

_____

_____

19. Describe five strategies to use when communicating with patients who have impaired hearing.

_____

_____

20. Describe three strategies to use when communicating with patients who have language barriers.

_____

_____

21. How should a medical assistant start the coaching process?_____

_____

_____

D. Coaching on Disease Prevention

1. List three common disease prevention coaching topics a medical assistant may provide._____

_____

_____

2. Describe cough etiquette._____

_____

_____

E. Coaching on Health Maintenance and Wellness

1. What is the purpose of self-exams? _____

_____

_____

2. Women with an average risk of breast cancer should start having yearly mammograms between age
   _____ and _____.

3. About half of men diagnosed with testicular cancer are between _____ and _____ years of age.

4. _____ is the most dangerous type of skin cancer.

5. List three risk factors for skin cancer. _____

_____

_____

6. List four symptoms of oral cancer._____

_____

_____

7. People age 18-39 years should have a blood pressure check every _____ to _____ years.

8. Adults with no history of high cholesterol should have it checked every _____ years.

9. Adults 45 years old and older with normal risk should have a stool screening test every _____ or _____ years depending on the test and a colonoscopy every _____ years.

10. A dental exam and cleaning are recommended _____.

11. For women ages 30-65, a Pap test is recommended every 5 years if the _____ test is also done.

12. Type 2 diabetes mellitus screening should be done every _____ years starting at age 18.

13. List three risk factors for hepatitis C. _____

    _____

    _____

14. An alcoholic drink is classified as a(n) _____ of beer, a(n) _____ of wine, or a(n) _____ of liquor.

15. List five common signs of drug abuse. _____

    _____

    _____

16. Intimate partner violence includes what behaviors? _____

    _____

    _____

17. Describe common signs of elder abuse and neglect for each of the following categories.

    a. Physical abuse _____

        _____

    b. Emotional abuse _____

        _____

    c. Neglect _____

        _____

F. Coaching on Diagnostic Tests

1. List two advantages of the Cologuard Stool DNA test over the guaiac fecal occult blood test. _____

    _____

    _____

    _____

2. A patient needs to undergo a CT scan that requires contrast medium.

    a. What questions should the medical assistant ask the patient? _____

    _____

    _____

    b. List common patient instructions. _____

    _____

    _____

3. A patient needs to undergo a magnetic resonance imaging (MRI).

    a. What questions should the medical assistant ask the patient? _____

    _____

    _____

    b. List common patient instructions. _____

    _____

    _____

4. A patient needs to undergo mammography.

    a. What questions should the medical assistant ask the patient? _____

    _____

    _____

    b. List common patient instructions. _____

    _____

    _____

5. A patient needs to have a Pap test. List common patient preparation instructions. _____

    _____

    _____

G. Coaching on Treatment Plans

1. What type of information do patients need to know when taking medications at home? _____

    _____

    _____

    _____

    _____

H. Care Coordination

1. Describe the goals of care coordination in the ambulatory care setting. _____
   _____
   _____

2. Name four advantages of care coordination. _____
   _____
   _____

3. Define *patient navigator*. _____
   _____
   _____
   _____

4. Describe the role of the medical assistant as a patient navigator. _____
   _____
   _____

5. For care coordination/patient navigation, with what areas could the medical assistant assist the patient?
   _____
   _____
   _____

6. Describe types of community resources._____
   _____
   _____
   _____

CERTIFICATION PREPARATION
Circle the correct answer.

1. Coaching provides patients with
   a. skills.
   b. knowledge.
   c. support and confidence.
   d. all of the above.

2. Providing patients with information on routine screenings and showing patients how to do self-exams is what type of coaching?
   a. Disease prevention
   b. Health maintenance
   c. Diagnostic tests
   d. Specific needs

3. Providing patients with information on hygiene practices, recommended vaccines, and nicotine cessation is what type of coaching?
   a. Disease prevention
   b. Health maintenance
   c. Diagnostic tests
   d. Specific needs

4. When a patient is experiencing sadness and uncertainty when grieving, what stage of Kübler-Ross' theory is the person in?
   a. Denial
   b. Anger
   c. Bargaining
   d. Depression

5. Language barriers are barriers to learning in the _____ domain.
   a. psychomotor
   b. affective
   c. cognitive
   d. a and c

6. According to Erikson's theory, an adolescent is in which stage?
   a. Identity versus role confusion
   b. Intimacy versus isolation
   c. Industry versus inferiority
   d. Generativity versus stagnation

7. What colorectal cancer screening test requires no patient preparation and consists of a computer analysis that checks the stool for cancer and precancerous cells?
   a. gFOBT
   b. FIT
   c. PET
   d. MD-sDNA

8. Which imaging procedure uses x-rays to create pictures of cross-sections of the patient's body?
   a. X-ray
   b. Computed tomography scan
   c. Magnetic resonance imaging
   d. Mammography

9. What diagnostic test provides an x-ray picture of the breasts and is used to find tumors?
   a. X-ray
   b. Computed tomography scan
   c. Magnetic resonance imaging
   d. Mammography

10. What diagnostic test uses high-frequency sound waves to create an image of the organs and structures?
    a. Ultrasound
    b. Computed tomography scan
    c. Magnetic resonance imaging
    d. Mammography

WORKPLACE APPLICATIONS

1. Working in family medicine, Suzanne works with people of all ages. Describe tips to remember when coaching/working with patients of the following ages.

   a. 1-year-old _____

   _____

   b. 2-year-old _____

   _____

   c. 5-year-old _____

   _____

   d. 8-year-old _____

   _____

   e. 14-year-old _____

   _____

f. 30-year-old _____

_____

g. 72-year-old _____

_____

_____

2. Suzanne is coaching a patient about the early warning signs of malignant melanoma. Describe the ABCDE rule.

_____

_____

_____

_____

INTERNET ACTIVITIES

1. Using the FDA website (www.fda.gov), research "disposal of unused medications" in the home environment. Create a poster, PowerPoint, or paper summarizing your research. Focus on these areas:
   a. Using authorized collectors for disposal (e.g., take-back programs)
   b. Disposal in household trash
   c. Disposing of fentanyl patches

2. Using the CDC website (www.cdc.gov), research recommended immunizations for children. Create a poster, PowerPoint, or paper summarizing your research. Focus on five recommended childhood immunizations and address the following for each:
   a. Name of immunization
   b. Why is it recommended or what does it prevent?
   c. Schedule of the vaccine (or the ages when a child should receive the immunization)
   d. Side effects of the vaccine

3. Using the CDC website (www.cdc.gov), research recommended immunizations. Create a poster, PowerPoint, or paper summarizing your research. Focus on immunizations prior to, during, and after pregnancy.
   a. What is recommended? Why is it recommended?
   b. What is not recommended?

Procedure 22.1   Coach a Patient on Disease Prevention

Name _____   Date _____   Score _____

Tasks: Coach a patient on the recommended vaccinations for his or her age. Adapt coaching for the patient's communication barriers and developmental life stage. Document the coaching in the patient's health record.

Scenario: You are working with Dr. David Kahn. You need to room Charles Johnson (date of birth [DOB]: 03/03/1958) and his record indicates he has not been seen in several years. Charles has a significant hearing loss and he communicates by signing. His wife interprets for him. You look in his health record and see that he is due for influenza, Td, and recombinant zoster (shingles) vaccines. Per the provider's request (order), you need to coach adult patients on potential vaccines they are due for during the initial rooming process.

Directions: Role-play this scenario with two other peers.

Equipment and Supplies:
- VIS (available at http://www.immunize.org/vis/)
- Patient's health record

Standard: Complete the procedure and all critical steps in _____ minutes with a minimum score of 85% within two attempts (*or as indicated by the instructor*).

Scoring: Divide the points earned by the total possible points. Failure to perform a critical step, indicated by an asterisk (*), results in grade no higher than an 84% (*or as indicated by the instructor*).

Time: Began_____ Ended_____ Total minutes: _____

Steps:	Point Value	Attempt 1	Attempt 2
1. Wash hands or use hand sanitizer.	5		
2. Greet the patient. Identify yourself. Verify the patient's identity with full name and date of birth. Explain what you will be doing.	10		
3. Arrange the chairs so the patient can see both you and the person signing. Speak slowly. Pause as needed to allow person signing to finish with the last statement. Look at the patient when communicating.	15		
4. Use simpler language when talking. Speak clearly. Communicate with dignity and respect. Allow time for the patient to respond. Listen to the patient's concerns.	15*		
5. Ask the patient if he has received vaccines somewhere else over the past few years.	5		
Scenario update: Patient has not seen any healthcare providers over the last few years. The only vaccines received were given in this facility. 6. Describe the vaccines that are due. Use the VIS for each vaccine as you coach the patient on the purpose of the vaccine.	15*		
Scenario update: The patient knows the shingles vaccine is not covered and costs more than $200. He refuses the shingles vaccines and he does not believe in getting the influenza vaccine. He is interested in getting the Td vaccine. 7. Ask the patient which vaccines he is interested in getting. If he refuses, be respectful of his choice. Any reason he gives for the refusal should be communicated to the provider.	15*		

8.	Document the coaching in the patient's health record. Include the provider's name, what was taught, how the patient responded, and any vaccines refused.	20			
	Total Points	100			

Documentation

Comments

CAAHEP Competencies	Step(s)
V.P.4.c. Coach patients regarding: disease prevention	6, 7
V.P.5.b. Coach patients appropriately considering: developmental life stage	4
V.P.5.c. Coach patients appropriately considering: communication barriers	3, 4
X.P.3. Document patient care accurately in the medical record	8
ABHES Competencies	**Step(s)**
5.d. Adapt care to address the developmental stages of life	4
8.h. Teach self-examination, disease management and health promotion	6
8.j. Make adaptations for patients with special needs (psychological or physical limitations)	3, 4
8.k. Make adaptations to care for patients across their lifespan	4

Procedure 22.2 Develop a List of Community Resources and Facilitate Referrals

Name _____ Date _____ Score _____

Tasks: As a patient navigator, develop a current list of community resources that meet the patient's health-care needs. Discuss the resources with the patient and facilitate referrals to the chosen resources.

Scenario 1: Robert Caudill (DOB: 10/31/1940) was just diagnosed with dementia. He currently lives with his daughter, Ruby, who works full-time. Ruby is feeling overwhelmed with being his only caregiver and realizes that she needs to find someone to care for her father while she is working.

Scenario 2: Leslie Green (DOB 08/03/03) just tested positive for pregnancy. She does not feel that she has a support system to help her make decisions.

Scenario 3: Ella Rainwater's husband of 30 years died suddenly 1 month ago. Ella (DOB: 07/11/1959) stated that she feels alone and has no one to talk to. Her daughter feels that she needs the support of others who have gone through the same thing.

Directions: Role-play these scenarios with another peer. The peer will be the family member or patient during the first part of the role-play and then the community resource agency representative during the second part.

Equipment and Supplies:
- Computer with internet or a telephone book
- Paper and pen
- Community Resource Referral Form (Work Product 22.1) or referral form
- Patient's health record

Standard: Complete the procedure and all critical steps in _____ minutes with a minimum score of 85% within two attempts (*or as indicated by the instructor*).

Scoring: Divide the points earned by the total possible points. Failure to perform a critical step, indicated by an asterisk (*), results in grade no higher than an 84% (*or as indicated by the instructor*).

Time: Began_____ Ended_____ Total minutes: _____

Steps:	Point Value	Attempt 1	Attempt 2
1. Using the scenario, identify the possible types of community resources that would assist each patient or family. Identify three different types of resources (e.g., medical equipment, support group) that would meet each patient's needs.	5		
2. Using the internet or the phone book, identify two local resources for each of the three kinds of resources (i.e., find two assisted living resources, two medical equipment suppliers, etc.). Make a list of six resources for the patient and family. Include the following: a. Organization's name b. Address and contact information c. Summary of the services provided d. Cost and other relevant information	30		

3.	*Role-play the scenario indicated by the instructor*: Provide the patient or family member with the list of six resources. Describe the services offered and any costs.	**15***		
4.	Allow the patient or family member time to review the services. Answer any questions.	**10**		
5.	Use professional, tactful verbal and nonverbal communication as you work with the patient or family member.	**10***		
6.	*Role-play making the community referral(s)*: Have the patient or family member decide on two or more services they are interested in. Complete the referral document (Work Product 22.1). Have the patient provide any additional information required on the form. Call the community resource agency and provide the referral information to the representative (a peer).	**20***		
7.	Document the patient education and the referrals in the health record.	**10**		
	Total Points	**100**		

Documentation

.

Comments

CAAHEP Competencies	Step(s)
V.P.9. Develop a current list of community resources related to patients' healthcare needs	1, 2
V.P.10. Facilitate referrals to community resources in the role of a patient navigator	3-6
X.P.3. Document patient care accurately in the medical record	7
ABHES Competencies	**Step(s)**
5. Human Relations b.3) List organizations and support groups that can assist patients and family members of patients experiencing terminal illnesses	1, 2
8.i. Identify community resources and Complementary and Alternative Medicine practices (CAM)	1, 2

Work Product 22.1   Community Resource Referral Form

To be used with Procedure 22.2.

Name _____   **Date** _____   **Score** _____

Patient's Name: Date of Birth:

Community Resource Information:

Agency: _____ Contact Name: _____

Address: _____ Phone number: _____

_____ Website: _____

Services Provided:

Agency: _____ Contact Name: _____

Address: _____ Phone number: _____

_____ Website: _____

Services Provided:

Agency: _____ Contact Name: _____

Address: _____ Phone number: _____

_____ Website: _____

Services Provided:

Agency: _____ Contact Name: _____

Address: _____ Phone number: _____

_____ Website: _____

Services Provided:

Nutrition and Health Promotion

CAAHEP Competencies	Assessment
IV.C.1.a. Describe dietary nutrients including: carbohydrates	Skills and Concepts – B. 3, 19; Certification Preparation – 1
IV.C.1.b. Describe dietary nutrients including: fat	Skills and Concepts – B. 19-22; Certification Preparation – 3
IV.C.1.c. Describe dietary nutrients including: protein	Skills and Concepts – B. 13-17, 19; Certification Preparation – 2
IV.C.1.d. Describe dietary nutrients including: minerals	Skills and Concepts – B. 26-28; Certification Preparation – 4
IV.C.1.e. Describe dietary nutrients including: electrolytes	Skills and Concepts – B. 26-28
IV.C.1.f. Describe dietary nutrients including: vitamins	Skills and Concepts – B. 29-38; Certification Preparation – 6
IV.C.1.g. Describe dietary nutrients including: fiber	Skills and Concepts – B. 9-12
IV.C.1.h. Describe dietary nutrients including: water	Skills and Concepts – B. 39-41
IV.C.2. Define the function of dietary supplements	Skills and Concepts – B. 12
IV.C.3.a. Identify the special dietary needs for: weight control	Skills and Concepts – E. 4-5
IV.C.3.b. Identify the special dietary needs for: diabetes	Skills and Concepts – E. 7-8; Certification Preparation – 7
IV.C.3.c. Identify the special dietary needs for: cardiovascular disease	Skills and Concepts – E. 10-13
IV.C.3.d. Identify the special dietary needs for: hypertension	Skills and Concepts – E. 9-11; Certification Preparation – 8
IV.C.3.e. Identify the special dietary needs for: cancer	Skills and Concepts – F. 6-7; Workplace Applications – 2
IV.C.3.f. Identify the special dietary needs for: lactose sensitivity	Skills and Concepts – E. 24-25
IV.C.3.g. Identify the special dietary needs for: gluten-free	Skills and Concepts – E. 22-23; Certification Preparation – 9

CAAHEP Competencies	Assessment
IV.C.3.h. Identify the special dietary needs for: food allergies	Skills and Concepts – E. 17-21
IV.P.1. Instruct a patient according to patient's special dietary needs	Procedure 23.1
IV.A.1. Show awareness of patient's concerns regarding a dietary change	Procedure 23.1

ABHES Competencies	Assessment
2. Anatomy and Physiology d. Apply a system of diet and nutrition 1) Explain the importance of diet and nutrition	Skills and Concepts – A. 1; B. 1
2.d.2) Educate patients regarding proper diet and nutrition guidelines	Procedure 23.1
2.d.3) Identify categories of patients that require special diets or diet modifications	Skills and Concepts – E. 3-4, 7, 9-12, 14-16, 22, 24-25; F. 1-7; Workplace Applications – 1-2

VOCABULARY REVIEW

Using the word pool on the right, find the correct word to match the definition. Write the word on the line after the definition.

Group A

1. The chemical process that occurs within a living organism to maintain life _____

2. A field of study that examines the substances in food that help us grow and stay healthy _____

3. Special proteins that speed up the chemical reactions in the body _____

4. Chemicals in food that the body uses for energy, growth, and development _____

5. Result when fats are broken down; used by the body for energy and tissue development _____

6. The process of smaller molecules being used to build larger molecules with the use of energy _____

7. The process of breaking down molecules into smaller molecules resulting in energy being released _____

8. Released during the digestion of protein foods in the intestines; carried by the blood to cells where they are used to make proteins _____

9. Results when carbohydrates are broken down; main sugar found in the blood and used as the main source of energy _____

10. A unit that measures how much energy is in a particular food _____

Word Pool
- fatty acids
- nutrition
- nutrients
- amino acids
- glucose
- calorie
- metabolism
- catabolism
- anabolism
- enzymes

Group B

1. The rate the body burns calories while the person is at rest
   _____

2. Nutrient used for energy and to regulate protein and fat metabolism
   _____

3. Cannot be made by the body and must be in the food eaten
   _____

4. Created by the body and do not need to be in food
   _____

5. Foods lacking vitamins, minerals, and fiber
   _____

6. A hormone produced by the beta cells in the pancreas; moves glucose into the cells so it can be used for energy
   _____

7. A nutrient that is broken down into amino acids
   _____

8. A hormone produced by the alpha cells in the pancreas; works on the liver to release glycogen and thereby prevent dangerously low blood glucose levels _____

9. Foods that have all the essential amino acids to support the body
   _____

10. Nutrients added back into a food after they were lost during food processing _____

Word Pool
- essential nutrients
- nonessential nutrients
- insulin
- carbohydrate
- nonnutrient-rich
- basal metabolic rate
- glucagon
- enriched
- complete proteins
- protein

Group C

1. Synthetic or natural substances found in food and supplements; may prevent or delay some types of cell damage
   _____

2. Providing information in a supportive environment that allows people to grow, change, or improve their situation
   _____

3. Average daily level of food intake needed to meet the nutrient requirements of most healthy people _____

4. The food and drink a person typically consumes when there are no dietary limitations _____

5. A rapidly progressing, life-threatening allergic reaction; characterized by hives, swelling of the mouth and airway, difficulty breathing, wheezing, and loss of consciousness
   _____

6. A credentialed healthcare professional who is trained in nutrition and is able to apply the information to the dietary needs of healthy and ill patients _____

7. Foods that do not contain all the essential amino acids
   _____

8. Nutrients are added to a food; these nutrients were never originally in the food _____

Word Pool
- regular diet
- anaphylaxis
- antioxidant
- coaching
- fortified
- incomplete proteins
- registered dietitian
- recommended dietary allowance

ABBREVIATIONS
Write out what each of the following abbreviations stands for.

1. BMR _____

2. GI _____

3. LDL _____

4. HDL _____

5. USDA _____

6. mg _____

7. DV _____

8. GERD _____

9. CDC _____

10. BMI _____

11. LAGB _____

12. FDA _____

13. DASH _____

14. AHA _____

SKILLS AND CONCEPTS
Answer the following questions. Write your answer on the line or in the space provided.

A. Metabolism

1. Describe the two phases of metabolism in your own words. _____

_____

2. List the three factors that affect the number of calories a person burns each day. _____

_____

_____

3. What happens with the unused calories in the body? _____

_____

_____

_____

B. Dietary Nutrients

1. Explain the difference between essential and nonessential nutrients in your own words._____

   _____

   _____

2. What is meant by the phrase *nutrient dense*?_____

   _____

3. Describe carbohydrates. Your answer should include what the body uses carbohydrates for and typical foods that contain this nutrient.

   _____

   _____

4. _____ increases the blood glucose level and _____ helps it move out of the bloodstream to the cells to be used for energy.

5. Glucose is also stored in the liver and muscles as _____.

6. When glycogen is released back into the blood, it increases the _____ levels.

7. Describe smart carbohydrate choices. _____

   _____

   _____

8. What is the glycemic index? _____

   _____

9. _____, a carbohydrate that passes through the digestive system and does not raise the blood glucose level.

10. Describe soluble fiber.

    a. What is soluble fiber? _____

       _____

    b. Describe the health benefits of soluble fiber._____

       _____

    c. List two nutrient-rich foods that contain soluble fiber. _____

       _____

11. Describe insoluble fiber.

    a. What is insoluble fiber? _____

       _____

b. List two nutrient-rich foods that contain insoluble fiber. _____

_____

12. What is the role of fiber supplements? _____

_____

13. Describe protein. What it is used for in the body?_____

_____

14. Describe the difference between essential and nonessential amino acids._____

_____

_____

15. Describe complete proteins and list three examples. _____

_____

_____

16. Describe incomplete proteins and list three examples._____

_____

17. Describe smart protein choices. _____

_____

_____

18. Where are omega-3 fatty acids found and what is their role? _____

_____

_____

19. List the number of calories provided by each: 1g of fat, protein, and carbohydrate._____

_____

_____

20. Describe how fat is used in the body. _____

_____

_____

21. Describe each of the following types of fats. Your answer should also include how it affects cholesterol and list two foods that contain that type of fat.

a. Saturated fats _____

_____

    b.   Unsaturated fats_____

_____

    c.   Trans-fatty acids_____

_____

22. What are triglycerides and how are they used in the body? _____

_____

23. What is cholesterol used for in the body? _____

_____

24. Where does cholesterol come from? _____

_____

25. _____ is considered bad cholesterol and _____ is considered good cholesterol and helps move the cholesterol from the tissues to the liver.

26. Describe the difference between minerals and electrolytes._____

_____

27. Describe major minerals (macrominerals) and trace minerals (microminerals) and give two examples of each.

_____

_____

28. For each of the following minerals, describe how they are used in the body and list two foods that contain the mineral.

    a.   Calcium _____

_____

    b.   Potassium _____

_____

    c.   Sodium _____

_____

    d.   Chloride_____

_____

    e.   Phosphorus_____

_____

    f.   Magnesium _____

_____

g. Iron_____

_____

29. Define *vitamins*. _____

_____

30. Discuss water-soluble vitamins. What are they? List two examples. What happens with extra in the body?

_____

_____

31. Discuss fat-soluble vitamins. What are they? List four examples. What happens with extra fat-soluble vitamin in the body?

_____

_____

32. A deficiency in vitamin A can cause _____.

33. _____ is made by the body after being in the sun.

34. _____ is made in the intestine and also comes from dark green and dark leafy vegetables. It helps blood clot.

35. A deficiency of thiamine (vitamin B_1) can cause _____.

36. A deficiency of niacin (vitamin B_3) can cause _____.

37. _____ works with vitamin B_{12} to help form blood cells. It is also important in pregnancy to prevent _____.

38. A deficiency of vitamin C can cause _____.

39. _____ makes up more than two-thirds of the body's weight and is the basis for the fluids in the body.

40. Describe the important roles water plays in the body. _____

_____

_____

41. Describe when we need to increase our water intake. _____

_____

_____

C. Dietary Guidelines

1. What is the focus of MyPlate?_____

_____

2. List the key messages of MyPlate. _____

_____

_____

3. What is the focus of the Dietary Guidelines published by the USDA? _____

_____

4. What is the current recommendation for sodium consumption for individuals 14 years and older?

_____

5. What is the current recommendation for alcohol consumption for men and women? _____

_____

D. Reading Food Labels

1. The _____ contains the nutritional information and the ingredient list.

2. Food labels provide information in both the _____ and the
_____, which reflects the % Daily Value (DV).

3. How are ingredients listed on the food label? _____

_____

4. _____ or _____ in the ingredient list indicate the presence of
trans-fats in the product.

E. Medically Ordered Diets

1. The provider will refer patient to a(n) _____ if the patient needs to make a dietary
change, which will be a lifestyle change (e.g., for diabetes or hypertension).

2. Describe the medical assistant's role with nutrition coaching. _____

_____

_____

3. Describe the following diets and indicate one reason why the patient may be on the diet.

a. Clear liquid diet _____

_____

_____

b. Full-liquid diet _____

_____

_____

c. Soft diet _____

_____

_____

d. Mechanical soft diet_____

_____

_____

e. Bland diet _____

_____

_____

4. What are the special dietary needs for weight control? (What must a person do to achieve and maintain a healthy weight?)

_____

_____

5. List four tips for people trying to achieve a healthy weight. _____

_____

_____

_____

6. _____ is the amount of food we eat and _____ is a standard measurement of food.

7. What are the special dietary needs for a person with diabetes? (What must this person monitor?)

_____

_____

8. Briefly describe the different diabetic eating plans that may be used by patients.

a. Exchange list system _____

_____

_____

b. "Create Your Plate" _____

_____

_____

c. Carbohydrate counting meal plan _____

_____

_____

9. What are the special dietary needs for a person with hypertension? (What must this person monitor?)

    _____

    _____

10. Describe how sodium affects the blood pressure. _____

    _____

    _____

11. What is the goal of the DASH eating plan? What conditions is it recommended for? _____

    _____

    _____

12. What are the special dietary needs for a person with cardiovascular disease? (Hint: review the Heart-Healthy Diet)

    _____

    _____

13. What is the AHA Eating Healthy Recommendation for:

    a. Protein? _____

        _____

    b. Grains?_____

        _____

    c. Oils? _____

        _____

14. What conditions are treated with a low-protein diet?_____

    _____

15. List conditions that are treated with a low-fiber diet. _____

    _____

    _____

16. List conditions that are treated with a high-fiber diet. _____

    _____

    _____

17. List the top eight food allergens. _____

    _____

    _____

18. Describe the special dietary needs for food allergies. (What does a person with a food allergy need to do?)

    _____

    _____

19. Describe the purpose of the elimination diet._____

    _____

    _____

20. Describe cross-reactivity with allergens._____

    _____

21. Describe oral allergy syndrome._____

    _____

22. People with _____ are put on a gluten-free diet.

23. Describe a gluten-free diet. (What is gluten? What foods need to be avoided?)_____

    _____

    _____

24. Describe lactose intolerance or sensitivity. _____

    _____

    _____

25. Describe the special dietary needs for those with lactose sensitivity. _____

    _____

    _____

F. Nutritional Needs for Various Populations

1. When is a child started on soft, puréed solid foods?_____

   _____

2. As an adult grows older, the metabolism _____ and the caloric needs

   _____.

3. What are the dietary recommendations for lactation (breastfeeding)? _____

   _____

4. What is the ketogenic diet and why might a person follow it? _____

   _____

5. When a person has HIV or AIDS, what are his or her special dietary needs?_____

_____

_____

6. Describe special dietary needs a person with cancer may have._____

_____

7. Describe nutritional tips for patients undergoing cancer treatments. _____

_____

_____

CERTIFICATION PREPARATION

Circle the correct answer.

1. What foods or beverages contain carbohydrates?
   a. Cookies, cakes, and other sweets
   b. Regular soda pop and milk products
   c. Breads and cereals
   d. All of the above

2. What foods contain protein?
   a. Fish, meat, and poultry
   b. Fruits and vegetables
   c. Tree nuts and legumes
   d. Both a and c

3. What foods contain fat?
   a. Fruits and vegetables
   b. Legumes
   c. Butter and cheese
   d. Rice and pasta

4. Which is not a mineral?
   a. Potassium
   b. Folate
   c. Calcium
   d. Copper

5. Which protect cells from free radicals and include vitamins A and C, lutein, and selenium?
   a. Antioxidants
   b. Minerals
   c. Vitamins
   d. Electrolytes

6. Which is a water-soluble vitamin?
   a. A
   b. B
   c. D
   d. E

7. What type of foods would be limited on a diabetic eating plan?
   a. Poultry and fish
   b. Breads and pastas
   c. Cakes and cookies
   d. b and c

8. What types of foods would be limited on a low-sodium diet for hypertension?
   a. Frozen dinners and canned foods
   b. Olives and pickles
   c. Soy sauce, ketchup, and mustard
   d. All of the above

9. What types of foods would be limited on a gluten-free diet?
   a. Oatmeal and rice
   b. Potatoes and corn
   c. Barley and wheat
   d. All of the above

10. What factors impact what foods a person purchases?
    a. Cost and convenience
    b. Background and culture
    c. Emotional comfort and routine
    d. All of the above

WORKPLACE APPLICATIONS

1. Working in family medicine, Kayla coaches people of all ages. Describe the nutritional needs for each of the following patients.

   a. 0- to 6-month-old _____

   _____

   b. 2-year-old _____

   _____

   c. 16-year-old female who has her menses _____

   _____

2. Kayla is coaching an older patient who is undergoing chemotherapy for cancer. The patient's mouth is extremely sore, which makes eating difficult. What tips could Kayla give this patient regarding nutrition and oral care?

   _____

   _____

   _____

3. A person with bulimia is usually at normal weight. What symptoms might another person see that may raise the suspicion of bulimia?

   _____

   _____

   _____

INTERNET ACTIVITIES

1. Using appropriate online resources, research a diet in this chapter. Create a poster, PowerPoint, or paper summarizing your research. Focus on these areas:
   a. What foods are included in the diet?
   b. Why is the diet typically ordered?

2. Using the tools on MyPlate website (www.choosemyplate.gov), track your food intake for 3 days. At the end of the 3 days, write a brief paper address these points:
   a. What are your dietary strengths? What did you do well?
   b. What are your dietary weaknesses? What do you need to work on?
   c. Select one weakness and plan how to improve that dietary issue.
   d. What was your overall impression of the tools you used on MyPlate website?

Procedure 23.1 Instruct a Patient on a Dietary Change

Name _____ Date _____ Score _____

Tasks: Instruct a patient on his special dietary needs. Show awareness of the patient's concerns regarding the dietary change. Document in the health record.

Equipment and Supplies:
- Patient's health record
- Heart-Healthy Diet brochure

Scenario: You are working with Dr. Angela Perez, a family practice provider. She just finished seeing Al Neviaser (date of birth [DOB]: 6/21/1968). Dr. Perez orders for Heart-Healthy Diet instructions to be given to the patient.

Standard: Complete the procedure and all critical steps in _____ minutes with a minimum score of 85% within two attempts (*or as indicated by the instructor*).

Scoring: Divide the points earned by the total possible points. Failure to perform a critical step, indicated by an asterisk (*), results in grade no higher than an 84% (*or as indicated by the instructor*).

Time: Began_____ Ended_____ Total minutes: _____

Steps:	Point Value	Attempt 1	Attempt 2
1. Using the scenario, role-play the situation with a peer. Assemble supplies needed for the provider's order. Ensure that the patient can read and understand the written materials. Verify the order if you have any questions.	5		
2. Greet the patient. Identify yourself. Verify the patient's identity with full name and date of birth. Explain the order from the provider. Answer any questions the patient may have about the procedure.	10		
3. Position yourself at the same level as the patient. Angle yourself towards the patient. Have a poised position.	5		
4. Accurately instruct the patient on the new diet. Use the written materials as you discuss the new eating plan.	15*		
5. Use words that the patient can understand. Refrain from jargon and medical terminology. Use professional verbal and nonverbal communication.	10		
Scenario Update: After going over the heart-healthy eating plan, Mr. Neviaser states he is not sure this diet is for him. He likes red meat and does not like to eat fish. He does not have a lot of money to buy expensive fresh fruits and vegetables. 6. Using therapeutic communication techniques (e.g., reflection, restatement, and summarizing), show the patient you are aware of his concerns. *(Refer to the Checklist for Affective Behaviors.)*	15*		
7. Based on the patient's concerns, provide food alternatives that would meet the eating plan requirements. *(Refer to the Checklist for Affective Behaviors.)*	15*		
8. Evaluate the patient's understanding of the teaching by asking the patient to summarize the eating plan or describe a day's worth of meals. Answer any questions the patient may have.	15		

9. Document the instruction in the patient's health record. Include the order, instruction given, written materials provided, and the patient's feedback.	10		
Total Points	100		

Checklist for Affective Behaviors

Affective Behavior	**Directions:** Check behaviors observed during the role-play.					
Awareness	**Negative, Unprofessional Behaviors**	**Attempt** 1	2	**Positive, Professional Behaviors**	**Attempt** 1	2
	Rude, discourteous			Pleasant and courteous		
	Disregarded the person's dignity and rights			Maintained the person's dignity and rights		
	Failed to clearly and/or professionally address the reason for the new diet			Clearly and professionally described the reason for the new diet		
	Failed to use therapeutic communication techniques (e.g., reflection, restating, clarifying, and summarizing) to verify patient's concerns			Used therapeutic communication techniques (e.g., reflection, restating, clarifying, and summarizing) to verify patient's concerns		
	Nonempathetic behaviors; failed to address patient's concerns			Showed empathy; addressed patient's concerns		
	Failed to clearly and/or professionally address the situation and/or patient's questions			Clearly and professionally addressed the situation and/or patient's questions		
	Failed to reassure patient or inappropriately reassured patient			Appropriately reassured patient		
	Negative nonverbal behaviors			Positive nonverbal behaviors		
	Other:			Other:		

Grading for Affective Behaviors		Point Value	Attempt 1	Attempt 2
Does not meet Expectation	• Response fails to show awareness of patient's concerns. • Student demonstrated more than two negative, unprofessional behaviors during the interaction.	0		
Needs Improvement	• Response fails to show awareness of patient's concerns. • Student demonstrated one or two negative, unprofessional behaviors during the interaction.	0		
Meets Expectation	• Response shows awareness of patient's concerns; no negative, unprofessional behaviors observed. • More practice is needed for behavior to appear natural and for student to appear comfortable and at ease.	15		

Occasionally Exceeds Expectation	• Response shows awareness of patient's concerns; no negative, unprofessional behaviors observed. • At times student appeared comfortable and at ease; but more practice is needed for behavior to become natural and consistent with a professional medical assistant.	15		
Always Exceeds Expectation	• Response shows awareness of patient's concerns; no negative, unprofessional behaviors observed. • Student's behaviors appeared natural and comfortable. Behaviors are consistent with a professional medical assistant.	15		

Documentation

Comments

CAAHEP Competencies	Step(s)
IV.P.1. Instruct a patient according to patient's special dietary needs	Entire procedure
IV.A.1. Show awareness of patient's concerns regarding a dietary change	6.7
ABHES Competencies	**Step(s)**
2.d.2) Educate patients regarding proper diet and nutrition guidelines	Entire procedure

Surgical Supplies and Instruments

CAAHEP	Assessments
III.C.3.b. Define the following as practiced within an ambulatory care setting: surgical asepsis	Skills and Concepts – F. 1
III.P.4. Prepare items for autoclaving 34.1	Procedure 24.1
III.P.5. Perform sterilization procedures 34.2	Procedure 24.2
ABHES	**Assessments**
8. Clinical Procedures a. Practice standard precautions and perform disinfection/sterilization techniques	Procedure 24.2

VOCABULARY REVIEW

Using the word pool on the right, find the correct word to match the definition. Write the word on the line after the definition.

Group A

1. An agent that causes partial or complete loss of sensation _____
2. A thick-walled, dormant form of bacteria that is very resistant to disinfection measures _____
3. To cut or separate tissue with a cutting instrument or scissors _____
4. A disease causing-organism _____
5. Localized collections of pus, which may be under the skin or deep in the body, that cause tissue destruction _____
6. A metal rod with a smooth, rounded tip that is placed in hollow instruments to reduce injury to body tissues during insertion _____
7. A liquid substance that dilutes or lessens the strength of a solution or mixture _____
8. Contraction of the muscles causing the narrowing of the inside tube of the vessel _____
9. A metal probe that is inserted into or passed through a catheter, needle, or tube used for clearing purposes or to facilitate passage into a body orifice _____
10. Not lasting, enduring, or permanent _____

Word Pool
- diluent
- pathogen
- transient
- spore
- anesthetic
- abscess
- vasoconstriction
- dissect
- stylus
- obturator

Group B

1. Capable of burning, corroding, or destroying living tissue _____

2. The act of scraping a body cavity with a surgical instrument such as a curette _____

3. Not permitting penetration _____

4. A recess in the upper part of the vagina caused by protrusion of the cervix into the vaginal wall _____

5. Allowing for penetration _____

6. Open condition of a body cavity or canal _____

7. The opening or widening of the circumference of a body orifice with a dilating instrument _____

8. Invasion of body tissues by microorganisms, which then multiply and damage tissues _____

9. A rigid tube that surrounds a blunt trocar or a sharp, pointed trocar, which is inserted into the body _____

Word Pool
- cannula
- fornix
- dilation
- curettage
- patency
- infection
- permeable
- impervious
- caustic

SKILLS AND CONCEPTS

Answer the following questions. Write your answer on the line or in the space provided.

A. Surgical Solutions and Medications

1. Explain the purpose of topical anesthetics and how they act. _____

_____

_____

_____

_____

_____

_____

_____

2. Why is epinephrine frequently an ingredient in a local anesthetic? _____

_____

_____

_____

_____

_____

3. Explain the purpose of additional surgical supplies that may be used in minor surgical procedures in the provider's office.

   _____

   _____

   _____

   _____

   _____

   _____

   _____

   _____

   _____

B. Surgical Instruments

Name the instruments pictured in the following figures.

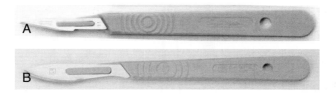

1. _____

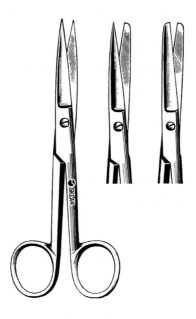

2. _____

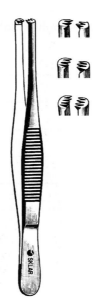

3. _____

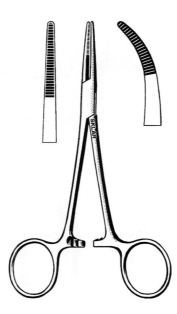

4. _____

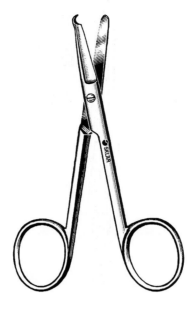

5. _____

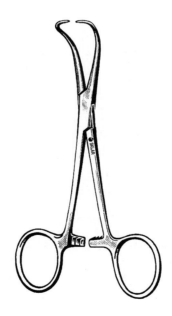

6. _____

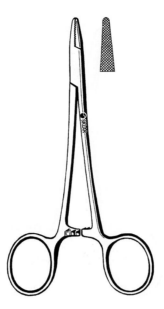

7. _____

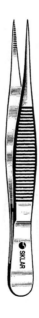

8. _____

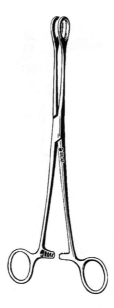

9. _____

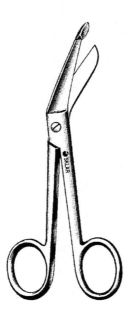

10. _____

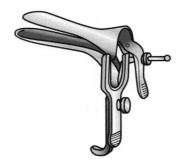

11. _____

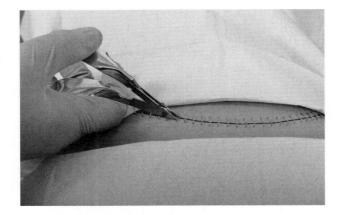

12. _____

C. Classifications of Surgical Instruments

1. List four groups of surgical instruments and give an example of each.

a. _____

_____

b. _____

_____

c. _____

_____

d. _____

_____

D. Specialty Instruments

Name the instruments pictured in the following figures.

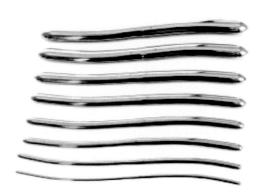

1. _____

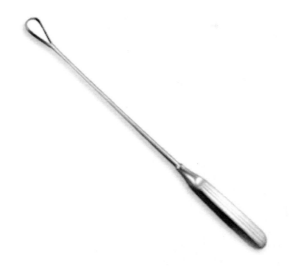

2. _____

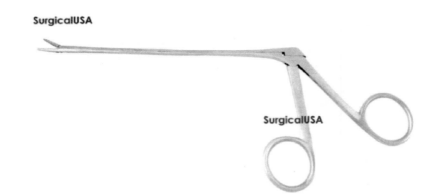

3. _____

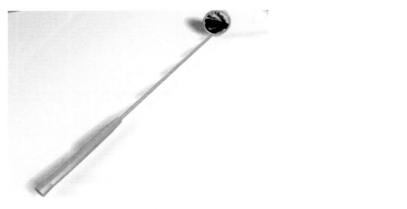

4. _____

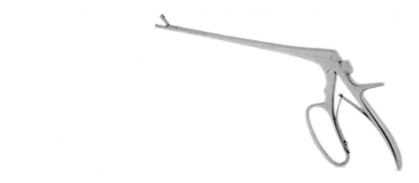

5. _____

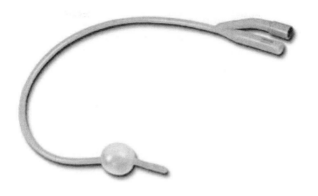

6. _____

E. Drapes, Sutures, and Needles

1. Summarize four advantages of tissue adhesives.

   a. _____

   _____

   b. _____

   _____

   c. _____

   _____

   d. _____

   _____

2. Explain the difference between absorbable and nonabsorbable sutures. When would each type of suture be used? Give an example of each.

   _____

   _____

   _____

   _____

   _____

   _____

   _____

   _____

F. Surgical Asepsis and Preparation of Surgical Instruments

1. Differentiate between medical asepsis and surgical asepsis. _____

   _____

   _____

   _____

   _____

2. Explain the following types of sterilization indicators. Which is considered the best method for checking whether instrument packs are being sterilized when autoclaved? What are the CDC recommendations for each type?

   a. Chemical _____

   _____

   _____

   _____

   _____

   _____

   _____

   _____

   b. Biologic _____

   _____

   _____

   _____

   _____

   _____

   _____

   _____

3. The medical assistant is responsible for making sure no problems occur with autoclave procedures. Describe what could be causing the following problems and how they could be prevented.

   a. Damp autoclave paper _____

   _____

   _____

   _____

   _____

b. Corroded instruments_____

_____

_____

_____

_____

c. Spotted or stained instruments _____

_____

_____

_____

_____

d. Steam leakage_____

_____

_____

_____

_____

e. Chamber door does not open _____

_____

_____

_____

_____

4. Describe what is meant by *event-related practices* when determining whether an autoclaved instrument pack is still sterile.

_____

_____

_____

_____

_____

_____

_____

_____

5. Explain quality-assurance logs related to sterilization procedures. _____

_____

_____

_____

_____

_____

CERTIFICATION PREPARATION

Circle the correct answer.

1. Choose the smallest diameter of suture strand.
   a. 0
   b. 5-0
   c. 5
   d. 1-0

2. The recommended way to clean sharp instruments is to
   a. use an ultrasonic cleaner.
   b. wear appropriate PPE.
   c. use the proper concentration of disinfectant.
   d. rinse instruments with sterile water before sterilizing.

3. The jaws of which instrument are shorter and stronger than hemostat jaws?
   a. Splinter forceps
   b. Towel forceps
   c. Needleholder
   d. Suture scissors

4. Which is one of the strongest nonabsorbable sutures?
   a. Dacron
   b. Vicryl
   c. Silk
   d. Maxon

5. _____ is the complete destruction of microorganisms and spores. This technique is mandatory for any procedure that invades the body's skin or tissues, such as surgery.
   a. Disinfection
   b. Sterilization
   c. Medical asepsis
   d. Surgical asepsis

6. The recommended temperature for sterilization in an autoclave is
   a. 98.6° F.
   b. 104° F.
   c. 121° C.
   d. 37.6° C.

7. What is the complete destruction of pathogens and spores?
   a. Sanitization
   b. Disinfection
   c. Sterilization
   d. Germicide

8. Which instrument would be damaged by the high temperature and steam under pressure of autoclaves and must be disinfected after each procedure?
   a. Endoscope used in an endoscopy
   b. Microscope used for microsurgery
   c. Electrosurgical tip used for electrosurgery
   d. Laser tip used for laser surgery

9. Which gynecologic instrument is used to remove polyps, secretions, and bits of placental tissue?
   a. Sims uterine curette
   b. Endocervical curette
   c. Schroeder uterine vulsellum forceps
   d. Both a and b

10. Which ophthalmologic and otolaryngologic instrument is used to remove foreign bodies or polyps?
    a. Krause nasal snare
    b. Hartmann "alligator" ear forceps
    c. "Buck" ear curette
    d. All of the above

WORKPLACE APPLICATIONS

1. Melissa, the medical assistant, is preparing instruments for the autoclave. What rules must she follow when wrapping the instruments?

   _____

   _____

   _____

   _____

2. Tony Carmini, 5 years old, was brought to the clinic today by his mother for treatment of a laceration above his right eyebrow. Rather than suturing the wound, the provider may decide to use either Steri-Strips or skin adhesive. Why are these suturing alternatives a good choice for this patient? Describe both skin closure materials in your answer.

   _____

   _____

   _____

   _____

3. Callie is working with a medical assistant student who is at WMFC for her practicum. What guidelines should Callie explain to the student about unloading the autoclave?

   _____

   _____

   _____

   _____

INTERNET ACTIVITIES

1. Using internet resources, research the use of surgical staples. Create a poster presentation, a PowerPoint presentation, or write a paper that summarizes your research. Include the following points in your project:
   a. What types of surgeries use staples to close a wound?
   b. How are they applied?
   c. How are they removed?

2. One of medical assistant's duties is to purchase supplies for minor office procedures. Search the internet for equipment and supplies typically needed to perform such procedures. Print a list of materials and prices. Share the information with your classmates. Did you find anything surprising?

Procedure 24.1   Wrap Instruments and Supplies for Sterilization in an Autoclave

Name _____ Date _____ Score _____

Task: To place dry, inspected, and sanitized supplies and instruments inside appropriate wrapping materials for sterilization and storage without contamination.

Equipment and Supplies:
- Dry, inspected, and sanitized instruments
- Double-ply autoclave paper
- Autoclave tape
- Sterilization strip
- Waterproof, felt-tipped pen
- Gloves (if part of office policy)

Standard: Complete the procedure and all critical steps in _____ minutes with a minimum score of 85% within two attempts (*or as indicated by the instructor*).

Scoring: Divide the points earned by the total possible points. Failure to perform a critical step, indicated by an asterisk (*), results in grade no higher than an 84% (*or as indicated by the instructor*).

Time: Began_____ Ended_____ Total minutes: _____

Steps:	Point Value	Attempt 1	Attempt 2
1. Wash or sanitize your hands. Collect and assemble already inspected, sanitized instruments to be wrapped. Gloves may be worn.	10		
2. Place the double-ply autoclave paper on a clean, flat surface.	10		
3. Place the instruments diagonally at the approximate center of the double-ply autoclave paper. Make sure the size of the square is large enough for the items.	15*		
4. Open any hinged instruments. If the instrument is sharp, its teeth or tip should be shielded with cotton or gauze.	15*		
5. Place a sterilization strip in the center of the pack to check for sterilization standards.	10		
6. Bring up the bottom corner of the wrap and fold back a portion of it.	10		
7. Repeat the previous step with each corner, making sure to turn back a portion each time.	10		
8. Fold the last flap over.	10		
9. Secure with autoclave tape and label the package with the date, including the year, contents, and your initials.	10		
Total Points	100		

Comments

CAAHEP Competencies	Step(s)
III.P.4. Prepare items for autoclaving	Entire procedure
ABHES Competencies	**Step(s)**
4.a. Identify appropriate procedures for sterilization of 1. Instruments 2. Surgical equipment 3. Surgical towels, drapes, or dressings	Entire procedure
4.c. Utilize proper instrument and tray packaging for sterilization	Entire procedure
8.a. Practice standard precautions and perform disinfection/sterilization techniques	Entire procedure

Procedure 24.2   Operate the Autoclave

Name _____ Date _____ Score _____

Task: To sterilize properly prepared supplies and instruments using the autoclave.

Equipment and Supplies:
- Autoclave
- Wrapped items ready to be sterilized
- Heat-resistant gloves

Standard: Complete the procedure and all critical steps in _____ minutes with a minimum score of 85% within two attempts (*or as indicated by the instructor*).

Scoring: Divide the points earned by the total possible points. Failure to perform a critical step, indicated by an asterisk (*), results in grade no higher than an 84% (*or as indicated by the instructor*).

Time: Began_____ Ended_____ Total minutes: _____

Steps:	Point Value	Attempt 1	Attempt 2
NOTE: *The specific instructions for operating an autoclave may vary based on the model number and manufacturer. Refer to the instructions that accompany the autoclave to be sure the appropriate steps are followed.*			
1. Check the water level in the reservoir and add distilled water as necessary.	5		
2. Turn the control to "Fill" to allow water to flow into the chamber. The water flows until you turn the control to its next position. Do not let the water overflow.	5		
3. Load the chamber with wrapped items, spacing them for maximum circulation and penetration.	10*		
4. Close and seal the door.	5		
5. Turn the control setting to "On" or "Autoclave" to start the cycle.	5		
6. Watch the gauges until the temperature gauge reaches at least 121°C (250°F) and the pressure gauge reaches 15 lbs. of pressure.	10*		
7. Set the timer for the desired time.	5		
8. At the end of the timed cycle, turn the control setting to "Vent."	5		
9. Wait for the pressure gauge to reach zero.	5		
10. Standing behind the autoclave door, carefully open the chamber door 1/4".	10		
11. Leave the autoclave control at "Vent" to continue releasing heat.	10		
12. Allow complete drying of all articles.	5		
13. Using heat-resistant gloves, remove the items from the chamber and place the sterilized packages on dry, covered shelves or open the autoclave door and allow the items to cool completely before removal and storage.	10		
14. Turn the control knob to "Off" and keep the door slightly ajar.	10		
Total Points	100		

Comments

CAAHEP Competencies	Step(s)
III.P.5. Perform sterilization procedures	Entire procedure
ABHES Competencies	**Step(s)**
4.b. Identify modes of sterilization 1. Autoclave	Entire procedure
1.d. List the general responsibilities and skills of the medical assistant	Entire procedure

Assisting with Surgical Procedures

chapter

25

CAAHEP	Assessments
I.P.8. Instruct and prepare a patient for a procedure or a treatment	Procedure 25.1, 25.7, 25.8
III.P.6. Prepare a sterile field	Procedure 25.3, 25.4, 25.6
III.P.7. Perform within a sterile field	Procedure 25.3, 25.4, 25.6
III.P.8. Perform wound care	Procedure 25.6, 25.7
III.P.9. Perform dressing change	Procedure 25.7
III.A.1. Recognize the implications for failure to comply with Center for Disease Control (CDC) regulations in healthcare settings	Procedure 25.7
V.A.4. Explain to a patient the rationale for performance of a procedure	Procedure 25.7
X.P.3. Document patient care accurately in the medical record	Procedure 25.6, 25.7, 25.8
ABHES	**Assessments**
1. General Orientation d. List the general responsibilities and skills of the medical assistant	All procedures
8. Clinical Procedures a. Practice standard precautions and perform disinfection/sterilization techniques	Procedure 25.2
8. Clinical Procedures e. Perform specialty procedures, including but not limited to minor surgery, cardiac, respiratory, OB-GYN, neurological, and gastroenterology	All procedures

VOCABULARY REVIEW

Using the word pool on the right, find the correct word to match the definition. Write the word on the line after the definition.

1. Keen watchfulness to detect danger _____

2. Early scar tissue that appears pale, contracted, and firm
    _____

3. Vapor, smoke, and particle debris produced by laser procedures
    _____

4. The stoppage of bleeding _____

5. Near; close together _____

Word Pool
- plume
- vigilance
- approximated
- hemostasis
- cicatrix

SKILLS AND CONCEPTS

Answer the following questions. Write your answer on the line or in the space provided.

A. Surgical Procedures

1. Describe the following common surgical procedures done in the provider's office.

    a. Electrosurgery _____

    _____

    _____

    _____

    b. Laser_____

    _____

    _____

    _____

    c. Microsurgery _____

    _____

    _____

    _____

    d. Endoscopic procedures_____

    _____

    _____

    _____

e. Cryosurgery _____

_____

_____

_____

B. Assisting with Surgical Procedures

1. Explain the importance of skin preparation and describe how it is done._____

_____

_____

_____

_____

_____

_____

2. Summarize the steps that must be taken to prepare a patient for surgery in the ambulatory care setting.

_____

_____

_____

_____

_____

_____

3. What must the patient understand before signing the informed consent form? _____

_____

_____

_____

_____

_____

4. When setting up a sterile field, the Mayo stand must first be _____.

5. What are the two most common sources of contamination when a sterile field is set up? _____

_____

_____

6. Describe the process of passing instruments to the provider. _____

   _____

   _____

   _____

7. When giving a patient postoperative instructions, what are the warning signs that the patient should report immediately?

   _____

   _____

C. Wound Care

1. Describe first and second intention healing and give an example of each. _____

   _____

   _____

   _____

   _____

2. Describe the differences between an incised wound and a lacerated wound and give an example of each.

   _____

   _____

   _____

3. Describe the four phases of wound healing._____

   _____

   _____

   _____

   _____

   _____

4. What are the reasons for applying a sterile dressing?

   a. _____

   b. _____

   c. _____

   d. _____

5. How is a bandage different from a dressing? _____

_____

_____

_____

_____

CERTIFICATION PREPARATION

Circle the correct answer.

1. For which postoperative condition should the patient call the provider's office?
   a. Redness around the operative site
   b. Fever or swelling
   c. Increasing or severe pain
   d. All of the above

2. The LEEP excisional procedure is considered
   a. endoscopy.
   b. laser surgery
   c. microsurgery
   d. electrosurgery

3. Which statement is *not* true about informed consent for surgery?
   a. The patient must provide his or her own witness for the signature.
   b. The patient must understand the potential risks and benefits of the surgery.
   c. The patient must understand the possible risks of any alternative treatment.
   d. The patient cannot give consent if he or she has received preoperative medication.

4. Which endoscope is rigid?
   a. Laparoscope
   b. Colonoscope
   c. Bronchoscope
   d. Gastroscope

5. Which wound passes through to a body organ or cavity?
   a. Incised wound
   b. Lacerated wound
   c. Puncture wound
   d. Penetrating wound

6. In which phase of wound healing is fibrin most involved?
   a. First phase
   b. Second phase
   c. Third phase
   d. Fourth phase

7. Which bandage material is superior for covering round, narrow surfaces such as fingers or toes?
   a. Plain roller gauze
   b. Wrinkled crepe-type roller bandage
   c. Elastic bandage
   d. Seamless tubular gauze bandage

8. Which is a violation of sterile technique?
   a. Holding a sterile article above waist level
   b. Facing a sterile field
   c. Reaching over a sterile field
   d. Placing a sterile item in the center of the a sterile field

9. The purpose of a sterile fenestrated drape is
   a. comfort and warmth for the provider.
   b. to provide a sterile area around the operative site.
   c. to prevent the patient from observing the operative site.
   d. to protect the patient's clothing from blood and other secretions.

10. Cryosurgery involves
    a. freezing temperatures.
    b. sound waves.
    c. x-rays.
    d. chemicals.

WORKPLACE APPLICATIONS

1. Minor surgical procedures such as the laser surgery are commonly done in Melissa's office. What is Melissa's role in a laser surgery?

   _____

   _____

   _____

   _____

2. The provider has ordered open wound healing for a patient with a traumatic injury. What does this mean? How does healing occur? What are some of the advantages of this type of healing process?

   _____

   _____

   _____

   _____

INTERNET ACTIVITIES

1. Using internet resources, research a procedure that is commonly performed in a primary care facility. Create a poster presentation, a PowerPoint presentation, or write a paper that summarizes your research. Include the following points in your project:
   a. Describe the procedure and the instruments needed.
   b. What preoperative patient preparation is needed?
   c. What would be the medical assistant's role in this procedure?

2. Using internet resources, research healthcare-associated infections. Create a poster presentation, a PowerPoint presentation, or write a paper that summarizes your research. Include the following points in your project:
   a. Describe what a healthcare-associated infection is.
   b. How is sterile technique connected to healthcare-associated infections?
   c. What can a medical assistant do to prevent healthcare-associated infections?

Procedure 25.1   Perform Skin Prep for Surgery

Name _____ Date _____ Score _____

Tasks: To prepare the patient's skin and remove hair from the surgical site to reduce the risk of wound contamination.

Equipment and Supplies:
- Disposable skin prep kit, or collect the following:
  - Gauze
  - Cotton-tipped applicators
  - Soap
  - Gloves
  - Electric clippers
  - Two small bowls
  - Antiseptic or antiseptic swabs (e.g., Betadine swabs)
  - Sterile normal saline solution
  - Optional: cotton balls, nail pick, scrub brush
- Sterile drape
- Biohazard waste container
- Biohazard sharps container
- Patient's health record

Standard: Complete the procedure and all critical steps in _____ minutes with a minimum score of 85% within two attempts (*or as indicated by the instructor*).

Scoring: Divide the points earned by the total possible points. Failure to perform a critical step, indicated by an asterisk (*), results in grade no higher than an 84% (*or as indicated by the instructor*).

Time: Began _____ Ended _____ Total minutes: _____

Steps:	Point Value	Attempt 1	Attempt 2
1. Wash hands or use hand sanitizer.	5		
2. Greet the patient. Identify yourself. Verify the patient's identity with full name and date of birth. Explain the procedure to be performed in a manner that is understood by the patient. Answer any questions the patient may have on the procedure.	5		
3. Ask the patient to remove any clothing that might interfere with exposure of the site and provide a gown if needed.	5		
4. Assist the patient into the proper position for site exposure. Provide a drape if necessary to protect the patient's privacy.	5		
5. Expose the site. Use a light if necessary.	5		
6. If hair is present, the area may need to be shaved. Put on gloves and shave the required area with electric clippers.	10		
7. While wearing gloves, open the skin prep pack and add the soap to the two bowls.	5		
8. Start at the incision site and begin washing with the soap on a gauze sponge in a circular motion, moving from the center to the edges of the area to be scrubbed.	10*		

9. After one complete wipe, discard the sponge and begin again with a new sponge soaked in the antiseptic solution.	**5**		
10. Repeat the process, using sufficient friction for 5 minutes (or follow office policy for the length of time required for a particular prep).	**5**		
11. Rinse the area with sterile normal saline solution.	**5**		
12. Dry the area, using the same circular technique with dry sponges. The area may be dried by blotting with a sterile towel.	**10***		
13. Paint on the antiseptic with the cotton-tipped applicators or gauze sponges, using the same circular technique and never returning to an area that has already been painted	**10**		
14. Place a sterile drape and/or towel over the area.	**5**		
15. Answer all the patient's questions to relieve anxiety about the upcoming surgical procedure.	**5**		
16. Document completion of the skin prep in the patient's health record.	**5**		
Total Points	**100**		

Documentation

Comments

CAAHEP Competencies	Step(s)
I.P.8. Instruct and prepare a patient for a procedure or treatment	Entire procedure
ABHES Competencies	**Step(s)**
8.e. Perform specialty procedures, including but not limited to minor surgery, cardiac, respiratory, OB-GYN, neurological, and gastroenterology	Entire procedure
1.d. List the general responsibilities and skills of the medical assistant	Entire procedure

Procedure 25.2   Perform a Surgical Hand Scrub

Name _____ Date _____ Score _____

Task: To scrub the hands with surgical soap using friction, running water, and a disposable sterile brush to sanitize the skin before assisting with any procedure that requires surgical asepsis.

Equipment and Supplies:
- Sink with foot, knee, or arm control for running water
- Surgical soap in a dispenser
- Towels (sterile towels if indicated by office policy)
- Nail file or orange stick
- Sterile disposable brush

Standard: Complete the procedure and all critical steps in _____ minutes with a minimum score of 85% within two attempts (*or as indicated by the instructor*).

Scoring: Divide the points earned by the total possible points. Failure to perform a critical step, indicated by an asterisk (*), results in grade no higher than an 84% (*or as indicated by the instructor*).

Time: Began_____ Ended_____ Total minutes: _____

Steps:	Point Value	Attempt 1	Attempt 2
1. Remove all jewelry.	5		
2. Roll long sleeves above the elbows.	5		
3. Inspect your fingernails for length and your hands for skin breaks.	5		
4. Turn on the faucet and regulate the water to a comfortable temperature, being careful to stand away from the sink to prevent contamination of clothing from contact with the sink or countertop.	5		
5. Keep your hands upright and held at or above waist level.	10*		
6. Clean your fingernails with a file, discard it (in most situations you will drop the file into the sink and discard it later to prevent contamination by lowering your hands and/or touching a waste receptacle), and rinse your hands under the faucet without touching the faucet or the inside of the sink basin.	5		
7. Allow the water to run over your hands from the fingertips to the elbows without moving the arm back and forth under the water.	5		
8. Apply surgical soap from the dispenser to the sterile brush (or use a prepared disposable brush) and start the scrub by scrubbing the palm of the hand in a circular fashion.	5		
9. Continue from the palm to the base of the thumb, then move on to the other fingers, scrubbing from the base, along each side, and across the nail, holding the fingertips upward and remembering to rub between the fingers. After the fingers have been completely scrubbed, clean the posterior surface of the hand in a circular fashion and then proceed to the wrist. The scrub process should take at least 5 minutes for each hand and arm.	10*		
10. Do not return to a clean area after you have moved to the next part of the hand.	5		

11. Wash the wrists and forearms in a circular fashion around the arm while holding your hands above waist level.	5		
12. Rinse the arms and forearms from the fingertips upward, holding the fingers up, without touching the faucet or the inside of the sink basin.	5		
13. Apply more solution without touching any dirty surface and repeat the scrub on the other side, remembering to wash and use friction between each finger with a firm, circular motion.	5		
14. Scrub all surfaces, being careful not to abrade your skin. The second hand and arm should take at least 5 minutes.	5		
15. Rinse thoroughly, keeping your hands up and above waist level. Discard the scrub brush without lowering the arms below the waist.	5		
16. Turn off the faucet with the foot, knee, or forearm lever, if available.	5		
17. Dry your hands with a sterile towel, being careful to keep the fingers pointing upward and your hands above the waist. Do not rub back and forth, dragging contaminants from the dirtier area of the upper arm down toward the hands. Use the opposite end of the towel for the other hand.	5		
18. Using a patting motion, continue to dry the forearms. Discard the towel and keep your hands up and above waist level.	5		
Total Points	**100**		

Comments

CAAHEP Competencies	Step(s)
III.P.3 Perform hand washing	Entire procedure
ABHES Competencies	**Step(s)**
1.d. List the general responsibilities and skills of the medical assistant	Entire procedure

Procedure 25.3   Prepare a Sterile Field; Use Transfer Forceps; Pour a Sterile Solution into a Sterile Field

Name _____ Date _____ Score _____

Tasks: To open a sterile instrument pack using correct aseptic technique and create a sterile field; move sterile items on a sterile field or transfer sterile items to a gloved team member; pour a sterile solution into a sterile stainless-steel bowl or container sitting at the edge of a sterile field.

Equipment and Supplies:
- A sterile instrument pack wrapped with autoclave paper that, when opened, will serve as a sterile table drape or field
- Mayo stand or countertop
- Disinfectant and gauze sponges or disinfectant wipes
- Sterile item to move or transfer
- Sterile wrapped transfer forceps
- Bottle of sterile solution
- Sterile bowl or container
- Sink or waste receptacle

Standard: Complete the procedure and all critical steps in _____ minutes with a minimum score of 85% within two attempts (*or as indicated by the instructor*).

Scoring: Divide the points earned by the total possible points. Failure to perform a critical step, indicated by an asterisk (*), results in grade no higher than an 84% (*or as indicated by the instructor*).

Time: Began_____ Ended_____ Total minutes: _____

Steps:	Point Value	Attempt 1	Attempt 2
1. Check that the Mayo stand or countertop is dust-free and clean. If it is not, disinfect and allow to air dry.	5		
2. Wash or sanitize your hands and make sure they are completely dry. If you will be assisting with a surgical procedure immediately after opening the sterile pack, perform the surgical hand scrub as explained in Procedure 25.2.	5		
3. Gather supplies. Check the label of the ordered solution. Check the solution name and the expiration date.	5		
4. If using an autoclaved pack, check the indicator tape for a color change.	5		
5. Open the outside cover. Position the package so that the outer envelope flap is at the top and with the tab facing you.	5		
6. Open the outermost flap. Next, open the first flap away from you. You can cross over the uncovered portion of the Mayo stand as it is not sterile. Do not cross over the pack.	5		
7. Open the second corner, pulling to side.	5		
8. Be careful to lift the flaps by touching only the small, folded-back tab and without touching or crossing over the inner surface of the pack or its contents. Open the remaining two corners of the pack.	10*		
9. You now have a sterile drape as a sterile field from which to work and for the distribution of additional sterile supplies and instruments.	5		

10. Open a package containing sterile transfer forceps. Using sterile technique, handle the sterile forceps by the ring handle only. Always point the forceps tips down.	5*		
11. Grasp an item on the sterile field with the sterile forceps, points down, and move it to its proper position for the procedure, making sure not to cross the sterile field with the hand or contaminated end of the forceps.	5		
12. Set the forceps aside after one-time use.	5		
13. Check the label of the ordered solution when first obtaining the solution.	5		
14. Check the label of the solution for the second time. Place your hand over the label and lift the bottle.	5		
15. Lift the cover of the bottle straight up and then slightly to one side; hold the cover in your nondominant hand facing downward.	5		
16. If the container does not have a double cap, before pouring the solution into the sterile container, pour off a small amount of the solution into a waste receptacle.	10*		
17. Tilt the bottle up to stop the pouring while it is still over the bowl.	5		
18. Check the label of the solution for the third time. Working away from the sterile field, replace the cap (or caps). Be careful not to touch and therefore contaminate the internal surface of the lid.	5		
Total Points	100		

Comments

CAAHEP Competencies	Step(s)
III.P.6. Prepare a sterile field	Entire procedure
III.P.7. Perform within a sterile field	Entire procedure
ABHES Competencies	**Step(s)**
1.d. List the general responsibilities and skills of the medical assistant	Entire procedure

Procedure 25.4   Two-Person Sterile Tray Setup

Name _____ Date _____ Score _____

Task: Perform a sterile tray setup for a cyst removal.

Equipment and Supplies:
- Sterile drape
- Sterile gloves
- In a sealed autoclave pouch; needle holder, operating scissor, tissue forceps, hemostatic forceps
- Suture material with needle
- Sterile 4x4s
- Disposable scalpel

Directions: This procedure involves two people. One person will be act as the nonsterile person and the other will have on sterile gloves and will place the items on the sterile tray.

Standard: Complete the procedure and all critical steps in _____ minutes with a minimum score of 85% within two attempts (*or as indicated by the instructor*).

Scoring: Divide the points earned by the total possible points. Failure to perform a critical step, indicated by an asterisk (*), results in grade no higher than an 84% (*or as indicated by the instructor*).

Time: Began_____ Ended_____ Total minutes: _____

Steps – Nonsterile person	Point Value	Attempt 1	Attempt 2
1. Check that the Mayo stand or countertop is dust-free and clean. If it is not, disinfect and allow to air dry.	5		
2. Wash or sanitize your hands and make sure they are completely dry. If you will be assisting with a surgical procedure immediately after opening the sterile pack, perform the surgical hand scrub as explained in Procedure 25.2.	5		
3. Place the package containing the sterile drape on flat surface near Mayo stand/tray. Check the integrity of the outer package. Open package without touching barrier field.	10		
4. Pick up the sterile drape, by the corner, as you move away from table and allow it to unfold without touching anything else. Drape it over the Mayo stand without crossing over the sterile field.	10		
5. Inspect the sterile 4x4 package for holes and tears; if seen, discard and start over. Slowly pull sides of peel pack of sterile 4x4s away from each other. Maintain control of item inside the package by only opening far enough for sterile person to grab item. Allow the sterile person to take the 4x4s. Inspect and discard wrapper.	10*		
6. Inspect the peel pack of suture for holes and tears; if seen, discard and start over. Slowly pull sides of peel pack of suture away from each other. Maintain control of item inside the package by only opening far enough for sterile person to grab item. Allow the sterile person to take the suture package. Inspect and discard wrapper.	10*		

7.	Inspect the peel pack of scalpel for holes and tears; if seen, discard and start over. Slowly pull sides of peel pack of scalpel away from each other. Maintain control of item inside the package by only opening far enough for sterile person to grab item. Allow the sterile person to take the scalpel. Inspect and discard wrapper.	10*		
8.	Inspect the peel pack of instruments for holes and tears; if seen, discard and start over. Slowly pull sides of peel pack of the instruments away from each other. Maintain control of item inside the package by only opening far enough for sterile person to grab item. Allow the sterile person to take all of the instruments. Inspect and discard wrapper.	10*		
Steps – Sterile person				
9.	Wash or sanitize your hands and make sure they are completely dry. If you will be assisting with a surgical procedure immediately after opening the sterile pack, perform the surgical hand scrub as explained in Procedure 25.2.	5		
10.	Remove items from peel pack and maintain sterile technique.	5		
11.	After nonsterile person has indicated that the peel pack has not been compromised, place item on sterile tray. Repeat for all items. Arrange items on sterile tray.	10		
12.	Maintain sterility of sterile field and sterile supplies.	10*		
	Total Points	100		

Comments

CAAHEP Competencies	Step(s)
III.P.6. Prepare a sterile field	Entire procedure
III.P.7. Perform within a sterile field	Entire procedure
ABHES Competencies	**Step(s)**
1.d. List the general responsibilities and skills of the medical assistant	Entire procedure

Procedure 25.5   Put on Sterile Gloves

Name _____   Date _____   Score _____

Task: To put on sterile gloves correctly before performing sterile procedures.

Equipment and Supplies:
• Pair of packaged sterile gloves in your size

Standard: Complete the procedure and all critical steps in _____ minutes with a minimum score of 85% within two attempts (*or as indicated by the instructor*).

Scoring: Divide the points earned by the total possible points. Failure to perform a critical step, indicated by an asterisk (*), results in grade no higher than an 84% (*or as indicated by the instructor*).

Time: Began_____ Ended_____ Total minutes: _____

Steps:	Point Value	Attempt 1	Attempt 2
1. Perform the surgical hand scrub as explained in Procedure 25.2 before putting on sterile gloves.	5		
2. Check that the Mayo stand or countertop is dust-free and clean. If it is not, disinfect and allow to air dry.	10		
3. Open package and remove the glove pack from the outer package. Place the glove pack on the Mayo stand or countertop. Open the glove pack, being careful not to cross over the open area in the middle of the pack. Remember, a 1-inch area around the perimeter of the glove wrapper is considered nonsterile.	5		
4. Glove your dominant hand first. With your nondominant hand, pick up the glove for your dominant hand with your thumb and forefinger, grabbing the edge of the folded cuff closest to you, which is the inside of the glove, being careful not to cross over the other sterile glove.	10*		
5. Lift the glove up and away from the sterile package.	10		
6. Hold your hands up and away from your body and slide the dominant hand into the glove.	10		
7. Leave the cuff folded.	10		
8. With your gloved dominant hand, pick up the second glove by slipping your gloved fingers under the cuff, extending the thumb up and away from the glove (thumbs up position), so that your gloved fingers touch only the outside of the second glove.	10*		
9. Slide your nondominant hand into the glove without touching the exterior of the glove or any part of the gloved hand.	10		
10. Still holding your hands away from you, unroll the cuff by slipping the fingers into the cuff and gently pulling up and out. Do not touch your bare arm or the internal surface of the glove with any part of the sterile glove.	10		
11. Now, slip your gloved fingers up under the first cuff and unroll it, using the same technique.	10		
Total Points	**100**		

Comments

.

ABHES Competencies	Step(s)
1.d. List the general responsibilities and skills of the medical assistant	Entire procedure

Procedure 25.6 Assisting with Minor Surgery

Name _____ Date _____ Score _____

Tasks: To maintain the sterile field and pass instruments in a prescribed sequence during a surgical procedure that involves the making of a surgical incision and the removal of tissue.

Equipment and Supplies:
- Open patient drape pack on the side counter
- Mayo stand covered with a sterile drape
- Packaged sterile gloves (two pairs)
- Needle and syringe for local anesthetic medication
- Vial of local anesthetic medication
- Alcohol wipes
- Sterile drape
- Disposable scalpel with No. 15 blade
- Tissue forceps
- Skin retractor
- Three hemostats
- Needleholder
- Supply of sterile gauze sponges
- Biohazard waste container
- Sharps container
- Needle with suture material
- Specimen cup
- Laboratory requisitions
- Patient's health record

Standard: Complete the procedure and all critical steps in _____ minutes with a minimum score of 85% within two attempts (*or as indicated by the instructor*).

Scoring: Divide the points earned by the total possible points. Failure to perform a critical step, indicated by an asterisk (*), results in grade no higher than an 84% (*or as indicated by the instructor*).

Time: Began_____ Ended_____ Total minutes: _____

Steps:	Point Value	Attempt 1	Attempt 2
1. Prep the patient's skin with surgical soap and antiseptic solution as explained in Procedure 25.1. Explain the prep procedure to the patient.	3*		
2. Perform the surgical hand scrub as explained in Procedure 25.2.	2		
3. Instruct and prepare the patient for the procedure. Explain the following: what will occur, what the patient should do during the procedure, how long the procedure will take, and what the patient will sense (e.g., feel, smell, etc.).	2*		
4. Position the Mayo stand near the patient and the operative site, making sure the patient understands not to touch the sterile field.	3		
5. Put on sterile gloves using surgical technique as explained in Procedure 25.5.	2		
6. Put on sterile gloves using surgical technique. Grasp the patient drape by holding one edge or corner in each hand.	3		

7.	Drape the surgical site without touching any part of the patient or the operating area with your gloved hands.	5		
8.	If the provider requests medication, such as a local anesthetic, a second circulating assistant holds the vial of local anesthetic so that the provider can read the label and wipes to the top of the vial with the alcohol wipe. The provider withdraws the desired amount using sterile technique.	5		
9.	The provider injects the local anesthetic and waits a few minutes for it to take effect.	2		
10.	Position yourself across from the provider. Arrange the sterile field. Check the placement location on the Mayo stand.	5		
11.	Keep all sharp equipment conspicuously placed on the sterile field.	5		
12.	Pass the scalpel, blade down and handle first, to the provider, or the provider will reach for it. The provider will take the scalpel with the thumb and forefinger in the position ready for use.	5		
13.	Pick up a tissue forceps by the tips and pass it to the provider to grasp a piece of the tissue to be excised.	5		
14.	Dispose of soiled sponges in the biohazard waste container, being careful to keep your hands above your waist and to avoid touching any nonsterile items	5		
15.	Hold clean sponges in your hand to pat or sponge the wound as needed.	3		
16.	Safely position the specimen (if any) where it will not be disturbed in a sterile container on the sterile field.	5		
17.	If there is a bleeding vessel or if a hemostat is requested, pass the hemostat in the manner described in step 13.	5		
18.	Continue to sponge blood from the wound site.	2		
19.	Retract the wound edge, as needed, with a skin retractor.	5		
20.	Continue to monitor the sterile field and assist the provider as needed.	3		
21.	Pass the needle and suture material to close the wound and apply a sterile dressing as requested	5		
22.	Monitor the patient and provide assistance as needed. Provide any patient education required.	5		
23.	Clean up the room. Place sharps in the sharps disposal container and other biohazardous material in the biohazard waste container. Discard other waste in regular waste container. Disinfect the areas used.	5		
24.	Collect the specimen using Standard Precautions, place it in a labeled specimen cup, and send it to the laboratory with the proper requisitions.	5		
25.	Wash hands or use hand sanitizer. Document the procedure, wound condition, and patient education given in the patient's health record.	5		
	Total Points	100		

Documentation

Comments

CAAHEP Competencies	Step(s)
I.P.8. Instruct and prepare a patient for a procedure or a treatment.	1, 3
III.P.6. Prepare a sterile field	4
III.P.7. Perform within a sterile field	Entire procedure
III.P.8. Perform wound care	21
III.P.10.a. Demonstrate proper disposal of biohazardous material: sharps	23
III.P.10.b. Demonstrate proper disposal of biohazardous material: regulated wastes	14, 23
X.P.3. Document patient care accurately in the medical record	25
XII.P.2.c. Demonstrate proper use of: sharps disposal containers	23
ABHES Competencies	**Step(s)**
1.d. List the general responsibilities and skills of the medical assistant	Entire procedure
9.c. Dispose of biohazardous materials	14, 23

Procedure 25.7   Apply a Sterile Dressing

Name _____   Date _____   Score _____

Tasks: Perform a dressing change; apply a sterile dressing while maintaining aseptic technique; instruct and prepare the patient for the procedure; explain the rationale for the procedure.

Equipment and Supplies:
- Gloves
- Biohazard waste container
- Sterile water or hydrogen peroxide (optional)
- Disposable ruler
- Culture swab
- Lab requisition, label, and plastic specimen bag for transport
- Sterile gloves
- Antiseptic swabs
- Sterile dressing and ABD pad
- Tape
- Mannequin with a wound
- Patient's record

Order: Change dressing and apply a sterile dressing. Culture wound drainage.

Scenario: Dr. Walden ordered a dressing change. You are to apply a sterile dressing after you obtain a culture of the wound drainage. As you are beginning the procedure, the patient asks you questions regarding PPE and the reason for the wound culture. You need to explain the rationale for wearing PPE and why a wound culture is obtained.

Directions: Role-play the scenario with a peer. The peer will be the patient and you are the medical assistant. After the role-play, the rest of the procedure is done on a mannequin.

Standard: Complete the procedure and all critical steps in _____ minutes with a minimum score of 85% within two attempts (*or as indicated by the instructor*).

Scoring: Divide the points earned by the total possible points. Failure to perform a critical step, indicated by an asterisk (*), results in grade no higher than an 84% (*or as indicated by the instructor*).

Time: Began_____ Ended_____ Total minutes: _____

Steps:	Point Value	Attempt 1	Attempt 2
1. Wash hands or use hand sanitizer. Assemble supplies on Mayo stand/tray and place biohazard waste container within easy reach.	2		
2. Greet the patient. Identify yourself. Verify the patient's identity with full name and date of birth. Verify the patient's allergies.	2		
3. Instruct and prepare the patient for the procedure. Explain the procedure to be performed in a manner that is understood by the patient. Explain the following: what will occur, what the patient should do during the procedure, how long the procedure will take, and what the patient will sense (e.g., feel, smell, etc.). Answer any questions the patient may have on the procedure.	3*		

Scenario update: The patient questions why you need to change gloves so much during the procedure. He also asks why the wound culture needs be done. 4. Based on the patient's questions, explain the reason for changing your gloves during the procedure and also for the wound culture. Demonstrate empathy and appropriate nonverbal communication when addressing the patient's questions and concerns. *(Refer to the Checklist for Affective Behaviors.)*	5*		
Scenario update: The rest of the steps can be done on a mannequin. 5. Put on gloves. Loosen tape on old bandage from edges to the middle, towards the wound. Remove bandage and dressing, one at a time. If dressing is stuck, use a small amount of sterile water or hydrogen peroxide to loosen.	3		
6. Check for drainage on the dressing and bandage. Note the color of the drainage. Measure any drainage using a disposable ruler, then discard everything in the biohazard waste container.	5*		
7. Assess the wound. If present, count the sutures or staples. Check if they are intact. Check the wound for signs of infection.	3*		
8. If the wound is open and/or redness or drainage is present: a. Culture the wound using a sterile swab (if ordered). Place in a culture transfer tube. Squeeze the tube to release formalin to preserve the specimen. b. Concisely and accurately report the relevant information (any issues with the wound or wound closures) to the provider. Ask the provider to check the wound before re-dressing.	5*		
9. Remove gloves and place in biohazard waste container.	5		
10. Wash hands or use hand sanitizer.	2		
11. Open and arrange sterile supplies in the order they will be used. Apply the principles of sterile technique.	5*		
12. Put on sterile gloves. State that the nondominant hand will be nonsterile and the dominant hand will be sterile.	5		
13. With the nondominant hand, pick up the antiseptic swab container. With the dominant hand, grasp an antiseptic swab without touching the package. Clean from center of wound to edge, use one roll of the swab and discard in waste container. Start with new swab where you left off with the previous swab. Continue until all the exudate is removed.	10*		
14. With the dominant hand, remove the sterile dressing without touching the package. Place the sterile dressing material over the wound and cover the wound completely.	10*		
15. With the dominant hand, place an ABD pad over the dressing as a bandage.	5		
16. Remove and discard the sterile gloves. Secure the bandage with tape.	5		
17. Provide patient education as needed for wound care.	5		
18. Complete the lab requisition for the culture. Put on gloves. Label the culture tube and place the culture tube in the plastic specimen bag for transport to the lab.	5		
19. Clean up the area. Discard all biohazardous waste in biohazard waste containers. Discard all other waste in the regular waste containers. Disinfect the tables.	3		

20. Remove gloves and dispose of them appropriately. Wash hands or use hand sanitizer.	**2**			
21. Using the patient's health record, document the following: wound appearance, number of intact sutures or staples (if present), the culture obtained, wound care performed, and the patient education provided.	**5***			
22. In the written response section, discuss the implication for failing to comply with CDC regulations in healthcare settings.	**5***			
Total Points	**100**			

Checklist for Affective Behaviors

Affective Behavior	**Directions:** Check behaviors observed during the role-play.					
Empathy	**Negative, Unprofessional Behaviors**	**Attempt**		**Positive, Professional Behaviors**	**Attempt**	
		1	**2**		**1**	**2**
	Unsupportive, uninterested, or uncaring			Demonstrated supportive, caring behaviors		
	Did not acknowledge or respond appropriately to the patient's emotional responses; cold, aloof, insensitive, indifferent, or unfeeling			Acknowledged and responded appropriately to the patient's concerns; showed sensitivity		
	Failed to reassure patient; did not respond to the patient's concerns			Reassured patient by repeating and responding to the patient's concerns		
	Used language that is hard to understand (e.g., slang, generational terms, medical terminology, too scientific)			Used language that the patient can understand		
	Failed to address the patient's questions; or answers to patient's questions were inappropriate			Answered the patient's questions appropriately		
	Other:			Other:		
Nonverbal Communication	Spoke in an artificial manner; tone, pitch, and/or volume were unprofessional			Used a natural tone, pitch, and volume when speaking		
	Failed to respond to the patient's nonverbal behaviors			Responded appropriately to patient's nonverbal behaviors		
	Used inappropriate gestures and/or facial expressions			Used appropriate gestures and facial expressions		
	Poor eye contact with patient			Proper eye contact with patient		
	Other:			Other:		

Grading		Point Value	Attempt 1	Attempt 2
Does not meet Expectation	• Response demonstrated inappropriate nonverbal communication, and/or lacks empathy. • Student demonstrated more than 2 negative, unprofessional behaviors during the interaction.	0		
Needs Improvement	• Response demonstrated inappropriate nonverbal communication, and/or lacks empathy. • Student demonstrated 1 or 2 negative, unprofessional behaviors during the interaction.	0		
Meets Expectation	• Response demonstrated appropriate nonverbal communication, and empathy; no negative, unprofessional behaviors observed. • More practice is needed for behavior to appear natural and for student to appear comfortable and at ease.	5		
Occasionally Exceeds Expectation	• Response demonstrated appropriate nonverbal communication, and empathy; no negative, unprofessional behaviors observed. • At times student appeared comfortable and at ease; but more practice is needed for behavior to become natural and consistent with a professional medical assistant.	5		
Always Exceeds Expectation	• Response demonstrated appropriate nonverbal communication, and empathy; no negative, unprofessional behaviors observed. • Student's behaviors appeared natural and comfortable. Behaviors are consistent with a professional medical assistant.	5		

Documentation

You fail to wear gloves when changing a patient's dressing. During the procedure, you got blood on your hands. Discuss the implication for failing to comply with CDC regulations in healthcare settings. Answer the following questions:

1. How might your actions (of not wearing gloves) impact the patient's health and safety? _____

_____

_____

_____

_____

_____

2. How might your actions (of not wearing gloves) impact your health and safety? _____

_____

_____

_____

_____

_____

_____

Comments

CAAHEP Competencies	Step(s)
I.P.8. Instruct and prepare a patient for a procedure or a treatment.	3
III.P.8. Perform wound care	Entire procedure
III.P.9. Perform dressing change	Entire procedure
III.P.10.b. Demonstrate proper disposal of biohazardous material: regulated wastes	6, 9, 19
III.A.I. Recognize the implications for failure to comply the Center for Disease Control (CDC) regulations in healthcare setting.	22
V.P.11. Report relevant information concisely and accurately.	8b
V.A.4. Explain to a patient the rationale for performance of a procedure	4
X.P.3. Document patient care accurately in the medical record	21
ABHES Competencies	**Step(s)**
1.d. List the general responsibilities and skills of the medical assistant	Entire procedure
8.e. Perform specialty procedures, including but not limited to minor surgery, cardiac, respiratory, OB-GYN, neurological, and gastroenterology	Entire procedure
9.c. Dispose of biohazardous materials	6, 9, 19

Procedure 25.8   Removal of Sutures and/or Surgical Staples

Name _____ Date _____ Score _____

Task: To remove sutures and/or surgical staples from a healed incision using sterile technique and without injuring the closed wound.

Equipment and Supplies:
Sterile suture removal kit containing the following:
- Suture removal scissors
- Gauze
- Thumb dressing forceps
- Steri-Strips or adhesive bandage strips (e.g., Band-Aids)
- Skin antiseptic swabs (e.g., Betadine swabs)
- Surgical staple remover with 4×4-inch gauze
- Biohazard waste container
- Biohazard sharps container
- Gloves
- Sterile gloves
- Patient's health record

Standard: Complete the procedure and all critical steps in _____ minutes with a minimum score of 85% within two attempts (*or as indicated by the instructor*).

Scoring: Divide the points earned by the total possible points. Failure to perform a critical step, indicated by an asterisk (*), results in grade no higher than an 84% (*or as indicated by the instructor*).

Time: Began_____ Ended_____ Total minutes: _____

Steps:	Point Value	Attempt 1	Attempt 2
1. Wash hands or use hand sanitizer. Assemble the necessary supplies.	5		
2. Greet the patient. Identify yourself. Verify the patient's identity with full name and date of birth. Explain the procedure to be performed in a manner that is understood by the patient. Answer any questions the patient may have on the procedure. Instruct the person to lie or sit still during the procedure.	10*		
3. Position the patient comfortably and support the sutured area.	5		
4. Place dry towels under the site.	5		
5. Check the incision line to make sure the wound edges are approximated and there are no signs of infection such as inflammation, edema, or drainage.	5		
6. Put on gloves. Using antiseptic swabs, cleanse the wound to remove exudate and destroy microorganisms around the sutures or staples. Clean the site from the inside out, starting at the top of the wound and working your way down. Use a new swab if the step must be repeated. Remove gloves and discard.	10*		
7. Open the suture or staple removal pack while maintaining the sterility of the contents.	10*		

8. Place sterile gauze next to the wound site.	**5**		
9. Put on sterile gloves.	**5**		
10. Remove the sutures or staples.	**5**		
11. Remove the gauze holding the sutures or staples. Dispose of sutures in the biohazard waste container. Dispose of staples in the biohazard sharps container.	**10***		
12. The provider may apply or may have you apply Steri-Strips or an adhesive bandage strip for added support, strength, and protection.	**5**		
13. Instruct the patient to keep the wound edges clean and dry and not to place excessive strain on the area.	**10**		
14. Document the procedure, wound condition, number of sutures or staples removed, whether a dressing or bandage was applied, and the instructions on wound care given to the patient.	**10**		
Total Points	**100**		

Documentation

Comments

CAAHEP Competencies	Step(s)
I.P.8. Instruct and prepare a patient for a procedure or a treatment	2
X.P.3. Document patient care accurately in the medical record	14
ABHES Competencies	**Step(s)**
1.d. List the general responsibilities and skills of the medical assistant	Entire procedure

Principles of Electrocardiography

chapter

26

CAAHEP Competencies	Assessment
I.P.2.a. Perform: electrocardiography	Procedure 26.1
I.P.8. Instruct and prepare a patient for a procedure or a treatment	Procedure 26.1, 26.2
I.A.2. Incorporate critical thinking skills when performing patient care	Procedure 26.1
I.A.3. Show awareness of a patient's concerns related to the procedure being performed	Procedure 26.1
VI.P.8. Perform routine maintenance of administrative or clinical equipment	Procedure 26.1
X.P.3. Document patient care accurately in the medical record	Procedure 26.1, 26.2

ABHES Competencies	Assessment
1. General Orientation d. List the general responsibilities and skills of the medical assistant	Skills and Concepts – A. 1, 2
8. Clinical Procedures d. Assist provider with specialty examination, including cardiac, respiratory, OB-GYN, neurological, and gastroenterology procedures	Procedure 26.1, 26.2
e. Perform specialty procedures, including but not limited to minor surgery, cardiac, respiratory, OB-GYN, neurological, and gastroenterology	Procedure 26.1, 26.2

VOCABULARY REVIEW

Using the word pool on the right, find the correct word to match the definition. Write the word on the line after the definition.

Group A

1. A complete heartbeat _____
2. Electricity is picked up by the electrodes and moves into this machine _____
3. A record or recording of electrical impulses of the heart as produced by an electrocardiograph _____
4. Adhesive patches that conduct electricity from the body to the ECG machine wires _____
5. The use of ultrasonic waves directed through the heart to study the structure and motion of the heart; the visual record produced is called an *echocardiogram* _____
6. During this phase, the heart is at rest and the atria fill with blood _____
7. A myocardial cell forms a strong connection to the next cells through these special junctions _____
8. During this phase, the heart is contracting _____
9. Pacemaker of the heart _____
10. A specialized internodal tract that takes the impulse to the left atria _____

Word Pool
- cardiac cycle
- intercalated discs
- systole
- electrocardiogram
- echocardiography
- electrocardiograph
- Bachmann's bundle
- sinoatrial node
- electrodes
- diastole

Group B

1. Resting state of the cell _____
2. Recovery state of the cell _____
3. An electrically charged atom or the smallest component of an element _____
4. The state when the impulse hits the cell _____
5. A substance, structure, or event that does not naturally occur in a situation _____
6. A straight line on an ECG tracing _____
7. Any movement away from the baseline in the tracing _____
8. A period of time between two points or events _____
9. Having two poles or electrical charges _____
10. An abnormal heart rate or rhythm _____
11. Having one pole or electrical charge _____
12. A pocket-sized tool used for measuring the height and width of the ECG waves and intervals _____

Word Pool
- depolarized state
- arrhythmia
- deflection
- artifact
- unipolar
- bipolar
- caliper
- polarized state
- repolarized stated
- interval
- ion
- isoelectric line

ABBREVIATIONS

Write out what each of the following abbreviations stands for.

1. ECG, EKG_____

2. AV _____

3. SL_____

4. O_2_____

5. CO_2 _____

6. SA _____

7. ECHO _____

8. RA _____

9. LA _____

10. LL _____

11. RL _____

12. aV _____

13. UV _____

14. EHR_____

15. ICS_____

16. PACs _____

17. PVCs _____

18. V-tach _____

19. V-fib _____

20. ICD _____

SKILLS AND CONCEPTS

Answer the following questions. Write your answer on the line or in the space provided.

A. Introduction

1. Describe the role of the medical assistant with cardiac procedures._____

_____

_____

_____

B. Cardiovascular System Review

1. The _____ chambers receive blood from the body and the _____ chambers pump blood out to the body.

2. The _____ divides the right and left sides of the heart.

3. Describe the location of the following valves.

    a. Tricuspid valve _____

    _____

    b. Pulmonary valve _____

    _____

    c. Bicuspid or mitral valve _____

    _____

    d. Aortic valve _____

    _____

4. Summarize the flow of the blood and include the valves, chambers, and major arteries and veins involved. Start with the three structures that empty the blood into the right atrium. Finish the flow with the aorta.

    _____

    _____

    _____

    _____

    _____

    _____

5. Summarize the conduction system of the heart. Describe the structures in order starting with the "pacemaker of the heart."

    _____

    _____

    _____

    _____

    _____

    _____

6. Describe the three states that the cardiac cells cycle through. Put the states in order starting with the resting state.

_____

_____

_____

_____

_____

_____

_____

C. ECG Tracing

1. Complete the table below. Add the following information to the columns:
   a. Summarized column: Write the chamber and the state of the cardiac cells (e.g., atrial repolarization)
   b. Conduction System column: Describe the movement of the impulse and list the structures involved (e.g., impulse moves from the SA node to the AV node)
   c. Mechanical Action column: Describe the contraction of chambers and the blood flow (e.g., atrial chambers contract, blood flows into the ventricles)

Waves	Summarized	Conduction System	Mechanical Action
P wave			
PR segment			
QRS complex			
Q wave			
R wave			
S wave			
ST segment			
T wave			
U wave			

2. What is an interval? _____

_____

_____

3. Describe the PR interval and the Q-T interval._____

_____

_____

D. 12-Lead ECG

1. _____ electrodes and lead wires create _____ leads or pictures.

2. The following questions refer to the bipolar or standard leads.

   a. What are names of the leads? _____

   _____

   b. The bipolar leads provide pictures of the _____ or _____ plane of the heart.

   c. What electrodes and lead wires are used to create the bipolar leads? _____

   _____

   d. If you see artifact on lead I, which two electrodes and lead wires should you look at?_____

   _____

   e. If you see artifact on lead II, which two electrodes and lead wires should you look at? _____

   _____

   f. If you see artifact on lead III, which two electrodes and lead wires should you look at? _____

   _____

   g. If you see artifact on leads I and III, which electrode and lead wire should you look at? _____

   _____

3. The following questions refer to the augmented leads.

   a. What are names of the leads? _____

   _____

   b. The augmented leads provide pictures of the _____ or _____ plane of the heart.

   c. What electrodes and lead wires are used to create the augmented leads?_____

   _____

   d. If you see artifact on lead aVR, which electrodes and lead wires should you look at? _____

   _____

4. The following questions refer to the chest or precordial leads.

   a. What are names of the leads? _____

   _____

   b. The chest leads provide pictures of the _____ plane of the heart.

   c. What electrodes and lead wires are used to create the chest leads? _____

   _____

   d. If you see artifact on lead V_2, which electrode(s) and lead wire(s) should you look at?_____

_____

E. ECG Supplies and Equipment

1. Describe the small and large boxes on the ECG paper. _____

_____

2. When a provider analyzes the ECG tracing, what tool is used to measure the wave forms?_____

_____

3. Describe how to handle and store thermal ECG paper. _____

_____

_____

4. The vertical lines on an ECG tracing are used to measure the _____ or _____ of the waveform.

5. The horizontal lines measure the _____.

6. When the paper speed (chart speed) is set at 25 mm/second, each small box is _____ seconds and each large box equals _____ seconds.

7. The _____ on electrodes helps pick up the electrical impulses.

8. Describe the following ECG machine settings and address the normal default and reasons to change the default.

   a. Chart speed_____

_____

   b. Gain or Sensitivity _____

_____

9. Describe the appearance of the standardization mark._____

_____

_____

F. ECG Procedure

1. Describe three ways the skin can be prepared for the electrodes._____

_____

_____

2. Complete the table by describing where the electrode should be placed.

Electrode	Placement
Right arm (RA)	
Left arm (LA)	
Right leg (RL)	
Left leg (LL)	
Chest V_1 (V_1)	
Chest V_2 (V_2)	
Chest V_3 (V_3)	
Chest V_4 (V_4)	
Chest V_5 (V_5)	
Chest V_6 (V_6)	

3. List four special situations that would require an electrode placement deviation. Also describe the new placement.

_____

_____

_____

_____

_____

4. The following questions relate to wandering baseline artifact.

   a. Describe the appearance of the artifact. _____

   _____

   b. Describe why the artifact occurs. _____

   _____

   _____

   c. Describe how a medical assistant can prevent the artifact. _____

   _____

   _____

5. The following questions relate to somatic tremor artifact.

   a. Describe the appearance of the artifact. _____

   _____

   b. Describe why the artifact occurs. _____

   _____

   _____

   c. Describe how a medical assistant can prevent the artifact. _____

   _____

   _____

6. The following questions relate to AC interference artifact.

   a. Describe the appearance of the artifact. _____

   _____

   b. Describe why the artifact occurs. _____

   _____

   c. Describe how a medical assistant can prevent the artifact. _____

   _____

   _____

7. The following questions relate to interrupted baseline artifact.

   a. Describe the appearance of the artifact. _____

   _____

   b. Describe why the artifact occurs. _____

   _____

   c. Describe how a medical assistant can prevent the artifact. _____

   _____

   _____

8. Describe the appearance of the following arrhythmias.

   a. Premature atrial contraction (PAC) _____

   _____

   b. Atrial flutter _____

   _____

   c. Third-degree heart block _____

_____

   d. Premature ventricular contractions (PVCs)_____

_____

G. Additional ECG Testing

1. Describe the preparations for an exercise stress test. _____

_____

_____

_____

2. Describe a Holter monitor test. _____

_____

3. Describe patient education required for the Holter monitor test. _____

_____

_____

_____

4. Describe the cardiac event recorder and discuss how the patient uses the recorder. _____

_____

_____

_____

CERTIFICATION PREPARATION
Circle the correct answer.

1. _____ is a deflection from the baseline.
   a. Interval
   b. Segment
   c. Complex
   d. Wave

2. What ECG wave or segment reflects atrial depolarization?
   a. P wave
   b. Q wave
   c. R and S waves
   d. T wave

3. What ECG wave or segment is a negative deflection and represents interventricular septal depolarization?
   a. P wave
   b. Q wave
   c. R and S waves
   d. T wave

4. What ECG wave or segment represents ventricular repolarization?
   a. P wave
   b. Q wave
   c. R and S waves
   d. T wave

5. _____ is signal distortion or unwanted, erratic movement of the stylus caused by outside interference.
   a. Interval
   b. Deflection
   c. Artifact
   d. Caliper

6. If AC interference artifact appears, what should the medical assistant do?
   a. Check to see if the electrodes and lead wires are attached.
   b. Turn on the muscle-tremor filter.
   c. Help the patient relax.
   d. Separate the lead wires so they do not overlap.

7. _____ is when the ventricles quiver uncontrollably. The patient has no pulse, and is not breathing.
   a. Ventricular fibrillation
   b. Third-degree heart block
   c. Ventricular tachycardia
   d. Atrial flutter

8. _____ results in the absence of a heartbeat.
   a. Ventricular fibrillation
   b. Asystole
   c. Ventricular tachycardia
   d. Premature ventricular contractions

9. Which test involves radioactive substance injected into a vein and a gamma camera used to take images of the blood flow; shows the blood flow into the heart muscle during rest and activity?
   a. Exercise stress test
   b. Implantable loop recorder
   c. Nuclear stress test
   d. Transtelephonic monitor

10. Which device is surgically implanted under the skin in the upper chest and continuously records the ECG for 2-3 years?
    a. Holter monitor
    b. Cardiac event recorder
    c. Transtelephonic monitoring
    d. Implantable loop recorder

WORKPLACE APPLICATIONS

1. Renee is performing an ECG on a patient. How might she prep the patient's skin so the electrodes will adhere?

   _____

   _____

   _____

2. Renee is performing an ECG on a patient. She notices that lead I has upward and downward movement of the waveform. What is occurring and how should she correct the problem?

   _____

   _____

   _____

3. Renee is performing an ECG on a patient. She notices many of the leads have jagged peaks with irregular heights and spacing. What is occurring and how should she correct the problem?

   _____

   _____

   _____

INTERNET ACTIVITIES

1. Using appropriate online resources, research a cardiac test discussed in the "Additional ECG Testing" section. Create a poster, PowerPoint presentation, or a paper and include at least two citations. Discuss the following topics:
    a. Description of the test
    b. Patient education and preparation

2. Using online resources, create an ECG brochure for patients. Include the following in the brochure:
    a. Purpose of the test
    b. Description of the test
    c. Patient instructions

3. Using online resources, research an abnormal rhythm mentioned in the chapter. Identify reasons for the rhythm and possible treatments. In a paper, PowerPoint presentation, or poster, summarize your research and cite your resources.

Procedure 26.1   Perform Electrocardiography

Name _____ Date _____ Score _____

Tasks: Perform electrocardiography and routine maintenance on the machine. Document the procedure in the patient's health record. Show awareness of a patient's concerns and incorporate critical thinking skills when performing patient care.

Equipment and Supplies:
- ECG machine
- Disposable electrodes
- ECG paper
- Alcohol pads
- Razor (optional)
- Gauze pads (optional)
- Patient gown or paper cape
- Tissue
- Disinfecting wipes
- Gloves
- Waste container
- Patient's health record

Standard: Complete the procedure and all critical steps in _____ minutes with a minimum score of 85% within two attempts (*or as indicated by the instructor*).

Scoring: Divide the points earned by the total possible points. Failure to perform a critical step, indicated by an asterisk (*), results in grade no higher than an 84% (*or as indicated by the instructor*).

Time: Began _____ Ended _____ Total minutes: _____

Steps:	Point Value	Attempt 1	Attempt 2
1. Wash hands or use hand sanitizer.	2		
2. Assemble equipment and supplies needed for the ECG procedure. Plug in and turn on the ECG machine. Verify that the standardization and chart/paper speed are correct.	3		
3. Greet the patient. Identify yourself. Verify the patient's identity with full name and date of birth. Explain the procedure to be performed in a manner that is understood by the patient. Answer any questions the patient may have on the procedure.	5*		
Scenario update: The patient states that he is really worried that something is wrong with his heart. The patient states he is really nervous about having an ECG. 4. Using therapeutic communication techniques (e.g., reflection, restatement, and summarizing), show the patient you are aware of his concerns. *(Refer to the Awareness - Checklist for Affective Behaviors.)*	5*		
5. Ask the patient to remove all clothing from the waist up, including undergarments, and put on the gown/cape so that the opening is in the front. Ask the patient if assistance is needed. If so, provide help. If not, leave the room and allow the patient time to change. When reentering the room, provide a courtesy knock on the door.	2		

6.	Assist the patient into a comfortable supine position on the exam table. Provide support for the legs and arms.	**3**	
7.	Identify the locations for the ECG electrodes on the chest. Prepare the skin. If the patient has a hairy chest, get the person's permission prior to shaving the areas (optional). Wipe each spot with alcohol and allow it to dry. Fold the gauze pad over your index finger and briskly rub the site to abrade the skin (optional).	**5***	
8.	Correctly apply the six chest electrodes. If using tab electrodes, tabs should be pointed towards the waist.	**10**	
9.	Identify the locations for the ECG electrodes on the extremities. Refer to the operating manual for arm electrode position if needed. Wipe each spot with alcohol and allow it to dry. Correctly apply the four limb electrodes to nonbony areas. If using tab electrodes, the lower leg tabs should point towards the waist. The arm/wrist tabs should be pointed towards the fingers.	**10**	
10.	Attach the correct lead wire to each of the electrodes. The wires should follow the natural contour of the body and not overlap other wires.	**10***	
11.	Enter the patient's data into the ECG machine. Identify any changes with the default settings, electrode position, or patient's position.	**3**	
12.	Double-check that the lead wires are in the correct position and attached to the electrodes. Make sure each electrode is attached to the skin. Take any corrective action necessary.	**5***	
13.	Instruct the patient to lie still and not to talk during the tracing. Tell the patient how long the tracing will take.	**5**	
14.	Verify that the filter(s) are on. Check the leads on the screen or monitor. Based on what is observed, use critical thinking skills and take any corrective action necessary. Run the tracing when the leads look clear and without artifact. *(Refer to the Critical Thinking - Checklist for Affective Behaviors.)*	**5***	
15.	Check the tracing for clarity, artifact, and abnormal life-threatening rhythms. Based on what is observed, use critical thinking skills and take any action necessary. *(Refer to the Critical Thinking - Checklist for Affective Behaviors.)*	**5***	
16.	Disconnect the lead wires and remove the electrodes. Wipe any reside from the patient's skin. Wash your hands or use hand sanitizer. Instruct the patient to get dressed. Ask the patient if assistance is needed. If so, help the patient to dress.	**5**	
17.	Provide the patient with information about following up with the provider. Complete any necessary actions with the ECG (e.g., upload to the electronic health record, mount and route to the provider).	**2**	
18.	Document accurately in the patient's health record. Indicate the provider ordering the test, what test was performed, how the patient tolerated the test, and what you did with the ECG tracing. You can also add any instructions you provided to the patient regarding follow-up.	**5**	
Scenario update: Perform routine machine maintenance by adding paper to ECG machine or printer. 19. Review the operator's manual on how to change the paper. Gather the new ream of ECG paper (or roll).	**5***	
20.	Open the machine. Remove the remaining paper and add the new paper per the steps in the manual.	**2**	

21. Apply gloves and disinfect the lead wires per the operator's manual. Disinfect the exam table. Clean up the work area. Remove the gloves. Wash your hands or use hand sanitizer.	3		
Total Points	100		

Checklist for Affective Behaviors

Affective Behavior	*Directions:* Check behaviors observed during the role-play.					
Critical Thinking	**Negative, Unprofessional Behaviors**	**Attempt**		**Positive, Professional Behaviors**	**Attempt**	
		1	**2**		**1**	**2**
	Coached or told of an issue or problem			Independently identified the problem or issue		
	Failed to ask relevant questions related to the condition			Asked appropriate questions to obtain the information required		
	Failed to consider alternatives; failed to ask questions that demonstrate understanding of principles/concepts			Willing to consider other alternatives; asked appropriate questions that showed understanding of principles/concepts		
	Failed to make an educated, logical judgment/decision			Made an educated, logical judgment/decision based on the protocol		
	Actions or lack of actions demonstrated unsafe practices and/or did not follow the protocol			Took appropriate actions based on observations; actions reflected principles of safe practice		
	Other:			Other:		

Awareness	Rude, discourteous			Pleasant and courteous		
	Disregarded the person's dignity and rights			Maintained the person's dignity and rights		
	Failed to clearly and/or professionally address the reason for the ECG			Clearly and professionally described the reason for the ECG		
	Failed to use therapeutic communication techniques (e.g., reflection, restating, clarifying, and summarizing) to verify patient's concerns			Used therapeutic communication techniques (e.g., reflection, restating, clarifying, and summarizing) to verify patient's concerns		
	Nonempathetic behaviors; failed to address patient's concerns			Shows empathy; addresses patient's concerns		
	Failed to clearly and/or professionally address the situation and/or patient's questions			Clearly and professionally addressed the situation and/or patient's questions		
	Failed to reassure patient or inappropriately reassured patient			Appropriately reassured patient.		
	Negative nonverbal behaviors			Positive nonverbal behaviors		
	Other:			Other:		

Grading for Affective Behaviors		**Point Value**	**Attempt 1**	**Attempt 2**
Does not meet Expectation	• Response fails to show awareness of patient's concerns or critical thinking skills. • Student demonstrated more than 2 negative, unprofessional behaviors during the interaction.	0		
Needs Improvement	• Response fails to show awareness of patient's concerns or critical thinking skills. • Student demonstrated 1 or 2 negative, unprofessional behaviors during the interaction.	0		
Meets Expectation	• Response demonstrates awareness of patient's concerns or critical thinking; no negative, unprofessional behaviors observed. • More practice is needed for behavior to appear natural and for student to appear comfortable and at ease.	5		
Occasionally Exceeds Expectation	• Response demonstrates awareness of patient's concerns or critical thinking; no negative, unprofessional behaviors observed. • At times student appeared comfortable and at ease; but more practice is needed for behavior to become natural and consistent with a professional medical assistant.	5		

Always Exceeds Expectation	• Response demonstrates awareness of patient's concerns or critical thinking; no negative, unprofessional behaviors observed. • Student's behaviors appeared natural and comfortable. Behaviors are consistent with a professional medical assistant.	5		

Documentation

Comments

CAAHEP Competencies	**Step(s)**
I.P.2.a. Perform: electrocardiography	1-18
I.P.8. Instruct and prepare a patient for a procedure or a treatment	3, 13
I.A.2. Incorporate critical thinking skills when performing patient care	14, 15
I.A.3. Show awareness of a patient's concerns related to the procedure being performed	4
VI.P.8. Perform routine maintenance of administrative or clinical equipment	19-21
X.P.3. Document patient care accurately in the medical record	18
ABHES Competencies	**Step(s)**
8.d. Assist provider with specialty examination, including cardiac, respiratory, OB-GYN, neurological, and gastroenterology procedures	Entire procedure
8.e. Perform specialty procedures, including but not limited to minor surgery, cardiac, respiratory, OB-GYN, neurological, and gastroenterology	Entire procedure

Procedure 26.2   Apply a Holter Monitor

Name _____ Date _____ Score _____

Tasks: Apply a Holter monitor and coach a patient on the procedure. Document the procedure in the patient's health record.

Equipment and Supplies:
- Holter monitor, new batteries, flash memory card (if required), carrying case, and operator's manual
- Disposable electrodes
- Razor
- Sharps container
- Alcohol pads
- Gauze pads (optional)
- Cloth nonallergenic tape (optional)
- Journal
- Waste container
- Patient's health record

Standard: Complete the procedure and all critical steps in _____ minutes with a minimum score of 85% within two attempts (*or as indicated by the instructor*).

Scoring: Divide the points earned by the total possible points. Failure to perform a critical step, indicated by an asterisk (*), results in grade no higher than an 84% (*or as indicated by the instructor*).

Time: Began_____ Ended_____ Total minutes: _____

Steps:	Point Value	Attempt 1	Attempt 2
1. Wash hands or use hand sanitizer.	5		
2. Assemble equipment and supplies needed for the procedure. Insert flash memory card if required. Insert new batteries into the monitor. Consult the operator's manual for the required amount and placement of electrodes.	5		
3. Greet the patient. Identify yourself. Verify the patient's identity with full name and date of birth. Explain the procedure to be performed in a manner that is understood by the patient. Answer any questions the patient may have on the procedure.	10		
4. Ask the patient to remove clothing from the waist up and to sit at the end of the exam table. Ask the patient if assistance is needed. If so, help. If not, leave the room and allow the patient time to change. When reentering the room, provide a courtesy knock on the door.	5		
5. Identify the locations for the electrodes and prepare the skin for the electrodes. Shave the area if the patient has a hairy chest. Wipe the area with the alcohol pad and allow it to dry. Fold the gauze pad over your index finger and briskly rub the site to abrade the skin.	10		
6. Snap the lead wire onto the electrode. Apply the electrodes to the sites as indicated by the manufacturer. Press firmly and make sure the entire electrode adheres completely to the skin	10		
7. Loop and tape down the wires on the chest.	5		

8.	Attach the patient cable to the monitor if required. Turn on the recorder and set as indicated by the manufacturer. Enter the patient data as indicated.	**10**		
9.	Have the patient get dressed. Assist as needed.	**10**		
10.	Coach the patient regarding making journal entries while wearing the monitor. Provide the required patient education.	**10**		
11.	Assist the patient in scheduling a return appointment in 24 hours. Provide the patient with contact information should a question arise.	**10**		
12.	Document accurately in the patient's health record. Indicate the provider ordering the test, the procedure done, patient education provided, and return appointment.	**10**		
	Total Points	**100**		

Documentation

Comments

CAAHEP Competencies	Step(s)
I.P.8. Instruct and prepare a patient for a procedure or a treatment	3, 10
X.P.3. Document patient care accurately in the medical record	12
ABHES Competencies	**Step(s)**
8.d. Assist provider with specialty examination, including cardiac, respiratory, OB-GYN, neurological, and gastroenterology procedures	Entire procedure
8.e. Perform specialty procedures, including but not limited to minor surgery, cardiac, respiratory, OB-GYN, neurological, and gastroenterology	Entire procedure

Medical Emergencies

CAAHEP Competencies	Assessment
I.C.13. List principles and steps of professional/provider CPR	Skills and Concepts – B. 19
I.C.14. Describe basic principles of first aid as they pertain to the ambulatory healthcare setting	Skills and Concepts – B. 6, 8, 13, 14, 16
I.P.13.a. Perform first aid procedures for: bleeding	Procedure 27.5
I.P.13.b. Perform first aid procedures for: diabetic coma or insulin shock	Procedure 27.1
I.P.13.c. Perform first aid procedures for: fractures	Procedure 27.5
I.P.13.d. Perform first aid procedures for: seizures	Procedure 27.3
I.P.13.e. Perform first aid procedures for: shock	Procedure 27.6
I.P.13.f. Perform first aid procedures for: syncope	Procedure 27.5
I.A.1. Incorporate critical thinking skills when performing patient assessment	Procedure 27.2
X.P.3. Document patient care accurately in the medical record	Procedure 27.1 through 27.6

ABHES Competencies	Assessment
8. Clinical Procedures g. Recognize and respond to medical office emergencies	Procedure 27.1 through 27.7

VOCABULARY REVIEW

Using the word pool on the right, find the correct word to match the definition. Write the word on the line after the definition.

Group A

1. A catheter that is inserted into the trachea through the mouth; provides a patent airway _____
2. Open _____
3. A term used in healthcare settings to indicate an emergency situation and summon the trained team to the scene

    _____
4. A rolling supply cart that contains emergency equipment

    _____
5. A patient without an appointment _____
6. The level and type of care an ordinary, prudent healthcare professional having the same training and experience in a similar practice would have provided under a similar situation

    _____
7. Contraction of the muscles causing the narrowing of the inside tube of the vessel _____
8. The application of manual chest compressions and ventilations (also called *rescue breathing*) to patients who are not breathing or do not have a pulse; also known as *basic life support* (BLS)

    _____
9. A written flow map to make triage decisions; based on answers to questions, the person moves through the map until a triage decision is made _____
10. To sort out and classify the injured; used in the military and emergency settings to determine the priority of a patient to be treated _____

Word Pool
- triage flow map
- triage
- walk-in patient
- crash cart
- vasoconstriction
- cardiopulmonary resuscitation (CPR)
- standard of care
- endotracheal (ET) tube
- code
- patent

Group B

1. Tissue death _____
2. Redness _____
3. Itching _____
4. A position on the person's side that helps to keep the airway open and clear _____
5. A sensation that causes someone to feel as though everything is spinning _____
6. A traumatic brain injury caused by a blow to the head

    _____
7. A sudden increase of electrical activity in one or more parts of the brain _____
8. Also called a *stroke* _____
9. Also called *over breathing*; a rapid and deep breathing

    _____
10. Fainting _____

Word Pool
- seizure
- pruritus
- recovery position
- concussion
- syncope
- cerebrovascular accident
- necrosis
- vertigo
- erythema
- hyperventilation

ABBREVIATIONS

Write out what each of the following abbreviations stands for.

1. CPR _____

2. ET _____

3. LPN _____

4. RN _____

5. IV _____

6. AED _____

7. PPE _____

8. %TBSA _____

9. IM _____

10. RICE _____

11. CVA _____

12. ED _____

13. MI _____

14. EAP _____

15. POTS _____

SKILLS AND CONCEPTS

Answer the following questions. Write your answer on the line or in the space provided.

A. Emergency Equipment and Supplies

1. The following questions relate to crash carts.

    a. How often should a crash cart be checked? _____

    b. Who should check the crash cart? _____

    c. Describe how to check crash cart supplies. _____

    _____

    _____

2. List the equipment required when a provider performs an endotracheal tube intubation. _____

    _____

    _____

3. The following statements relate to common medications found on crash carts.

    a. _____ is used for bradycardia and will increase the heart rate.

    b. _____ is used for seizures.

    c. _____ is used for anaphylaxis, severe asthma, and cardiac arrest.

    d. _____ is an antihistamine that is used for allergic reactions.

    e. _____, a hormone that simulates the liver to release glucose into the blood, is given for hypoglycemia.

    f. _____ is used for opioid overdoses.

4. Describe the Broselow tape and Broselow ColorCode Cart. _____

    _____

    _____

B. Handling Emergencies

1. What is the role of the medical assistant with emergency situations? _____

    _____

2. Describe first aid procedures for the following conditions.

    a. Frostbite_____

    _____

    b. Hypothermia _____

    _____

    c. Heat cramps _____

    _____

    d. Heat exhaustion _____

    _____

    e. Heat stroke _____

    _____

    f. Minor burns _____

    _____

    g. Major burns _____

    _____

3. List six signs and symptoms of poisoning. _____

_____

4. Describe first aid procedures for poisoning. _____

_____

_____

5. Describe first aid procedures for severe allergic reactions. _____

_____

_____

6. What is the first aid procedure in the ambulatory care facility for an animal bite? _____

_____

7. What types of screening questions should a medical assistant ask a patient who is calling regarding an animal bite?

_____

_____

8. What is the first aid procedure for a foreign body in the eye and what is done in the ambulatory care facility?

_____

_____

9. _____ is called *severe hypoglycemia* or *insulin reaction*.

10. _____ is called *severe hyperglycemia*.

11. List five symptoms of hypoglycemia and two symptoms of severe hypoglycemia. _____

_____

_____

12. List five symptoms of hyperglycemia and two symptoms of diabetic ketoacidosis. _____

_____

_____

13. What are first aid procedures and additional treatments for insulin shock in a conscious and unconscious individual?

_____

_____

_____

_____

_____

14. Describe how to splint an injured extremity. _____

_____

_____

15. Why is a cold pack applied to a musculoskeletal injury? _____

_____

16. For the following scenarios, the patient is in the ambulatory care facility. Describe first aid that the medical assistant should provide.

a. A patient gets dizzy. _____

_____

_____

b. A patient has seizure-like activity. _____

_____

_____

c. A patient is confused and not making sense; has left arm and leg weakness and facial drooping.

_____

_____

d. A patient is having an asthma attack. _____

_____

_____

e. A patient faints. _____

_____

_____

f. A patient is bleeding from a gash on her arm. There is no obvious debris in the wound._____

_____

_____

17. A patient goes into shock. What is the typical treatment in the ambulatory care facility? _____

_____

_____

18. A patient has chest pain and left arm pain. What is the typical treatment in the ambulatory care facility?

_____

_____

19. Using Procedure 27.7, summarize the steps and principles involved with rescue breathing, CPR, and using the AED machine.

_____

_____

_____

_____

_____

_____

_____

CERTIFICATION PREPARATION

Circle the correct answer.

1. What is considered a mild heat-related illness that causes muscle pains and spasms due to electrolyte imbalance?
   a. Heat stroke
   b. Heat exhaustion
   c. Heat cramps
   d. Hypothermia

2. What is considered a partial-thickness burn?
   a. First-degree burn
   b. Second-degree burn
   c. Third-degree burn
   d. Fourth-degree burn

3. Which type of burn causes erythema, tenderness, and physical sensitivity, but no scar development occurs?
   a. First-degree burn
   b. Second-degree burn
   c. Third-degree burn
   d. Fourth-degree burn

4. An adult has burns on his back, left arm and hand, and left foot and leg. Using the Rule of Nines, estimate the percentage of total burn surface area.
   a. 18%
   b. 27%
   c. 36%
   d. 45%

5. Which animal is not a common carrier of rabies?
   a. Guinea pig
   b. Raccoon
   c. Bat
   d. Fox

6. What is a symptom of a concussion?
   a. Confusion and amnesia
   b. Ringing in the ears
   c. Temporary loss of consciousness right after the incident
   d. All of the above

7. What is a symptom of a cerebrovascular accident?
   a. Confusion and speech difficulty
   b. Numbness of the face, arm, or leg
   c. Problem seeing in one or both eyes
   d. All of the above

8. What is not a sign of a partial airway obstruction?
   a. Forceful or weak coughing
   b. Bluish skin color
   c. Labored, noisy, or gasping breathing
   d. Panicked appearance, extreme anxiety, or agitation

9. What is a possible cause of syncope?
   a. Dehydration
   b. Standing up too quickly
   c. Drop in blood glucose
   d. All of the above

10. What is not a typical symptom of a shock?
    a. Anxiety and agitation
    b. Chest pain
    c. Nausea
    d. Diaphoresis

WORKPLACE APPLICATIONS

1. A medical assistant suspects a patient is starting to have an allergic reaction. What should the medical assistant do? What will the provider order? How should the medication be administered?

   _____

   _____

   _____

2. Gabe was rooming Mr. Smith, who stated, "I think I am having a heart attack." What are the common symptoms of a myocardial infarction (MI)?

   _____

   _____

   _____

3. Dr. Walden ordered nitroglycerin for Mr. Smith. How does nitroglycerin work in the body? _____

   _____

   _____

   _____

INTERNET ACTIVITIES

1. Using online resources, research one of the following conditions: seizures, cerebrovascular accident, asthmatic attack, and MI. Create a poster presentation, a PowerPoint presentation, or write a paper summarizing your research. Include the following points in your project:
   a. Description of the condition
   b. Etiology
   c. Signs and symptoms
   d. Diagnostic procedures
   e. Treatments

2. Using online resources, research a condition listed in #1. Create a patient education flyer based on your research. Include the following points in your flyer:
   a. Description of the condition
   b. Risks factors
   c. Warning signs and symptoms
   d. Actions the individual should take when experiencing the signs and symptoms

3. Research the following medications: diphenhydramine, epinephrine, glucagon, naloxone, and nitroglycerin. Using a reliable online drug resource, identify for each medication:
   a. Reasons for use
   b. Desired effects
   c. Side effects
   d. Adverse reactions

   Write a short paper addressing each of these four areas for each medication.

Procedure 27.1 Provide First Aid for a Patient with Insulin Shock

Name _____ Date _____ Score _____

Task: Provide first aid to an individual with hypoglycemia.

Background Information: A blood glucose test should be done to find out how low the patient is. After 15 minutes of the person eating/drinking the sugary food, the glucose test should be taken. If below 70 mg/dL, give additional sugary food/drink and repeat the glucose test in 15 minutes. Continue until the blood glucose level is 70 or over.

Scenario: You are working with Dr. Martin, a family practice provider. Maude Crawford arrives for her appointment.

Directions: Read the scenario and role-play the situation with a peer. The peer will be the patient and you are the medical assistant.

Equipment and Supplies:
- Sugary drink (4 oz. fruit juice or regular soda) or three glucose tablets
- Patient's health record

Standard: Complete the procedure and all critical steps in _____ minutes with a minimum score of 85% within two attempts (*or as indicated by the instructor*).

Scoring: Divide the points earned by the total possible points. Failure to perform a critical step, indicated by an asterisk (*), results in grade no higher than an 84% (*or as indicated by the instructor*).

Time: Began_____ Ended_____ Total minutes: _____

Steps:	Point Value	Attempt 1	Attempt 2
1. Wash hands or use hand sanitizer.	5		
2. Greet the patient. Identify yourself. Verify the patient's identity with full name and date of birth.	15		
Scenario update: Mrs. Crawford has diabetes and states that she thinks she has low blood sugar. She has blurry vision, tremors, and a headache. She asks you for something to eat. According to the facility's policy, you check her blood glucose level and it is 48 mg/dL. 3. Obtain a sugary drink or a fast-acting sugary food. Indicate how much to give to the patient.	20*		
Scenario update: After 15 minutes, her blood glucose level is 59 mg/dL. You notify the provider while a coworker stays with the patient. 4. Describe follow up care for the patient.	40		
Scenario update: After 15 minutes, her blood glucose level is 82 mg/dL. You notified the provider. 5. Document the situation. Include the blood glucose levels, your actions, the provider notified, and the patient's response.	20		
Total Points	**100**		

Documentation

Comments

CAAHEP Competencies	Step(s)
I.P.13.b. Perform first aid procedures for: diabetic coma or insulin shock	Entire procedure
X.P.3. Document patient care accurately in the medical record	5
ABHES Competencies	**Step(s)**
8. g. Recognize and respond to medical office emergencies	Entire procedure

Procedure 27.2 Incorporate Critical Thinking Skills When Performing Patient Assessment

Name _____ Date _____ Score _____

Task: Use critical thinking skills while performing a patient assessment regarding a neurologic emergency.

Scenario: You are working with Dr. Martin, a family practice provider. Maude Crawford's daughter called concerned about her mother. She stated that Maude fell and hit her head. She was "knocked out" for about a minute. She has been acting differently since the fall. You need to follow the "Emergency Phone Protocol" for your clinic.

Directions: Role-play the scenario with a peer. The peer will be the daughter and you will be the medical assistant. The peer can make up information regarding the scenario. Your instructor will be the provider.

WMFM Clinic – Neurologic Emergency Phone Protocol:

Obtain the patient's name, date of birth, signs/symptoms, and the history of the situation. After call, document situation, symptoms, and action in the patient's health record.

With the following concerns, send the patient to the emergency department via the ambulance immediately.
- Seizure lasting 3 or more minutes
- Passing out or fainting; dizziness or weakness that doesn't go away
- Sudden or unusual headache that starts suddenly
- Unable to see or speak; sudden confusion
- Neck or spine injury
- Injuries that cause loss of feeling or inability to move
- Head injury with passing out, fainting, or confusion

With the following concerns, schedule a visit for the same day. If no appointments are available, consult the triage nurse or the provider regarding the situation.
- Headache/migraine
- Nonemergent neurologic concern

Equipment and Supplies:
- Patient's health record
- Paper and pen
- Emergency Phone Protocol for clinic

Standard: Complete the procedure and all critical steps in _____ minutes with a minimum score of 85% within two attempts (*or as indicated by the instructor*).

Scoring: Divide the points earned by the total possible points. Failure to perform a critical step, indicated by an asterisk (*), results in grade no higher than an 84% (*or as indicated by the instructor*).

Time: Began_____ Ended_____ Total minutes: _____

Steps:	Point Value	Attempt 1	Attempt 2
1. Write five questions that can be asked to obtain additional information on the patient's signs and symptoms.	20*		
Scenario update: Role-play the scenario with a peer. 2. Obtain the patient's name and date of birth.	10		
3. Write down the patient's information obtained.	20		
4. Using critical thinking skills, ask appropriate questions to obtain information about the patient's condition. *(Refer to* the *Checklist for Affective Behaviors.)*	15*		
5. Follow the protocol to determine what actions to take. *(Refer to* the *Checklist for Affective Behaviors.)*	15*		
6. Instruct the caller on what should be done.	10		
7. Document the call in the patient's health record. Include the caller's name, the patient's condition (e.g., signs, symptoms, and concerns), name of the protocol used, information given to the caller, and the provider who was notified.	10		
Total Points	100		

Checklist for Affective Behaviors

Affective Behavior	Directions: *Check behaviors observed during the role-play.*					
Critical Thinking	**Negative, Unprofessional Behaviors**	**Attempt**		**Positive, Professional Behaviors**	**Attempt**	
		1	**2**		**1**	**2**
	Coached or told of an issue or problem			Independently identified the problem or issue		
	Failed to ask relevant questions related to the condition			Asked appropriate questions to obtain the information required		
	Failed to consider alternatives; failed to ask questions that demonstrate understanding of principles/concepts			Willing to consider other alternatives; asked appropriate questions that showed understanding of principles/concepts		
	Failed to make an educated, logical judgment/decision; actions or lack of actions demonstrated unsafe practices and/or do not follow the protocol			Made an educated, logical judgment/decision based on the protocol; actions reflected principles of safe practice		
	Other:			Other:		

Grading for Affective Behaviors		Point Value	Attempt 1	Attempt 2
Does not meet Expectation	• Response fails to show critical thinking. • Student demonstrated more than 2 negative, unprofessional behaviors during the interaction.	0		
Needs Improvement	• Response fails to show critical thinking. • Student demonstrated 1 or 2 negative, unprofessional behaviors during the interaction.	0		
Meets Expectation	• Response demonstrates critical thinking; no negative, unprofessional behaviors observed. • More practice is needed for behavior to appear natural and for student to appear comfortable and at ease.	15		
Occasionally Exceeds Expectation	• Response demonstrates critical thinking; no negative, unprofessional behaviors observed. • At times student appeared comfortable and at ease; but more practice is needed for behavior to become natural and consistent with a professional medical assistant.	15		
Always Exceeds Expectation	• Response demonstrates critical thinking; no negative, unprofessional behaviors observed. • Student's behaviors appeared natural and comfortable. Behaviors are consistent with a professional medical assistant.	15		

Questions to ask

Documentation

Comments

CAAHEP Competencies	Step(s)
I.A.1. Incorporate critical thinking skills when performing patient assessment	Entire role-play
X.P.3. Document patient care accurately in the medical record	9
ABHES Competencies	**Step(s)**
8.g. Recognize and respond to medical office emergencies	Entire procedure

Procedure 27.3   Provide First Aid for a Patient with Seizure Activity

Name _____ Date _____ Score _____

Tasks: Provide first aid to an individual having seizure activity and document in the health record.

Scenario: You are working with Dr. Martin, a family practice provider. Walter Biller arrives for his appointment.

Directions: Read the scenario and role-play the situation with a peer. The peer will be the patient and you are the medical assistant.

Equipment and Supplies:
- Watch
- Folded towel, blanket, or coat
- Patient's health record
- Gloves and other personal protective equipment (as required)

Standard: Complete the procedure and all critical steps in _____ minutes with a minimum score of 85% within two attempts (*or as indicated by the instructor*).

Scoring: Divide the points earned by the total possible points. Failure to perform a critical step, indicated by an asterisk (*), results in grade no higher than an 84% (*or as indicated by the instructor*).

Time: Began_____ Ended_____ Total minutes: _____

Steps:	Point Value	Attempt 1	Attempt 2
1. Wash hands or use hand sanitizer.	5		
2. Greet the patient. Identify yourself. Verify the patient's identity with full name and date of birth.	10		
Scenario update: While you are getting Mr. Biller's health history, he starts to have seizure activity. 3. Lower the patient to the floor and note the time when the seizure started. Gently raise the chin to tilt the head back slightly to open the airway.	15		
4. Yell for help while moving the patient into the recovery position.	15		
5. Check his pulse rate and respiration rate.	15		
6. Apply gloves and other personal protective equipment as needed.	10		
7. Clear any hard or sharp items away from the patient. Place a soft folded towel, blanket, or coat under the patient's head.	10		
8. Remove the patient's glasses (if on) and loosen any constrictive clothing around the neck. Stay with the person until he or she is fully awake and continue to monitor the respiration and pulse rates.	10		
9. Document the first aid measures you provided in the order that they occurred. In addition, document the seizure activity seen, length of the episode, and the provider notified.	10		
Total Points	**100**		

Documentation

Comments

CAAHEP Competencies	Step(s)
I.P.13.d. Perform first aid procedures for: seizures	Entire procedure
X.P.3. Document patient care accurately in the medical record	9
ABHES Competencies	**Step(s)**
8.g. Recognize and respond to medical office emergencies	Entire procedure

Procedure 27.4   Provide First Aid for a Choking Patient

Name _____ Date _____ Score _____

Tasks: Provide first aid to a conscious adult who is choking. Document in the health record.

Scenario: You are working with Dr. Martin, a family practice provider. As you return from lunch, you notice that an adult visitor is having an issue. It appears that she had been eating fast food and now she is holding her neck with both hands. She appears to be panicking.

Directions: Read the scenario and role-play the situation with a peer. The peer will be the visitor and you are the medical assistant.

Equipment and Supplies:
- Patient's health record
- Gloves
- Mannequin

Standard: Complete the procedure and all critical steps in _____ minutes with a minimum score of 85% within two attempts (*or as indicated by the instructor*).

Scoring: Divide the points earned by the total possible points. Failure to perform a critical step, indicated by an asterisk (*), results in grade no higher than an 84% (*or as indicated by the instructor*).

Time: Began_____ Ended_____ Total minutes: _____

Steps:	Point Value	Attempt 1	Attempt 2
1. Approach the person and ask, "Are you choking?"	**10**		
Scenario update: She nods her head yes and cannot speak. She is standing. 2. Yell for help. Wear gloves if available. Stand behind the victim with your feet slightly apart. Reach your arms around the person's waist.	**15***		
3. Make a fist and place it just above the person's navel. Make sure your thumb side is next to the person. Grasp the fist tightly with your other hand. *Note: Do not do abdominal thrusts on your peer.*	**15***		
Scenario update: The next steps must be done on a mannequin. 4. With the correct hand position, make quick, upward and inward thrusts with your fist. Do five abdominal thrusts before doing back blows.	**15***		
5. Stand behind the person and wrap one arm around the person's upper body. Position the person so he or she is bent forward with the chest parallel to the ground.	**15**		
6. Use the heel of your other hand to give a firm blow between the shoulder blades. Check to see if the object dislodges. If not, continue by giving another four back blows.	**10**		
7. Continue to give five abdominal thrusts followed by five back blows until the object is dislodged or the person loses consciousness. *Note:* If the person faints or loses consciousness, lower the person to the floor. Call 911 (or the local emergency number) or have someone else call. Begin CPR starting with chest compressions. Check to see if the item is in the airway. Only remove it if it is loose.	**10**		

Scenario update: After two sets, she coughs out a piece of food. She can now talk. 8. Arrange for the person to be seen by the provider. Document the first aid measures you provided in the order that they occurred.	**10**		
Total Points	**100**		

Documentation

Comments

ABHES Competencies	Step(s)
8.g. Recognize and respond to medical office emergencies	Entire procedure

Procedure 27.5 Provide First Aid for a Patient With a Bleeding Wound, Fracture, and Syncope

Name _____ Date _____ Score _____

Tasks: Provide first aid to an individual with a suspected fracture, a bleeding wound, and syncope. Document the first aid you provide.

Scenario: You are returning from lunch and see a person fall at the entrance of the healthcare facility. He is an older man and is complaining of pain in his right lower arm. His arm looks deformed and is bleeding. You call for help. A provider comes, and coworkers bring supplies. The provider tells you to care for the wound and splint the arm before moving the individual. You have a coworker helping you.

Directions: Read the scenario and role-play the situation with two peers. One peer will be the patient and the other peer will be a coworker. You will be the medical assistant.

Equipment and Supplies:
- Gloves
- Sterile gauze
- Bandage
- Splinting material (e.g., SAM splint)
- Coban wrap or gauze roll

Standard: Complete the procedure and all critical steps in _____ minutes with a minimum score of 85% within two attempts (*or as indicated by the instructor*).

Scoring: Divide the points earned by the total possible points. Failure to perform a critical step, indicated by an asterisk (*), results in grade no higher than an 84% (*or as indicated by the instructor*).

Time: Began_____ Ended_____ Total minutes: _____

Steps:	Point Value	Attempt 1	Attempt 2
1. Wash hands or use hand sanitizer if possible. Identify yourself to the patient. Obtain the patient's name and date of birth as you put on gloves.	10		
2. Using sterile gauze, apply direct pressure over the wound to stop the bleeding. Make sure to immobilize the injured arm as you apply pressure. If possible, elevate the arm to help slow the bleeding. If the blood seeps through the gauze, apply another layer of gauze on the initial one. Continue with the direct pressure until the bleeding stops.	15*		
3. Once the bleeding has stopped, cover the dressing with a bandage. Remember to immobilize the injured arm as you work.	10		
Scenario update: As you apply the bandage to the injured arm, the patient states he does not feel good. He says he feels dizzy and thinks he is going to pass out. Your peer takes over by supporting his arm, and the man faints. He is still breathing and has a pulse. 4. Position the patient on his back. Continue to check his respirations and pulse rates.	15*		
5. Loosen any constrictive clothing around the neck and chest. Raise the legs above the heart level (about 12 inches).	15*		

Scenario update: After a few minutes, he starts to come around. He jokes that blood makes him faint. As he is lying on his back talking with you, you need to splint his injured arm. 6. Use the splint material and shape it to the injured arm. Do not straighten the arm. Apply the splint beyond the joint above and the joint below the injury.	**15***		
7. Use Coban or a gauze roll to secure the splint in place. Encourage the patient to hold the injured arm against his chest as he moves.	**10***		
8. Document the first aid measures you provided in the order that they occurred. Indicate the provider was at the scene.	**10**		
Total Points	**100**		

Documentation

Comments

CAAHEP Competencies	**Step(s)**
I.P.13.a. Perform first aid procedures for: bleeding	2, 3
I.P.13.c. Perform first aid procedures for: fractures	6, 7
I.P.13.f. Perform first aid procedures for: syncope	4, 5
X.P.3. Document patient care accurately in the medical record	8
ABHES Competencies	**Step(s)**
8.g. Recognize and respond to medical office emergencies	Entire procedure

Procedure 27.6   Provide First Aid for a Patient With Shock

Name _____ Date _____ Score _____

Tasks: Provide first aid to an individual who is in shock. Document the first aid you provide.

Scenarios: You are working with Dr. Julie Walden. The administrative medical assistant at the reception desk notifies you that Robert Caudill (date of birth [DOB] 10/31/1940) is here and looks very ill. You bring the patient and his wife immediately back to the procedure room, as it is the only available room. He asks to move to the exam table and you assist him as he transfers to the table. You obtain his vital signs, which are: P: 92, R: 26, BP 72/48, and T: 103.2° F

Directions: Role-play the scenario with two peers. One peer will be the patient and the other peer will be the wife. You will be the medical assistant.

Equipment and Supplies:
- Stethoscope
- Watch
- Pen
- Sphygmomanometer (blood pressure cuff)
- Pillows, blankets, or small stool to help elevate the feet
- Exam table

Standard: Complete the procedure and all critical steps in _____ minutes with a minimum score of 85% within two attempts (*or as indicated by the instructor*).

Scoring: Divide the points earned by the total possible points. Failure to perform a critical step, indicated by an asterisk (*), results in grade no higher than an 84% (*or as indicated by the instructor*).

Time: Began_____ Ended_____ Total minutes: _____

Steps:	Point Value	Attempt 1	Attempt 2
1. Call for help. Monitor the patient's breathing and pulse until the provider arrives.	10		
Scenario update: The provider examines the patient and suspects septic shock. You administer 2 L of oxygen per nasal cannula as the provider ordered. The triage RN inserts an IV and administers IV fluids. The provider directs another medical assistant to call 911. 2. Raise the patient's legs 12 inches.	15*		
3. Make sure the patient's head is flat on the bed.	10*		
4. Loosen the person's clothing. Make sure the clothing does not restrict the neck and chest area.	15*		
5. Obtain a pulse rate, respiration rate, and blood pressure. Continue to monitor the patient's airway, pulse rate, and respiration rate.	15		
6. While monitoring the patient, speak calmly with the patient. Use a gentle tone of voice. Demonstrate a calming body language (e.g., do not appear scared, rushed, or out of control).	15		
7. Talk calmly with the patient's wife and explain what is occurring. Answer any questions the wife may have.	10		

8.	Document the first aid measures you provided in the order that they occurred. Indicate which provider examined the patient. In addition, document the administration of oxygen and the vital signs obtained.	**10**		
	Total Points	**100**		

Documentation

Comments

CAAHEP Competencies	Step(s)
I.P.13.e. Perform first aid procedures for: shock	Entire procedure
X.P.3. Document patient care accurately in the medical record	8
ABHES Competencies	**Step(s)**
8.g. Recognize and respond to medical office emergencies	Entire procedure

Procedure 27.7   Provide Rescue Breathing, Cardiopulmonary Resuscitation (CPR), and Automated External Defibrillator (AED)

Name _____ Date _____ Score _____

Tasks: Perform rescue breathing and CPR. Use the AED machine.

Scenario: You are out jogging and find a person on the ground. No one is around.

Directions: Role-play the scenario with a peer. The peer will be the person on the ground.

Equipment and Supplies:
- AED machine with adult pads
- Barrier ventilation device
- Mannequin
- Gloves (if available)

Standard: Complete the procedure and all critical steps in _____ minutes with a minimum score of 85% within two attempts (*or as indicated by the instructor*).

Scoring: Divide the points earned by the total possible points. Failure to perform a critical step, indicated by an asterisk (*), results in grade no higher than an 84% (*or as indicated by the instructor*).

Time: Began_____ Ended_____ Total minutes: _____

Steps:	Point Value	Attempt 1	Attempt 2
1. Check the scene for safety. Is it safe to approach and provide help to the victim?	5		
2. Check the person's response. Tap the individual on the shoulder and shout, "Are you all right?" Pause for a few moments for a response.	5		
Scenario update: There is no response from the individual. A bystander comes up and you direct that person to find an AED machine. 3. Call 911 and answer the questions from the dispatcher.	10		
4. Put on gloves if available. Roll the person over if the person is face down. Roll the person as an entire unit, supporting the head, neck and back. Open the airway and assess the respirations and the pulse for 5-10 seconds. **Note:** Occasional gasping is not considered breathing. • Person is breathing and has a pulse: If no head, neck, or spinal injury is suspected, then place the patient in the recovery position. • Person is not breathing and has a pulse: Give ventilations and monitor pulse. • Person is not breathing and has no pulse: Give CPR starting with compressions.	10*		

Anudeth Paul

Scenario update: The individual has a weak pulse and is not breathing. (Use a mannequin for the following steps.) 5. Use a barrier device if available. Pinch the person's nose and give each rescue breath over 1 second. Watch for the chest to rise. Give the appropriate amount of ventilations for the person's age. Continue to monitor the pulse as you give rescue breaths. *Note:* For a situation in which a person had been choking, look in the mouth before giving a rescue breath. If you see the object, sweep it out with your finger. You can also provide nose ventilation, if the mouth is injured. Stoma ventilation must be done if the person has a stoma (in the throat area).	**10***		
Scenario update: When you check the pulse again, there is no pulse. 6. Place your hands at the correct location on the chest. Bring your shoulders directly over the victim's sternum as you compress downward. Keep your elbows locked.	**10**		
7. Give 30 compressions at the appropriate depth. Give 100-120 compressions per minute.	**10***		
8. Give two ventilations and watch for the chest to rise. Continue with the cycle.	**10***		
Scenario update: After two cycles, a bystander brings an AED, but does not know how to use it. The bystander also does not know CPR. You need to stop the CPR and use the AED. 9. Turn on the AED and follow the directions. Attach the AED pads to the individuals' bare dry chest. Attach the pads to the machine if required. *Note:* Make sure to remove any medication patches and medication residue from the chest before operating applying the pads.	**10***		
10. Have everyone stand back from the patient by announcing "Stand clear." Push the analyze button and allow the machine to analyze the heartbeat.	**10***		

11. Follow the prompts on the AED machine.
  a. If a shock is advised, announce, "Stand clear" and make sure no one is touching the individual. Press the shock button. After the shock do CPR for 2 minutes starting with compressions. Continue following the prompts until the emergency responders arrive.
  b. If a shock is not advised, continue doing CPR for 2 minutes starting with compressions. Continue following the prompts until the emergency responders arrive.
	10*		

Total Points	**100**		

Comments

ABHES Competencies	Step(s)
8.g. Recognize and respond to medical office emergencies	Entire procedure

Principles of Pharmacology

CAAHEP Competencies	Assessment
I.C.11.a. Identify the classifications of medications including: indications for use	Certification Preparation – 9; Workplace Applications – 1; Internet Activities – 3e
I.C.11.b. Identify the classifications of medications including: desired effects	Certification Preparation – 10; Workplace Applications – 1; Internet Activities – 3f
I.C.11.c. Identify the classifications of medications including: side effects	Workplace Applications – 2; Internet Activities – 3h
I.C.11.d. Identify the classifications of medications including: adverse reactions	Workplace Applications – 2; Internet Activities – 3i
IV.C.2. Define the function of dietary supplements	Skills and Concepts – C. 3

ABHES Competencies	Assessment
1. General Orientation d. List the general responsibilities and skills of the medical assistant	Skills and Concepts – A. 1-2
1.f. Comply with federal, state, and local health laws and regulations as they relate to healthcare settings	Skills and Concepts – C. 6-7, 9, 11
6. Pharmacology a. Identify drug classification, usual dose, side effects and contraindications of the top most commonly used medications.	Workplace Applications – 1-2; Internet Activities – 3
6.c. 1) Identify parts of prescriptions	Skills and Concepts – F. 2-3
6.c. 2) Identify appropriate abbreviations that are accepted in prescription writing	Abbreviations – 16, 18-24, 27-48; Procedure 28.1
6.c. 3) Comply with legal aspects of creating prescriptions, including federal and state laws	Skills and Concepts – F. 4-6; Procedure 28.1
6.d. Properly utilize the Physician's Desk Reference (PDR), drug handbooks, and other drug references to identify a drug's classification, usual dosage, usual side effects, and contraindications	Internet Activities – 3

Anandeep Kaur

VOCABULARY REVIEW

Using the word pool on the right, find the correct word to match the definition. Write the word on the line after the definition.

Group A

1. The study of drug absorption, distribution, metabolism, and excretion in the body ___pharmacokinetics___
2. The study of the properties, actions, and uses of drugs ___pharmacology___
3. A drug that reduces or eliminates pain ___analgesic___
4. A drug that destroys or inhibits the growth of bacteria ___antibiotic___
5. Unpleasant effects of a drug in addition to the desired or therapeutic effect ___side effects___
6. A drug that prevents or alleviates heart arrhythmias ___antiarrhythmic___
7. Harmful and deadly effects of a medication that can develop due to the buildup of medication or byproducts in the body ___toxicity___
8. A substance (i.e., medication or chemical) that prevent the clotting of blood ___anticoagulant___
9. A substance that inhibits the growth of microorganisms on living tissue ___antiseptic___
10. The means by which a drug enters the body ___route___

Word Pool
- antiarrhythmic
- anticoagulant
- antiseptic
- antibiotic
- analgesic
- side effects
- pharmacology
- toxicity
- route
- pharmacokinetics

Group B

1. Medications that are administered in an inactive form ___prodrugs___
2. A series of chemical processes whereby enzymes change drugs in the body ___metabolism___
3. Tissues that slowly release the drug into the bloodstream and keep the blood levels from decreasing too rapidly ___reservoirs___
4. A medication that prevents or reduces inflammation ___Antiinflammatory___
5. The movement of metabolites out of the body ___excretion___
6. The movement of absorbed drug from the blood to the body tissues ___distribution___
7. Route of administration where the drug is placed under the tongue to dissolve ___sublingual___
8. Route of administration where the drug is placed between the cheek and the gums to dissolve ___buccal___
9. The movement of drug from the site of administration to the bloodstream ___absorption___
10. Route of medication where the medication is injected just below the skin ___subcutaneous___

Word Pool
- antiinflammatory
- reservoirs
- excretion
- absorption
- distribution
- metabolism
- prodrugs
- buccal
- sublingual
- subcutaneous

Group C

1. A medication that slows down the cell's activity
   depressing
2. Byproducts of drug metabolism _metabolites_
3. A medication that increases the cell's activity
   stimulants
4. Desired effects _therapeutic effects_
5. A higher initial dose of medication _loading dose_
6. A medication that kills cells or disrupts parts of cells
   destroying
7. Unexpected or life-threatening reaction _adverse reactions_
8. Medical doctors who have been specially trained to diagnose and treat patients with mental, emotional, and behavioral conditions
   psychiatrists
9. A disease that occurs when a person cannot stop or limit the use of a drug, even after negative consequences have been experienced _addiction_
10. Is reached when the blood concentration of a medication is high enough for the therapeutic effect to occur
    therapeutic range

Word Pool
- psychiatrists
- loading dose
- destroying
- adverse reaction
- metabolites
- addiction
- depressing
- stimulating
- therapeutic range
- therapeutic effects

Group D

1. Information that appears on the drug label and addresses serious or life-threatening risks _boxed warning_
2. Comparing a document with another document to ensure that they are consistent _reconciling_
3. Conditions or diseases for which the drug is used
   indication
4. A medication order given in person or over the phone
   verbal order
5. Directions given by a provider for a specific medication to be administered to a patient _medication order_
6. Reasons or conditions that make administration of the drug improper or undesirable _contraindications_
7. A written order by a provider to the pharmacist
   prescription
8. An identifier assigned by the Centers for Medicare and Medicaid Services (CMS) that classifies the healthcare provider by license and medical specialties _NPI_
9. Indicates the greatest amount of medication a person should have within a 24-hour period _Maximum dosage_
10. Physical characteristics of a medication (e.g., tablet and suspension) _medication form_

Word Pool
- contraindications
- indication
- form
- verbal order
- medication order
- prescription
- National Provider Identifier
- maximum dosage
- boxed warning
- reconciling

ABBREVIATIONS

Write out what each of the following abbreviations stands for.

1. IV _Intravenous_
2. ID _Intradermal_
3. NAS _Nasal_
4. subcut _Subcutaneous_
5. PO _by mouth_
6. ung _Ointment_
7. soln, sol. _solution_
8. cap _capsule_
9. tinct _tincture_
10. IM _Intramuscular_
11. C _Celsius_
12. F _Fahrenheit_
13. m _meter_
14. cm _centimeter_
15. mm _millimeter_
16. tab(s) _tablet(s)_
17. kg _kilogram_
18. g _gram_
19. mg _milligram_
20. mcg _microgram_
21. gr _grain_
22. gtt(s) _drop(s)_
23. L _Liter_
24. mL _milliliter_
25. lb _pound_
26. fl oz _fluid ounce_
27. qt _quart_
28. pt _pint_
29. Tbs, tbsp _tablespoon_

30. tsp ___ teaspoon
31. AM, a.m. ___ Morning
32. PM, p.m. ___ Afternoon
33. pc ___ after meal
34. ac ___ before meal
35. ad lib ___ as ~~its~~ desired
36. d ___ day
37. noc, noct ___ night
38. hr, h ___ hour
39. p̄ ___ after
40. min ___ minute
41. qh ___ every hour
42. prn ___ as needed
43. q4h ___ every 4 hours
44. q6h ___ every 6 hours
45. qam ___ every morning
46. tid ___ three times a day
47. bid ___ twice a day
48. qid ___ four times a day
49. STAT ___ Immediately
50. ASA ___ Aspirin
51. K ___ Potassium
52. Fe ___ Iron
53. NS ___ Normal Saline
54. MOM ___ Milk of Magnesia
55. NSAID ___ Non-steriod Anti-Inflammatory Drug
56. PPD ___ Purified Protein Derivative
57. OTC ___ Over the Counter
58. aq ___ water
59. med ___ medicine
60. NKA ___ no known allergies

61. NKDA _No known Drug allergies_
62. NPO _Nothing by mouth_
63. āa _of each (used in prescription)_
64. c̄ _with_
65. s̄ _without_
66. pt _patient_
67. qs _quantity sufficient_
68. Rx _take_
69. Sig _give the following directions_
70. VO _Verbal Order_
71. x _times_

SKILLS AND CONCEPTS

Answer the following questions. Write your answer on the line or in the space provided.

A. Introduction

1. Explain why medical assistants need to know about medications. _Because in ambulatory care, setting, MA deals with medication from history taking to administring medication MA have general understanding of drugs._

2. Describe what medical assistants need to know about medications. _They need to know how to pronouce medication names, they must know how to give medications, typically, side effects and the dose to give_

B. Pharmacology Basics

1. List the natural sources of drugs and give one example for each. _① An antiarrythmic medication comes from pulm flower ② Nicotine comes from tobacco leaves._

2. List two advantages to synthetic medications. _____
   ① Its cheaper to produce
   ② The quantity of synethetic medication can also be controlled._

3. Describe the eight uses of drugs and list one example for each use. ① Prevention :- used to prevent ② Treatment :- relieve symptoms ③ Diagnosis :- use to monitor condition ④ Cure :- eliminate disease ⑤ Contraceptive :- prevent pregnancy ⑥ Health maintaince :- enhance health ⑦ Palliative :- don't cure, but improve ⑧ Replacement :- used to increase blood levels.

4. Describe the four parts of pharmacokinetics. ① Absorption :- movement of drug from site of administrive to the bloodstream. ② Distribution :- Absorbed drug from blood to body tissue ③ Metabolism :- series of chemical process ④ Excretion :- movement of metabolities out of body.

5. Describe the effect of the blood-brain barrier to the distribution of medication. Allow certain fat-soluble medications to pass into cerbeaspinal fluid & brain.

6. Describe why only limited medications can be given to a woman who is pregnant. Because most of the medications lead to fotal death and may also alter the fotal development.

7. Explain why different routes affect the dose of medication given. Oral medications are absorbed in stomach or intestines. Blood containing absorbed digestive nutrients & drugs pass through hepatic portal vein & it circulates to rest of body.

8. __Prodrugs__ are medications that are administrated in an inactive form and change into the active form during the metabolic process.

9. Where does most drug metabolism occur? What populations have issues metabolizing medications and are at risk for toxicity?

   Most drug metabolism occurs in liver, Young or children, older adults may have issues.

10. Most metabolites are excreted through the _large intestine_ and _kidneys_ .

11. Describe why medications are limited when a female is breastfeeding her baby. Most drug references indicate if medications pass into breast milk because it alter the baby is health.

12. List all ways drugs are excreted by the body. Large Intestine, kidneys sweat, exhale air, saliva and breast milk.

13. What three populations are at risk for the buildup of metabolic drug byproducts in the body? Young children, older adults and those with kidney disease

14. Describe the four main drug actions. ① Depressing — slow down cell activity. 2) Stimulating :- Increase cell's activity. 3) Destroying ;- kill cells 4) Replacing substances:- substance required by body given medication

15. Pharmacogenics. is the study of how genetic factors influence a person's metabolic response to a specific medication.

16. Describe six factors that influence drug action. ① Age:- Infants have problem with metabolism ② Body sex :- A person side affects amount of drug ③ Gender:- women more fatty than man ④ Generic:- can effect how person response to drug ⑤ Disease:- kidney disease alter drug action ⑥ Diet:- certain food can affects.

17. Explain why a provider may prescribe a loading dose. Your answer should also include the advantage of giving a loading dose of medication.
To help to quickly increase the medication level in blood.

18. Drug allergy occurs when a person develops antibodies against a specific drug.

19. Anaphylaxis is extreme hypersensitivity to a specific drug (antigen) and can cause life-threatening symptoms.

20. List four symptoms of anaphylaxis.
Swelling of mouth, difficult breathing, wheezing, death.

21. Idiosyncrasy is a peculiar response to a certain drug.

22. When prior doses of medications are not excreted before the next dose is given, Cumulative effect can occur.

23. The buildup of medication or byproducts in the body can lead to toxicity, which is harmful and possibly fatal.

C. Drug Legislation and the Ambulatory Care Setting

1. Describe the activities *prescribe, administer,* and *dispense.* Include who can perform each of these activities.

    Prescribe :- To order a medication as treatment for a condition
    Administer :- Give a prescribed dose of medication to patient.
    Dispense :- Give a supply of medication that patient
    will take at a later time.

2. Describe the Food, Drug, and Cosmetic Act. Who enforces the act? Food, Drug, and
   Cosmetic Act is enforced by Food and Drug
   Administration (FDA).

3. Define the function of dietary supplements. To provide nutrients that are
   not obtained in the foods we eat and drink.

4. Describe the Controlled Substance Act. Who enforces the act? The Drug Enforcement
   Agency (DEA) enforces the Controlled Substance
   Act.

5. Briefly describe the schedule of controlled substances. It divided into five
   schedules. These schedules are arranged from the
   greatest to the least abuse potential.

6. What is the DEA registration number? How long is it good for? Each provider have
   unique number. The DEA number is good for
   3 years.

7. Discuss how controlled substances are to be stored. Controlled substances have
   a paper trail. This record start with manufacter
   and ends when medication is dispensed or
   administered.

8. Discuss storage of medications (in general). Refers to package inserts
   for specific storage information. Store medication
   in a cool, dry location.

9. Discuss the importance of keeping inventory records of controlled substances. Your answer should also include the importance of reconciling the log and the length of time the logs need to be kept.

Periodic reconciling of the log is important to identify missing medications. An inventory off all controlled substances must done annually. It kept for 2 years.

10. What is meant by *diversion* of controlled substances? Diversion means using medication for personal reasons.

11. If a medical assistant suspects the diversion of controlled substances, discuss what must occur. Important to notify provider of supervisor,

D. Drug Names

1. The ___brand___ name or ___trade___ name is assigned by the manufacturer and no other company can use that name.

2. The ___Generic___ name is assigned by the U.S. Adopted Name Council.

3. The ___Chemical___ name represents the exact formula of the medication.

4. The ___Official___ name is used to list the medication in the U.S. Pharmacopeia and in the National Formulary (USP-NP).

5. Two companies make the exact same medication. What names would both companies use? What name(s) would be unique for each company?

Some will market medication under brand name and others will use generic name. Medication have different with inactive ingredients,

E. Drug Reference Information

1. Name resources that can be used to learn more about medications. An old classic, PDR, was a very large book that contained a comprehensive collection of package insert information,

2. Define the following terms.

   a. Dosage _Specific the route, dose, and timing of the medication._

   b. Indication _Conditions or diseases for which the drug is used._

   c. Contraindications _Reasons that make administration of the drug improper._

   d. Precautions _Indicates necessary actions._

   e. Adverse reactions _undesirable experiences associated with medication._

   f. Interactions _Include food and beverages that interect with medication._

   g. Action _How the drug provide therapeutic results in the body._

F. Types of Medication Orders

1. What information must the provider give for a medication order? _Patient's name and DOB, Medication name, dose, and route._

2. Describe the four parts of a prescription. _Superscription, inscription, Signature and subscription._

3. List the information that must be included for all prescriptions. _Superscription; means take, Medication name and strength, direction To patient regarding dose g directions to pharmacist._

4. Describe how prescriptions for schedule II/IIN medications are handled. _The provider needs to call in order to give medication._

5. Describe how prescriptions for schedule III/III N and IV medications are handled. _____

It required a form to fill. These are written on a prescription pad or in electronic message.

6. Describe how prescriptions for schedule V medications are handled._____

These medication don't required anything. We can get it over-the-counter.

CERTIFICATION PREPARATION

Circle the correct answer.

1. The rate of medication absorption is influenced by the
   a. blood flow to the absorption area.
   b. route.
   c. conditions at the site of the absorption.
   d. all of the above.

2. Which statement is true regarding metabolism?
   a. Most drug metabolism occurs in the liver.
   b. Young children, older adults, and those with kidney disease have issues metabolizing medications.
   c. Prodrugs change to inactive forms of drugs during metabolism.
   d. a and c

3. _____ means one drug reduces or blocks the effect of another drug.
   a. Toxicity
   b. Synergism
   c. Antagonism
   d. Potentiation

4. _____ means one drug increases the effect of the second drug.
   a. Toxicity
   b. Synergism
   c. Antagonism
   d. Potentiation

5. _____ means to give a prescribed dose of medication to a patient.
   a. Dispense
   b. Administer
   c. Prescribe
   d. Treatment

6. What is the classification of amoxicillin?
   a. Analgesic
   b. Antianxiety
   c. Antibiotic
   d. Antidepressant

7. What is the classification of atenolol?
   a. Antianxiety
   b. Anticonvulsant
   c. Antidepressant
   d. Antihypertensive

8. What is the classification of albuterol?
   a. Cholesterol-lowering agent
   b. Bronchodilator
   c. Corticosteroid
   d. Antihypertensive

9. Which classification of medication increases urinary output and lowers blood pressure?
   a. Laxative
   b. Corticosteroid
   c. Antihypertensive
   d. Diuretic

10. What is the action of an antiemetic?
    a. Treats depression
    b. Reduces nausea and vomiting
    c. Treats bacterial infections
    d. Reduces blood glucose level

WORKPLACE APPLICATIONS

1. Using Table 28.4, Information on Commonly Prescribed Medications, complete the table. Identify the indications for use and the desired effects for the medication classifications listed.

Medication Classification	Indications for Use	Desired Effects
Analgesics		
Antianxiety		
Antiarrhythmic		
Antibiotics		
Anticoagulants		
Anticonvulsants		
Antidepressants		
Antihistamines		
Antihyperglycemics (noninsulin)		
Antihypertensives		
Antiplatelets		
Bronchodilators		
Cholesterol-lowering agents		
Corticosteroids (oral)		
Diuretics		
Muscle relaxants		
Stimulants		

2. Using Table 28.4, Information on Commonly Prescribed Medications, complete the table. Identify the two side effects and two adverse reactions for the following medication classifications.

Class	Generic Name	Side Effects	Adverse Reaction
Analgesics (narcotic)	hydrocodone/ acetaminophen		
Anti-Alzheimer	memantine		
Antianxiety (benzodiazepines)	alprazolam		
Antiarrhythmics	digoxin		
Antibiotics (penicillin)	amoxicillin		
Anticoagulants	warfarin		
Anticonvulsants	gabapentin		
Antidepressant (SSRIs)	escitalopram		
Antihistamines	promethazine		
Antihyperglycemics	metformin		
Antihypertensive	valsartan		
Bronchodilators	albuterol		
Cholesterol-lowering agents	atorvastatin		
Diuretics	furosemide		
Proton-pump inhibitors	omeprazole		

INTERNET ACTIVITIES

1. Using online resources, identify four reliable websites that can be used for medication information. Cite the websites.

2. Using the internet, research the Prescribers' Digital Reference website (www.pdr.net) or the MedlinePlus website (medlineplus.gov). Summarize the following points in a paper, PowerPoint Presentation, or in a poster.
   a. What types of drug information are available?
   b. How can a medical assistant use this website?
   c. What resources are available on this website?

3. Using appropriate online drug reference resources, research one medication from 12 different classifications listed in Table 28.3. The medications should not be listed on Table 28.4. Cite your references. In a paper, PowerPoint presentation, or poster, address the following points for each of the 12 medications:
   a. Generic name
   b. Trade names (in the U.S. only)
   c. Usual adult dose
   d. Classification
   e. Indication for use
   f. Desired effects
   g. Contraindications (list two or more)
   h. Side effects (list five or more)
   i. Adverse reactions (list three or more)

Procedure 28.1 Prepare a Prescription

Name _____ Date _____ Score _____

Tasks: Prepare prescriptions using a prescription refill protocol. Use approved abbreviations.

Scenario: You received a call from Noemi Rodriguez (DOB 11/04/1971). She is requesting refills on three of her prescriptions from Jean Burke, NP. She saw Jean Burke 10 months ago. Noemi has NKA. She is doing well with the prescriptions and has no concerns. You determine it is time for refills. Her prescriptions include Coumadin 5 mg, 1 tablet orally daily; Tenormin 50 mg, 1 tablet orally daily; and Plendil 5 mg, 1 tablet orally daily.

Prescription Refill Protocol
Walden-Martin Family Medicine Clinic

Description: A Certified Medical Assistant (CMA) can refill current hypertensive medications that fall within the guidelines of this protocol.

Step 1	Step 2	
For medications to be refilled, the following points need to be addressed.	**Qualifying Medications**	**Prescription Refill**
• Has the person seen the provider within the last year? • Is the prescription for a hypertensive, hyperlipidemia, or hyperthyroidism medication, a current prescription? • Is the person free of concerns or complications due to the medication? • Is it time for a refill? (The medical assistant must verify that it is time for a refill.) If the answers to the above questions are all YES, then proceed to Step 2. If any of the answers to the above questions are NO, then schedule the person for an appointment with the provider.	amlodipine amlodipine/benazepril atenolol atenolol/chlorthalidone benazepril captopril diltiazem enalapril felodipine fosinopril irbesartan isradipine lisinopril losartan nifedipine quinapril ramipril	Extend the current prescription for 6 months. Instruct patient that in 6 months: • A visit to the provider will be required • Blood pressure reading will be required • Lab work may be required

Equipment and Supplies:
- SimChart for the Medical Office (SCMO) or paper prescriptions (Work Product 28.1) and pen
- Prescription refill protocol
- Drug reference book or online resource

Standard: Complete the procedure and all critical steps in _____ minutes with a minimum score of 85% within two attempts (*or as indicated by the instructor*).

Scoring: Divide the points earned by the total possible points. Failure to perform a critical step, indicated by an asterisk (*), results in grade no higher than an 84% (*or as indicated by the instructor*).

Time: Began _____ Ended _____ Total minutes: _____

Steps:	Point Value	Attempt 1	Attempt 2
1. Using the scenario, look up the generic medication names using the drug reference book or online resource.	10		
2. Read the prescription refill protocol. Compare the generic names to the list of medications given. Identify medication(s) that meet the protocol.	10		
3. Prepare prescription(s) for refill according to the protocol using SCMO or paper prescriptions. a. Using SCMO: Search for the patient. Verify the date of birth before selecting the patient. On the INFO PANEL, select Phone Encounter. Complete the fields on the Create New Encounter window and save. Check the box beside the No known allergy statement on the allergy screen and save. Select Order Entry from the Record dropdown list and select Add in the Out-of-office section. b. Using paper prescriptions: Add in the patient's complete name, date of birth, and address.	20		
4. Using the information in the scenario, complete the prescription information on either the paper prescription or in the SCMO fields. Use only approved abbreviations.	20		
5. Complete any additional prescription(s) as needed by the prescription refill protocol.	30		
6. Review the prescriptions for any errors. Void the prescription and redo if needed. **Note**: After the provider signs the prescriptions and depending on the facility's policy, the medical assistant may need to document the refill in the health record. This cannot be done until the provider approves the prescriptions.	10		
Total Points	100		

Comments

ABHES Competencies	Step(s)
6.c.2) Identify appropriate abbreviations that are accepted in prescription writing	4
6.c.3) Comply with legal aspects of creating prescriptions, including federal and state laws	Entire procedure

Work Product 28.1   Prescriptions
To be used with Procedure 28.1.

Walden-Martin Family Medical Clinic
1234 AnyStreet, AnyTown, AnyState, 12345
Phone: 123-123-1234 Fax: 123-123-5678

Jean Burke NP, Family Nurse Practitioner

Patient: _____   DOB: _____

Address: _____   Date: _____

R℞

Route:

Sig:

Disp:

Refills:

❑   Generics permitted

_____
Jean Burke, NP
NPI#:1234567891

Walden-Martin Family Medical Clinic
1234 AnyStreet, AnyTown, AnyState, 12345
Phone: 123-123-1234 Fax: 123-123-5678

Jean Burke NP, Family Nurse Practitioner

Patient: _____   DOB: _____

Address: _____   Date: _____

R℞

Route:

Sig:

Disp:

Refills:

❑   Generics permitted

_____
Jean Burke, NP
NPI#:1234567891

Walden-Martin Family Medical Clinic
1234 AnyStreet, AnyTown, AnyState, 12345
Phone: 123-123-1234 Fax: 123-123-5678

Jean Burke NP, Family Nurse Practitioner

Patient: _____   DOB: _____

Address: _____   Date: _____

℞

Route:

Sig:

Disp:

Refills:

❏   Generics permitted

_____
Jean Burke, NP
NPI#:1234567891

Pharmacology Math

CAAHEP Competencies	Assessment
II.C.1. Demonstrate knowledge of basic math computations	Math for Medications – C. to K.; Certification Preparation – 1-10
II.C.2. Apply mathematical computations to solve equations	Math for Medications – C. to K.; Certification Preparation – 1-10
II.C.3.a. Define basic units of measurement in: the metric system	Math for Medications – D. 1-13; Certification Preparation – 5
II.C.3.b. Define basic units of measurement in: the household system	Math for Medications – C. 1-8; Certification Preparation – 1
II.C.4. Convert among measurement systems	Math for Medications – C. 9-40, D. 14-28; Certification Preparation – 2-4
II.C.5. Identify abbreviations and symbols used in calculating medication dosages	Abbreviations – 1-17
II.P.1. Calculate proper dosages of medication for administration	Procedure 29.1

ABHES Competencies	Assessment
6. Pharmacology b. Demonstrate accurate occupational math and metric conversions for proper medication administration	Math for Medications – A. to K.

VOCABULARY REVIEW

Using the word pool on the right, find the correct word to match the definition. Write the word on the line after the definition.

1. Holds a specified quantity of medication in a single-use container
   _____

2. The number obtained by multiplying two or more numbers together _____

3. A grant from the government that gives a creator (or manufacturer) of an invention the sole right to produce, use, and sell the product for a set period of time _____

4. A tablet with a groove on the surface, used for splitting it in half
   _____

5. The sole right to market an approved medication granted by the FDA _____

6. The quantity of medication to be administered at one time
   _____

Word Pool
- exclusivity
- dosage
- product
- unit-dose packaging
- patent
- scored tablet

ABBREVIATIONS

Write out what each of the following abbreviations stands for.

1. C_____
2. F_____
3. m _____
4. cm _____
5. mm _____
6. kg_____
7. g_____
8. mg _____
9. mcg _____
10. gtt(s) _____
11. L_____
12. mL _____
13. fl oz _____
14. qt _____
15. pt _____
16. Tbs, tbsp _____
17. tsp _____

SKILLS AND CONCEPTS
Answer the following questions. Write your answer on the line or in the space provided.

A. Drug Labels

1. Explain the difference between the brand name and the generic name. _____

   _____

   _____

   _____

2. _____ is the amount of drug in the unit dose.

3. _____ indicated the batch of drug the medication came from.

4. The _____ is a unique 10-digit number indicating the product and is required by federal law to be on all prescription and nonprescription medication packages and inserts in the U.S.

MATH FOR MEDICATIONS
Answer the following questions. Write your answer on the line or in the space provided. Write your answers following the healthcare rules with writing numbers.

A. Rounding Numbers
Round the following numbers to the nearest tenth.

1. 2.367 = _____
2. 102.65 = _____
3. 2.634 = _____
4. 1.98 = _____
5. 0.658 = _____
6. 42.212 = _____
7. 3.09 = _____
8. 2.096 = _____
9. 9.98 = _____
10. 37.788 = _____
11. 12.456 = _____
12. 4.22 = _____

B. Roman Numerals
Write the number or Roman numeral on the line.

1. vi = _____
2. iiss = _____
3. x = _____
4. ivss = _____
5. iii = _____
6. ix = _____
7. 7 = _____
8. 3.5 = _____
9. 6.5 = _____
10. 9.5= _____
11. 5 = _____
12. 3 = _____

C. Household System
Define the basic units of measurement by writing the equivalent on the line.

1. 1 kg = _____ lb
2. 1 Tbs = _____ mL

3. 5 mL = _____ tsp

4. 1 oz = _____ mL

5. 1 oz = _____ tsp

6. 1 lb = _____ oz

7. 3 tsp = _____ Tbs

8. 1 oz = _____ Tbs

Determine the equivalents.

9. 9 tsp = _____ Tbs

10. 15 Tbs = _____ mL

11. 12 Tbs = _____ tsp

12. 45 mL= _____ Tbs

13. 90 mL = _____ oz

14. 5.5 oz = _____ Tbs

15. 3 oz = _____ mL

16. 21 Tbs = _____ oz

17. 8 tsp = _____ mL

18. 4 oz = _____ tsp

19. 55 mL = _____ tsp

20. 36 tsp = _____ oz

Solve the problems below using the lb and kg equivalents. Round your answer to the nearest tenth.

21. 24 kg = _____ lb

22. 34 kg = _____ lb

23. 52 lb = _____ kg

24. 67.58 lb = _____ kg

25. 58.9 kg = _____ lb

26. 189 kg = _____ lb

27. 310 lb = _____ kg

28. 78.9 lb = _____ kg

29. 108 kg = _____ lb

30. 56.7 kg = _____ lb

31. 123 lb = _____ kg

32. 222 lb = _____ kg

Solve the problems below using the oz and lb equivalents. Round your answer to the nearest tenth.

33. 13 oz = _____ lb

34. 9 oz = _____ lb

35. 15 oz = _____ lb

36. 10 oz = _____ lb

Solve the problems below using the oz and lb equivalents. Round the following to the nearest hundredth.

37. 3 oz = _____ lb

38. 2 oz = _____ lb

39. 7 oz = _____ lb

40. 5 oz = _____ lb

D. Metric System
Write the answer on the line.

1. In the metric system, _____ is measured in liters.

2. In the metric system, _____ is measured in meters.

3. In the metric system, _____ is measured in grams.

Define the basic units of measurement by writing the equivalent on the line.

4. 1 L = _____ mL

5. 1 L = _____ cc

6. 1 mL = _____ cc

7. 1 mg = _____ mcg

8. 1 m = _____ cm

9. 1 m = _____ mm

10. 1 cm = _____ mm

11. 1 g = _____ mg

12. 1 g = _____ mcg

13. 1 kg = _____ g

Solve the problems below using metric equivalents. Do not round your answers.

14. 2 kg = _____ g

15. 2.3 g = _____ mg

16. 5500 g = _____ kg

17. 6758 mg= _____ g

18. 3.1 g = _____ mg

19. 90 mL = _____ cc

20. 230 cm = _____ m

21. 31 cc = _____ mL

22. 5 m = _____ cm

23. 5.7 kg = _____ g

24. 108 mL = _____ L

25. 3456 mm = _____ m

26. 123 L = _____ mL

27. 0.05 m = _____ mm

28. 270 mcg = _____ mg

E. Temperature Conversion
Solve the problems below using the F and C conversions. Round your answer to the nearest tenth.

1. 124° F = _____ ° C

2. 96.3° F = _____ ° C

3. 39.6° C = _____ ° F

4. 123° C = _____ ° F

5. 103.6° F = _____ ° C

6. 48.9° F = _____ ° C

7. 32.9° C = _____ ° F

8. 85.7° C = _____ ° F

9. 98.6° F = _____ ° C

10. 230° F = _____ ° C

11. 66.4° C = _____ ° F

12. 101.2° C = _____ ° F

F. Quantity Needed for a Specific Time Period
Solve the problems. Label your answers.

1. **Prescription:** XYZ medication 200 mg, 5 tabs bid x 6 days. How many tablets will be dispensed from the pharmacy? _____

2. **Prescription:** XYZ medication 250 mg, 2 tabs qid x 14 days. How many tablets will be dispensed from the pharmacy? _____

3. **Prescription:** XYZ medication 50 mg, 3 tabs bid x 10 days. How many tablets will be dispensed from the pharmacy? _____

4. **Prescription:** XYZ medication 70 mg, 4 tabs tid x 3 days. How many tablets will be dispensed from the pharmacy? _____

5. **Prescription:** XYZ medication 40 mg, 6 tabs bid x 7 days. How many tablets will be dispensed from the pharmacy? _____

6. **Prescription:** XYZ medication 90 mg, 3 tabs qid x 20 days. How many tablets will be dispensed from the pharmacy_____

7. **Prescription:** XYZ medication 75 mg, 4 tabs bid x 14 days. How many tablets will be dispensed from the pharmacy? _____

8. **Prescription:** XYZ medication 100 mg, 2 tabs tid x 5 days. How many tablets will be dispensed from the pharmacy? _____

9. **Prescription:** XYZ medication 400 mg, 3 tabs bid x 8 days. How many tablets will be dispensed from the pharmacy? _____

10. **Prescription:** XYZ medication 300 mg, 3 tabs qid x 14 days. How many tablets will be dispensed from the pharmacy? _____

G. Number of Tablets per Dose
Solve the problems and round your answer to the nearest tenth. Label your answers.

1. **Order:** ABC 175 mg po. **Stock:** ABC 350 mg po scored tablets. How many tablets will the patient take per dose? _____

2. **Order:** ABC 120 mcg po. **Stock:** ABC 80 mcg po scored tablets. How many tablets will the patient take per dose? _____

3. **Order:** ABC 185 mg po. **Stock:** ABC 370 mg po scored tablets. How many tablets will the patient take per dose? _____

4. **Order:** ABC 80 mg po. **Stock:** ABC 32 mg po scored tablets. How many tablets will the patient take per dose? _____

5. **Order:** ABC 125 mg po. **Stock:** ABC 25 mg po scored tablets. How many tablets will the patient take per dose? _____

6. **Order:** ABC 2.25 mg po. **Stock:** ABC 4.5 mg po scored tablets. How many tablets will the patient take per dose? _____

7. **Order:** ABC 195 mg po. **Stock:** ABC 65 mg po scored tablets. How many tablets will the patient take per dose? _____

8. **Order:** ABC 180 mg po. **Stock:** ABC 45 mg po scored tablets. How many tablets will the patient take per dose? _____

9. **Order:** ABC 45 mcg po. **Stock:** ABC 90 mcg po scored tablets. How many tablets will the patient take per dose? _____

10. **Order:** ABC 50 mg po. **Stock:** ABC 12.5 mg po scored tablets. How many tablets will the patient take per dose? _____

H. Liquid Medication Dose with Matching Labels
Solve the problems and round your answer to the nearest tenth. Label your answers.

1. **Order:** ABC 2200 units. **Stock:** ABC 2600 units/mL. How many mL will you give?
    _____

2. **Order:** ABC 8 mg. **Stock:** ABC 25 mg/3 mL. How many mL will you give? _____

3. **Order:** ABC 130 mg. **Stock:** ABC 250 mg/mL. How many mL will you give? _____

4. **Order:** ABC 75 mcg. **Stock:** ABC 125 mcg/2 mL. How many mL will you give?

    _____

5. **Order:** ABC 80 mg. **Stock:** ABC 50 mg/mL. How many mL will you give? _____

6. **Order:** ABC 60 mg. **Stock:** ABC 100 mg/mL. How many mL will you give? _____

7. **Order:** ABC 250 units. **Stock:** ABC 180 units/mL. How many mL will you give?

    _____

8. **Order:** ABC 85 mg. **Stock:** ABC 130 mg/mL. How many mL will you give? _____

9. **Order:** ABC 800 mg. **Stock:** ABC 1500 mg/2 mL. How many mL will you give?

    _____

10. **Order:** ABC 40 mg. **Stock:** ABC 200 mg/2 mL. How many mL will you give? _____

11. **Order:** ABC 100 mg. **Stock:** ABC 60 mg/mL. How many mL will you give? _____

12. **Order:** ABC 70 mg. **Stock:** ABC 40 mg/mL. How many mL will you give? _____

I. Liquid Medication Dose with Non-Matching Labels

Solve the problems and round your answer to the nearest tenth. Label your answers.

1. **Order:** ABC 1700 mg. **Stock:** ABC 2.8 g/3 mL. How many mL will you give? _____

2. **Order:** ABC 1 g. **Stock:** ABC 2500 mg/2 mL. How many mL will you give? _____

3. **Order:** ABC 120 mg. **Stock:** ABC 1 g/2 mL. How many mL will you give? _____

4. **Order:** ABC 750 mg. **Stock:** ABC 1.2 g/2 mL. How many mL will you give? _____

5. **Order:** ABC 800 mg. **Stock:** ABC 5 g/5 mL. How many mL will you give? _____

6. **Order:** ABC 2.3 g. **Stock:** ABC 1500 mg/mL. How many mL will you give? _____

7. **Order:** ABC 800 mg. **Stock:** ABC 2 g/mL. How many mL will you give? _____

8. **Order:** ABC 450 mg. **Stock:** ABC 1.2 g/3 mL. How many mL will you give? _____

9. **Order:** ABC 550 mg. **Stock:** ABC 1.2 g/2 mL. How many mL will you give? _____

10. **Order:** ABC 400 mg. **Stock:** ABC 2 g/4 mL. How many mL will you give? _____

11. **Order:** ABC 760 mg. **Stock:** ABC 3 g/2 mL. How many mL will you give? _____

12. **Order:** ABC 1.2 g. **Stock:** ABC 900 mg/mL. How many mL will you give? _____

J. Solution Dose

Solve the problems and round your answer to the nearest tenth. Label your answers.

1. **Order:** ABC 50 mg. **Stock:** ABC 4% solution. How many mL will you give? _____

2. **Order:** ABC 300 mg. **Stock:** ABC 15% solution. How many mL will you give? _____

3. **Order:** ABC 80 mg. **Stock:** ABC 6% solution. How many mL will you give? _____

4. **Order:** ABC 60 mg. **Stock:** ABC 5% solution. How many mL will you give? _____

5. **Order:** ABC 30 mg. **Stock:** ABC 4% solution. How many mL will you give? _____

6. **Order:** ABC 48 mg. **Stock:** ABC 3% solution. How many mL will give? _____

7. **Order:** ABC 65 mg. **Stock:** ABC 8% solution. How many mL will you give? _____

8. **Order:** ABC 80 mg. **Stock:** ABC 10% solution. How many mL will you give? _____

9. **Order:** ABC 67 mg. **Stock:** ABC 4% solution. How many mL will you give? _____

10. **Order:** ABC 25 mg. **Stock:** ABC 4% solution. How many mL will you give? _____

11. **Order:** ABC 35 mg. **Stock:** ABC 2% solution. How many mL will you give? _____

12. **Order:** ABC 230 mg. **Stock:** ABC 15% solution. How many mL will you give? _____

K. Pediatric Doses

Solve the problems. Remember to round to the nearest thousandth when working through the problem and round your final answer to the nearest tenth. Label your answers.

1. **Patient's wt:** 60 lb **Medication order:** 0.5 mg/kg **Stock medication:** 10 mg/mL. How many mL will you give? _____

2. **Patient's wt:** 122 lb **Medication order:** 3 mg/kg **Stock medication:** 180 mg/mL. How many mL will you give? _____

3. **Patient's wt:** 66 lb **Medication order:** 0.6 mg/kg **Stock medication:** 50 mg/2 mL. How many mL will you give? _____

4. **Patient's wt:** 82 lb **Medication order:** 1.2 mg/kg **Stock medication:** 80 mg/2 mL. How many mL will you give? _____

5. **Patient's wt:** 78 lb **Medication order:** 0.5 mg/kg **Stock medication:** 10 mg/mL. How many mL will you give? _____

6. **Patient's wt:** 59 lb **Medication order:** 1.5 mg/kg **Stock medication:** 30 mg/mL. How many mL will you give? _____

7. **Patient's wt:** 48 lb **Medication order:** 0.8 mg/kg **Stock medication:** 60 mg/2 mL. How many mL will you give? _____

8. **Patient's wt:** 39 lb **Medication order:** 0.4 mg/kg **Stock medication:** 6 mg/mL. How many mL will you give? _____

9. **Patient's wt:** 96 lb **Medication order:** 1.7 mg/kg **Stock medication:** 90 mg/2 mL. How many mL will you give? _____

10. **Patient's wt:** 66 lb **Medication order:** 0.8 mg/kg **Stock medication:** 40 mg/2 mL. How many mL will you give? _____

11. **Patient's wt:** 98 lb **Medication order:** 0.2 mg/kg **Stock medication:** 20 mg/mL. How many mL will you give? _____

12. **Patient's wt:** 68 lb **Medication order:** 0.6 mg/kg **Stock medication:** 50 mg/mL. How many mL will you give? _____

READING SYRINGES

For each picture, write what each line is equal to in column A. Then indicate the readings for B, C, and D in the columns. Label your answers and follow the healthcare rules when writing numbers (see textbook Chapter 29, Pharmacology Math). Note: All syringes without the word "unit" are calibrated in mL.

	Syringe Pictures	A	B	C	D
1.					
2.					
3.					
4.					
5.					
6.					

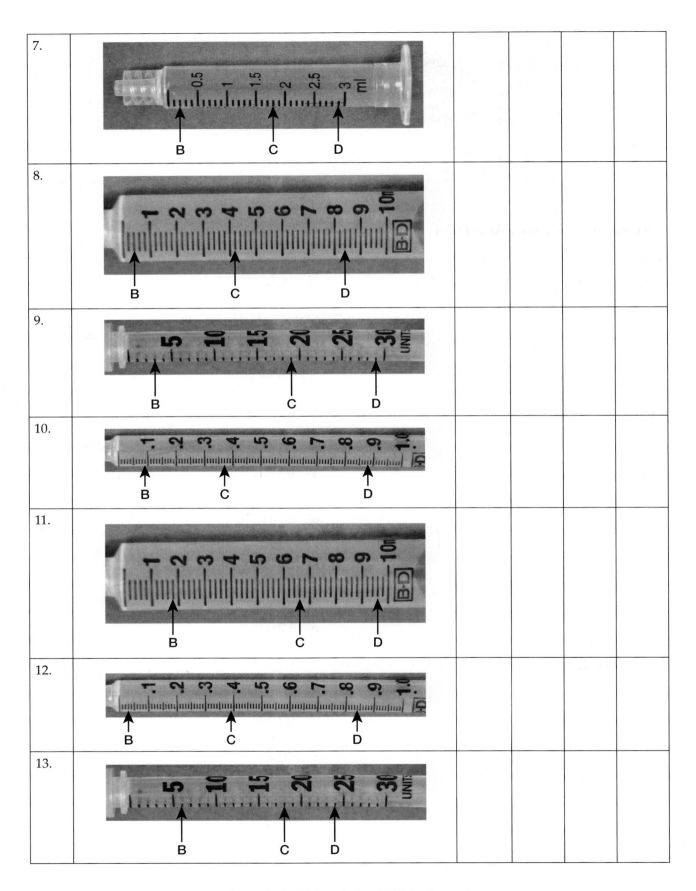

| 14. | 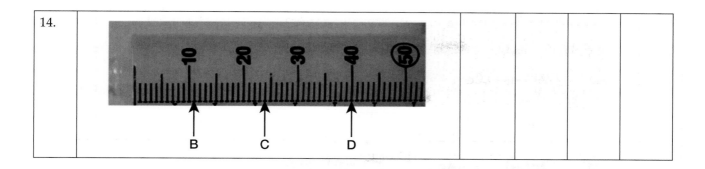 | | | | |

CERTIFICATION PREPARATION

Round answers to the nearest tenth. Circle the correct answer.

1. 12 tsp = _____ Tbs
   a. 36
   b. 24
   c. 3
   d. 4

2. 5 oz = ___ mL
   a. 150
   b. 50
   c. 25
   d. 10

3. 63.5 kg = _____ lb
   a. 28.9
   b. 29
   c. 139.7
   d. 140

4. 220.2 lb = _____ kg
   a. 484
   b. 484.4
   c. 100
   d. 100.1

5. 8632 mg = _____ g
   a. 86.32
   b. 8.632
   c. 863.2
   d. 0.8632

6. 23° C = _____ ° F
   a. 99
   b. 44.8
   c. 73.4
   d. −16.2

7. Order: ABC 240 mcg po. Stock: ABC 160 mcg po scored tablets. How many tablets will the patient take per dose?
   a. 2 tablets
   b. 1.5 tablets
   c. 0.7 tablet
   d. 0.5 tablet

8. Order: ABC 20 mg. Stock: ABC 30 mg/2 mL. How many mL will you give?
   a. 0.7 mL
   b. 1.3 mL
   c. 0.6 mL
   d. 1.5 mL

9. Order: ABC 1.5 g. Stock: ABC 2500 mg/2 mL. How many mL will you give?
   a. 1 mL
   b. 0.1
   c. 0.6 mL
   d. 1.2 mL

10. Patient's wt: 64 lb. Medication order: 0.8 mg/kg. Stock medication: 60 mg/2 mL. How many mL will you give?
    a. 1.7 mL
    b. 0.8 mL
    c. 0.9 mL
    d. 0.4 mL

WORKPLACE APPLICATIONS

1. A child weighs 48 lb and Dr. Walden ordered 0.3 mg/kg. The medication label states 20 mg/mL. How many mL will you give? _____

2. A child weighs 32 lb and Dr. Walden ordered 0.2 mg/kg. The medication label states 4 mg/mL. How many mL will you give? _____

3. A child weighs 23 lb and Dr. Walden ordered 0.3 mg/kg. The medication label states 10 mg/mL. How many mL will you give? _____

INTERNET ACTIVITIES

1. Using appropriate online resources, research medication errors in healthcare facilities. Create a poster, PowerPoint presentation, or a paper and include at least two citations. Discuss the following topics:
   a. Leading causes of medication errors
   b. How can a medical assistant prevent medication errors?

Procedure 29.1 Calculate Proper Dosages of Medication for Administration

Name _____ Date _____ Score _____

Tasks: Calculate dosages for oral medication, injectable medication, and dosages for children.

Orders:
- Order 1: Dr. Martin orders ABC medication 135 mg. Stock bottle reads: 45 mg scored tablets
- Order 2: Dr. Martin orders ABC medication 650 mg. Stock bottle reads: 1300 mg scored tablets
- Order 3: Dr. Martin orders XYZ medication 430 mg IM. Stock bottle reads: 1000 mg/2 mL
- Order 4: Dr. Martin orders XYZ medication 680 mg IM. Stock bottle reads: 1200 mg/mL
- Order 5: Dr. Martin orders MNO medication 3 mg/kg IM. Child weighs 53 pounds. Stock bottle reads: 125 mg/mL
- Order 6: Dr. Martin orders MNO medication 5 mg/kg IM. Child weighs 71 pounds. Stock bottle reads: 225 mg/mL

Equipment and Supplies:
- Provider's order
- Paper and pencil
- Calculator (optional per instructor)

Standard: Complete the procedure and all critical steps in _____ minutes with a minimum score of 85% within two attempts (*or as indicated by the instructor*).

Scoring: Divide the points earned by the total possible points. Failure to perform a critical step, indicated by an asterisk (*), results in grade no higher than an 84% (*or as indicated by the instructor*).

Time: Began_____ Ended_____ Total minutes: _____

Steps:	Point Value	Attempt 1	Attempt 2
1. Using Order 1, calculate the number of tablets to give the patient. Label your answer.	10*		
2. Using Order 2, calculate the number of tablets to give the patient. Label your answer.	10*		
3. Using Order 3, calculate the amount in milliliters to give the patient. Round your answer to the nearest tenth. Label your answer.	15*		
4. Using Order 4, calculate the amount in milliliters to give the patient. Round your answer to the nearest tenth. Label your answer.	15*		
5. Using Order 5, calculate the amount in milliliters to give the patient. Round your answer to the nearest tenth. Label your answer.	20*		
6. Using Order 6, calculate the amount in milliliters to give the patient. Round your answer to the nearest tenth. Label your answer.	20*		
7. Double-check your answers to ensure the correct dose will be given.	10		
Total Points	**100**		

Comments

CAAHEP Competencies	Step(s)
II.P.1. Calculate proper dosages of medication for administration	Entire procedure
ABHES Competencies	**Step(s)**
6.b. Demonstrate accurate occupational math and metric conversions for proper medication administration	Entire procedure

Administering Medications

CAAHEP Competencies	Assessment
I.P.4.a. Verify the rules of medication administration: right patient	Procedure 30.1, 30.7 through 30.10
I.P.4.b. Verify the rules of medication administration: right medication	Procedure 30.1 through 30.10
I.P.4.c. Verify the rules of medication administration: right dose	Procedure 30.1 through 30.10
I.P.4.d. Verify the rules of medication administration: right route	Procedure 30.1 through 30.10
I.P.4.e. Verify the rules of medication administration: right time	Procedure 30.1 through 30.10
I.P.4.f. Verify the rules of medication administration: right documentation	Procedure 30.1, 30.7 through 30.10
I.P.5. Select proper sites for administering parenteral medication	Procedure 30.7 through 30.10
I.P.6. Administer oral medications	Procedure 30.1
I.P.7. Administer parenteral (excluding IV) medications	Procedure 30.7 through 30.10
II.P.1. Calculate proper dosages of medication for administration	Procedure 30.1
III.P.2. Select appropriate barrier/personal protective equipment.	Procedure 30.7 through 30.10
III.P.10.a. Demonstrate proper disposal of biohazardous material: sharps	Procedure 30.7 through 30.10
X.P.3. Document patient care accurately in the medical record	Procedure 30.1, 30.7 through 30.10
XII.P.2.c. Demonstrate proper use of: sharps disposal containers	Procedure 30.2, 30.3, 30.5, 30.7 through 30.10

ABHES Competencies	Assessment
4. Medical Law and Ethics a. Follow documentation guidelines	Procedure 30.1, 30.7 through 30.10
8. Clinical Procedures a. Practice standard precautions and perform disinfection/sterilization techniques	Procedure 30.7 through 30.10
8.f. Prepare and administer oral and parenteral medications and monitor intravenous (IV) infusions	Procedure 30.1 through 30.10

VOCABULARY REVIEW

Using the word pool on the right, find the correct word to match the definition. Write the word on the line after the definition.

Group A

1. The means by which a drug enters the body
   Route

2. Physical characteristics of a medication (e.g., tablet, suspension)
   form

3. Solid form of medication formed by compressed powdered medication; may be coated *tablet*

4. Medication in a hard or soft gelatin shell
   Capsule

5. Passes through the acidic environment of the stomach and breaks down in the base environment of the intestines
   enteric Coated

6. Solid form of medicine that is placed on the tongue and breaks down in the presence of saliva *fast - dissolving tablet*

7. Coated, oval medication tablet *Caplet*

8. A notched tablet which can be split into half with a pill cutter (or splitter) *Scored tablet*

9. Flat, round form containing active medication and sweetened flavoring; dissolves on the tongue *lozenge*

10. A solid form containing the active medication and an antacid
    Buffered

Word Pool
- caplet 7
- capsule 4
- tablet
- form 2
- enteric coated 5
- scored tablet 8
- buffered 10
- lozenge 9
- fast-dissolving tablet 6
- route 1

Group B

1. Semisolid, greasy drug preparation that is thicker and less penetrating than ointments ___paste___
2. Active medication mixed in an oil base and used in the rectum, urethra, or vagina ___suppository___
3. A sugar and water solution that contains flavoring and medicinal substance ___syrup___
4. Semisolid drug preparation made of active medication, oil and water ___cream___
5. A vaginal suppository ___pessary___
6. Very potent solution of alcohol or alcohol and water and the active medicine ___tincture___
7. A suspension of oil and water ___emulsion___
8. Route of medication when medication is placed under the tongue ___sublingual___
9. Route of medication when medication is placed between the cheek and the gums ___buccal___
10. Route of medication when medication is placed on the skin and absorbed into the bloodstream ___transdermal___

Word Pool
- transdermal 10
- pessary 5
- sublingual 8
- cream 4
- tincture 6
- buccal 9
- paste 1
- syrup 3
- emulsion
- suppository 2

Group C

1. Medication that affects the area where it was applied ___local___
2. Medication that affects the entire body ___systemic___
3. Route of medication when medication is applied to a mucous membrane or the skin ___topical___
4. Poured medication drop by drop ___instilled___
5. Administration by injection, infusion, or implantation ___parenteral route___
6. Part of the needle that attaches or screws onto the syringe ___hub___
7. Administration within a muscle ___intramuscular___
8. To bathe or flush open wounds or body cavities ___irrigation___
9. Administration beneath the skin ___subcutaneous___
10. Administration within the dermis ___intradermal___

Word Pool
- parenteral route
- subcutaneous
- instilled
- irrigation
- intradermal
- local
- topical
- hub
- intramuscular
- systemic

Group D

1. Another name for 0.9% sodium chloride ___Normal saline___

2. A type of needle that automatically covers after the injection ___passive safety needle___

3. Part of the needle where the needle attaches ___hilt___

4. Resistance to flow ___viscosity___

5. Slanted end of the needle shaft ___bevel___

6. Number indicating the size of the lumen of a needle ___gauge___

7. Hollow space inside the needle ___lumen___

8. Type of needle that requires the healthcare professional to activate the safety device ___active safety needle___

9. Solid particles that settle out of a liquid ___precipitate___

10. To withdraw fluid using suction ___aspirate___

Word Pool
- viscosity
- aspirate
- precipitate
- gauge
- hilt
- normal saline
- active safety needle
- passive safety needle
- lumen
- bevel

Group E

1. A dried substance (powder) that has been restored to a fluid form so it can be injected ___reconstitued___

2. A liquid substance that dilutes or lessens the strength of a solution or mixture ___diluent___

3. A severe allergic reaction that can be life-threatening ___anaphylaxis___

4. A tense, pale elevation of the skin ___wheal___

5. A raised, hardened area of the skin ___induration___

6. Redness ___erythema___

Word Pool
- anaphylaxis
- erythema
- induration
- diluent
- wheal
- reconstituted

ABBREVIATIONS

Write out what each of the following abbreviations stands for.

1. EHR ___Electronic Health Record___
2. VIS ___Vaccine Information Statement___
3. OTC ___Over the Counter___
4. po ___oral route or by mouth___
5. SL ___Sublingual___
6. MDI ___Metered-Dose Inhaler___
7. IM ___Intramuscular___
8. subcut ___Subcutaneous___
9. ID ___Intradermal___
10. IV ___Intravenous___
11. G ___Gauge___
12. OSHA ___Occupational Safety and Health Administration___
13. TST ___Tuberculin Skin Test___
14. HIV ___Human Immunodeficiency Virus___
15. BCG ___Bacillus Calmette-Guerin___
16. PPD ___Purified Protein Derivative___
17. TB ___Tuberculosis___
18. NTM ___Nontuberculous Mycobacteria___
19. QFT-GIT ___Quantiferon Gold In-Tube Test___
20. T-Spot ___T-Spot TB test___
21. MMR ___Measles Mumps Rubella___
22. CDC ___Centers of Disease Control and Prevention___
23. Td ___Tetanus diphtheria___
24. Tdap ___Tetanus diptheria with Pertussis___

SKILLS AND CONCEPTS

Answer the following questions. Write your answer on the line or in the space provided.

A. Nine Rights of Medication Administration

1. Using the table, list the Rights of Medication Administration. Then explain how the medical assistant should verify or perform the check.

When it is done	Right	How is this achieved?
Completed when preparing medications	Right Medication	Check medication three times to ensure correct name and form.
	Right Dose	Calculate how many tablets to give.
	Right Route	Check three times
	Right Time	Review patient's vaccination history and person age.
Completed with the patient prior to administration	Right Patient	Ask full name and date of birth.
	Right Education	Give the name of medication and who order and explain effects.
	Right to Refuse	Do not pressure the patient, Respect their decision.
	Right Technique	Ask patient to rate the pain. Obtain vital signs.
Done after giving the medication	Right Documentation	Put on PHR system.

2. Describe when the medication label is checked against the order. We have to do three times during preparation process.

3. Explain why it is important to do an activity between each check. It helps to ensure that you have right medication

4. Describe live virus vaccines and list two examples of vaccines. The microorganism is alive but attenuated in laboratory. Ex- MMR, Varicella

5. Describe five reasons a person may not be able to get a live virus vaccine. _____

    • were vaccinated with another live virus vaccine.
    • Pregnant or may become pregnant.
    • Receiving chemotherapy.

6. List what a medical assistant must document when giving a VIS to a patient. _____

    • The edition date of VIS.
    • The date of VIS was provided and Administrated.

B. Forms of Medications

1. Complete the medication forms table with at least five examples in each column.

Solid	Semisolid	Liquid – Solutions
Tablet	Ointment	Tincture
Chewable tablet	Cream	Fluid extract
Caplet	Suppository	Spirit
Capsule		Syrup
Scored tablet		Elixir
		Liquid – Suspensions
		Lotion
		Emulsion
		Gel
		Aerosol

2. List two forms of medications that cannot be crushed, chewed, or cut. Also describe what can happen to the patient if the medication is crushed, chewed, or cut.

    Slow - or entered - released tablet - It results in overdose.
    Enteric - coated tablet - may cause stomach distress

3. Describe the difference between a solution and a suspension. _____

    when medication dissolve in liquid called solution.
    Suspension - when medication cannot dissolve in liquid.

C. Routes of Medication

1. Complete the following table by entering the abbreviation, description, and precautions or special techniques for each route.

Route	Description	Precautions/Special Techniques
Oral	Medication taken by oral route (po).	• straw used for liquid medication • Oral medication not followed by water immed
Sublingual	Placed under tongue	• Do not eat or smoke. • Do not chew or swallow.
Buccal	Placed between cheek and gum	• Water can be taken prior to medication. • Cheeks used for buccal medication.
Transdermal	Placed on the skin	• Write date and time • wear disposable gloves.
Topical	Apply drug to mucus membrane	• Wear gloves • Rub creams gently into skin
Vaginal	Tablets, creams, and foam into the vagina.	• wear gloves • Insert medications like suppositories using a finger.
Rectal	Insert into the rectum	• Teach a patient about insert suppositories. • Disposable gloves
Nasal	Drug given through nose.	• Wear gloves. • Blow their nose prior to recieve medication.
Ocular	Instilled into eye	• Do not touch eye with tip • Always keep applicator sterile.
Otic	Instilled into the ear	• If an applicator ~~sterile~~ contaminated, discard the container.

2. Complete the following table by entering the abbreviation and description for each route.

Route	Abbreviation	Description
Intramuscular	IM	Administration within a muscle
Subcutaneous	Subcut	administration beneath the skin
Intradermal	ID	administration within the dermis
Intravenous	IV	administration within the vein

D. Needles and Syringes

1. Describe the two measurements each needle has and explain the importance of each when giving an injection.

Each needle has two measurements :- gauge and the length. The higher the gauge number, the smaller the lumen.

2. What is the purpose of safety needles? To reduce the risk of needlesticks after an injection.

3. Describe the difference between passive and active safety needles. Passive is designed so that needle automatically covered after injection. Active requires healthcare to activate safety device.

4. Describe when it is safe to recap needles and when you never recap needles. Needles can be recapped until they are used on same patient. Never recap any needle that has been used on patient.

E. Preparing Parenteral Medication

1. Describe four reasons to discard parenteral medication. • medication looks abnormal in color • medication expired • medication no longer sterile • If have abnormal precipitate.

2. Describe an ampule and explain why an ampule is used for medication. A single dose of medication. Because it contains medication more than patients needs.

3. Explain why a filter needle is used when working with an ampule. To aspirate the medication into the syringe.

4. Describe a vial. A plastic or glass container with rubber stopper that is covered by a cap.

5. Describe the difference between a single-dose vial and a multidose vial. Multidose contains many doses of medication and single dose used only for one patient.

6. How long are multidose vials good for? 28 days.

7. Since vials are under pressure, describe what you need to do before drawing out liquid. You need to aid into the vial before you draw out amount of liquid you need.

8. Describe the four major steps in reconstituting powdered medication and withdrawing a dose of the medication.

    • Remove air from powder • Withdraw liquid from diluent vial.
    • Mix liquid with powdered medication • Add in air

9. Insulin is measured in ___units___.

10. Insulins like NPH are ___Suspensions___ and require ___mixing___ before withdrawing the medication.

F. Giving Parenteral Medications

1. Describe advantages of parenteral medication administration. It is useful when patient has gastrointestinal distress or unconscious.

2. Describe disadvantages of parenteral medication administration. • Pain with injection
    • Risk of injection
    • Unpredictable absorption rate of poor circulation

3. When selecting a site for an injection, list considerations the medical assistant must think about.
    • Never give injection near bones.
    • Avoid abrasions, lesions, wounds, bruises.

4. Describe four ways to decrease the pain and anxiety of an injection. • Give sugar-coated medicine
    • Apply topical anesthic skin refricant or cream.
    • Talk with patient.

5. What should the medical assistant do if the needle breaks off during the injection? Pull out the needle, if it is visible. If not visibe mark it and ask for help.

6. What should the medical assistant do if the bone is hit when doing an intramuscular injection?
    Pull the needle out about ¼ inch.

7. List signs and symptoms of anaphylaxis. Anxiety, warm feeling
    • Shortness of breath, dysphea
    • Pain & vomiting

8. If the medical assistant suspects the patient is having an anaphylactic reaction, what should the medical assistant do?

   After inject, put patient in waiting room for 15 minutes,

9. What is the first-line medication used for anaphylaxis?

   Epinephrine

G. Intradermal Injections

1. Answer the following regarding performing an intradermal injection.

   a. What size needle would be used? *1/4 to 5/8 inch — 25-27 gauge*

   b. What is the maximum volume of medication given? *0.1 ml*

   c. What is the angle of the needle when administering the medication? *15° angle*

   d. What must be done to the site while inserting the needle? *Pull the skin*

   e. Where are the most common sites? *forearm, upper arm and back*

2. When doing a TST, how large must the wheal be? If the wheal is not that size, what must occur?

   The wheal must measure 6 to 10 mm in diameter or test repeated.

3. If a TST needs to be repeated on the same arm, the sites need to be separated by at least ___ *0.1 ml* ___.

4. Answer the following regarding reading TSTs.

   a. The patient must return within ___ *48 to 72 hours* ___ for the reading.

   b. If the test is read before or after this time, the results are ___ *invalidates* ___.

   c. The medical assistant must check the patient health record for the location and then palpates the site for a(n) ___ *induration* ___.

   d. If present, the measurement is taken in ___ *millimeters* ___.

   e. The ___ *erythema* ___ (redness) is not measured.

   f. The medical assistant indicates the measurement in the documentation. The provider uses the ___ *test results* ___ and the ___ *patient history* ___ to determine if the patient has tuberculosis.

5. Define a false-positive TST reaction and list three reasons for the reaction. _Means person may not have reacted to the test._
• Weak immune system • very old TB infection • Incorrect administration

6. Define a false-negative TST reaction and list six reasons for the reaction. _____
The person reacted to the test.
• Lung infection • Incorrect administer • Previous vaccine

7. List three reasons a TST would be contraindicated in a patient. _____

_____

8. With a two-step TST, when can the second test be placed? _when body "forgets" to react to TST._

9. Describe the TST process for new healthcare students and professionals and the yearly follow-up.
It require two-step TST.

_____

10. If a patient has a positive TST according to the provider, what is the typical follow-up? _It gave additional tests to determine if person has TB._

11. Regarding the approved tuberculin blood tests:

a. Name two FDA-approved tests. _QFT-GIT and T-SPOT_

_____

b. Discuss the advantage of the tuberculin blood test over the two-step TST. _It will show the accurate result._

c. Discuss the results of the tuberculin blood tests and the usual interpretation (or meaning of the results).
Positive – The person has been infected with TB.
Negative – It is unlikely the person has TB.

H. Subcutaneous Injections

1. Answer the following regarding performing a subcut injection.

a. What size needle would be used? _25 gauge_

_____

b. What is the maximum volume of medication given? _0.5 – 1.5ml_

_____

c. What is the angle of the needle when administering the medication? _____

_____ 45° angle.

d. What must be done to the site while inserting the needle? Pinch up the tissue with index finger and thumb of nondominant hand.

e. What site is used for vaccines for patients younger than 1 year of age? _____

_____ Anterior thigh.

f. What site(s) is used for vaccines for patients older than 1 year of age? _____

_____ Upper outer arm or anterior angle.

2. Describe how to find the subcut injection sites.

a. Abdominal site Have the patient remove the clothing in that area. The site is located below the costal margins to the iliac crests.

b. Outer posterior aspect of the upper arm site Expose the arm. The outer posterior site extends from 3 inches above elbow to about 3 finger beneath below acromion process

c. Anterior aspect of the thigh site Place one hand above the knee and other hand below the greater trochanter. The site is the middle one-third of the thigh,

I. Intramuscular Injections

1. There are more ___blood vessel___ in the muscles; thus, absorption is ___faster___ than in the subcutaneous layer.

2. For medications given by IM injection, ___aqueous___ medications should be given with a higher-gauge needle than that used for ___oil-based___ medications

3. Fill in the table regarding information on performing an IM injection on an adult.

	Deltoid	Vastus Lateralis	Ventrogluteal
Needle length and gauge ranges	5/8 — 1 inch Adults :- 1½ inch	Children 22-25 G Adult :- 18-21 G	
Administration technique	90° angle		
Maximum volume	1 ml		1-11 year - 2ml 12+ = 3 ml

4. Fill in the table regarding information on performing an IM injection on children.

	Deltoid	Vastus Lateralis	Ventrogluteal
Needle length	1-11 years:	0 days to 12 years:	0 days to 12 years:
Gauge ranges	22-25g	22-25G	22-25G

5. Describe the aspiration procedure, including when it is done and how to do it. Once needle is in the site, the medical assistant should pull back on the plunger for 5 seconds and check the barrel of the syringe.

6. Describe the air lock technique, including when it is done and the purpose for doing it. Remove the bubbles in the syringe and measure the exact amount of medication needed. Once these steps done, add 0.2 to 0.5 ml of air into syringe.

7. Describe the Z-track technique, including when it is done and the purpose for doing it. For Z-track technique, the skin is pulled laterally with medical assistant non-dominant hand.

8. Describe how to find the IM injection sites.

   a. Deltoid site Place a finger on acromion process and then 2 finger from that. The top of the site is 1 to 2 inches below acromion process.

   b. Vastus lateralis site You will need to create a rectangle. Think about dividing the thigh into three sections. Place one hand above knee and other hand below greater trochanter.

   c. Ventrogluteal site Place the palm on patient greater trochanter. Your finger needs to point forward the head. Position index and middle finger to make triangle

CERTIFICATION PREPARATION

Circle the correct answer.

1. When providing the "right education" prior to medication administration, what must the medical assistant do?
   a. Give the name of the medication and who ordered the medication
   b. Give the desired effect or action and common side effects of the medication
   c. Verify the patient's allergies
   d. All of the above

2. What medication form can be crushed prior to administration?
   a. Caplet
   b. Scored tablet
   c. Extended-release tablet
   d. a and b only

3. What is not proper procedure when administering buccal medications?
   a. Always use the same cheek.
   b. Give water immediately after administering the medication.
   c. Allow smoking and eating just prior to administration of the medication.
   d. None of the above are proper procedure.

4. The parenteral route is administration by:
   a. implantation.
   b. infusion.
   c. injection.
   d. all of the above.

5. Which syringe and needle would be most appropriate for a TST?
   a. 3 mL syringe; 1/2 inch, 25-gauge needle
   b. 3 mL syringe; 5/8 inch, 21-gauge needle
   c. 1 mL syringe; 3/8 inch, 27-gauge needle
   d. 1 mL syringe; 1/2 inch, 23-gauge needle

6. What is true regarding TST?
   a. A TST and a live virus vaccine can be given on the same day.
   b. A TST can be given 2-3 weeks after a live virus vaccine.
   c. A live virus vaccine does not impact the TST results.
   d. Options a and b are true.

7. Which syringe and needle would be most appropriate for an adult subcutaneous 90-degree injection?
   a. 3 mL syringe; 1/2 inch, 25-gauge needle
   b. 3 mL syringe; 5/8 inch, 21-gauge needle
   c. 1 mL syringe; 3/8 inch, 27-gauge needle
   d. 1 mL syringe; 1/2 inch, 23-gauge needle

8. When giving an IM vaccine injection to an 8-month-old child, what site is used?
   a. Deltoid
   b. Vastus lateralis
   c. Ventrogluteal
   d. a and b only

9. Which syringe and needle would be most appropriate to use when giving a deltoid IM injection to an adult male weighing 180 pounds?
   a. 3 mL syringe; 5/8 inch, 25-gauge needle
   b. 3 mL syringe; 1 1/4 inch, 22-gauge needle
   c. 1 mL syringe; 1 inch, 20-gauge needle
   d. 1 mL syringe; 1 inch, 27-gauge needle

10. Which syringe and needle would be most appropriate to use when giving a deltoid IM injection to 5-year-old child?
    a. 3 mL syringe; 5/8 inch, 20-gauge needle
    b. 3 mL syringe; 1 1/4 inch, 22-gauge needle
    c. 3 mL syringe; 5/8 inch, 23-gauge needle
    d. 1 mL syringe; 1 inch, 27-gauge needle

WORKPLACE APPLICATIONS

1. You are giving an analgesic to a patient. You need to obtain the patient's pain level rating before you give the medication. Describe how you would explain a 0 to 10 pain scale to an adult.

   _____

   _____

   _____

2. The patient states, "I am a recovering alcoholic." Explain why it is important for the medical assistant to communicate this information to the provider.

   _____

   _____

3. A patient needs a two-step TST. The patient asks Gabe why one test is not "good enough." Describe how Gabe would answer the patient.

   _____

   _____

   _____

INTERNET ACTIVITIES

1. Using the CDC website (www.cdc.gov), research two routine Vaccine Information Statements (VIS). In a paper, PowerPoint presentation, or poster, address the following points:
   a. For each VIS:
      i. Name the vaccine.
      ii. Discuss why to get the vaccine.
      iii. Indicate who should get the vaccine.
      iv. List the situations when the vaccine should not be given.
      v. Describe the risks from the vaccine, including the common, uncommon, and very rare problems.
   b. Describe severe allergic reactions and what should be done.

2. Using the CDC website (www.cdc.gov), search for "vaccines and immunization." Go to Vaccine and Immunization home page and then click on link for healthcare providers. Review the materials and tools available to healthcare professionals. Create a paper, PowerPoint Presentation, or poster and summarize your findings.

3. Using the CDC website (www.cdc.gov), search for "travelers health." Review the materials and tools available to travelers and healthcare professionals. Create a paper, PowerPoint Presentation, or poster and summarize your findings.

Procedure 30.1 Administering Oral Medications

Name _____ Date _____ Score _____

Tasks: Calculate the dose to give. Prepare a liquid and a solid medication and administer medications to a patient. Document medication administration.

Equipment and Supplies:
- Provider's orders
- Patient's health record
- Drug reference information
- Liquid medication and a solid medication (use drug labels shown)
- Paper cup
- Plastic medication cup
- Marker
- Medication tray
- Glass of water

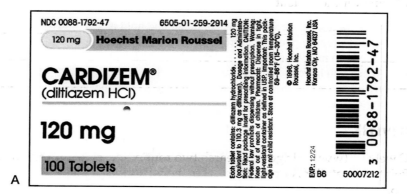

A

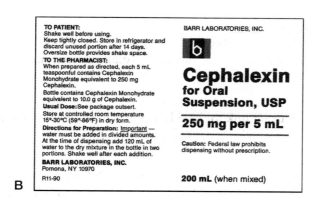

B

(From Brown M, Mulholland JM: *Drug calculations: process and problei practice*, ed 9, St. Louis, 2012.)

Orders: Diltiazem 240 mg po and cephalexin suspension 375 mg po.

Standard: Complete the procedure and all critical steps in _____ minutes with a minimum score of 85% within two attempts (*or as indicated by the instructor*).

Scoring: Divide the points earned by the total possible points. Failure to perform a critical step, indicated by an asterisk (*), results in grade no higher than an 84% (*or as indicated by the instructor*).

Time: Began_____ Ended_____ Total minutes: _____

Steps:	Point Value	Attempt 1	Attempt 2
1. Using the drug reference information and the orders, review the information on the medications.	5		
2. Using the orders and the drug labels shown, calculate the amount of medication you need to give. Verify the right doses with the instructor. Verify if it is the right time for the order if that applies.	10*		
3. Wash hands or use hand sanitizer. Select the right medications from the storage area. Check each medication label against the order. Check for the right name, form, and route. Check the expiration date to make sure the drug has not expired.	5*		
4. Assemble the supplies required to prepare the medications. Using the marker, write the medication name and dose on the appropriate cups.	5		
5. Perform the second medication check. Check each medication label against the order. Check for the right name, form, and route.	5*		
6. For the solid medication: Remove the cover of the container and hold it so the inside is facing up. Carefully pour the correct number of tablets into the cover. If you pour too many into the cover, pour the extra tablets back into the bottle. When you have the correct number of tablets in the cover, pour them from the cover into the paper cup. Place the cover on the container. Make sure not to contaminate the inside of the container or the cover.	10*		
7. For liquid medication: a. Place the plastic medication cup on a high, even surface. Uncover the bottle and place the cover on the counter, making sure the inside is facing up. Place your palm over the medication label. Position yourself so you are eye level with the medication cup. b. Pour the medication into the cup until the lowest point of the meniscus is at the correct measurement needed. c. If too much medication is poured into the cup, flush the extra down the sink. Replace the cover on the bottle without contaminating the inside of the cover or bottle.	10*		
8. Place the medication cups on the medication tray. Clean up the area.	5		
9. Perform the third medication check. Check each medication label against the order. Check for the right name, form, and route. Verify that the amount of medication in each cup is correct according to the order.	5*		
10. Prior to entering the exam room, knock on the door and wait a moment. Greet the patient. Identify yourself. Verify the patient's identity with full name and date of birth. Make sure the patient's information matches the order and the record. Explain what you are going to do.	10*		
11. Provide the right education to the patient. Explain the medication ordered, the desired effect, common side effects, and identify the provider who ordered it. Answer any questions the patient may have. Use language the patient can understand. Ask the patient if he or she has any allergies. If the patient refuses the medication, notify the provider.	10		
12. Perform the right technique. Do any assessments required prior to giving the medication. If the patient can have water with the medication, have water available.	5		

13. Allow the patient to take the medication in his or her hand or use the cup. Stay with the patient until the medication has been taken.	**5**		
14. Document the procedure in the health record. Include assessments done; allergies; teaching or instructions provided; the name of the provider who ordered the medication; the medication's name, dose, and route; and how the patient tolerated the medication. For vaccines and controlled substances, add the lot number, the expiration date, and the manufacturer number.	**10***		
Total Points	**100**		

Documentation

Comments

CAAHEP Competencies	Step(s)
I.P.4.a. Verify the rules of medication administration: right patient	10
I.P.4.b. Verify the rules of medication administration: right medication	3, 5, 9
I.P.4.c. Verify the rules of medication administration: right dose	2, 6, 7, 9
I.P.4.d. Verify the rules of medication administration: right route	3, 5, 9
I.P.4.e. Verify the rules of medication administration: right time	2
I.P.4.f. Verify the rules of medication administration: right documentation	14
I.P.6. Administer oral medications	Entire procedure
II.P.1. Calculate proper dosages of medication for administration	2
X.P.3. Document patient care accurately in the medical record	14
ABHES Competencies	**Step(s)**
4.a. Follow documentation guidelines	14
8.f. Prepare and administer oral and parenteral medications and monitor intravenous (IV) infusions	Entire procedure

Procedure 30.2 Prepare Medication from an Ampule

Name _____ Date _____ Score _____

Task: Prepare medication from an ampule.

Equipment and Supplies:
- Provider's order
- Ampule of medication
- Gauze or ampule breaker
- Alcohol wipes
- Filter needle and hypodermic safety needle
- 3 mL syringe
- Biohazard sharps container
- Waste container
- Drug reference information
- Marker

Order: 0.9% sodium chloride 0.7 mL IM

Standard: Complete the procedure and all critical steps in _____ minutes with a minimum score of 85% within two attempts (*or as indicated by the instructor*).

Scoring: Divide the points earned by the total possible points. Failure to perform a critical step, indicated by an asterisk (*), results in grade no higher than an 84% (*or as indicated by the instructor*).

Time: Began_____ Ended_____ Total minutes: _____

Steps:	Point Value	Attempt 1	Attempt 2
1. Wash hands or use hand sanitizer. Using the drug reference information and the order, review the information on the medication if needed. Clarify any questions you have with the provider.	5		
2. Select the right medication from the storage area. Check the medication label against the order. Check for the right name, form, and route. Check the expiration date to make sure the drug has not expired. Verify the right dose and the right time.	5*		
3. Assemble the supplies required for the procedure.	5		
4. Perform the second medication check. Check the medication label against the order. Check for the right name, form, dose, and route.	5*		
5. Attach the filter needle to the syringe. Using a marker, label the syringe with the medication name.	5*		
6. Gently tap the medication from the head of the ampule or hold the ampule securely, upright in your hand. Quickly move your hand downward. After all the medication has drained into the body of the ampule, wipe the neck with an alcohol wipe.	5		

7.	Place the ampule breaker over the head of the ampule (following the directions from the manufacturer) or wrap the neck with gauze. Hold the body with your nondominant hand. With your dominant hand, firmly hold the head (or breaker) between your first two fingers and thumb. Quickly snap off the head of the ampule, making sure it breaks away from your body and others.	**10***		
8.	Discard the breaker or gauze with the ampule head in a biohazard sharps container.	**5**		
9.	Place the ampule on a flat surface. Uncover the filter needle and insert the needle into the ampule without contaminating the needle. Keeping the bevel in the medication, pull the plunger upward, aspirating the medication into the syringe. Tilt the ampule as you remove all the medication.	**10**		
10.	Recap the needle using the one-hand scoop technique. Perform the third medication check. Check the medication label against the order. Check for the right name, form, and route. Discard the ampule in the biohazard sharps container.	**5***		
11.	Remove the filter needle and attach a new needle without contaminating the unit. Discard the filter needle in the biohazard sharps container.	**5***		
12.	Hold the syringe in a vertical position with the uncapped needle pointed upward. Tap the barrel carefully with the fingertips or a pen to move the air bubbles up to the top of the barrel. Once all the air bubbles are at the top, push the plunger slowly to the correct calibration marking for the ordered dose. Recap the needle.	**10***		
13.	Double-check the dose of medication measured against the order. Make sure no air bubbles are in the syringe.	**10***		
14.	Maintain the sterility of the medication and the needle throughout the procedure.	**10***		
15.	Clean up the work area. Packaging and other waste should be discarded in the waste container.	**5**		
	Total Points	**100**		

Comments

CAAHEP Competencies	Step(s)
I.P.4.b. Verify the rules of medication administration: right medication	2, 4, 10
I.P.4.c. Verify the rules of medication administration: right dose	2, 4, 12, 13
I.P.4.d. Verify the rules of medication administration: right route	2, 4, 10
I.P.4.e. Verify the rules of medication administration: right time	2
XII.P.2.c. Demonstrate proper use of: sharps disposal containers	10, 11
ABHES Competencies	**Step(s)**
8.f. Prepare and administer oral and parenteral medications and monitor intravenous (IV) infusions	Entire procedure

Procedure 30.3   Prepare Medication Using a Prefilled Sterile Cartridge

Name _____ Date _____ Score _____

Tasks: Prepare medication using a prefilled sterile cartridge. Discard a prefilled sterile cartridge with a reusable holder.

Equipment and Supplies:
- Provider's order
- Prefilled sterile cartridge
- Hypodermic safety needle (if needed)
- Carpuject cartridge holder
- Biohazard sharps container
- Waste container
- Drug reference information

Order: 0.9% sodium chloride 1.6 mL IM

Standard: Complete the procedure and all critical steps in _____ minutes with a minimum score of 85% within two attempts (*or as indicated by the instructor*).

Scoring: Divide the points earned by the total possible points. Failure to perform a critical step, indicated by an asterisk (*), results in grade no higher than an 84% (*or as indicated by the instructor*).

Time: Began_____ Ended_____ Total minutes: _____

Steps:	Point Value	Attempt 1	Attempt 2
1. Wash hands or use hand sanitizer. Using the drug reference information and the order, review the information on the medication if needed. Clarify any questions you have with the provider.	5		
2. Select the right medication from the storage area. Check the medication label against the order. Check for the right name, form, and route. Check the expiration date to make sure the drug has not expired. Verify the right dose and the right time.	5*		
3. Assemble the supplies required for the procedure.	5		
4. Perform the second medication check. Check the medication label against the order. Check for the right name, form, dose, and route.	5*		
5. Break the seal. With one hand on the needle cover and the other on the barrel of the prefilled cartridge, move your hands together until you hear a pop. If needed, remove the cover on the cartridge and attach a covered needle.	5		
6. Hold the Carpuject holder so the opening (for the barrel) is facing up. Pull the plunger rod out until it clicks. Turn the blue lock until it clicks. This should increase the space between the blue lock and the flange.	10		
7. Insert the cartridge into the Carpuject holder. To secure the cartridge, turn the blue lock on the Carpuject holder until it clicks. The space between the blue lock and the flange should decrease. Turn the white plunger rod until it screws onto the rubber stopper.	10*		

8.	Remove the cover. Hold the syringe unit in a vertical position with the uncapped needle or tip pointed upward. Tap the barrel carefully with the fingertips or a pen to move the air bubbles up to the top of the barrel. Once all the air bubbles are at the top, push the plunger slowly to the correct calibration marking for the ordered dose.	10*		
9.	Recap the needle using the one-hand scoop technique. Perform the third medication check. Check the medication label against the order. Check for the right name, form, and route.	10*		
10.	Double-check the dose of medication measured against the order. Make sure no air bubbles are in the syringe.	5*		
11.	Maintain the sterility of the medication and the needle throughout the procedure.	10		
12.	After "giving" the injection, unscrew the plunger rod and pull out until it clicks. Turn the blue lock until it clicks. The space between the blue lock and the flange should increase in size.	5		
13.	Carefully invert the Carpuject holder over a biohazard sharps container to discard the cartridge. Hold the Carpuject holder firmly so it does not end up in the sharps container.	10*		
14.	Disinfect the Carpuject holder. Clean up the work area. Waste should be put in the waste container.	5		
	Total Points	**100**		

Comments

CAAHEP Competencies	Step(s)
I.P.4.b. Verify the rules of medication administration: right medication	2, 4, 9
I.P.4.c. Verify the rules of medication administration: right dose	2, 4, 8, 10
I.P.4.d. Verify the rules of medication administration: right route	2, 4, 9
I.P.4.e. Verify the rules of medication administration: right time	2
XII.P.2.c. Demonstrate proper use of: sharps disposal containers	13
ABHES Competencies	**Step(s)**
8.f. Prepare and administer oral and parenteral medications and monitor intravenous (IV) infusions	Entire procedure

Procedure 30.4   Prepare Medication from a Vial

Name _____ Date _____ Score _____

Task: Prepare medication from a vial.

Equipment and Supplies:
- Provider's order
- Vial of medication
- Alcohol wipes
- Hypodermic safety needle and 3 mL syringe or needle/syringe unit
- Biohazard sharps container
- Waste container
- Drug reference information
- Marker

Order: 0.9% sodium chloride 1.2 mL IM

Standard: Complete the procedure and all critical steps in _____ minutes with a minimum score of 85% within two attempts (*or as indicated by the instructor*).

Scoring: Divide the points earned by the total possible points. Failure to perform a critical step, indicated by an asterisk (*), results in grade no higher than an 84% (*or as indicated by the instructor*).

Time: Began _____ Ended _____ Total minutes: _____

Steps:	Point Value	Attempt 1	Attempt 2
1. Wash hands or use hand sanitizer. Using the drug reference information and the order, review the information on the medication if needed. Clarify any questions you have with the provider.	5		
2. Select the right medication from the storage area. Check the medication label against the order. Check for the right name, form, and route. Check the expiration date to make sure the drug has not expired. Verify the right dose and the right time.	5*		
3. Assemble the supplies required for the procedure.	5		
4. Perform the second medication check. Check the medication label against the order. Check for the right name, form, dose, and route.	5*		
5. Open the syringe and needle. Tighten the preassembled syringe and needle unit (if needed) or attach the needle to the syringe. Using a marker, label the syringe with the medication name.	5		
6. Mix the medication by rolling it with your hands if needed. Remove cap on the vial (if present). Clean the rubber stopper with an alcohol wipe. Let the stopper dry.	5*		
7. With the syringe in a vertical position, pull the syringe plunger down. Draw up an amount of air equal to the amount of medication ordered.	5*		
8. Hold the vial firmly against a flat surface. Insert the needle into the center of the dried rubber stopper. Inject the aspirated air above the fluid in the vial.	5		

9.	With the palm of your nondominant hand facing upward, grasp the vial between your middle and index finger. Keeping the syringe unit in the vial, pick up and invert them. Use your thumb, ring, and little fingers of your nondominant hand to stabilize the syringe in the vial.	**10**		
10.	With the syringe at eye level, pull the plunger down using your dominant hand. Fill the syringe with more medication than what was ordered.	**10**		
11.	Continue to hold the vial/needle/syringe unit in a vertical position (with the needle pointing upward) with your nondominant hand. With your dominant hand, either use your fingers or a pen to tap the bubbles to the top of the barrel.	**5**		
12.	Once all the air bubbles are at the top, push the plunger slowly to the correct calibration marking for the ordered dose.	**10***		
13.	Double-check that no air bubbles are in the syringe and the right dose was measured. If everything is correct, remove the vial from the syringe/needle unit.	**5***		
14.	Use the one-hand scoop technique to cover the needle. Perform the third medication check. Check each medication label against the order. Check for the right name, form, and route.	**5***		
15.	Maintain the sterility of the medication and the needle throughout the procedure.	**10***		
16.	Clean up the work area.	**5**		
	Total Points	**100**		

Comments

CAAHEP Competencies	**Step(s)**
I.P.4.b. Verify the rules of medication administration: right medication	2, 4, 14
I.P.4.c. Verify the rules of medication administration: right dose	2, 4, 13
I.P.4.d. Verify the rules of medication administration: right route	2, 4, 14
I.P.4.e. Verify the rules of medication administration: right time	2
ABHES Competencies	**Step(s)**
8.f. Prepare and administer oral and parenteral medications and monitor intravenous (IV) infusions	Entire procedure

Procedure 30.5   Reconstituting Powdered Medication

Name _____ Date _____ Score _____

Tasks: Reconstitute powdered medication and prepare the dose of medication.

Equipment and Supplies:
- Provider's order
- Vial of powdered medication
- Vial of diluent
- Alcohol wipes
- Two hypodermic syringes (a 3 mL and a larger syringe)
- Two hypodermic safety needles
- Biohazard sharps container
- Waste container
- Drug reference information
- Marker

Order: (Powdered medication name) 0.5 mL IM or use the order provided by the instructor.

Standard: Complete the procedure and all critical steps in _____ minutes with a minimum score of 85% within two attempts (*or as indicated by the instructor*).

Scoring: Divide the points earned by the total possible points. Failure to perform a critical step, indicated by an asterisk (*), results in grade no higher than an 84% (*or as indicated by the instructor*).

Time: Began_____ Ended_____ Total minutes: _____

Steps:	Point Value	Attempt 1	Attempt 2
1. Wash hands or use hand sanitizer. Using the drug reference information and the order, review the information on the medication if needed. Clarify any questions you have with the provider.	2		
2. Select the right medication from the storage area. Check the medication label against the order. Check for the right name, form, and route. Check the expiration date to make sure the vials are not expired. Verify the right dose and the right time. Read the medication label to determine the correct diluent. Obtain the diluent and check the name, route, and expiration date.	5*		
3. Assemble the supplies required for the procedure. If needed, calculate the dose of medication required.	3		
4. Perform the second medication check. Check the medication labels against the order and directions for reconstituting the powder. Check for the right name, form, and route.	5*		
5. Open and assemble the syringes and needles Using a marker, label the 3 mL syringe with the medication name.	2		
6. Remove the caps on the vials. Clean the rubber stoppers with an alcohol wipe. Let the stoppers dry.	3*		
7. With the powdered medication vial on a firm surface, insert the needle of the largest volume syringe unit. Make sure the tip stays out of the powder. Pull back on the plunger and withdraw air equal to the amount of diluent that must be added. Pull the needle/syringe out of the stopper.	5*		

8.	Using the syringe with the aspirated air (equal to the amount of diluent needed), insert the needle into the center of the dried rubber stopper of the diluent vial. Push the air into the vial, but do not force the air into the vial. Make sure the needle is not in the fluid.	**5**		
9.	With the palm of your nondominant hand facing upward, grasp the vial between your middle and index fingers. Keeping the syringe unit in the vial, pick up and invert them. Use your thumb, ring, and little fingers of your nondominant hand to stabilize the syringe in the vial. Pull down on the plunger until you have more diluent than what you need.	**5**		
10.	Continue to hold the vial/needle/syringe unit in a vertical position (with the needle pointing upward) with your nondominant hand. With your dominant hand, use either your fingers or a pen to tap the bubbles to the top of the barrel.	**5**		
11.	Once all the air bubbles are at the top, push the plunger slowly to the correct calibration marking for the ordered dose. Keep the syringe at eye level.	**5***		
12.	Double-check that no air bubbles are in the syringe and the right dose was measured. If everything is correct, remove the vial from the syringe/needle unit.	**5***		
13.	Using an alcohol wipe, clean the rubber stopper of the powdered medication vial. With the vial flat on a hard surface, insert the needle into the dried stopper. Push the diluent into the vial. If resistance is met, take your finger off the plunger, and allow air to fill in the syringe. Gradually work all the diluent into the vial. Withdraw the needle from the vial and discard the needle and syringe in the biohazard sharps container.	**5***		
14.	Gently mix the vial by rolling it in your palms. Mix the medication until all the powder has dissolved.	**2**		
15.	Clean the rubber stopper of the powdered medication vial with an alcohol wipe. Let the stopper dry. With the second syringe in a vertical position, pull the syringe plunger down. Draw up an amount of air equal to the amount of medication ordered.	**3***		
16.	Hold the vial firmly against a flat surface. Insert the needle into the center of the dried rubber stopper. Inject the aspirated air above the fluid in the vial.	**2**		
17.	With the palm of your nondominant hand facing upward, grasp the vial between your middle and index fingers. Keeping the syringe unit in the vial, pick up and invert them. Use your thumb, ring, and little fingers of your nondominant hand to stabilize the syringe in the vial.	**3**		
18.	With the syringe at eye level, pull the plunger down using your dominant hand. Fill the syringe with more medication than what was ordered.	**5**		
19.	Continue to hold the vial/needle/syringe unit in a vertical position (with the needle pointing upward) with your nondominant hand. With your dominant hand, use either your fingers or a pen to tap the bubbles to the top of the barrel.	**5**		
20.	Once all the air bubbles are at the top, push the plunger slowly to the correct calibration marking for the ordered dose.	**5***		
21.	Double-check that no air bubbles are in the syringe and the right dose was measured. If everything is correct, remove the vial from the syringe/needle unit.	**5***		

22. Use the one-hand scoop technique to cover the needle. Perform the third medication check. Check each medication label against the order. Check for the right name, form, and route.	5*		
23. Maintain the sterility of the medication and the needle throughout the procedure.	5		
24. If medication is in a multidose vial, label the vial with the expiration date, diluent added, and your initials. Clean up the work area. Put the packaging and other waste in the waste container. Discard the vial(s) in the biohazard waste container.	5		
Total Points	100		

Comments

CAAHEP Competencies	Step(s)
I.P.4.b. Verify the rules of medication administration: right medication	2, 4, 22
I.P.4.c. Verify the rules of medication administration: right dose	2, 20, 21
I.P.4.d. Verify the rules of medication administration: right route	2, 4, 22
I.P.4.e. Verify the rules of medication administration: right time	2
XII.P.2.c. Demonstrate proper use of: sharps disposal containers	13, 24
ABHES Competencies	**Step(s)**
8.f. Prepare and administer oral and parenteral medications and monitor intravenous (IV) infusions	Entire procedure

Procedure 30.6   Mixing Two Insulins

Name _____   Date _____   Score _____

Task: Mix two types of insulin in one syringe.

Equipment and Supplies:
- Provider's order
- Regular insulin vial
- NPH insulin vial
- Alcohol wipes
- Insulin needle and syringe unit
- Biohazard sharps container
- Waste container
- Drug reference information
- Marker

Order: Regular insulin 16 units mixed with NPH insulin 30 units subcut.

Standard: Complete the procedure and all critical steps in _____ minutes with a minimum score of 85% within two attempts (*or as indicated by the instructor*).

Scoring: Divide the points earned by the total possible points. Failure to perform a critical step, indicated by an asterisk (*), results in grade no higher than an 84% (*or as indicated by the instructor*).

Time: Began_____ Ended_____ Total minutes: _____

Steps:	Point Value	Attempt 1	Attempt 2
1. Wash hands or use hand sanitizer. Using the drug reference information and the order, review the information on the medication if needed. Clarify any questions you have with the provider	5		
2. Select the right medications from the storage area. Check the medication labels against the order. Check for the right name, form, and route. Check the expiration date to make sure the vials are not expired. Verify the right dose and the right time.	5*		
3. Assemble the supplies required for the procedure. If the insulin is cold, roll the vials in your hands to warm the medication.	5		
4. Perform the second medication check. Check the medication labels against the order. Check for the right name, form, and route.	5*		
5. Open and assemble the syringe and needle. Using a marker, label the syringe with the medication name. Mix the NPH insulin by rolling the vial in your hands. If present, remove the metal or plastic caps on the vials. Clean the rubber stoppers with an alcohol wipe. Let the stoppers dry.	10*		
6. With the syringe in a vertical position, pull the syringe plunger down. Draw up an amount of air equal to the amount of NPH insulin ordered. With the NPH vial on a firm surface, insert the needle in the rubber stopper. Inject the air into the NPH vial, keeping the needle tip out of the medication. Withdraw the needle from the stopper.	5		
7. With the syringe in a vertical position, pull the syringe plunger down. Draw up an amount of air equal to the amount of Regular insulin ordered. With the Regular vial on a firm surface, insert the needle in the rubber stopper. Inject the air into the Regular vial, keeping the needle tip out of the medication.	5		

8.	With the palm of your nondominant hand facing upward, grasp the vial between your middle and index finger. Keeping the syringe unit in the vial, pick up and invert them. Use your thumb, ring, and little fingers of your nondominant hand to stabilize the syringe in the vial. Pull down on the plunger until you have more Regular insulin than what you need.	5		
9.	Continue to hold the vial/needle/syringe unit in a vertical position (with the needle pointing upward) with your nondominant hand. With your dominant hand, use either your fingers or a pen to tap the bubbles to the top of the barrel.	5		
10.	Once all the air bubbles are at the top, push the plunger slowly to the correct calibration marking for the ordered dose. Keep the syringe at eye level.	5*		
11.	Double-check that no air bubbles are in the syringe and the right dose was measured. If everything is correct, remove the vial from the syringe/needle unit.	5*		
12.	Using an alcohol wipe, wipe the rubber stopper of the NPH vial. Calculate the total amount of insulin that needs to be given.	5*		
13.	With the NPH vial flat on a hard surface, insert the needle into the dried stopper. With the palm of your nondominant hand facing upward, grasp the vial between your middle and index fingers. Keeping the syringe unit in the vial, pick up and invert them. Use your thumb, ring, and little fingers of your nondominant hand to stabilize the syringe in the vial. Pull down on the plunger until the rubber stopper reaches the calibration mark required. Do not withdraw any extra NPH insulin.	10*		
14.	Double-check that no air bubbles are in the syringe and the right dose was measured. If everything is correct, remove the vial from the syringe/needle unit.	5*		
15.	Use the one-hand scoop technique to cover the needle. Perform the third medication check. Check each medication label against the order. Check for the right name, form, and route.	5*		
16.	Maintain the sterility of the medication and the needle throughout the procedure.	10*		
17.	Clean up the work area. Put the packaging and other waste in the waste container. Place the insulin vials back in their storage location.	5		
	Total Points	100		

Comments

CAAHEP Competencies	Step(s)
I.P.4.b. Verify the rules of medication administration: right medication	2, 4, 15
I.P.4.c. Verify the rules of medication administration: right dose	2, 10, 11, 13, 14
I.P.4.d. Verify the rules of medication administration: right route	2, 4, 15
I.P.4.e. Verify the rules of medication administration: right time	2
ABHES Competencies	**Step(s)**
8.f. Prepare and administer oral and parenteral medications and monitor intravenous (IV) infusions	Entire procedure

Procedure 30.7 Administer an Intradermal Injection

Name _____ Date _____ Score _____

Tasks: Prepare medication from a vial, administer an intradermal injection, read the tuberculin skin test, and document in the health record.

Equipment and Supplies:
- Provider's order
- Patient's health record
- Vial of medication
- Alcohol wipes
- 1 mL syringe with 1/4 to 5/8 inch, 25- to 27-gauge safety needle
- Bandage (if per facility's policy)
- Medication tray
- Biohazard sharps container
- Waste container
- Drug reference information
- Gloves
- Marker and pen
- Millimeter ruler

Order: Tuberculin purified protein derivative (PPD) (5 tuberculin units) 0.1 mL ID

Standard: Complete the procedure and all critical steps in _____ minutes with a minimum score of 85% within two attempts (*or as indicated by the instructor*).

Scoring: Divide the points earned by the total possible points. Failure to perform a critical step, indicated by an asterisk (*), results in grade no higher than an 84% (*or as indicated by the instructor*).

Time: Began_____ Ended_____ Total minutes: _____

Steps:	Point Value	Attempt 1	Attempt 2
1. Wash hands or use hand sanitizer. Using the drug reference information and the order, review the information on the medication if needed. Clarify any questions you have with the provider.	2		
2. Select the right medication from the storage area. Check the medication label against the order. Check for the right name, form, and route. Check the expiration date to make sure the drug has not expired. Verify the right dose and the right time.	2*		
3. Assemble the supplies required for the procedure. Perform the second medication check. Check the medication label against the order. Check for the right name, form, dose, and route.	3*		
4. Open the syringe and needle. Tighten the preassembled syringe and needle unit (if needed) or attach the needle to the syringe. Using a marker, label the syringe with the medication name. Mix the medication by rolling it with your hands if needed. Remove cap on the vial (if present). Clean the rubber stopper with an alcohol wipe. Let the stopper dry. Using the syringe, draw up an amount of air equal to the amount of medication ordered. Then insert the needle into the vial and inject the air.	5		

5. With the palm of your nondominant hand facing upward, grasp the vial between your middle and index finger. Keeping the syringe unit in the vial, pick up and invert them. Use your thumb, ring, and little fingers of your nondominant hand to stabilize the syringe in the vial.	**3**		
6. With the syringe at eye level, pull the plunger down using your dominant hand. Fill the syringe with more medication than what was ordered. Tap the bubbles. Once all the air bubbles are at the top, push the plunger slowly to the correct calibration marking for the ordered dose.	**5***		
7. Double-check that no air bubbles are in the syringe and the right dose was measured. If everything is correct, remove the vial from the syringe/needle unit. Use the one-hand scoop technique to cover the needle. Perform the third medication check. Check each medication label against the order. Check for the right name, form, and route. Place syringe on a medication tray and clean up the work area.	**5***		
8. Maintain the sterility of the medication and the needle throughout the procedure.	**5***		
9. Prior to entering the exam room, knock on the door and wait a moment. Greet the patient. Identify yourself. Verify the patient's identity with full name and date of birth. Make sure the patient's information matches the order and the record. Explain what you are going to do.	**5***		
10. Provide the right education to the patient. Explain the medication ordered, the desired effect, and common side effects; also identify the provider who ordered it. Answer any questions the patient may have. Use language the patient can understand. Ask the patient if he or she has any allergies. If the patient refuses the medication, notify the provider.	**5**		
11. Perform the right technique. Ask the patient the following questions: • Can the patient return in 48-72 hours for the reading? • Has the patient ever had BCG? • Has the patient ever had a TB skin test? If yes, did the patient have a reaction to it?	**5**		
12. Use hand sanitizer and put on gloves.	**2***		
13. Have the patient extend a forearm. With the palm facing upward, identify an appropriate site for an injection. The site should be 2-4 inches below the elbow. Loosen the cap on the needle, but still protect the needle from contamination. Open the alcohol wipes.	**3***		
14. Place your nondominant hand to the side of the site, pulling the skin taut. Another option is to place your nondominant hand on the back of the patient's forearm, pulling the skin taut	**3**		
15. Cleanse the site with an alcohol wipe using a circular motion. Move from the center outward, using some friction to help clean the site. Create about a 2-inch circle at the site. Let the site dry while continuing to hold the area.	**5***		
16. Pick up the syringe and tip it to remove the cover. Grasp the syringe in your dominant hand, using your thumb and index finger. Make sure to have no fingers under the syringe. Ensure that the bevel is up.	**3**		
17. Using a 5- to 15-degree angle, slowly insert the needle until the bevel is covered with skin. Carefully lower the syringe to the skin, and hold it steady with your dominant hand.	**5**		

18. Carefully move your nondominant hand to the plunger. Slowly and steadily inject the medication by pressing on the plunger. If a 6-10 mm wheal does not appear, repeat the test at least 2 inches from the site.	5		
19. Double-check the barrel of the syringe to make sure all the medication was administered. Withdraw the needle. Activate the needle's safety device with one hand.	5*		
20. Discard the needle/syringe in a biohazard sharps container. Make sure to put the needle in first.	3*		
21. Do not massage the area. According to the facility's policy, if the person is wearing a light-colored shirt with long sleeves, offer a bandage. Place the bandage on loosely to just absorb any blood from the site.	2		
22. Observe the patient for any adverse reactions. Clean up the area. Discard the waste in the waste container. Sanitize your hands.	2		
23. Document the procedure in the health record. Include assessments done, allergies, teaching or instructions provided, the provider ordering the medication, the medication name, dose, route, and how the patient tolerated the medication. Also include the manufacturer, the lot number, and the expiration date of the vial.	5*		
Scenario update: Patient returns for the reading. 24. Check the health record to identify the location of the test. Greet the patient. Identify yourself. Verify the patient's identity with full name and date of birth. Make sure the patient's information matches the order and the record. Explain what you are going to do.	2*		
25. Palpate the site for an induration. If an induration is felt, ask the patient if you can write on his or her arm. Using a ballpoint pen, draw a line toward the induration from the outer edge of the arm. Repeat on the other side. Another option is to palpate the induration to find the edge and mark the edge with a pen. Repeat on the other side. Using a millimeter ruler, accurately measure the distance between the two points.	5		
26. Document the reading in the patient's health record. Include the reason for the patient's visit, the test site, the size of the induration in millimeters, and the provider notified.	5*		
Total Points	100		

Documentation

Comments

CAAHEP Competencies	Step(s)
I.P.4.a. Verify the rules of medication administration: right patient	9
I.P.4.b. Verify the rules of medication administration: right medication	2, 3, 7
I.P.4.c. Verify the rules of medication administration: right dose	2, 3, 6, 7
I.P.4.d. Verify the rules of medication administration: right route	2, 3, 7
I.P.4.e. Verify the rules of medication administration: right time	2
I.P.4.f. Verify the rules of medication administration: right documentation	23
I.P.5. Select proper sites for administering parenteral medication	13
I.P.7. Administer parenteral (excluding IV) medications	Entire procedure
III.P.2. Select appropriate barrier/personal protective equipment.	12
III.P.10.a. Demonstrate proper disposal of biohazardous material: sharps	20
X.P.3. Document patient care accurately in the medical record	23, 26
XII.P.2.c. Demonstrate proper use of: sharps disposal containers	20
ABHES Competencies	**Step(s)**
4.a. Follow documentation guidelines	23, 26
8.a. Practice standard precautions and perform disinfection/sterilization techniques	12
8.f. Prepare and administer oral and parenteral medications and monitor intravenous (IV) infusions	Entire procedure

Procedure 30.8   Administer a Subcutaneous Injection

Name _____ Date _____ Score _____

Tasks: Prepare medication from a vial, administer a subcutaneous injection, and document the medication administration in the health record.

Equipment and Supplies:
- Provider's order
- Patient's health record
- Vial of medication
- Alcohol wipes
- 3 mL syringe with 5/8-inch or 1/2-inch 25-gauge needle
- Gauze
- Bandage
- Medication tray
- Biohazard sharps container
- Waste container
- Drug reference information
- VIS for polio vaccine (IPV) (optional)
- Gloves
- Marker

Scenario: Dr. Martin ordered polio vaccine (IPV) 0.5 mL subcut for Johnny Parker (DOB 06/15/2010). (Vial information: ABC Manufacturer, Lot 1234, expires 1 year from today.)

Standard: Complete the procedure and all critical steps in _____ minutes with a minimum score of 85% within two attempts (*or as indicated by the instructor*).

Scoring: Divide the points earned by the total possible points. Failure to perform a critical step, indicated by an asterisk (*), results in grade no higher than an 84% (*or as indicated by the instructor*).

Time: Began_____ Ended_____ Total minutes: _____

Steps:	Point Value	Attempt 1	Attempt 2
1. Wash hands or use hand sanitizer. Using the drug reference information and the order, review the information on the medication if needed. Clarify any questions you have with the provider.	2		
2. Select the right medication from the storage area. Check the medication label against the order. Check for the right name, form, and route. Check the expiration date to make sure the drug has not expired. Verify the right dose and the right time.	2*		
3. Assemble the supplies required for the procedure. Perform the second medication check. Check the medication label against the order. Check for the right name, form, dose, and route.	3*		
4. Open the syringe and needle. Tighten the preassembled syringe and needle unit (if needed) or attach the needle to the syringe. Using a marker, label the syringe with the medication name. Mix the medication by rolling it with your hands if needed. Remove cap on the vial (if present). Clean the rubber stopper with an alcohol wipe. Let the stopper dry. Using the syringe, draw up an amount of air equal to the amount of medication ordered. Then insert the needle into the vial and inject the air.	5		

5. With the palm of your nondominant hand facing upward, grasp the vial between your middle and index finger. Keeping the syringe unit in the vial, pick up and invert them. Use your thumb, ring, and little fingers of your nondominant hand to stabilize the syringe in the vial.	**3**		
6. With the syringe at eye level, pull the plunger down using your dominant hand. Fill the syringe with more medication than what was ordered. Tap the bubbles. Once all the air bubbles are at the top, push the plunger slowly to the correct calibration marking for the ordered dose.	**5***		
7. Double-check that no air bubbles are in the syringe and the right dose was measured. If everything is correct, remove the vial from the syringe/needle unit. Use the one-hand scoop technique to cover the needle. Perform the third medication check. Check each medication label against the order. Check for the right name, form, and route. Place syringe on a medication tray and clean up the work area.	**5***		
8. Maintain the sterility of the medication and the needle throughout the procedure.	**5***		
9. *(Peer will play the parent.)* Prior to entering the exam room, knock on the door and wait a moment. Greet the patient. Identify yourself. Verify the patient's identity with full name and date of birth. Make sure the patient's information matches the order and the record. Explain what you are going to do.	**5***		
10. Provide the right education to the parent/patient. Explain the medication ordered, the desired effect, and common side effects; also identify the provider who ordered it. Answer any questions the patient may have. Use language the patient can understand. Ask the patient if he or she has any allergies. If the patient refuses the medication, notify the provider.	**5**		
11. Use hand sanitizer and put on gloves.	**5***		
12. Loosen the cap on the needle, but still protect the needle from contamination. Open the alcohol wipes. Have gauze and a bandage available.	**5**		
13. *(Peer will play the patient.)* Find the injection site.	**5***		
14. Cleanse the site with an alcohol wipe using a circular motion. Move from the center outward, using some friction to help clean the site. Create about a 2-inch circle at the site. Let the site dry.	**5***		
15. Perform the right technique. Place a gauze between index and middle finger of your nondominant hand. With that hand, use your index finger and thumb to pinch up at the cleansed area.	**5**		
16. Pick up the syringe and tip it to remove the cover. Hold the syringe between the thumb and index finger of your dominant hand. Quickly and smoothly insert the needle into the site at a 45- or 90-degree angle, depending on the needle size. Insert the entire needle. Make sure the needle tip is not pointed toward your nondominant hand.	**5**		
17. One-hand option: Continue to pinch the site. Securely grasp the syringe between the fingers of your dominant hand. With your dominant hand, aspirate if required, and then push the plunger to inject the medication. Two-hand option: Release the pinch and with the nondominant hand, aspirate if required, and then push the plunger to inject the medication.	**5**		
18. Inject the medication at the rate of 1 mL over 10 seconds. Ensure all the medication has been injected before pulling out the needle in the same angle of entry. Release the pinch if using the one-hand option.	**5**		

19. Activate the needle's safety device with one hand while the other hand covers the site with gauze. Gently apply pressure at the site to stop any bleeding. Apply a bandage if the patient requests it.	5*		
20. Discard the needle/syringe in a biohazard sharps container. Make sure to put the needle goes into the sharps container first.	5*		
21. Observe the patient for any adverse reactions. Clean up the area. Discard the waste in the waste container. Sanitize your hands.	5		
22. Document the procedure in the health record. Include assessments done; allergies; teaching or instructions provided; the name of the provider who ordered the medication; the medication's name, dose, and route; and how the patient tolerated the medication. Also include the manufacturer, the lot number, and the expiration date for the vaccines and controlled substances.	5*		
Total Points	100		

Documentation

Comments

CAAHEP Competencies	Step(s)
I.P.4.a. Verify the rules of medication administration: right patient	9
I.P.4.b. Verify the rules of medication administration: right medication	2, 3, 7
I.P.4.c. Verify the rules of medication administration: right dose	2, 3, 6, 7
I.P.4.d. Verify the rules of medication administration: right route	2, 3, 7
I.P.4.e. Verify the rules of medication administration: right time	2
I.P.4.f. Verify the rules of medication administration: right documentation	22
I.P.5. Select proper sites for administering parenteral medication	13
I.P.7. Administer parenteral (excluding IV) medications	Entire procedure
III.P.2. Select appropriate barrier/personal protective equipment.	11
III.P.10.a. Demonstrate proper disposal of biohazardous material: sharps	20
X.P.3. Document patient care accurately in the medical record	22
XII.P.2.c. Demonstrate proper use of: sharps disposal containers	20
ABHES Competencies	**Step(s)**
8.a. Practice standard precautions and perform disinfection/sterilization techniques	11
8.f. Prepare and administer oral and parenteral medications and monitor intravenous (IV) infusions	Entire procedure

Procedure 30.9   Administer an Intramuscular Injection

Name _____ Date _____ Score _____

Tasks: Prepare medication from a vial, administer an intramuscular injection, and document the medication administration in the health record.

Equipment and Supplies:
- Provider's order
- Patient's health record
- Vial of medication
- Alcohol wipes
- 3 mL syringe
- 22- to 25-gauge, 1- to 1½-inch needle
- Gauze
- Bandage
- Medication tray
- Biohazard sharps container
- Waste container
- Drug reference information
- VIS for influenza vaccine (optional)
- Gloves
- Marker

Scenario: Dr. Martin ordered influenza vaccine (IIV) 0.5 mL IM for Erma Willis (DOB 12/09/1947). (Vial information: MN Manufacturer, Lot 7845, expires 1 year from today.)

Standard: Complete the procedure and all critical steps in _____ minutes with a minimum score of 85% within two attempts (*or as indicated by the instructor*).

Scoring: Divide the points earned by the total possible points. Failure to perform a critical step, indicated by an asterisk (*), results in grade no higher than an 84% (*or as indicated by the instructor*).

Time: Began_____ Ended_____ Total minutes: _____

Steps:	Point Value	Attempt 1	Attempt 2
1. Wash hands or use hand sanitizer. Using the drug reference information and the order, review the information on the medication if needed. Clarify any questions you have with the provider.	2		
2. Select the right medication from the storage area. Check the medication label against the order. Check for the right name, form, and route. Check the expiration date to make sure the drug has not expired. Verify the right dose and the right time.	2*		
3. Assemble the supplies required for the procedure. Perform the second medication check. Check the medication label against the order. Check for the right name, form, dose, and route.	3*		

4.	Open the syringe and needle. Tighten the preassembled syringe and needle unit (if needed) or attach the needle to the syringe. Using a marker, label the syringe with the medication name. Mix the medication by rolling it with your hands if needed. Remove cap on the vial (if present). Clean the rubber stopper with an alcohol wipe. Let the stopper dry. Using the syringe, draw up an amount of air equal to the amount of medication ordered. Then insert the needle into the vial and inject the air.	**5**		
5.	With the palm of your nondominant hand facing upward, grasp the vial between your middle and index finger. Keeping the syringe unit in the vial, pick up and invert them. Use your thumb, ring, and little fingers of your nondominant hand to stabilize the syringe in the vial.	**3**		
6.	With the syringe at eye level, pull the plunger down using your dominant hand. Fill the syringe with more medication than what was ordered. Tap the bubbles. Once all the air bubbles are at the top, push the plunger slowly to the correct calibration marking for the ordered dose.	**5***		
7.	Double-check that no air bubbles are in the syringe and the right dose was measured. If everything is correct, remove the vial from the syringe/needle unit. Use the one-hand scoop technique to cover the needle. Perform the third medication check. Check each medication label against the order. Check for the right name, form, and route. Place syringe on a medication tray and clean up the work area.	**5***		
8.	Maintain the sterility of the medication and the needle throughout the procedure.	**5***		
9.	Prior to entering the exam room, knock on the door and wait a moment. Greet the patient. Identify yourself. Verify the patient's identity with full name and date of birth. Make sure the patient's information matches the order and the record. Explain what you are going to do.	**5***		
10.	Provide the right education to the patient. Explain the medication ordered, the desired effect, and common side effects; also identify the provider who ordered it. Answer any questions the patient may have. Use language the patient can understand. Ask the patient if he or she has any allergies. If the patient refuses the medication, notify the provider.	**5**		
11.	Use hand sanitizer and put on gloves.	**5***		
12.	Loosen the cap on the needle, but still protect the needle from contamination. Open the alcohol wipes. Have gauze and a bandage available.	**5**		
13.	Find the site using the landmarks.	**5***		
14.	Cleanse the site with an alcohol wipe using a circular motion. Move from the center outward, using some friction to help clean the site. Create about a 2-inch circle at the site. Let the site dry.	**5***		
15.	Perform the right technique. Place a gauze between index and middle finger of your nondominant hand. With that hand, stretch or flatten the site. Hold the site.	**5**		
16.	Pick up the syringe and tip it to remove the cover. Hold the syringe like a dart with your dominant hand. Quickly and smoothly insert the needle into the site using a 90-degree angle. Insert the entire needle.	**5**		

17. <u>One-hand option</u>: Continue to hold the site. Securely grasp the syringe between the fingers of your dominant hand. Place your thumb under the plunger edge, and push the plunger out farther to aspirate. <u>Two-hand option</u>: Move your nondominant hand to the plunger. Pull the plunger out farther to aspirate.	**5**		
18. Aspirate for 5 seconds, and check the barrel for blood. If blood is seen, pull out the needle and discard it. Restart the procedure. If no blood is seen, inject the medication at a rate of about 10 seconds per milliliter. Ensure that all the medication has been injected. Wait 10 seconds before withdrawing the needle and letting go with your nondominant hand.	**5**		
19. Activate the needle's safety device with one hand while the other hand covers the site with gauze. Gently apply pressure at the site to stop any bleeding. Apply a bandage if the patient requests it.	**5***		
20. Discard the needle/syringe in a biohazard sharps container. Make sure to put the needle in first.	**5***		
21. Observe the patient for any adverse reactions. Clean up the area. Discard the waste in the waste container. Sanitize your hands.	**5**		
22. Document the procedure in the health record. Include assessments done; allergies; teaching or instructions provided; the name of the provider who ordered the medication; the medication's name, dose, and route; and how the patient tolerated the medication. Also include the manufacturer, the lot number, and the expiration date for the vaccines and controlled substances.	**5***		
Total Points	**100**		

Documentation

Comments

CAAHEP Competencies	Step(s)
I.P.4.a. Verify the rules of medication administration: right patient	9
I.P.4.b. Verify the rules of medication administration: right medication	2, 3, 7
I.P.4.c. Verify the rules of medication administration: right dose	2, 3, 6, 7
I.P.4.d. Verify the rules of medication administration: right route	2, 3, 7
I.P.4.e. Verify the rules of medication administration: right time	2
I.P.4.f. Verify the rules of medication administration: right documentation	22
I.P.5. Select proper sites for administering parenteral medication	13
I.P.7. Administer parenteral (excluding IV) medications	Entire procedure
III.P.2. Select appropriate barrier/personal protective equipment.	11
III.P.10.a. Demonstrate proper disposal of biohazardous material: sharps	20
X.P.3. Document patient care accurately in the medical record	22
XII.P.2.c. Demonstrate proper use of: sharps disposal containers	20
ABHES Competencies	**Step(s)**
8.a. Practice standard precautions and perform disinfection/sterilization techniques	11
8.f. Prepare and administer oral and parenteral medications and monitor intravenous (IV) infusions	Entire procedure

Procedure 30.10 Administer an Intramuscular Injection using the Z-track Technique

Name _____ Date _____ Score _____

Tasks: Prepare medication from a vial, administer an intramuscular injection, and document the medication administration in the health record.

Equipment and Supplies:
- Provider's order
- Patient's health record
- Vial of medication
- Alcohol wipes
- 3 mL syringe
- 22- to 25-gauge, 1- to 1½-inch needle
- Gauze
- Bandage
- Medication tray
- Biohazard sharps container
- Waste container
- Drug reference information
- Gloves
- Marker

Scenario: Dr. Martin ordered iron dextran 0.5 mL IM for Erma Willis (DOB 12/09/1947). (Vial information: FE Manufacturer, Lot 625, expires 1 year from today).

Standard: Complete the procedure and all critical steps in _____ minutes with a minimum score of 85% within two attempts (*or as indicated by the instructor*).

Scoring: Divide the points earned by the total possible points. Failure to perform a critical step, indicated by an asterisk (*), results in grade no higher than an 84% (*or as indicated by the instructor*).

Time: Began_____ Ended_____ Total minutes: _____

Steps:	Point Value	Attempt 1	Attempt 2
1. Wash hands or use hand sanitizer. Using the drug reference information and the order, review the information on the medication if needed. Clarify any questions you have with the provider.	2		
2. Select the right medication from the storage area. Check the medication label against the order. Check for the right name, form, and route. Check the expiration date to make sure the drug has not expired. Verify the right dose and the right time.	2*		
3. Assemble the supplies required for the procedure. Perform the second medication check. Check the medication label against the order. Check for the right name, form, dose, and route.	3*		

4.	Open the syringe and needle. Tighten the preassembled syringe and needle unit (if needed) or attach the needle to the syringe. Using a marker, label the syringe with the medication name. Mix the medication by rolling it with your hands if needed. Remove cap on the vial (if present). Clean the rubber stopper with an alcohol wipe. Let the stopper dry. Using the syringe, draw up an amount of air equal to the amount of medication ordered. Then insert the needle into the vial and inject the air.	**5**		
5.	With the palm of your nondominant hand facing upward, grasp the vial between your middle and index finger. Keeping the syringe unit in the vial, pick up and invert them. Use your thumb, ring, and little fingers of your nondominant hand to stabilize the syringe in the vial.	**3**		
6.	With the syringe at eye level, pull the plunger down using your dominant hand. Fill the syringe with more medication than what was ordered. Tap the bubbles. Once all the air bubbles are at the top, push the plunger slowly to the correct calibration marking for the ordered dose.	**5***		
7.	Double-check that no air bubbles are in the syringe and the right dose was measured. If everything is correct, remove the vial from the syringe/needle unit. Use the one-hand scoop technique to cover the needle. Perform the third medication check. Check each medication label against the order. Check for the right name, form, and route. Place syringe on a medication tray and clean up the work area.	**5***		
8.	Maintain the sterility of the medication and the needle throughout the procedure.	**5***		
9.	Prior to entering the exam room, knock on the door and wait a moment. Greet the patient. Identify yourself. Verify the patient's identity with full name and date of birth. Make sure the patient's information matches the order and the record. Explain what you are going to do.	**5***		
10.	Provide the right education to the patient. Explain the medication ordered, the desired effect, and common side effects; also identify the provider who ordered it. Answer any questions the patient may have. Use language the patient can understand. Ask the patient if he or she has any allergies. If the patient refuses the medication, notify the provider.	**5**		
11.	Use hand sanitizer and put on gloves.	**5***		
12.	Loosen the cap on the needle, but still protect the needle from contamination. Open the alcohol wipes. Have gauze and a bandage available.	**5**		
13.	Find the site using the landmarks.	**5***		
14.	Perform the right technique. Place a gauze between index and middle finger of your nondominant hand. Displace the tissue using your nondominant hand.	**5**		
15.	Cleanse the site with an alcohol wipe using a circular motion. Move from the center outward, using some friction to help clean the site. Create about a 2-inch circle at the site. Let the site dry while continuing to hold the area.	**5***		
16.	Pick up the syringe and tip it to remove the cover. Hold the syringe like a dart with your dominant hand. Quickly and smoothly insert the needle into the site at a 90-degree angle. Insert the entire needle.	**5**		
17.	Continue to hold the site. Securely grasp the syringe between the fingers of your dominant hand. Place your thumb under the plunger edge and push the plunger out farther to aspirate.	**5**		

18. Aspirate for 5 seconds and check the barrel for blood. If blood is seen, pull out the needle and discard. Restart the procedure. If no blood is seen, inject the medication at a rate of about 10 seconds per mL. Ensure all the medication has been injected. Wait 10 seconds before withdrawing the needle and letting go with your nondominant hand.	5		
19. Activate the needle's safety device with one hand while the other hand covers the site with gauze. Gently apply pressure at the site to stop any bleeding. Apply a bandage if the patient requests it.	5*		
20. Discard the needle/syringe in a biohazard sharps container. Make sure to put the needle in first.	5*		
21. Observe the patient for any adverse reactions. Clean up the area. Discard the waste in the waste container. Sanitize your hands.	5		
22. Document the procedure in the health record. Include assessments done, allergies, teaching or instructions provided, the provider who ordered the medication, the medication's name, dose, and route, and how the patient tolerated the medication. Also include the manufacturer, the lot number, and the expiration date for the vaccines and controlled substances.	5*		
Total Points	100		

Documentation

Comments

CAAHEP Competencies	Step(s)
I.P.4.a. Verify the rules of medication administration: right patient	9
I.P.4.b. Verify the rules of medication administration: right medication	2, 3, 7
I.P.4.c. Verify the rules of medication administration: right dose	2, 3, 6, 7
I.P.4.d. Verify the rules of medication administration: right route	2, 3, 7
I.P.4.e. Verify the rules of medication administration: right time	2
I.P.4.f. Verify the rules of medication administration: right documentation	22
I.P.5. Select proper sites for administering parenteral medication	13
I.P.7. Administer parenteral (excluding IV) medications	Entire procedure
III.P.2. Select appropriate barrier/personal protective equipment.	11
III.P.10.a. Demonstrate proper disposal of biohazardous material: sharps	20
X.P.3. Document patient care accurately in the medical record	22
XII.P.2.c. Demonstrate proper use of: sharps disposal containers	20
ABHES Competencies	**Step(s)**
8.a. Practice standard precautions and perform disinfection/sterilization techniques	11
8.f. Prepare and administer oral and parenteral medications and monitor intravenous (IV) infusions	Entire procedure

Ophthalmology and Otolaryngology

chapter
31

CAAHEP Competencies	Assessment
I.C.4. List major organs in each body system	Skills and Concepts – A. 1-5
I.C.5. Identify the anatomical location of major organs in each body system	Skills and Concepts – A. 1-5
I.C.6. Compare structure and function of the human body across the life span	Skills and Concepts – E. 1, 5, 6, F. 1, 2
I.C.7. Describe the normal function of each body system	Skills and Concepts – B. 1-6, D. 1
I.C.8.a. Identify common pathology related to each body system including: signs	Skills and Concepts – E. 2, 5c, d, F. 4c, d
I.C.8.b. Identify common pathology related to each body system including: symptoms	Skills and Concepts – E. 2, 5c, d, F. 4c, d
I.C.8.c. Identify common pathology related to each body system including: etiology	Skills and Concepts – E. 5b, F. 4b
I.C.9.a. Analyze pathology for each body system including: diagnostic measures	Skills and Concepts – E. 5e, F. 4e
I.C.9.b. Analyze pathology for each body system including: treatment modalities	Skills and Concepts– E. 5f, F. 4f
V.C.10. Define medical terms and abbreviations related to all body systems	Vocabulary Review – 1-30; Abbreviations – 1-12
I.P.4.a. Verify the rules of medication administration: right patient	Procedures 31.4, 31.5, 31.6, 31.7
I.P.4.b. Verify the rules of medication administration: right medication	Procedures 31.4, 31.5, 31.6, 31.7
I.P.4.c. Verify the rules of medication administration: right dose	Procedures 31.4, 31.5, 31.7
I.P.4.d. Verify the rules of medication administration: right route	Procedures 31.4, 31.5, 31.6, 31.7
I.P.4.e. Verify the rules of medication administration: right time	Procedures 31.4, 31.5, 31.7
I.P.4.f. Verify the rules of medication administration: right documentation	Procedures 31.4, 31.5, 31.6, 31.7
X.P.3. Document patient care accurately in the medical record	Procedures 31.4, 31.5, 31.6, 31.7

CAAHEP Competencies	Assessment
I.P.8. Instruct and prepare a patient for a procedure or a treatment	Procedures 31.1, 31.2, 31.3, 31.4, 31.5, 31.6, 31.7
I.P.9. Assist provider with a patient exam	Procedures 31.1, 31.2, 31.3, 31.4
I.P.3. Perform patient screening using established protocols	Procedures 31.1, 31.2, 31.3

ABHES Competencies	Assessment
2. Anatomy and Physiology a. List all body systems and their structures and functions	Skills and Concepts – A. 1-5, B. 1-6, D. 1
b. Describe common diseases, symptoms, and etiologies as they apply to each system	Skills and Concepts – E. 2, 5b, c, d, F. 4b, c, d
c. Identify diagnostic and treatment modalities as they relate to each body system	Skills and Concepts – E. 2, 5e, f, F. 4e, f
3. Medical Terminology c. Apply medical terminology for each specialty	Vocabulary Review – A. 1-10, B. 1-10, C. 1-9
d. Define and use medical abbreviations when appropriate and acceptable	Abbreviations – 1-12
4. Medical Law and Ethics a. Follow documentation guidelines	Procedures 31.1 – 31.7
8. Clinical Procedures a. Practice standard precautions and perform disinfection/sterilization techniques	Procedures 31.4, 31.5, 31.6, 31.7
c. Assist provider with general/physical examination	Procedures 31.1, 31.2, 31.3

VOCABULARY REVIEW

Using the word pool on the right, find the correct word to match the definition. Write the word on the line after the definition.

Amandeep Kaur

Group A

1. A state of rest or balance due to the equal action of opposing forces ___equilibrium___
2. The lowest part of the brain, continuous with the top of the spinal cord ___medulla oblongata___
3. Having (blood) vessels that conduct or circulate liquids (blood) ___vascular___
4. The region of the cerebral cortex that receives auditory data ___auditory cortex___
5. Relating to balance when moving at an angle or rotating ___Dynamic equilibrium___
6. Involving the sensory nerves, especially as they affect hearing ___sensorineural___
7. Involving, relating, or seeing with both eyes ___Binocular___
8. Relating to balance when moving in a straight line ___static equilibrium___
9. The middle part of the brain through which sensory impulses pass to reach the cerebral cortex ___thalamus___
10. Having two outward curving surfaces on a lens ___biconvex___

Word Pool
- binocular
- vascular
- biconvex
- sensorineural
- equilibrium
- dynamic equilibrium
- static equilibrium
- medulla oblongata
- thalamus
- auditory cortex

Group B

1. An instrument used to measure intraocular pressure ___Tonometer___
2. A medicine or substance capable of damaging cranial nerve VIII or the organs of hearing and balance ___ototoxic___
3. A sound in one or both ears such as buzzing, ringing, or whistling, occurring without an external stimulus ___tinnitus___
4. Used to diagnose glaucoma and inspect ocular movement ___gonioscopy___
5. An excessive discharge of sebum from the sebaceous glands, forming greasy scales or crusty areas on the body ___seborrhea___
6. Capable of being heard ___audible___
7. Extreme sensitivity to light ___photophobia___
8. Any substance or medication that causes constriction of the pupil ___miotic___
9. A condition where the ossicles of the middle ear become fused and act as a single unit instead of individual bones, which restricts their movement and results in conductive hearing loss ___otosclerosis___
10. Dull or dim vision, with no apparent organic defect ___amblyopia___

Word Pool
- audible
- amblyopia
- photophobia
- tonometer
- gonioscopy
- miotic
- otosclerosis
- ototoxic
- tinnitus
- seborrhea

Group C

1. Dizziness; abnormal sensations of movement when there is none
_____vertigo_____

2. The unit of measurement used in hearing examinations; a wave frequency equal to 1 cycle per second _____hertz_____

3. A medicated eye drop that dilates the pupil and enhances visualization of the eye structures _____mydriatic_____

4. Characterized by the formation and/or discharge of pus
_____suppurative_____

5. To turn the eyelid inside out; this typically is done by the provider to inspect the area for foreign bodies _____everts_____

6. Allied healthcare professional who specializes in evaluation of hearing function, detection of hearing impairment, and determination of the anatomic site of impairment
_____audiologist_____

7. A usually chronic, recurrent skin disease marked by bright red patches covered with silvery scales _____psoriasis_____

8. A thin, watery, serum-like drainage _____serous_____

9. The lens of the eye flattens to adjust to something seen at a distance or thickens for close vision; process where the lens flattens or thickens its shape _____accommodation_____

Word Pool
- psoriasis
- suppurative
- vertigo
- accommodation
- mydriatic
- hertz
- audiologist
- serous
- everts

ABBREVIATIONS

Write out what each of the following abbreviations stands for.

1. AD _____Right Ear_____
2. ENT _____Ear, Nose, Throat_____
3. AK _____Astigmatic Keratotomy_____
4. OAE _____Otoacoustic Emissions_____
5. EOM _____Extraocular Movement_____
6. TM _____Tympanic Movement_____
7. IOL _____Intraocular lens_____
8. UNHS _____Universal Newborn Hearing Screening_____
9. LASIK _____laser-assisted in situ Keratomileusis_____
10. MY _____Myopia_____
11. PDR _____Proliferative diabetic Retinopathy_____
12. VA _____Visual Acuity_____

SKILLS AND CONCEPTS

A. Anatomy of the Eye

1. List and describe the three layers of the eyeball. _____
    outer :- contain white, opaque sclera, transparent cornea
    Middle :- Choroid, Iris, ciliary body
    Inner :- Retina, lens

2. List and describe the two light-sensitive neurons located on the retina. _____
    rods :- highly sensitive to light and can function in dim light.
    Cones :- function in bright light and detect color

3. There is a natural blind spot in our vision where the _____ _optic disk_ _____ is located.

4. Describe the function of the vitreous humor. _____
    It maintains the shape of posterior eye.

5. Describe the function of the aqueous humor. _____
    It helps maintain normal pressure within the eye

B. Physiology of the Eye

1. A visual impulse begins with the passage of light through the _____ _cornea_ _____, where light is
    _____ _refracted_ _____.

2. The _____ _ciliary muscle_ _____ adjusts the curvature of the _____ _lens_ _____ to again refract
    light rays so that they pass onto the _____ _retina_ _____.

3. Focused light triggers the photoreceptor cells called _____ _rods_ _____ and
    _____ _cones_ _____.

4. Light energy is converted into a(n) _____ _electrical impulse_

5. The electrical impulse is sent through the _____ _optic nerve_ _____ to the _____ _visual cortex_ _____ of
    the brain.

6. The brain interprets the light impulses and a picture is created that we perceive as
    _____ _sight_ _____.

C. Anatomy of the Ear

1. List the three structures of the outer ear. _____
    _____ _Auricle, external auditory canal_ _____

2. The three bones of the middle ear are called the _____ _ossicles_ _____

3. Give the scientific and common names of the three bones of the middle ear. _____
   _Malleus, Incus, Stapes_____

4. List the three structures of the inner ear._____
   _Cochlea, Semicircular canals, vestibule_____

5. Earwax or cerumen is secreted by modified sweat glands in the _external auditory canal_

6. Which structure helps equalize the pressure between the middle ear and the throat? _____
   _Eustachian tube_____

7. The ossicles transmit bone-conducted sound waves through the middle ear to the
   _____ _oval window_

8. Sound waves travel through the fluid of the inner ear as _____ _vibrations_ _____.

9. Located within the cochlea, the _____ _organ of corti_ contains receptors for sound.

10. Semicircular canals detect _____ _dynamic_ _____ equilibrium, and the vestibule detects
    _____ _static_ _____ equilibrium.

D. Physiology of the Ear

1. Briefly describe the physiology of the ear. _Hearing starts with the soundwaves reaching_
   the tympanic membrane. to vibrate, which causes the ossicles
   to transmit the waves to oval window. In cochlea eight nerve
   transmit ~~waves~~ auditory impulse to medulla oblongata which
   then travel to thalmus,

E. Disorders of the Eye

1. List and describe the four major types of refractive errors of the eye. _____
   Myopia;- when a person can see near object but not far object.
   hyperopia;- when a person see far object, not near object.
   presbyopia;- loss of vision due to age.
   astigmatism;- a condition where a point object incident on
   cornea is not focused to form a point image, after refraction.

2. List some common signs and symptoms of refractive errors. _____
   Squinting, frequent rubbing, headaches, blurred vision,
   fading of words at reading level.

3. List some common treatments for refractive errors. _____

eye glasses, contact lens, Lasik surgery

_____

_____

4. Write out a definition in your own words for each term or condition listed below.

   a. Strabismus failure of eyes to track together.

   _____

   b. Nystagmus constant, involuntary movement of one or both
   eyes

   c. Hordeolum localized, purulent infection of sebaceous gland
   of the eyelid

   d. Keratitis Inflammation of the cornea.

   _____

   e. Conjunctivitis Inflammation of the conjunctiva

   _____

   f. Nyctalopia Inability to see in dim light or at night

   _____

5. The following relate to cataracts.

   a. Describe cataracts. A clouding of the normal lens of the eye.

   _____

   b. List the cause (etiology) of cataracts. _____
   • Injury to eye, exposure to heat or radiation.

   c. List two signs of cataracts. (Signs are objective and can be measured or observed by others.)
   Decreased visual acuity and lens opacities.

   d. List two symptoms of cataracts. (Symptoms are subjective and can only be perceived by the patient.)
   • difficulty with night vision – increased sensitivity to light or glare.

   e. List one diagnostic procedure used for cataracts._____
   A slit lamp procedure.

   f. List one treatment commonly prescribed by the provider._____
   surgical removal of the lens.

6. Briefly describe glaucoma.

It is characterized by increased intraocular pressure, which damages the optic nerve and cause blindness of left untreated.

7. Briefly describe macular degeneration.

It is a problem with retina of eye. It happens when aging cause damage to the macule.

F. Disorders of the Ear

1. Describe the difference between conductive hearing impairment and sensorineural hearing impairment.

Conductive hearing loss occurs when something interferes with the transmission of sound from outer, middle ear to inner ear. Sensorineural hearing loss occurs from damage to the auditory nerve or to the hair cells in the inner ear.

2. Write a definition of *presbycusis* in your own words.

Loss of hearing due to age.

3. Write out a definition in your own words for each term or condition listed below.

a. Tinnitus *ringing of the ears*

b. Otitis externa *inflammation of external ear*

c. Mastoiditis *Infection of the mastoid process*

d. Otitis media *Inflammation of middle ear*

4. The following relate to Meniere's disease.

a. Describe Meniere's disease. *It is a chronic progressive condition that effect labyrinth.*

b. List the cause (etiology) of Meniere's disease. _Trauma, abnormal hormones, infections._

c. List a sign of Meniere's disease. (Signs are objective and can be measured or observed by others.)
hearing loss, vertigo and tinnitus.

d. List two symptoms of Meniere's disease. (Symptoms are subjective and can only be perceived by the patient.)
~~vert~~ preceding attack of vertigo, hearing loss, sensation of aural pressure

e. List two diagnostic procedures used for Meniere's disease. _ENG, MRI, CT scan_

f. List treatments commonly ordered by the provider for Meniere's disease. _salt restricted diet, diuretics and antihistamines._

G. The Medical Assistant's Role in Ophthalmology and Otolaryngology Procedures

1. Define the acronym _PERRLA_. _It stands for pupil equalities doctor should review during an eye exam. The list includes Pupils, Equal, Round, Reactive, Light, Accomadation._

2. Write out a definition in your own words for each term or condition listed below.

a. Blepharoptosis _dropping of the upper eyelid_

b. Exophthalmia _abnormal protrusion of the eyeball_

c. Snellen alphabetical chart _to check the visual acuity_

d. Ishihara color vision test _to check the colors._

e. Weber hearing test _a tunning fork is placed in the middle of the head and make sure both ears are equal_

f. Rinne hearing test _evalutes bone conduction verses air conduction of sound in one ear at a time with a tuning fork._

3. Briefly describe audiometric testing. _____

It is used to measure lowest intensity of sound an individual can hear.

4. List the types of treatments a medical assistant might help with in ophthalmology. _____

Patient who is tested for glasses, undergoing surgery & laser correction.

5. List the types of treatments a medical assistant might help with in otolaryngology. _____

Ear irrigation, instilling abc medication

CERTIFICATION PREPARATION
Circle the correct answer.

1. What is buzzing, ringing, or whistling in the ear(s), occurring without an external stimulus?
   a. Vertigo
   b. Presbycusis
   c. Tinnitus
   d. Astigmatism

2. Which is part of the anterior surface of the eye?
   a. Retina
   b. Lens
   c. Optic disc
   d. Macula lutea

3. The colored portion of the eye is called the
   a. iris.
   b. pupil.
   c. retina.
   d. none of the above.

4. What is the term used for a drooping upper eyelid?
   a. Hordeolum
   b. Blepharedema
   c. Keratitis
   d. Blepharoptosis

5. Which structures are located in the middle ear?
   a. Pinna, external auditory canal, tympanic membrane
   b. Semicircular canals, vestibule, cochlea
   c. Malleus, incus, stapes
   d. Oval window, eustachian tube, vestibule

6. The organ of Corti is located in the
   a. middle ear.
   b. semicircular canal.
   c. cochlea.
   d. vestibule.

7. Which could be a sign or symptom of glaucoma?
   a. Mild headaches
   b. Impaired adaptation to the dark
   c. Loss of peripheral vision, often called *tunnel vision*
   d. All of the above

8. Macular degeneration is most commonly diagnosed after age
   a. 45.
   b. 55.
   c. 65.
   d. 75.

9. What is the term for age-related hearing loss?
   a. Presbycusis
   b. Otosclerosis
   c. Otitis media
   d. Paracusis

10. Which condition could be diagnosed in an older adult patient?
    a. Macular degeneration
    b. Glaucoma
    c. Presbycusis
    d. All of the above

WORKPLACE APPLICATIONS

1. Rosie greets her patient, Harry, age 10, and his mother. Harry loves to swim in the pond on the family farm, but recently he has been having pain in his right ear and some discharge of clear fluid. It has been hard for Harry to sleep the last few days because he normally sleeps on his right side. Given this very limited information, what possible condition(s) could cause these signs and symptoms?

   _____

   _____

2. Rosie is reviewing eye and ear diseases and disorders as part of a continuing education course. Briefly describe the following diagnostic procedures:

   a. Visual acuity test _____

   _____

   b. Tonometry _____

   _____

   c. Audiometry _____

   _____

   d. Speech audiometry _____

   _____

3. Patrick Kachajian has been diagnosed with color blindness.

   a. Describe color blindness. _____

   _____

   b. Briefly describe the signs and symptoms of color blindness. _____

   _____

   c. What test is used to diagnose color blindness? _____

   _____

INTERNET ACTIVITIES

1. Using online resources, research a test used for diagnosing an eye or ear disease. Create a poster presentation, a PowerPoint presentation, or a written paper summarizing your research. Include the following points in your project:
   a. Description of the test
   b. Any contraindications for the test
   c. Patient preparation for the test
   d. What occurs during the test

2. Using online resources, research an eye or ear disease or disorder. Create a poster presentation, a PowerPoint presentation, or a written paper summarizing your research. Include the following points in your project:
   a. Description of the disease
   b. Etiology
   c. Signs and symptoms
   d. Diagnostic procedures
   e. Treatments
   f. Prognosis
   g. Prevention

3. Using online resources, research the effect that diet can have on the management of Meniere's disease. In a one-page paper, summarize the information that you found.

Procedure 31.1   Measuring Distance Visual Acuity

Name _____ Date _____ Score _____

Task: To determine the patient's degree of visual clarity at a measured distance of 20 feet using the Snellen chart.

Equipment and Supplies:
- Patient's health record
- Provider's order
- Snellen eye chart
- Disposable eye occluder or an alcohol wipe to clean the occluder before use
- Pen or pencil and paper

Standard: Complete the procedure and all critical steps in _____ minutes with a minimum score of 85% within two attempts (*or as indicated by the instructor*).

Scoring: Divide the points earned by the total possible points. Failure to perform a critical step, indicated by an asterisk (*), results in grade no higher than an 84% (*or as indicated by the instructor*).

Time: Began_____ Ended_____ Total minutes: _____

Steps:	Point Value	Attempt 1	Attempt 2
1. Wash hands or use hand sanitizer.	5		
2. Prepare the area. Make sure the room is well lit and that a distance marker is 20 feet from the chart.	5		
3. Greet the patient. Identify yourself. Verify the patient's identity with full name and date of birth. Explain the procedure to be performed in a manner that is understood by the patient. Answer any questions the patient may have on the procedure. Instruct the patient not to squint during the test because this temporarily improves vision. The patient should not have an opportunity to study the chart before the test is given. If the patient wears corrective lenses, they should be worn during the test.	5		
4. Position the patient in a standing or sitting position at the 20-foot marker.	10		
5. Check that the Snellen chart is positioned at the patient's eye level.	5		
6. If the occluder is not disposable, disinfect it before the procedure starts. Then instruct the patient to cover the left eye with the occluder and to keep both eyes open throughout the test to prevent squinting.	5		
7. Stand beside the chart and point to each row as the patient reads it aloud, starting with the 20/70 row.	5*		
8. Proceed down the rows of the chart until the smallest row the patient can read with a maximum of two errors is reached. If one or two letters are missed, the outcome is recorded with a minus sign and the number of errors (e.g., 20/40–2). If more than two errors are made, the previous line should be documented.	10*		
9. Record any of the patient's reactions while reading the chart.	10		
10. Repeat the procedure with the left eye, covering the right eye.	10		
11. Repeat the procedure with both eyes uncovered.	10		

12. Disinfect the occluder, if it is not disposable, and wash hands or use hand sanitizer.	**10**		
13. Document the procedure in the patient's record, including the date and time, visual acuity results, and any reactions by the patient. Also record whether corrective lenses were worn.	**10**		
Total Points	**100**		

Comments

CAAHEP Competencies	Step(s)
I.P.8. Instruct and prepare a patient for a procedure or a treatment	3
I.P.9. Assist provider with a patient exam	Entire procedure
I.P.3. Perform patient screening using established protocols	Entire procedure

Procedure 31.2 Assess Color Acuity Using the Ishihara Test

Name _____ Date _____ Score _____

Task: To assess a patient's color acuity correctly and record the results.

Equipment and Supplies:
- Patient's health record
- Provider's order
- Room with natural light if possible
- Ishihara color plate book
- Pen, pencil, and paper
- Watch with a second hand

Standard: Complete the procedure and all critical steps in _____ minutes with a minimum score of 85% within two attempts (*or as indicated by the instructor*).

Scoring: Divide the points earned by the total possible points. Failure to perform a critical step, indicated by an asterisk (*), results in grade no higher than an 84% (*or as indicated by the instructor*).

Time: Began_____ Ended_____ Total minutes: _____

Steps:	Point Value	Attempt 1	Attempt 2
1. Assemble the equipment and prepare the room for testing. The room should be quiet and illuminated with natural light.	10		
2. Greet the patient. Identify yourself. Verify the patient's identity with full name and date of birth. Explain the procedure to be performed in a manner that is understood by the patient. Answer any questions the patient may have on the procedure. Use a practice card during the explanation and make sure the patient understands that he or she has 3 seconds to identify each plate.	10		
3. Hold up the first plate at a right angle to the patient's line of vision and 30 inches from the patient. Be sure both of the patient's eyes are kept open during the test	15*		
4. Ask the patient to tell you the number on the plate. Record the plate number and the patient's answer	15		
5. Continue this sequence until all 11 plates have been read. If the patient cannot identify the number on the plate, place an X in the record for that plate number.	15		
6. Include any unusual symptoms such as eye rubbing, squinting, or excessive blinking in your record.	15		
7. Place the book back in its cardboard sleeve and return it to its storage space.	10		
8. Document the procedure in the patient's health record, including the date and time, the testing results, and any patient symptoms shown during the test.	10		
Total Points	100		

Comments

CAAHEP Competencies	Step(s)
I.P.8. Instruct and prepare a patient for a procedure or a treatment	2
I.P.9. Assist provider with a patient exam	Entire procedure
I.P.3. Perform patient screening using established protocols	Entire procedure
ABHES Competencies	**Step(s)**
8.c. Assist provider with general/physical examination	Entire procedure

Procedure 31.3   Measuring Hearing Acuity with an Audiometer

Name _____ Date _____ Score _____

Task: To perform audiometric testing of hearing acuity.

Equipment and Supplies:
- Patient's health record
- Provider's order
- Audiometer with adjustable headphones and graph paper
- Quiet area

Standard: Complete the procedure and all critical steps in _____ minutes with a minimum score of 85% within two attempts (*or as indicated by the instructor*).

Scoring: Divide the points earned by the total possible points. Failure to perform a critical step, indicated by an asterisk (*), results in grade no higher than an 84% (*or as indicated by the instructor*).

Time: Began_____ Ended_____ Total minutes: _____

Steps:	Point Value	Attempt 1	Attempt 2
1. Wash hands or use hand sanitizer, assemble the equipment, and bring the patient into a quiet area.	10		
2. Greet the patient. Identify yourself. Verify the patient's identity with full name and date of birth. Explain the procedure to be performed in a manner that is understood by the patient. Answer any questions the patient may have on the procedure.	10		
3. Explain that the audiometer measures whether the patient can hear various sound wave frequencies through the headphones. Each ear is tested separately. When the patient hears a frequency, he or she should raise a hand or push the button to signal the medical assistant.	10		
4. Place the headphones over the patient's ears, making sure they are adjusted for comfort.	10		
5. The audiometer tests each ear separately, starting at a low frequency. If the results are not automatically recorded by the machine, the medical assistant documents the patient's response to the frequencies on a graph or audiogram. Results for the left ear are marked with an X, and those for the right ear are marked with an O.	10*		
6. Frequencies are increased gradually to test the patient's ability to hear. Each response by the patient is documented.	10		
7. After one ear has been tested, the other ear is then tested, and the results are documented.	10		
8. The results are given to the provider for interpretation or downloaded into the patient's electronic health record for the provider to review.	10		
9. The equipment is sanitized and disinfected according to the manufacturer's guidelines.	10		
10. Wash hands or use hand sanitizer.	10		
Total Points	100		

Comments

CAAHEP Competencies	Step(s)
I.P.8. Instruct and prepare a patient for a procedure or a treatment	2, 3
I.P.9. Assist provider with a patient exam	Entire procedure
I.P.3. Perform patient screening using established protocols	Entire procedure
ABHES Competencies	**Step(s)**
8.c. Assist provider with general/physical examination	Entire procedure

Procedure 31.4   Irrigate a Patient's Eye

Name _____   Date _____   Score _____

Tasks: Irrigate a patient's eye and document patient care.

Equipment and Supplies:
- Provider's order
- Patient health record
- Drug reference information
- Sterile ophthalmic irrigation solution and supplies
- Disposable waterproof pad and towels
- Basin
- Sterile gauze
- Gloves

Standard: Complete the procedure and all critical steps in _____ minutes with a minimum score of 85% within two attempts (*or as indicated by the instructor*).

Scoring: Divide the points earned by the total possible points. Failure to perform a critical step, indicated by an asterisk (*), results in grade no higher than an 84% (*or as indicated by the instructor*).

Time: Began_____ Ended_____ Total minutes: _____

Steps:	Point Value	Attempt 1	Attempt 2
1. Wash hands or use hand sanitizer.	5		
2. Select the right medication (fluid) from the storage area. Check the medication label against the order. Check for the right name, form, and route. Check the expiration date to make sure the fluid is not expired. Verify the right dose and the right time.	5*		
3. Using the drug reference information and the order, review the information on the medication.	5		
4. Perform the second medication check. Check the medication label against the order. Check for the right name, form, dose, and route.	5*		
5. Assemble the supplies required for the procedure.	5		
6. Perform the third medication check. Check the medication label against the order. Check for the right name, form, dose, and route.	5*		
7. Prior to entering the exam room, knock on the door and give it a moment. Greet the patient. Identify yourself. Verify the patient's identity with full name and date of birth. Make sure the patient's information matches the order and the record.	10*		
8. Provide the right education to the patient. Explain the procedure ordered, provider ordering the procedure, the desired effect, and common side effects. Answer any questions the patient may have. Use language the patient can understand. Ask the patient if he or she has any allergies. If the patient refuses the procedure, notify the provider.	10		

9. Using room-temperature fluid, set up the equipment. If using an IV bag, prime or run fluid through the tubing. If using a prepackaged solution, remove the cover. If using a bulb syringe, pour the required fluid into a basin. Remember to palm the label. Draw the solution into the bulb syringe.	**5**		
10. Assist the patient into a sitting or supine position. Have the patient remove glasses or contact lens. Ask the patient to turn the head towards the side of the affected eye. Place the disposable waterproof pad over the patient's neck and shoulder. Place or have the patient hold the drainage basin next to the affected eye.	**5**		
11. Put on gloves. Moisten a gauze pad with the irrigation fluid. Using the gauze, clean the eyelid from the inner to outer canthus. Discard the gauze after each wipe.	**5**		
12. Perform the right technique. With your nondominant hand, separate and hold the eyelids using the index finger and thumb. With the dominant hand, hold the irrigation equipment on or near the bridge of the nose.	**5***		
13. Direct the solution towards the lower conjunctiva of the inner canthus. Allow a steady flow of solution to slowly flush the eye from the inner to the outer canthus. Do not touch the tip of the irrigation equipment to the eye.	**10***		
14. Continue until the ordered amount of fluid has flushed the eye. Dry the eyelid with sterile gauze, moving from the inner to outer canthus.	**5**		
15. Help the patient into a comfortable position. Clean up the area. Remove gloves and wash hands or use hand sanitizer.	**5**		
16. Document the procedure in the health record. Include allergies, teaching or instructions provided, the provider ordering the irrigation, the fluid used for the irrigation, the amount used, the site, and how the patient tolerated the procedure.	**10***		
Total Points	**100**		

Documentation

Comments

CAAHEP Competencies	Step(s)
I.P.4.a. Verify the rules of medication administration: right patient	7
I.P.4.b. Verify the rules of medication administration: right medication	2, 4, 6
I.P.4.c. Verify the rules of medication administration: right dose	2, 4, 6
I.P.4.d. Verify the rules of medication administration: right route	2, 4, 6
I.P.4.e. Verify the rules of medication administration: right time	2
I.P.4.f. Verify the rules of medication administration: right documentation	16
III.P.2. Select appropriate barrier/personal protective equipment.	11
X.P.3. Document patient care accurately in the medical record	16
I.P.8. Instruct and prepare a patient for a procedure or a treatment	8
ABHES Competencies	**Step(s)**
8.a. Practice standard precautions and perform disinfection/sterilization techniques	11

Procedure 31.5   Instill an Eye Medication

Name _____ Date _____ Score _____

Tasks: Instill an eye drop or ointment and document medication administration.

Equipment and Supplies:
- Provider's order
- Patient health record
- Drug reference information
- Sterile ophthalmic eye drops or ointment
- Sterile gauze
- Gloves

Standard: Complete the procedure and all critical steps in _____ minutes with a minimum score of 85% within two attempts (*or as indicated by the instructor*).

Scoring: Divide the points earned by the total possible points. Failure to perform a critical step, indicated by an asterisk (*), results in grade no higher than an 84% (*or as indicated by the instructor*).

Time: Began_____ Ended_____ Total minutes: _____

Steps:	Point Value	Attempt 1	Attempt 2
1. Wash hands or use hand sanitizer.	5		
2. Select the right medication from the storage area. Check the medication label against the order. Check for the right name, form, and route. Check the expiration date to make sure the drug is not expired. Verify the right dose and the right time.	5*		
3. Using the drug reference information and the order, review the information on the medication.	5		
4. Perform the second medication check. Check the medication label against the order. Check for the right name, form, dose, and route.	5*		
5. Assemble the supplies required for the procedure.	10		
6. Perform the third medication check. Check the medication label against the order. Check for the right name, form, dose, and route.	10*		
7. Prior to entering the exam room, knock on the door and give it a moment. Greet the patient. Identify yourself. Verify the patient's identity with full name and date of birth. Make sure the patient's information matches the order and the record.	10*		
8. Provide the right education to the patient. Explain the medication ordered, provider ordering the medication, the desired effect, and common side effects. Answer any questions the patient may have. Use language the patient can understand. Ask the patient if he or she has any allergies. If the patient refuses the medication, notify the provider.	10		
9. Assist the patient into a sitting or supine position. Ask the patient to tilt the head backward and look up.	5		
10. Put on gloves. If crusting or draining is present on the eyelid, gently wash the area from the inner to outer canthus. Discard the gauze after each wipe. Dry the area.	10		

11. Perform the right technique. With your nondominant hand holding a sterile gauze, pull the lower conjunctival sac downward creating a pocket for the medication. Instruct the patient to look up. 　a. For the eye drops: with your dominant hand, hold the bottle or the dropper ¾ inch away from the conjunctival sac. Drop the required number of drops into the eye. If the drop misses the eye or the patient blinks, wipe the liquid on the skin and repeat the drop. Have the person gently press against the inner corner of the eye and the nose bone for 1 minute. Have the person keep the eye closed for 2-3 minutes after the administration of the drop. 　b. For eye ointment: with the dominant hand, hold the ointment container above the lower lid. Working from inner to outer canthus, apply a small layer of ointment along the inner lower lid margin. Have the patient close the eye and rub the eyelid in a circular motion. Wipe up any extra ointment.	10*		
12. Help the patient into a comfortable position. Clean up the area. Remove gloves and wash hands or use hand sanitizer.	5		
13. Document the procedure in the health record. Include allergies; teaching or instructions provided; the provider ordering the medication; the medication name, dose, route; and how the patient tolerated the medication.	10*		
Total Points	100		

Documentation

Comments

CAAHEP Competencies	Step(s)
I.P.4.a. Verify the rules of medication administration: right patient	7
I.P.4.b. Verify the rules of medication administration: right medication	2, 4, 6
I.P.4.c. Verify the rules of medication administration: right dose	2, 4, 6
I.P.4.d. Verify the rules of medication administration: right route	2, 4, 6
I.P.4.e. Verify the rules of medication administration: right time	2
I.P.4.f. Verify the rules of medication administration: right documentation	13
III.P.2. Select appropriate barrier/personal protective equipment.	10
X.P.3. Document patient care accurately in the medical record	13
I.P.8. Instruct and prepare a patient for a procedure or a treatment	8
ABHES Competencies	**Step(s)**
8.a. Practice standard precautions and perform disinfection/ sterilization techniques	10

Procedure 31.6 Irrigate a Patient's Ear

Name _____ Date _____ Score _____

Tasks: Irrigate a patient's ear and document patient care.

Equipment and Supplies:
- Provider's order
- Patient health record
- Ear wash basin
- Elephant ear wash system (or other ear wash system)
- Disposable waterproof pad and towels
- Thermometer (optional)
- Otoscope and disposable speculum (optional)
- Gauze
- Gloves
- Sterile water or saline
- Waste container

Order: Irrigate left ear with warm sterile water.

Standard: Complete the procedure and all critical steps in _____ minutes with a minimum score of 85% within two attempts (*or as indicated by the instructor*).

Scoring: Divide the points earned by the total possible points. Failure to perform a critical step, indicated by an asterisk (*), results in grade no higher than an 84% (*or as indicated by the instructor*).

Time: Began_____ Ended_____ Total minutes: _____

Steps:	Point Value	Attempt 1	Attempt 2
1. Wash hands or use hand sanitizer.	5		
2. Select the right medication (fluid) from the storage area. Check the medication label against the order. Check for the right name and route; check the expiration date.	5*		
3. Assemble the equipment and supplies needed. Perform the second medication check. Check the medication (fluid) name and route against the order.	5*		
4. Clean up the work area and perform the third medication check. Check the medication (fluid) name and route against the order.	5*		
5. Prior to entering the exam room, knock on the door and give it a moment. Greet the patient. Identify yourself. Verify the patient's identity with full name and date of birth. Make sure the patient's information matches the order and the record.	5*		
6. Provide the right education to the patient. Explain the procedure ordered, provider ordering the procedure, the desired effect, and common side effects of ear irrigations. Answer any questions the patient may have. Use language the patient can understand. If the patient refuses the procedure, notify the provider.	5		

7.	Prepare the equipment. Warm the irrigating solution to body temperature (98.6° F [check with a thermometer]) or until it is lukewarm. Lukewarm is neither hot nor cold. Fill the spray bottle with the fluid. Attach the disposal tip to the nozzle on the hose. If another type of ear wash system is being used, prepare the equipment and the fluid.	5		
8.	Assist the patient into a sitting position. Wrap a waterproof pad around the person's shoulder, protecting the clothing. Have a towel available for the patient if needed. Have the patient tilt his or her head towards the affected ear. Have the patient hold the ear wash basin under the affected ear.	10		
9.	Put on gloves. Using gauze, wipe any debris from the outer ear.	10		
10.	Insert the disposable tip gently into the ear. Do not insert too far since it could injure the canal. If possible, gently pull the pinna up and back if the patient is older than age 3. For patients younger than 3, pull the pinna down and back.	5*		
11.	Keeping the tubing straight, spray the fluid in the ear canal. Aim the fluid towards the top of the ear canal.	5		
12.	Continue irrigating until the solution is used, the maximum time has been reached, the desired result is achieved, or the patient has problems with the procedure. Empty the ear wash basin when it fills. Observe the fluid for any substances (i.e., cerumen).	5		
13.	Dry the outside of the ear with gauze. If facility procedure indicates, use otoscope to observe canal. Attach the speculum to the otoscope. Straighten the ear canal by pulling the appropriate direction on the pinna. Gently insert the otoscope. Observe the canal.	5		
14.	Place a clean, absorbent towel on the examination table. Have the patient rest quietly with the head turned to the irrigated side while you wait for the provider to return to check the affected ear.	10*		
15.	Clean up the work area. Remove your gloves and dispose in the waste container. Sanitize your hands.	5		
16.	Document the procedure in the health record. Include teaching or instructions provided, the provider ordering the irrigation, the fluid used for the irrigation, the amount used, the site, and how the patient tolerated the procedure.	10*		
	Total Points	100		

Documentation

Comments

CAAHEP Competencies	Step(s)
I.P.4.a. Verify the rules of medication administration: right patient	5
I.P.4.b. Verify the rules of medication administration: right medication	2, 3, 4
I.P.4.d. Verify the rules of medication administration: right route	2, 3, 4
I.P.4.f. Verify the rules of medication administration: right documentation	16
III.P.2. Select appropriate barrier/personal protective equipment.	9
X.P.3. Document patient care accurately in the medical record	16
I.P.8. Instruct and prepare a patient for a procedure or a treatment	6
ABHES Competencies	**Step(s)**
8.a. Practice standard precautions and perform disinfection/ sterilization techniques	9

Procedure 31.7   Instill Ear Drops

Name _____ Date _____ Score _____

Tasks: Instill ear drops and document medication administration.

Equipment and Supplies:
- Provider's order
- Patient health record
- Drug reference information
- Otic drops
- Gauze
- Gloves

Standard: Complete the procedure and all critical steps in _____ minutes with a minimum score of 85% within two attempts (*or as indicated by the instructor*).

Scoring: Divide the points earned by the total possible points. Failure to perform a critical step, indicated by an asterisk (*), results in grade no higher than an 84% (*or as indicated by the instructor*).

Time: Began_____ Ended_____ Total minutes: _____

Steps:	Point Value	Attempt 1	Attempt 2
1. Wash hands or use hand sanitizer.	5		
2. Select the right medication from the storage area. Check the medication label against the order. Check for the right name, form, and route. Check the expiration date to make sure the drug is not expired. Verify the right dose and the right time.	5*		
3. Using the drug reference information and the order, review the information on the medication.	5		
4. Perform the second medication check. Check the medication label against the order. Check for the right name, form, dose, and route.	5*		
5. Assemble the supplies required for the procedure.	5		
6. Perform the third medication check. Check the medication label against the order. Check for the right name, form, dose, and route.	5*		
7. Prior to entering the exam room, knock on the door and give it a moment. Greet the patient. Identify yourself. Verify the patient's identity with full name and date of birth. Make sure the patient's information matches the order and the record.	10*		
8. Provide the right education to the patient. Explain the medication ordered, provider ordering the medication, the desired effect, and common side effects. Answer any questions the patient may have. Use language the patient can understand. Ask the patient if he or she has any allergies. If the patient refuses the medication, notify the provider.	10		
9. Assist the patient into a sitting position or in a side-lying position on the unaffected side.	5		
10. Warm the medication bottle with your hands if needed. The drops should be at room temperature. Shake the medication if needed. Put on gloves.	5		

11. Perform the right technique. Have the patient tilt his/her head so the affected ear is upward. If cerumen or drainage is blocking the canal, gently remove it with a cotton-tipped application.	5		
12. Remove the cover of the bottle. With your nondominant hand, gently pull the pinna up and back if the patient is older than age 3. This straightens the external auditory canal. For patients younger than 3, pull the pinna down and back.	5		
13. Hold the dropper firmly in your dominant hand. Place the tip of the dropper about ½ inch above the ear canal. Be sure not to contaminate the dropper by touching it to the patient. Carefully drop the required number of drops in the patient's ear. Replace the cover.	10*		
14. Have the patient keep the ear facing up for 3-5 minutes, depending on the medication.	5		
15. Help the patient into a comfortable position. Clean up the area. Remove gloves and wash hands or use hand sanitizer.	5		
16. Document the procedure in the health record. Include allergies; teaching or instructions provided; the provider ordering the medication; the medication name, dose, route; and how the patient tolerated the medication.	10*		
Total Points	**100**		

Documentation

Comments

CAAHEP Competencies	Step(s)
I.P.4.a. Verify the rules of medication administration: right patient	7
I.P.4.b. Verify the rules of medication administration: right medication	2, 4, 6
I.P.4.c. Verify the rules of medication administration: right dose	2, 4, 6
I.P.4.d. Verify the rules of medication administration: right route	2, 4, 6
I.P.4.e. Verify the rules of medication administration: right time	2
I.P.4.f. Verify the rules of medication administration: right documentation	16
III.P.2. Select appropriate barrier/personal protective equipment.	10
X.P.3. Document patient care accurately in the medical record	16
I.P.8. Instruct and prepare a patient for a procedure or a treatment	8
ABHES Competencies	**Step(s)**
8.a. Practice standard precautions and perform disinfection/sterilization techniques	10

Amardeep Kaur
Removal of small section from a activated

Dermatology

CAAHEP Competencies	Assessment
I.C.4. List major organs in each body system	Skills and Concepts – A. 2-9
I.C.5. Identify the anatomical location of major organs in each body system	Skills and Concepts – A. 2-9
I.C.6. Compare structure and function of the human body across the life span	Skills and Concepts – B. 7
I.C.7. Describe the normal function of each body system	Skills and Concepts – A. 1-9, B. 1-7
I.C.8.a. Identify common pathology related to each body system including: signs	Skills and Concepts – C. 1-2, 3c, d
I.C.8.b. Identify common pathology related to each body system including: symptoms	Skills and Concepts – C. 1-2, 3c, d
I.C.8.c. Identify common pathology related to each body system including: etiology	Skills and Concepts – C. 3b
I.C.9.a. Analyze pathology for each body system including: diagnostic measures	Skills and Concepts – C. 3e, 6
I.C.9.b. Analyze pathology for each body system including: treatment modalities	Skills and Concepts – C. 3f, 8, 13
V.C.10. Define medical terms and abbreviations related to all body systems	Vocabulary Review – A. 1-10, B. 1-11; Abbreviations – 1-9
ABHES Competencies	**Assessment**
2. Anatomy and Physiology a. List all body systems and their structures and functions	Skills and Concepts – A. 1-9, B. 1-7
b. Describe common diseases, symptoms, and etiologies as they apply to each system	Skills and Concepts – C. 1-2, 3b, c, d
c. Identify diagnostic and treatment modalities as they relate to each body system	Skills and Concepts – C. 1-2, 3e, f, 6, 8, 13
3. Medical Terminology c. Apply medical terminology for each specialty	Vocabulary Review – A. 1-10, B. 1-11
d. Define and use medical abbreviations when appropriate and acceptable	Abbreviations – 1-9

VOCABULARY REVIEW

Using the word pool on the right, find the correct word to match the definition. Write the word on the line after the definition.

Amandeep Kaur

Group A

Word Pool
- pathogen
- synthesis
- epithelial cells
- strata
- basal
- melanocytes
- collagen
- elastin
- excoriated
- glomerulonephritis

1. To strip off or remove the skin from an area
    excoriated

2. Naturally or artificially formed layers of material, usually multiple layers _strata_

3. The most abundant structural protein found in skin and other connective tissues; provides strength and cushioning to many parts of the body _collagen_

4. Kidney disease affecting the capillaries of the nephron (glomeruli); characterized by albuminuria, edema, and hypertension
    glomerulonephritis

5. Form cellular sheets that cover surfaces, both inside and outside the body; cells are closely packed, take on different shapes, and strongly stick to each other _epithelial cells_

6. A highly elastic protein in connective tissue that allows tissues to resume their shape after stretching or contracting; found abundantly in the dermis of the skin _elastin_

7. Cells of the stratum germinativum that produce a brownish pigment called *melanin*; melanin gives skin its color
    melanocytes

8. A disease-causing organism _pathogen_

9. Bottom layer _basal_

10. Formation of a chemical compound from simpler compounds or elements _synthesis_

Group B

1. A reddish pigment that results from the breakdown of red blood cells in the liver _____ bilirubin _____

2. Discoloration of the skin caused by the escape of blood into the tissues from ruptured blood vessels; typically caused by bruising _____ ecchymosis _____

3. Lack of skin pigmentation, especially in patches _____ leukoderma _____

4. The technique of exposing tissue to extreme cold to produce a well-defined area of cell destruction _____ cryosurgery _____

5. A descriptive term for things or conditions that threaten life or well-being; the opposite of benign _____ malignment _____

6. Tiny openings in the surface of the skin that allow gases, liquids, or microscopic particles to pass _____ pores _____

7. A yellow discoloration of the skin and mucous membranes caused by deposits of bile _____ jaundice _____

8. Enlargement due to an abnormal multiplication of cells _____ hyperplasia _____

9. Very small, round hemorrhage in the skin or mucous membrane _____ petechiae _____

10. Not transparent; cloudy or murky _____ opaque _____

11. A noncancerous condition, not malignant, harmless _____ benign _____

Word Pool
- hyperplasia
- opaque
- benign
- malignant
- leukoderma
- jaundice
- bilirubin
- petechiae
- ecchymosis
- cryosurgery
- pores

ABBREVIATIONS

Write out what each of the following abbreviations stands for.

1. UV _____ Ultraviolet light _____
2. HPV _____ Human Papillomavirus _____
3. HSV-1 _____ Herpes Simplex Virus type 1 _____
4. OTC _____ Over the counter drugs _____
5. TIM _____ Topical Immunomodulators _____
6. PDT _____ Photodynamic Therapy _____
7. KS _____ Kaposi Sarcoma _____
8. SLE _____ Systemic Lupus Erythematosus _____
9. PUVA _____ Psoralen Plus ultraviolet A light Therapy _____

SKILLS AND CONCEPTS

Answer the following questions. Write your answer on the line or in the space provided.

A. Anatomy of the Integumentary System

1. What are the five functions of the integumentary system? Which is the most important? _Regulate temperature_
   Protection, excretion, Sensory organ activity, synthesis of vitamin D.
   most important is the sensory organ.

2. The upper layer of the skin is the ____epidermis____, and the lower layer of the skin is the
   ____dermis____.

3. Where are new skin cells formed in the epidermis? _Basal layer of the epidermis_

4. Describe what happens as a new epidermal cell moves from the basal layer of the epidermis to the upper layer of the epidermis?
   Cytoplasm then replaced with keratin. Once it done, it
   is called Keratinocytes

5. Write a brief definition of *dermal papillae*.
   It is define as the part where two layers of skin meet.

6. If the dermal-epidermal junction is damaged by a burn, irritation, abrasion, or friction, what may develop at the site of the damage?
   a blister formed

7. Name the two types of sweat glands. Where are they located in the skin and throughout the body?
   Eccrine and apocrine. Eccrine glands found over most of
   the body. Apocrine glands can found in the pubic
   and underarm areas.

8. Subcutaneous tissue is made up of what two types of tissue? ____
   Loose connective tissue and adipose fat.

B. Physiology of the Integumentary System

1. Describe how skin helps protect the body. _The keratin in our skin cells protects_
   us from excessive fluid loss and dehydration. Finally, melanin
   in the epidermis of the skin protects body from UV light

2. Describe how skin functions as a sensory organ. _The skin has many sensory_
   receptors. This allows us to respond to the environment
   and make appropriate changes to keep ourselves from harm

3. List the four types of sensory receptors located throughout the skin. _____

Pain, pressure, heat, cold _____

4. Describe how skin aids the body in temperature regulation. _skin have thermoregulator._
when we are cold, it constricts blood vessel close to skin.
This preserve body heat. When we are hot, it can
produce sweat that evaporates and cool us off. This is all
part of homeostasis.

5. Describe how skin aids the body in excretion. Give three examples of substances that the skin can excrete.

The body can regulate amount of sweat produced
and the chemical content of the sweat. We
excrete three substances: sweat, water,
electrolytes.

6. In your own words, describe how the skin helps in the process of vitamin D synthesis. _When skin_
is exposed to the sun's UV rays, it manufactures a
vitamin D precursor molecule. The molecule is carried
to liver and kidneys by way of the blood. The precursor
molecule is then converted by to the active form of vitamin D
that body can use.

7. Describe the differences in integumentary system diseases and disorders as we age. _Skin changes_
are most visible sign of aging. As age increased, people
gets wrinkles and sagging skin. There is also change
in connective tissue which reduce the skin's
strength and elasticity.

C. Diseases and Disorders of the Integumentary System

1. List common signs of skin diseases and disorders. _____

Skin lesion, scale, flaky skin surface.
_____
_____
_____

2. List a common symptom of skin diseases and disorders. _____

Itching q weeping, or bleeding lesions, blisters

3. The following relate to acne vulgaris.

   a. Describe acne vulgaris. A skin condition that occurs when a hair follicle becomes plugged with oil and dead skin cells.

   b. List the cause (etiology) of acne vulgaris. excess oil production, pores clogged with dead skin cells and oil, bacterial Infection,

   c. List three signs of acne vulgaris. (Signs are objective and can be measured or observed by others.)
   large, painful nodules, cystic acne, papules,

   d. List one symptom of acne vulgaris. (Symptoms are subjective and can only be perceived by the patient.)
   whiteheads and blackhead,

   e. List one diagnostic procedure used for acne vulgaris. Skin test, physical exam

   f. List one treatment commonly ordered by the provider and two home care treatments that can be used for acne vulgaris.
   Facewash, ~~topic~~

4. Describe rosacea in your own words. ~~Rosea~~ Rosacea is a chronic disease seen most frequently in women between the ages of 30 to 60.

5. Describe cellulitis in your own words. Inflammation of the skin or cells,

6. How are fungal infections diagnosed by a provider? Blood tests are used to diagnose fungal infection,

7. What virus causes warts? Human Papillomavirus (HPV)

8. How is a herpes simplex-1 (HSV-1) infection treated? It can treated by anti-viral medication such as acyclovir (Zovirax), docosanol (Abreva) etc.

9. What are two common parasites that can infest the skin? _____

   Scabies, Pediculosis.

10. Eczema is also known by another name, atopic dermatitis

11. Describe psoriasis in your own words. _____

    An autoimmune which can affect the life cycle of skin

12. Is psoriasis contagious?   YES   (NO)

13. How is discoid lupus erythematosus treated? _____

    Cortiseal cream or ointment maybe used with an injection.

14. Describe the "rule of nines" regarding burns. The rule of nines is a tool used to estimate a burn's percentage of your total skin. It divides your body into sections by multiples of 9% each.

15. Define the four degrees of burns. • First degree:- It damage epidermis.
    • second degree:- It damage first and second layer of skin and blister forms.
    • third degree:- Burn that damage epidermis, dermis and subcutaneous tissue.
    • four degree:- Burn that extends beyond subcutaneous into muscle and bone.

16. What are the three most common types of skin cancer?_____

    Basal Cell Carcinoma, squamous cell carcinoma, Melanoma

D. Role of the Medical Assistant in Dermatology

1. Define *diascope*. A glass plate held firmly against the skin to permit observation of changes produced in underlying areas when pressure is applied.

2. Define the following types of biopsy procedures.

Excision biopsy _removal of mole_

Punch biopsy _removal of a small section from a designated location in the lesion._

Shave biopsy _Performed with a razored by cutting or shaving off the growth or lesion for a thin specimen_

3. Describe how first- and second-degree burns are treated. _In first degree burn, place a cool wet compress on the area. Apply petroleum jelly. In 2nd degree, immerse the area in cool water atleast 10 min._

4. What is the purpose of Mohs surgery? _The purpose of Mohs surgery to remove cancer._

5. Describe PUVA therapy and how it is used in dermatology. _This therapy is used to treat number of different skin diseases. Psoralin gel is applied to affected area for 10 minutes before exposure to UVA._

6. List four appearance-modification procedures performed in dermatology. _Chemical peel dermabrasion laser, resurfacing, botox, injections._

CERTIFICATION PREPARATION

Circle the correct answer.

1. Which is/are accessory structures of the integumentary system?
   a. Hair
   b. Nails
   c. Sweat glands
   d. All of the above ⟵ circled

2. What is the main function of the integumentary system?
   a. Body movement
   b. pH balance
   c. Protection
   d. All of the above ⟵ circled

3. _____ is a hard protein material that enhances the skin by making it waterproof, abrasion-resistant, and able to retain moisture.
   a. Keratin ⟵ circled
   b. Sebum
   c. Melanin
   d. Collagen

4. Peg-like projections that help fasten the dermis and epidermis together are called
   a. elastin.
   b. pores.
   c. dermal papillae. ⟵ circled
   d. stratified epithelium.

5. Which is a sign of melanoma?
   a. A mole that changes in color, size, feel, or that bleeds
   b. A firm, red nodule on the skin
   c. A flat, flesh-colored or brown scar-like lesion
   d. A flat lesion with a scaly or crusted surface

6. What vitamin is synthesized in the skin?
   a. A
   b. B_3
   c. C
   d. D

7. Which disease is a common fungal infection?
   a. Decubitus ulcer
   b. Eczema
   c. Psoriasis
   d. Dermatophytosis

8. Which condition would *not* be found on a child's skin?
   a. Eczema
   b. Birth marks
   c. Melanoma
   d. Freckles

9. Atopic dermatitis is also known as
   a. vitiligo.
   b. seborrheic dermatitis.
   c. psoriasis.
   d. eczema.

10. What is a burn in which only the first and second layers of the skin (epidermis and part of the dermis) are affected?
    a. Fourth-degree burn
    b. Vitiligo
    c. Second-degree burn
    d. Psoriasis

WORKPLACE APPLICATIONS

1. A young mother calls in and says that she is concerned about her school-age son. She got a note from school saying that another student in his class has head lice. She has checked her son's hair and skin, following directions from the school note. The mother found what she thinks are a few nits in his hair.

   a. Which laboratory test will confirm a diagnosis of head lice (pediculosis)? _____

   _____

   b. What organisms can cause pediculosis? _____

   c. What type of preventive measure can be taken to guard against acquiring a lice infestation? _____

   _____

   _____

2. Mai is going over a patient chart in preparation for a follow-up visit with the provider. The patient had a cold injury recently: frostbite on her fingers. Mai was reviewing the signs and symptoms of frostbite. List the signs and symptoms of superficial and deep frostbite.

   _____

   _____

   _____

   _____

3. Helen Rodney is a 42-year-old woman in good health. She had suffered with acne vulgaris when she was in her late teens into her early 30s. Helen has acne scars that she has decided to treat at the dermatologist. She is going to have dermabrasion today. Describe in your own words what a dermabrasion procedure is like. Describe the usual precautions that must be taken by providers and medical assistants during this procedure.

_____

_____

_____

_____

_____

INTERNET ACTIVITIES

1. Using online resources, research a test used to diagnose an integumentary system disease. Create a poster presentation, a PowerPoint presentation, or a written paper summarizing your research. Include the following points in your project:
   a. Description of the test
   b. Any contraindications for the test
   c. Patient preparation for the test
   d. What occurs during the test

2. Using online resources, research a skin disease or condition. Create a poster presentation, a PowerPoint presentation, or a written paper summarizing your research. Include the following points in your project:
   a. Description of the disease
   b. Etiology
   c. Signs and symptoms
   d. Diagnostic procedures
   e. Treatments
   f. Prognosis
   g. Prevention

3. Using online resources, research the effect of diet on the management of psoriasis. In a one-page paper, summarize the information that you found.

Allergy and Infectious Disease

chapter 33

CAAHEP Competencies	Assessment
I.C.4. List major organs in each body system	Skills and Concepts – A. 2-8
I.C.5. Identify the anatomical location of major organs in each body system	Vocabulary Review – A. 6, 8; Skills and Concepts – A. 2-4, B. 7-9; Certification Preparation – 2, 9
I.C.6. Compare structure and function of the human body across the life span	Skills and Concepts – C. 11; Certification Preparation – 10
I.C.7. Describe the normal function of each body system	Skills and Concepts – A. 1, B. 1-5, 7-10, 12
I.C.8.a. Identify common pathology related to each body system including: signs	Skills and Concepts – C. 1, 4c, 5c, 8; Certification Preparation – 7, 8; Workplace Applications – 3; Internet Activities – 2
I.C.8.b. Identify common pathology related to each body system including: symptoms	Skills and Concepts – C. 1, 4c, 5c, 8; Certification Preparation – 7, 8; Workplace Applications – 3; Internet Activities – 2
I.C.8.c. Identify common pathology related to each body system including: etiology	Skills and Concepts – C. 1, 4b, 5b, 8; Certification Preparation – 6, 8; Internet Activities – 2
I.C.9.a. Analyze pathology for each body system including: diagnostic measures	Skills and Concepts – C. 2, 4d, 5d, 9, D. 2; Internet Activities – 1, 2
I.C.9.b. Analyze pathology for each body system including: treatment modalities	Skills and Concepts – C. 3, 4e, 5e, 9, D. 4; Internet Activities – 2
I.C.10. Identify CLIA-waived tests associated with common diseases	Skills and Concepts – C. 2, 4d, 5d, 9; Certification Preparation – 4
V.C.10. Define medical terms and abbreviations related to all body systems	Vocabulary Review – A. 1-10, B. 1-12; Abbreviations – 1-25

ABHES Competencies	Assessment
2. Anatomy and Physiology a. List all body systems and their structures and functions	Skills and Concepts – A. 1-8, B. 1-5, 7-10, 12
b. Describe common diseases, symptoms, and etiologies as they apply to each system	Skills and Concepts – C. 1, 4b, c, 5b, c, 8; Certification Preparation – 6-8; Workplace Applications – 3; Internet Activities – 2
c. Identify diagnostic and treatment modalities as they relate to each body system	Skills and Concepts – C. 2, 4d, e, 5d, e, 9, D. 2, 4; Internet Activities – 1, 2

ABHES Competencies	Assessment
3. Medical Terminology	Vocabulary Review – A. 1-10, B. 1-12
c. Apply medical terminology for each specialty	
d. Define and use medical abbreviations when appropriate and acceptable	Abbreviations – 1-25

VOCABULARY REVIEW

Group A

1. A type of white blood cell that has a large, round nucleus that is surrounded by a thin layer of agranular cytoplasm

   _____

2. The cellular material that fills the area between the nucleus and the cell membrane; contains the organelles of the cell

   _____

3. Disease-causing organisms _____

4. Any living organisms of microscopic size; examples include bacteria, protozoa, fungi, parasites, and helminths; some definitions include viruses, which are not alive

   _____

5. A pathology characterized by redness, swelling, pain, tenderness, heat, and disturbed function of an area of the body; especially a reaction of tissues to injury _____

6. A clear, yellowish fluid containing white blood cells in a liquid similar to plasma; comes from the tissues of the body and is moved through the lymphatic vessels and the bloodstream

   _____

7. Large white blood cells that live in the tissues; they engulf foreign particles, microorganisms, and cell debris

   _____

8. Small masses of lymphatic tissue found mostly in the ileum of the small intestine; they are an important part of the immune system because they monitor intestinal bacteria populations and prevent the growth of pathogenic bacteria in the intestines

   _____

9. Agranulocyte that engulfs foreign particles, microorganisms, and cell debris in the blood _____

10. The internal environment of the body that is compatible with life; a steady state that is created by all the body systems working together to provide a consistent, unvarying internal environment

    _____

Word Pool
- homeostasis
- pathogens
- lymph
- Peyer patches
- monocyte
- lymphocyte
- macrophage
- microorganism
- cytoplasm
- inflammation

Group B

1. Special proteins that speed up a chemical reaction in the body
   _____

2. A substance that stimulates the production of an antibody when introduced into the body; includes toxins, bacteria, viruses, and other foreign substances _____

3. The production of exact copies of a complex molecule, such as DNA _____

4. The total collection of microorganisms and their genetic material present on or in the human body or a specific site in the human body _____

5. Protein substances produced in the blood or tissues in response to a specific antigen that destroys or weakens the antigen; part of the immune system _____

6. Undifferentiated cells that can become specialized cells in the body _____

7. The ability to live _____

8. A contraction of muscles that causes narrowing of the inside tube of a vessel _____

9. Movements or processes caused by an automatic response that doesn't require thought _____

10. To distinguish one thing from another; to make a distinction between items _____

11. Complete or whole; not altered; unbroken
    _____

12. A substance or structure that can be passed through, especially by liquids or gases _____

Word Pool
- permeable
- differentiate
- intact
- reflexes
- enzymes
- vasoconstriction
- viability
- replication
- stem cells
- antigen
- antibody
- microbiome

ABBREVIATIONS

Write out what each of the following abbreviations stands for.

1. WBC _____

2. NK _____

3. HDN _____

4. SLE _____

5. TB _____

6. DTP _____

7. MMR _____

8. ANA _____

9. CBC _____

10. CMP _____

11. CRP _____

12. ESR _____

13. MRI _____

14. AIDS _____

15. HIV _____

16. ELISA _____

17. MGUS _____

18. AML _____

19. GAS _____

20. HAV _____

21. HBV _____

22. HCV _____

23. HDV _____

24. HEV _____

25. PPE _____

SKILLS AND CONCEPTS

Answer the following questions. Write your answer on the line or in the space provided.

A. Anatomy of the Lymphatic and Immune Systems

1. List four lymphatic and immune system functions in the body._____

   _____

   _____

2. Describe lymph in your own words. _____

   _____

   _____

3. List the structures of the lymphatic system. _____

   _____

   _____

4. _____ are large white blood cells that are called _____ when they enter tissues.

5. The chemical messengers of the immune system are _____.

6. List the granular white blood cells. _____

   _____

7. List the agranular white blood cells. _____

   _____

8. Name the two types of lymphocytes that are part of specific immunity. _____

   _____

B. Immune System Levels of Defense

1. Describe the primary function of the immune system. _____

   _____

2. Define *nonspecific immunity*. _____

   _____

   _____

3. Describe the first line of defense. _____

   _____

   _____

   _____

   _____

   _____

4. List the five protective measures of the second line of defense. _____

   _____

   _____

   _____

5. Briefly describe the five ways nonspecific immunity and specific immunity differ. _____

   _____

   _____

   _____

   _____

6. List the five classes of immunoglobulins. _____

   _____

   _____

7. Describe humoral immunity and the cells it involves. _____

_____

_____

_____

_____

8. Briefly describe what antibodies do in the body._____

_____

_____

_____

9. Briefly describe cell-mediated immunity. _____

_____

_____

_____

_____

_____

10. List the four different types of T cells and briefly describe them._____

_____

_____

_____

_____

11. _____ is an immune response that causes tissue damage in the host. It is an excessive response to a stimulus or foreign agent.

12. Compare active immunity and passive immunity. _____

_____

_____

_____

_____

_____

C. Diseases and Disorders of the Immune and Lymphatic Systems

1. List common signs and symptoms of immune and lymphatic system diseases and disorders. _____

    _____

    _____

2. List three common CLIA-waived tests used to diagnose lymphatic and immune system conditions.

    _____

3. What are common treatments for autoimmune diseases and disorders? _____

    _____

    _____

    _____

    _____

4. The following relate to HIV / AIDS.

    a. Describe HIV / AIDS. _____

        _____

        _____

        _____

    b. List the cause (etiology) of HIV / AIDS. _____

        _____

    c. List three signs or symptoms of HIV / AIDS. _____

        _____

        _____

    d. List one diagnostic procedure used for HIV / AIDS. _____

        _____

    e. List one prescribed treatment commonly ordered by the provider. _____

        _____

5. The following relate to Hodgkin's lymphoma.

    a. Describe Hodgkin's lymphoma. _____

        _____

        _____

        _____

b. List the cause (etiology) of Hodgkin's lymphoma._____

_____

_____

c. List three signs or symptoms of Hodgkin's lymphoma. _____

_____

_____

d. List two diagnostic procedures used for Hodgkin's lymphoma._____

_____

_____

e. List treatments commonly ordered by the provider for Hodgkin's lymphoma._____

_____

_____

6. List the types of viral hepatitis that are transmitted via the fecal-oral route, and those that are blood-borne pathogens.

_____

_____

7. Why should anyone who is sexually active be tested for STIs?_____

_____

_____

8. What are common signs and symptoms of strep throat? _____

_____

9. Describe how influenza is diagnosed and treated. _____

_____

_____

10. What are possible complications of infectious mononucleosis? _____

_____

_____

11. Describe the differences in lymphatic and immune system diseases and disorders as we age._____

_____

_____

_____

D. The Medical Assistant's Role in Allergy and Infectious Disease Procedures

1. Describe the difference between an allergy and a sensitivity. _____

   _____

   _____

2. List the four types of skin testing for allergies. _____

   _____

3. What PPE should be worn during an examination or specimen collection from a patient with a possible respiratory infection?

   _____

4. List common over-the-counter (OTC) medications for allergy relief._____

   _____

   _____

5. Describe how you would properly prepare an allergen injection and care for the patient after the injection.

   _____

   _____

   _____

6. Why is it important to educate your patient about proper hand hygiene if he or she has a respiratory infection?

   _____

   _____

   _____

CERTIFICATION PREPARATION

Circle the correct answer.

1. Which is a granulocyte in the blood?
   a. Neutrophil
   b. Eosinophil
   c. Lymphocyte
   d. Both a and b

2. A monocyte lives in the bloodstream. Where does a macrophage live?
   a. In the bloodstream
   b. In the tissues
   c. Only in the intestines
   d. None of the above

3. What is the main function of the immune system in the body?
   a. To recognize self and destroy anything foreign
   b. To recognize self and recognize foreign
   c. To recognize foreign and preserve foreign
   d. None of the above

4. Which is a CLIA-waived test?
   a. ESR
   b. CRP
   c. CMP
   d. All of the above

5. _____ is/are a collection of WBCs, dead WBCs, bacteria, and tissue cells.
   a. Inflammation
   b. Pyrexia
   c. Pus
   d. Peyer patches

6. EBV causes what condition?
   a. Influenza
   b. Infectious mononucleosis
   c. Strep throat
   d. RSV infections

7. Which could be a sign or symptom of an auto-immune disease?
   a. Skin changes, rashes, or lesions
   b. Low-grade fever and fatigue
   c. Joint pain
   d. All of the above

8. AIDS is caused by which virus?
   a. HIV
   b. Hepatitis B virus
   c. Herpes simplex-1
   d. Epstein-Barr virus

9. Where are Peyer patches located in the body?
   a. Intestines
   b. Brain
   c. Liver
   d. All internal organs

10. Which conditions could be seen in a young child?
    a. Multiple myeloma
    b. Leukemia
    c. Allergies to food
    d. Both b and c

WORKPLACE APPLICATIONS

1. Julia rooms a new patient, Robert, and his mother. Robert is 8 years old and was having an adventure in the woods near his house. About a day later, Robert developed a rash and itching on his legs. His mother suspects poison ivy is to blame. A reaction to poison ivy would be what type of hypersensitivity reaction?

   _____

2. Julia is reviewing STIs as part of a continuing education course. Briefly describe the following STIs' common signs and symptoms for males and females.

   a. Syphilis _____

   _____

   b. Chlamydia _____

   _____

3. Monica Green was recently diagnosed with influenza.

   a. What is the cause of influenza? _____

   _____

   b. Briefly describe the signs and symptoms of influenza. _____

   _____

INTERNET ACTIVITIES

1. Using online resources, research a test used for diagnosing a lymphatic or immune system disease. Create a poster presentation, a PowerPoint presentation, or a written paper summarizing your research. Include the following points in your project:
   a. Description of the test
   b. Any contraindications for the test
   c. Patient preparation for the test
   d. What occurs during the test

2. Using online resources, research a lymphatic or immune system disease or condition. Create a poster presentation, a PowerPoint presentation, or a written paper summarizing your research. Include the following points in your project:
   a. Description of the disease
   b. Etiology
   c. Signs and symptoms
   d. Diagnostic procedures
   e. Treatments
   f. Prognosis
   g. Prevention

3. Using online resources, research the effect that diet can have on the management of autoimmune disorders. In a one-page paper, summarize the information that you found.

Gastroenterology

CAAHEP Competencies	Assessment
I.C.4. List major organs in each body system	Skills and Concepts – A. 1,2
I.C.5. Identify the anatomical location of major organs in each body system	Skills and Concepts – A. 3
I.C.6. Compare structure and function of the human body across the life span	Skills and Concepts – A. 19; Certification Preparation – 10
I.C.7. Describe the normal function of each body system	Skills and Concepts – A. 5, 7-9, 11, 12, 14-18, B. 1-8
I.C.8.a. Identify common pathology related to each body system including: signs	Skills and Concepts – C. 12, 18c, 20c; Certification Preparation – 7; Workplace Application – 1-3
I.C.8.b. Identify common pathology related to each body system including: symptoms	Skills and Concepts – C. 12, 18d, 20c; Workplace Application – 1-3
I.C.8.c. Identify common pathology related to each body system including: etiology	Skills and Concepts – C. 14, 18b, 20b, 21; Certification Preparation – 8; Workplace Application – 2, 3
I.C.9.a. Analyze pathology for each body system including: diagnostic measures	Skills and Concepts – C. 15, 18e, 20d; Workplace Application – 1, 2; Internet Activities – 4
I.C.9.b. Analyze pathology for each body system including: treatment modalities	Skills and Concepts – C. 16; Workplace Application – 2, 4
I.C.10. Identify CLIA-waived tests associated with common diseases	Skills and Concepts – C. 18e, 20d; Certification Preparation – 4
I.P.10. Perform a quality control measure	Procedure 34.3
I.A.1. Incorporate critical thinking skills when performing patient assessment	Procedure 34.1
V.C.10. Define medical terms and abbreviations related to all body systems	Vocabulary Review – A. 1-8, B. 1-8; Abbreviations – 1-30
V.P.4.b. Coach patients regarding: health maintenance	Procedure 34.2, 34.4
V.P.5.b. Coach patients appropriately considering: developmental life stage	Procedure 34.2
X.P.3. Document patient care accurately in the medical record	Procedure 34.1, 34.2, 34.3, 34.4

ABHES Competencies	Assessment
2. Anatomy and Physiology a. List all body systems and their structures and functions	Skills and Concepts – A. 1-3, 5, 7-9, 11, 12, 14-18, B. 1-8
2.b. Describe common diseases, symptoms, and etiologies as they apply to each system	Skills and Concepts – C. 12, 18bcd, 20bc; Certification Preparation – 7; Workplace Application – 1-3
2.c. Identify diagnostic and treatment modalities as they relate to each body system	Skills and Concepts – C. 15, 16, 18e, 20d; Workplace Application – 1, 2, 4; Internet Activities – 4
3. Medical Terminology c. Apply medical terminology for each specialty	Vocabulary Review – A. 1-8, B. 1-8
3.d. Define and use medical abbreviations when appropriate and acceptable	Abbreviations – 1-30
8.e. Perform specialty procedures, including but not limited to minor surgery, cardiac, respiratory, OB-GYN, neurological, and gastroenterology	Procedure 34.2, 34.3, 34.4
9. Medical Laboratory Procedures a. Practice quality control	Procedure 34.3

VOCABULARY REVIEW

Using the word pool on the right, find the correct word to match the definition. Write the word on the line after the definition.

Amandeep Kaur

Group A

1. Folds in the wall of the organ; when the organ (e.g., stomach, bladder, uterus) fills or needs to expand, the ability to unfold is due to ___rugae___

2. Secreted by the parietal cells of the stomach; necessary for the absorption of vitamin B_{12} to prevent pernicious anemia ___intrinsic factor___

3. Wave-like movement from alternating contraction and relaxation of a tubular structure (e.g., intestine), which propels the contents forward ___peristalsis___

4. A mucus-producing membrane that lines tracts and structures of the body (e.g., GI tract, respiratory tract); also called *mucosa* ___mucous membrane___

5. A glandular secretion released through a duct ___exocrine___

6. The cavity, channel, or open space within a tube or tubular organ ___lumen___

7. Lid-like structure over the glottis that prevents food and liquids from entering the trachea when swallowing occurs ___epiglottis___

8. A circular muscle that either constricts and closes the opening or relaxes and allows substances to pass through the opening ___sphincter___

Word Pool
- epiglottis
- mucous membrane
- sphincter
- rugae
- intrinsic factor
- lumen
- peristalsis
- exocrine

Amandeep Kaur

Group B

1. Surgical removal of all or part of an organ
   resection

2. A surgical procedure where the large intestine is brought though the abdominal wall, creating either a temporary or permanent opening (stoma) to allow stool to pass out of the body
   colostomy

3. Pain is felt when the pressure on the abdomen is released
   rebound pain

4. Hidden or unseen _occult_

5. A glandular secretion that is released into the blood or lymph directly (does not go through a duct) _endocrine_

6. Kidney disorder that can occur after a digestive infection with *E. coli*, Shigella, or Salmonella; red blood cells are destroyed and block the kidneys' filtering system causing acute kidney failure
   Hemolytic uremic syndrome

7. When a substance suspends tiny droplets of one liquid into a second liquid; this allows mixing two liquids that usually do not mix well such as oil and water _emulsifies_

8. Sticky substance made of mucus, food particles, and bacteria that builds up on the exposed part of the tooth
   plaque

Word Pool
- emulsifies
- endocrine
- plaque
- rebound pain
- resection
- colostomy
- hemolytic uremic syndrome
- occult

ABBREVIATIONS

Write out what each of the following abbreviations stands for.

1. GI _Gastrointestinal_
2. UES _Upper Esophageal Sphincter_
3. LES _Lower Esophageal Sphincter_
4. CCK _Cholecystokinin_
5. GER _Gastroesophageal reflux_
6. GERD _Gastroesophageal Reflux Disease_
7. EGD _Esophagogastroduodenoscopy_
8. HAV _Hepatitis A Virus_
9. PPI _Proton Pump Inhibitor_
10. CVS _Cyclic Vomiting Sampling_
11. CBC _Complete Blood Count_
12. HCV _Hepatitis C Virus_
13. IPAA _Ileal Pouch Anal Anatomosis_
14. IBS _Irritable Bowel Syndrome_

15. SIBO _Small Intestinal Bacterial Overgrowth_
16. HIDA scan _Hepatobiliary Iminodiacetic Acid_
17. ERCP _Endoscopic Retrograde Cholangiopancreatography_
18. NSAID _Non-Steriodel Anti-Inflammatory Drug_
19. HBV _Hepatitis B Virus_
20. IBD _Inflammatory Bowel Disease_
21. HDV _Hepatitis D Virus_
22. FOBT _Fecal Occult Blood test_
23. IVIg _Intravenous Immunoglobulin_
24. NAFLD _Non alcoholic fatty liver disease_
25. DRE _Digital Rectal Examination_
26. MT-sDNA _Multi-targeted Stool DNA test_
27. HEV _Hepatitis E Virus_
28. gFOBT _guaiaic fecal Occult Blood test_
29. FIT _Fecal Immunochemical Test_
30. UGI _Upper Gastrointestinal Series_

SKILLS AND CONCEPTS

Answer the following questions. Write your answer on the line or in the space provided.

A. Anatomy of the Gastrointestinal System

1. List the structures of the gastrointestinal system. _Mouth, Pharynx, esophagus, Stomach, Small Intestine, Large Intestine_

2. List the accessory organs of the gastrointestinal system. _Salivary glands, Gall bladder, Liver, Pancreas_

3. Most of the gastrointestinal system organs and accessory organs are located in which cavity of the body? _Ventral Cavity,_

4. List the three sections of the pharynx. _Nasopharynx, Oropharynx, Laryngopharynx._

5. Describe how the sphincters at the top and bottom of the esophagus function. _The Upper esophageal sphincter stops air from entering the esophagus. Lower esophagel sphincter prevents stomach contents from moving up into esophagus._

6. List the three sections of the stomach. _Fundus, Body, Pylorus._

7. Which structure allows the stomach to expand when it unfolds? _Rugae_

8. The mixture created in the stomach that consists of gastric juices and ingested food is called _Chyme_.

9. Besides being a good reservoir and secreting gastric juices, the stomach has additional roles. List two below.
It produce ghrelin and it also produce gastrin.

10. List the three sections of the small intestine. _Duodenum, Jejuneum, Ileum_

11. The small intestine contains _villi_, which are small structures that are vital to proper nutrient absorption.

12. The valve that is found between the small and large intestines is called the _ileoucal valve_

13. List the sections of the large intestine. _sigmoid colon, rectum Cecum, ascending colon, transverse colon, descending colon,_

14. Where is vitamin K synthesized in the gastrointestinal tract? _Large Intestine_

15. List the three main functions of saliva. _• It helps to moist food • It helps in swallowing • It contain enzyme to break down starches_

16. List the additional functions of the liver beyond the gastrointestinal tract. _It produce plasma proteins, break down old or damaged blood cells, break down proteins and fats and produce energy, produces bile._

17. Explain the function of the gallbladder. _The bile produced by liver. The Gall baller stores the bile._

18. List the enzymes created and excreted from the pancreas. _Trypsin, chymotrypsin, amylase, Lipase._

19. Briefly describe the changes in the gastrointestinal system over a life span. _____

Changes to the gastrointestinal system generally consist of a decrease or slowing of functions and an increased risk of digestive tract disorders.

B. Physiology of the Gastrointestinal System

Write your own definition of the terms below.

1. Digestion _Breakdown of food in order of for nutrient absorption to occur._

2. Absorption _Small intestine nutrient molecules absorbed into bloodstream from the small intestine._

3. Ingestion _taking food and liquid into the body._

4. Excretion _eliminating indigestible waste._

5. Write a description of mechanical digestion in your own words._____

Physical breakdown of food.

6. Write a description of chemical digestion in your own words._____

Enzymatic breakdown of food in the stomach after mastication.

7. The ___lacteal___ in the villus of the small intestine absorbs ___lipids___ and the cardiovascular capillaries absorb ___glucose___ and ___amino acids___ .

8. The large intestine reabsorbs ___water___ and ___electrolytes___ to prevent dehydration.

C. Disorders of the Gastrointestinal System

Write a definition in your own words for each term listed below.

1. Constipation _Inability to produce bowel movements._

2. Diarrhea Loose, watery bowel movements.

3. Flatus Gas from the intestine pass through the anus.

4. Pyrosis Heartburn

5. Hematemesis Vomiting blood.

6. Gingivitis gum disease

7. Volvulus twisting of the GI tract

8. Cirrhosis Liver disease

9. Jaundice yellow skin.

10. Halitosis bad breath.

11. Describe a cleft lip and a cleft palate.

    a. Cleft lip when the lip tissue doesn't fuse before birth.

    b. Cleft palate The failure of the palate to close during the early development of the fetus.

12. What are signs and symptoms of gastroesophageal reflux disease (GERD)?
    Belching, heartburn, nausea, regurgitation.

13. Describe a hiatal hernia. when section of upper stomach pushes through an opening of diaphrem into the chest.

14. What is the causative agent of peptic ulcers?
    Helicobacter pylori.

15. How is peptic ulcer diagnosed?
    Urea Breath test, Endoscopy, biopsy of the stomach.

16. How is a peptic ulcer treated? _____

Antibiotic, H2 blocker, lining protectant.

17. Describe the following disorders of the esophagus and stomach.

a. Achalasia _When muscles of the lower esophagus doesnot relax._

b. Esophageal varices _enlarged veins in the esophagus rupture._

c. Dumping syndrome _Rapid gastric emptying._

d. Gastritis _Inflammation of the stomach._

e. Gastroparesis _delay in gastric emptying._

18. The following relate to appendicitis.

a. Describe acute appendicitis. _Inflammation of the appendix._

b. List the cause (etiology) of acute appendicitis. _Blockage in the appendix which can increase pressure._

c. List three signs of acute appendicitis. (Signs are objective and can be measured or observed by others.)

Low fever, vomiting, diarrhea.

d. List two symptoms of acute appendicitis. (Symptoms are subjective and can only be perceived by the patient.)

Pain in the LRQ, Inability to pass gas

e. List one diagnostic procedure used for acute appendicitis. _CBC test_

f. List two treatments commonly ordered by the provider for acute appendicitis. _____

Antibiotics and appendectomy

19. Describe celiac disease. _____

Autoimmune disorder which damage the small intestine by eating food with gluten.

20. The following relate to diverticulitis.

    a. Describe diverticulitis. _Inflammation of the diverticula._

    b. List the cause (etiology) of diverticulitis. _age, Obesity, smoking, lack of exercise, low fiber diets, high animal protein diets._

    c. List three signs and symptoms of diverticulitis. _Constant LLQ pain, nausea, Diarrhea._

    d. List two diagnostic procedures used for diverticulitis. _CT scan, Blood and urine tests._

21. List two bacteria and two viruses that can cause foodborne illnesses. _Bacteria :- Shigella, E. coli_ _Virus :- Norovirus, Hepatitis A_

22. Describe the three different types of hernia below.

    a. Femoral _Bulge below the groin in upper thigh_

    b. Inguinal _Bulge forms in the groin and may extent into the scrotum._

    c. Umbilical _muscle around the umbilicus doesn't close at birth._

23. List two chronic conditions that are included in inflammatory bowel disease. _Ulcerative Colitis and Crohn's disease_

24. Disorders of the accessory organs of the gastrointestinal system include:

    a. Cholelithiasis is also known as _gallstones_

    b. A chronic liver disease where liver cells are replaced with scar tissue _cirrhosis_

    c. An inflammation of the liver _Hepatitis_

    d. An inflammation of the pancreas _Pancreatitis_

D. The Medical Assistant's Role in Gastrointestinal Procedures

Define the following terms or acronyms.

1. Striae ___stretch marks___
2. Petechiae ___Small bruise___
3. Occult ___hidden___
4. Colonoscopy ___exam to see the colon___
5. Antacids ___medicine to neutralize the stomach acid.___
6. Antiemetics ___medicine to prevent or reduce vomiting.___
7. Laxatives ___Producing bowel movement.___
8. Proton-pump inhibitors ___medicine used to reduce the amount of stomach acid.___

CERTIFICATION PREPARATION

Circle the correct answer.

1. Which is/are an accessory structure(s) of the digestive system?
   a. Liver
   b. Pancreas
   c. Large intestine
   d. Both a and b *(circled)*

2. What is the proper order of the sections of the pharynx from top down?
   a. Nasopharynx-laryngopharynx-oropharynx
   b. Oropharynx-laryngopharynx-nasopharynx
   c. Nasopharynx-oropharynx-laryngopharynx *(circled)*
   d. Laryngopharynx-nasopharynx-oropharynx

3. What is/are the main function(s) of the gastro-intestinal system?
   a. Digest and absorb nutrients
   b. Ingestion of food
   c. Elimination of waste products
   d. All of the above *(circled)*

4. Which is a CLIA-waived test?
   a. Fecal occult blood test *(circled)*
   b. CT scan
   c. Tissue biopsy
   d. Ova and parasite testing

5. _____ are ring-like muscles that appear throughout the digestive system to keep chyme moving in one direction through the organs.
   a. Sphincter *(circled)*
   b. Arrector pili
   c. Pylorus
   d. Cecum

6. Which is the enzyme secreted by the pancreas to digest carbohydrates and starches?
   a. Lipase
   b. Protease
   c. Amylase *(circled)*
   d. Pepsin

7. Which is a sign of Crohn's disease?
   a. Abdominal pain
   b. Diarrhea with loose stools, possibly blood or mucus in stool *(circled)*
   c. Nausea
   d. Fatigue and lethargy

8. Peptic ulcers can be caused by which bacteria?
   a. *Staphylococcus aureus*
   b. *Helicobacter pylori* *(circled)*
   c. Herpes virus
   d. All of the above

9. Which is an inflammation of the liver?
   a. Cholelithiasis
   b. Pancreatitis
   c. Diverticulitis
   d. Hepatitis *(circled)*

10. Which condition could be seen in an older adult patient?
    a. GERD
    b. Cancer of the stomach
    c. Diverticulitis
    d. All of the above *(circled)*

WORKPLACE APPLICATION

1. Martha calls into Walden-Martin Family Medical (WMFM) Clinic and speaks to Samuel. She is wondering if she should come in and see a provider because she has been having recurring pain in the upper-right quadrant of her abdomen. The pain can be intense, but then subsides. Sometimes she feels nauseous.

   a. With this limited information, what three conditions could cause these types of symptoms?

   _____

   _____

   _____

   b. What diagnostic tests may be useful in determining the cause of the pain? _____

   _____

   _____

2. Samuel is going over a pamphlet with a patient who has hemorrhoids. The patient asks Samuel to answer a few questions.

   a. What is a hemorrhoid? _____

   _____

   _____

   _____

   b. The pamphlet states that the patient should eat a diet rich in fiber. What foods are recommended for a diet rich in fiber?

   _____

   _____

3. Emily Stark is planning a trip to Mexico to get away from the cold upper-Midwest winter. Her provider has recommended that she get a hepatitis A vaccine before her trip.

   a. How is hepatitis A acquired?_____

   _____

   _____

   b. Briefly describe the signs and symptoms of hepatitis A._____

   _____

   _____

   _____

   _____

INTERNET ACTIVITIES

1. Using online resources, research a test used for diagnosing a gastrointestinal system disease. Create a poster presentation, a PowerPoint presentation, or a written paper summarizing your research. Include the following points in your project:
    a. Description of the test
    b. Any contraindications for the test
    c. Patient preparation for the test
    d. What occurs during the test

2. Using online resources, research a gastrointestinal system disease or condition. Create a poster presentation, a PowerPoint presentation, or a written paper summarizing your research. Include the following points in your project:
    a. Description of the disease
    b. Etiology
    c. Signs and symptoms
    d. Diagnostic procedures
    e. Treatments
    f. Prognosis
    g. Prevention

3. Using online resources, research the effect that diet can have on the management of Crohn's disease. In a one-page paper, summarize the information that you found.

4. Using Table 34.5, Medication Classifications, select two generic medications from each of the following classifications: antacids and laxatives. Using a reliable online drug resource, identify for each medication:
    a. Reasons for use
    b. Desired effects
    c. Side effects
    d. Adverse reactions

    Write a short paper addressing each of these four areas for each medication.

Procedure 34.1 Use Critical Thinking when Performing Patient Screening

Name _____ Date _____ Score _____

Tasks: Incorporate critical thinking skills when performing patient assessment. Document the patient's history and chief complaint.

Scenario 1: You work at Walden-Martin Family Medical (WMFM) Clinic. A patient calls and states that she or he has had nausea, vomiting, diarrhea, and abdominal pain for 3 days. You need to gather the patient's information before talking with the provider per the facility's policy.

Scenario 2: You work at WMFM Clinic. A patient calls and states that she or he has had vomiting and constipation for 4 days. You need to gather the patient's information before talking with the provider per the facility's policy.

Directions: Role-play the scenario with a peer, who is the patient. Your instructor is the provider.

Equipment and Supplies:
- Phone log and pen
- Patient's health record
- Phone

Standard: Complete the procedure and all critical steps in _____ minutes with a minimum score of 85% within two attempts (*or as indicated by the instructor*).

Scoring: Divide the points earned by the total possible points. Failure to perform a critical step, indicated by an asterisk (*), results in grade no higher than an 84% (*or as indicated by the instructor*).

Time: Began_____ Ended_____ Total minutes: _____

Steps:	Point Value	Attempt 1	Attempt 2
1. Answer the telephone by the third ring, speaking directly into the mouthpiece or headset. Speak distinctly, using a pleasant tone and expression, at a moderate rate, and with sufficient volume.	10		
2. Greet the caller, identify the facility and yourself, and offer to help the caller.	10		
3. Verify the identity of the caller and his or her date of birth; access the patient's record. Note the patient's phone number in case you are disconnected.	5		
4. Determine the caller's needs using therapeutic communication skills.	10		
5. Upon learning the patient's complaint, use critical thinking skills and ask appropriate questions to obtain information about the patient's condition for the provider. Identify the onset, frequency, and duration of the complaint. If related to pain, identify the exact location, quality (e.g., sharp, dull, stabbing), and rating (using a 0-10 pain scale). Identify significant history and factors that increase or decrease the complaint. (*Refer to the Checklist for Affective Behaviors.*)	30*		

Scenario update: You know the provider is available and the patient is willing to be put on hold as you talk with the provider. 6. Discuss the patient's information with the provider. Present the information accurately and logically.	**20**		
7. Upon returning to the phone, give the patient the information from the provider. Conclude the phone call.	**5**		
8. Document the patient interaction, including the patient's medical history, the provider notified, and the information relayed to the patient.	**10**		
Total Points	**100**		

Checklist for Affective Behaviors

Affective Behavior	**Directions:** *Check behaviors observed during the role-play.*					
Critical Thinking	**Negative, Unprofessional Behaviors**	**Attempt** 1	2	**Positive, Professional Behaviors**	**Attempt** 1	2
	Coached or told of an issue or problem			Independently identified the problem or issue		
	Failed to ask relevant questions related to the condition			Asked appropriate questions to obtain the information required		
	Failed to consider alternatives; failed to ask questions that demonstrated understanding of principles/concepts			Willing to consider other alternatives; asked appropriate questions that showed understanding of principles/concepts		
	Failed to make an educated, logical judgment/decision; actions or lack of actions demonstrated unsafe practices and/or did not follow the protocol			Made an educated, logical judgment/decision based on the protocol; actions reflected principles of safe practice		
	Other:			Other:		

Grading for Affective Behaviors		Point Value	Attempt 1	Attempt 2
Does not meet Expectation	• Response fails to show critical thinking. • Student demonstrated more than 2 negative, unprofessional behaviors during the interaction.	0		
Needs Improvement	• Response fails to show critical thinking. • Student demonstrated 1 or 2 negative, unprofessional behaviors during the interaction.	0		
Meets Expectation	• Response demonstrates critical thinking; no negative, unprofessional behaviors observed. • More practice is needed for behavior to appear natural and for student to appear comfortable and at ease.	30		
Occasionally Exceeds Expectation	• Response demonstrates critical thinking; no negative, unprofessional behaviors observed. • At times student appeared comfortable and at ease; but more practice is needed for behavior to become natural and consistent with a professional medical assistant.	30		
Always Exceeds Expectation	• Response demonstrates critical thinking; no negative, unprofessional behaviors observed. • Student's behaviors appeared natural and comfortable. Behaviors are consistent with a professional medical assistant.	30		

Phone Log

Date: _____ Time: _____ Caller: _____

Documentation

Comments

CAAHEP Competencies	Step(s)
I.A.1. Incorporate critical thinking skills when performing patient assessment	5
X.P.3. Document patient care accurately in the medical record	8

Procedure 34.2 Coach Patient on Health Maintenance: Guaiac Fecal Occult Blood Test

Name _____ Date _____ Score _____

Tasks: Coach a patient on the guaiac fecal occult blood test (gFOBT), while considering the patient's developmental life stage. Document the coaching in the health record.

Background: When coaching patients, it is important to consider their developmental life stage. When working with older adults, it is important to communicate with dignity and respect. Use simpler language. Speak clearly and allow time for the patient to respond. It is important to find out what they know about the topic and respectfully correct any inaccuracies. Make sure to listen to their concerns and provide resources as needed.

Scenario: You work at WMFM Clinic. You are working with Dr. David Kahn, who asked you to coach Charles Johnson (date of birth [DOB] 03/03/1958) on the gFOBT. He is to receive three Hemoccult cards for stool smears.

Directions: Role-play the scenario with a peer, who is the patient. Your instructor is the provider. Use the following as the patient instructions:

Patient Instructions for Guaiac Fecal Occult Blood Test

To prepare for the test, avoid the following for 3 days prior to the test and while collecting the sample(s):
- Aspirin and nonsteroidal antiinflammatory drugs (NSAIDs) (e.g., ibuprofen and naproxen)
- More than 250 mg of vitamin C daily from supplements and foods (e.g., fruit and fruit juices)
- Red meats (e.g., pork, beef, and lamb)
- Horseradish, cantaloupe, raw turnips, broccoli, cauliflower, red radishes, and parsnips
- Antacids
- Antidiarrheal medications
- Iron supplements

To store cards and collect the specimens:
- Keep the Hemoccult test cards in their envelopes (if given that way). Keep the cards at room temperature, away from heat, light, chemicals, children, and pets.
- Prepare the card by writing your name, age, and address on the front of the card, if they are not prelabeled by the provider.
- Before collecting the sample, write the date on the front of the card.
- Prepare to collect the stool, using one of these three ways:
  - Either use a clean disposable container.
  - If given a flushable collection tissue with the Hemoccult card, unfold the tissue paper. Float it on the surface of the toilet water. The edges will stick to the side of the bowl and your stool will fall on the tissue. Sometimes water will collect on the tissue and this is fine.
  - Apply plastic wrap to the bowl.
- Remove the Hemoccult test card from the envelope and place it with the applicator stick in a dry location in the bathroom. Do not get them wet.
- Open the large flap on the front of the card. Sometimes there is a blue discoloration on the squares marked A and B, but this will not affect the test results.
- After collecting the stool, use the applicator stick and place a thin smear of stool in the square marked A.
- Do the same thing for the square marked B but take a sample from another part of the stool. Wrap the applicator stick in toilet paper and discard in the wastebasket. Empty the stool in the toilet and flush.
- Close the flap on the Hemoccult test card and insert the front flap under the tab. Store the card in the envelope until you have completed collecting all the samples. Keep the card in a cool dark place. Do not place it in a plastic bag or in the refrigerator.
- Wash your hands well with soap and water.
- Repeat these directions on days 2 and 3.
- Return the Hemoccult cards to the provider or the laboratory. If you are to mail the cards back, allow the last Hemoccult card to dry overnight. Then place the cards in the special mailing pouch you received and seal. Return the cards immediately.

Equipment and Supplies:
- Hemoccult test kit (Hemoccult cards, applicator sticks, and if available flushable collection tissue)
- Patient instructions
- Patient's health record
- Pen

Standard: Complete the procedure and all critical steps in _____ minutes with a minimum score of 85% within two attempts (*or as indicated by the instructor*).

Scoring: Divide the points earned by the total possible points. Failure to perform a critical step, indicated by an asterisk (*), results in grade no higher than an 84% (*or as indicated by the instructor*).

Time: Began_____ Ended_____ Total minutes: _____

Steps:	Point Value	Attempt 1	Attempt 2
1. Wash hands or use hand sanitizer.	10		
2. Greet the patient. Identify yourself. Verify the patient's identity with full name and date of birth. Explain what you will be doing.	10		
3. Use simpler language when talking. Speak clearly. Communicate with dignity and respect. Allow time for the patient to respond. Listen to the patient's concerns.	15*		
4. Ask the patient if he has ever taken a guaiac fecal occult blood test. If so, ask him what he remembers about it.	10		
5. Discuss the purpose of the test and the supplies needed (e.g., Hemoccult cards, applicator kits, and if available, flushable collection tissue). Show the supplies to the patient.	10		
6. Discuss how the patient needs to prepare for the tests and refer to the written instructions.	15		
7. Discuss how the patient should collect and return the Hemoccult cards. Use the written directions when coaching the patient. Write the patient's name, date of birth, and address on the Hemoccult cards if required by the agency.	10		
8. Ask the patient to teach back the preparation and the collection to you. Clarify any misconceptions or inaccuracies. Answer any questions the patient may have.	10		
9. Document the coaching in the patient's health record. Include the provider's name, what was taught, how the patient responded, and indicate the supplies and written directions sent home with the patient.	10		
Total Points	100		

Documentation

Comments

CAAHEP Competencies	Step(s)
V.P.4.b. Coach patients regarding: health maintenance	Entire procedure
V.P.5.b. Coach patients appropriately considering: developmental life stage	3
X.P.3. Document patient care accurately in the medical record	9
ABHES Competencies	**Step(s)**
8.e. Perform specialty procedures, including but not limited to minor surgery, cardiac, respiratory, OB-GYN, neurological, and gastroenterology	Entire procedure

Procedure 34.3   Developing a Hemoccult Card and Performing Quality Control

Name _____ Date _____ Score _____

Tasks: Test a stool specimen using a Hemoccult card and perform a quality control test. Document the test results in the patient's health record.

Scenario: Charles Johnson (DOB 03/03/1958) returns his Hemoccult card(s). Dr. David Kahn is his provider. You need to develop (test) the sample.

Equipment and Supplies:
- Hemoccult card with stool smear applied
- Hemoccult developer
- Gloves
- Timer
- Biohazard waste container
- Waste container
- Patient's health record

Standard: Complete the procedure and all critical steps in _____ minutes with a minimum score of 85% within two attempts (*or as indicated by the instructor*).

Scoring: Divide the points earned by the total possible points. Failure to perform a critical step, indicated by an asterisk (*), results in grade no higher than an 84% (*or as indicated by the instructor*).

Time: Began_____ Ended_____ Total minutes: _____

Steps:	Point Value	Attempt 1	Attempt 2
1. Wash hands or use hand sanitizer. Put on gloves.	10		
2. Identify when the specimen was applied and if testing can be done.	10		
3. Open the back of the card and apply two drops of the Hemoccult developer to the guaiac paper directly over each smear.	15		
4. Within 60 seconds, read the result accurately.	10		
5. Perform quality control on the card by applying one drop of the Hemoccult developer between the positive and negative Performance Monitors area.	10*		
6. Within 10 seconds, accurately read the results.	10*		
7. Discard the Hemoccult card in the biohazard bag. Clean up the area. Remove gloves and discard in the waste container.	10		
8. Wash hands or use hand sanitizer.	10		
9. Document the test result and the provider notified in the patient's health record.	15		
Total Points	100		

Documentation

Comments

CAAHEP Competencies	Step(s)
I.P.10. Perform a quality control measure	5, 6
X.P.3. Document patient care accurately in the medical record	9
ABHES Competencies	**Step(s)**
8.e. Perform specialty procedures, including but not limited to minor surgery, cardiac, respiratory, OB-GYN, neurological, and gastroenterology	Entire procedure

Procedure 34.4   Coach Patient on Health Maintenance: Colonoscopy

Name _____ Date _____ Score _____

Tasks: Coach a patient on colonoscopy preparation. Document the coaching in the health record.

Scenario: You work at WMFM Clinic. You are working with Dr. David Kahn, who has asked you to coach Charles Johnson (DOB 03/03/1958) on the colonoscopy preparation. Dr. Kahn wants Charles to take his antihypertensive medication the morning of the procedure, 1 hour after finishing the preparation solution.

    The ambulatory surgical center requires that Charles not drink anything 2 hours before the procedure. He needs to arrive 90 minutes before the procedure, which is scheduled at 11 AM. He will be receiving IV sedation during the procedure and will need a driver to take him home.

Directions: Role-play the scenario with a peer, who is the patient. Your instructor is the provider. Use the following as the patient instructions:

Dietary preparations:
- Two days before the procedure: Do not take fiber supplements or eat foods high in fiber (e.g., nuts, seeds, whole grains, and raw or cooked fruits and vegetables).
- One day before the procedure:
  - Do not eat solid foods, just drink clear liquids (e.g., broth, gelatin, coffee, tea, clear juice, popsicles, and sports drinks). Do not drink red liquids or eat red gelatin. Do not drink or eat dairy products or alcohol.
- On the day of the procedure:
  - Do not eat solid foods. Stop drinking clear liquids at least 2 hours before the procedure or as indicated by the provider.

Colon cleansing:
- Usually a split-dose preparation. The first dose of the preparation solution (e.g., GoLYTELY, Colyte) is taken the evening before the procedure. The second dose is taken the next morning and must be complete at least 2 hours before the procedure.
- How the patient will feel: Usually within 1 hour of starting the preparation solution, liquid stools can occur and continue until 2 hours after completing the solution. Chills, headache, cramping, weakness, nausea, vomiting, and bloating can occur when taking the solution. Drinking the preparation slower can help decrease the severe vomiting and cramping.

Postprocedure instructions:
- Do not drive. Plan to have someone bring you home.

Equipment and Supplies:
- Patient instructions
- Patient's health record

Standard: Complete the procedure and all critical steps in _____ minutes with a minimum score of 85% within two attempts (*or as indicated by the instructor*).

Scoring: Divide the points earned by the total possible points. Failure to perform a critical step, indicated by an asterisk (*), results in grade no higher than an 84% (*or as indicated by the instructor*).

Time: Began_____ Ended_____ Total minutes: _____

Steps:	Point Value	Attempt 1	Attempt 2
1. Wash hands or use hand sanitizer.	10		
2. Greet the patient. Identify yourself. Verify the patient's identity with full name and date of birth. Explain what you will be doing.	10		
3. Use simpler language when talking. Speak clearly. Communicate with dignity and respect. Allow time for the patient to respond. Listen to the patient's concerns.	15*		
4. Ask the patient if he has ever had a colonoscopy. If so, ask him what he remembers about it.	15		
5. Discuss the purpose of the colonoscopy and the preparation involved. Refer to the written instructions that the patient will be taking home.	20		
6. Ask the patient to teach back the preparation to you. Clarify any misconceptions or inaccuracies. Answer any questions the patient may have. Give the patient a phone number to call if he has questions.	15		
7. Document the coaching in the patient's health record. Include the provider's name, what was taught, how the patient responded, and any written directions (including appointment information) sent home with the patient.	15		
Total Points	100		

Documentation

Comments

CAAHEP Competencies	Step(s)
V.P.4.b. Coach patients regarding: health maintenance	Entire procedure
X.P.3. Document patient care accurately in the medical record	7
ABHES Competencies	**Step(s)**
8.e. Perform specialty procedures, including but not limited to minor surgery, cardiac, respiratory, OB-GYN, neurological, and gastroenterology	Entire procedure

Orthopedics and Rheumatology

CAAHEP Competencies	Assessment
I.C.4. List major organs in each body system	Skills and Concepts – A-E
I.C.5. Identify the anatomical location of major organs in each body system	Skills and Concepts – B. 4, D. 2; Certification Preparation – 1, 4
I.C.6. Compare structure and function of the human body across the life span	Skills and Concepts – D. 2; Certification Preparation – 2
I.C.7. Describe the normal function of each body system	Skills and Concepts – A. 1, B. 4-6, C. 1-6, D. 1-4
I.C.8.a. Identify common pathology related to each body system including: signs	Skills and Concepts – F. 1, 4c, 5c, 6c; Internet Activities – 2, 3
I.C.8.b. Identify common pathology related to each body system including: symptoms	Skills and Concepts – F. 1, 4c, 5c, 6c; Internet Activities – 2, 3
I.C.8.c. Identify common pathology related to each body system including: etiology	Skills and Concepts – F. 2, 4b, 5b, 6b; Certification Preparation – 5, 6; Workplace Application – 1; Internet Activities – 2, 3
I.C.9.a. Analyze pathology for each body system including: diagnostic measures	Skills and Concepts – F. 3, 4d, 5d, 6d, G. 1, H. 1, I. 1; Workplace Application – 1, 2; Internet Activities – 1, 2, 3
I.C.9.b. Analyze pathology for each body system including: treatment modalities	Skills and Concepts – F. 4e, 6e, J. 1-6, L. 1-10, M. 1-8; Certification Preparation – 7-10; Workplace Application – 2, 3, 4
I.C.10. Identify CLIA-waived tests associated with common diseases	Skills and Concepts – F. 3; Certification Preparation – 3
V.C.10. Define medical terms and abbreviations related to all body systems	Vocabulary Review – A. 1-10, B. 1-10, C. 1-7; Abbreviations – 1-25; Skills and Concepts – L. 8, 10
I.P.8. Instruct and prepare a patient for a procedure or a treatment	Procedure 35.1-35.7
X.P.3. Document patient care accurately in the medical record	Procedure 35.1-35.7
V.P.5.b. Coach patients appropriately considering: developmental life stage	Procedure 35.5
V.P.5.c. Coach patients appropriately considering: communication barriers	Procedure 35.6
V.P.4.d. Coach patients regarding: treatment plan	Procedure 35.1-35.7

ABHES Competencies	Assessment
2. Anatomy and Physiology	
a. List all body systems and their structures and functions	Skills and Concepts – A-E
2.b. Describe common diseases, symptoms, and etiologies as they apply to each system	Skills and Concepts – F. 1, 2, 4b, 4c, 5b, 5c, 6b, 6c; Certification Preparation – 5, 6; Workplace Application – 1; Internet Activities – 2, 3
2,c. Identify diagnostic and treatment modalities as they relate to each body system	Skills and Concepts – F. 3, 4e, 4d, 5d, 6d, 6e, G. 1, H. 1, I. 1, J. 1-6, L. 1-10, M. 1-8; Certification Preparation – 7-10; Workplace Application – 1, 2, 3; Internet Activities – 2, 3, 4
3. Medical Terminology	
c. Apply medical terminology for each specialty	Vocabulary Review – A. 1-10, B. 1-10, C. 1-7
3. d. Define and use medical abbreviations when appropriate and acceptable	Abbreviations – 1-25; Skills and Concepts – L. 10, 12
4. Medical Law and Ethics a. Follow documentation guidelines	Procedure 35.1-35.7
5. Human Relations d. Adapt care to address the developmental stages of life	Procedure 35.5
8. Clinical Procedures h. Teach self-examination, disease management and health promotion	Procedure 35.1-35.7
8.j. Make adaptations for patients with special needs (psychological or physical limitations)	Procedure 35.6
8.k. Make adaptations to care for patients across their lifespan	Procedure 35.5, 35.6

VOCABULARY REVIEW

Using the word pool on the right, find the correct word to match the definition. Write the word on the line after the definition.

Hmandeep Kaur

Group A

1. A series of small irregular-shaped bones that form the backbone or spine ___vertrebrae___
2. The formation of the blood cells and platelets ___hematopoiesis___
3. Connective tissue that attaches muscles to bone ___tendon___
4. The three small bones of the middle ear (malleus, incus, and stapes) ___ossicles___
5. Supportive connective tissue that connects bones at a joint ___ligament___
6. Bone cells that break down bone ___osteoclasts___
7. A therapeutic treatment for a disorder ___modalities___
8. Flexible connective tissue that covers the ends of many bones at the joint ___cartilage___
9. An immune response against a person's own tissues, cells, or cell parts, leading to the deterioration of tissue ___autoimmune___
10. Bone-forming cells ___osteoblasts___

Word Pool
- autoimmune
- modalities
- osteoblasts
- cartilage
- tendon
- ligament
- osteoclasts
- hematopoiesis
- ossicles
- vertebrae

Group B

1. A serious condition that involves increased pressure, usually in the muscles; which leads to compromised blood flow and muscle and nerve damage ___compartment syndrome___
2. A quality or characteristic of a material that allows another substance to pass through it ___permeability___
3. A point of communication between two cells ___Synapse___
4. Tough, fibrous covering of the muscles ___fascia___
5. A high-energy molecule found in every cell that supplies large amounts of energy for various biochemical processes ___ATP___
6. Category of medication used to prevent or treat seizures ___anticonvulsants___
7. Process of viewing living tissue that has been removed for the purpose of diagnosis and/or treatment ___biopsy___
8. Increase in the reactivity of the skin to sunlight or ultraviolet radiation ___photosensitivity___
9. Category of medication used to relieve pain ___Analgesic___
10. Category of medication or a chemical substance that prevents clotting of blood ___anticoagulant___

Word Pool
- synapse
- permeability
- ATP
- compartment syndrome
- analgesic
- anticoagulant
- anticonvulsants
- biopsy
- fascia
- photosensitivity

Group C

1. Contraction of a muscle causing a narrowing of the inside tube of a vessel _Vasoconstriction_
2. Category of medication used to suppress the immune system _immunosuppressants_
3. The standing position when using crutches; crutch tips are 4-6 inches to the side and front of each foot _tripod position_
4. Adhesive patches that conduct electricity from the body to machine wires _electrode_
5. The partial or complete disappearance of the clinical and subjective characteristics of a chronic or malignant disease _remission_
6. A temporary or permanent surgically created opening used for drainage (i.e., urine, stool) _stoma_
7. A usually chronic, recurrent skin disease marked by bright red patches covered with silvery scales _psoriasis_

Word Pool
- psoriasis
- remission
- immunosuppressants
- stoma
- vasoconstriction
- electrode
- tripod position

ABBREVIATIONS

Write out what each of the following abbreviations stands for.

1. ATP _Adenosine Triphosphate_
2. TENS _Transcutaneous Electrical Nerve Stimulation_
3. EMG _Electromyography_
4. ROM _Range Of Motion_
5. NMJ _Neuromuscular Junction_
6. ACh _Acetylcholine_
7. ORIF _Open Reduction and Internal Fixation_
8. WPI _Whole Person Impairment_
9. SS _Serotonin Syndrome_
10. RA _Rheumatoid Arthritis_
11. JA _Juvenile Arthritis_
12. DJD _Degenerative Joint Disease_
13. MD _Muscular Dystrophy_
14. CK _Creatine Kinase_
15. RLS _Restless Legs Syndrome_
16. WED _Willis-Ekbom Disease_
17. PLMD _Periodic Limb Movement Disorder_

18. ADL _Activity of Daily Living_
19. CSMT _Color, sensation, motion, temperature_
20. RICE _Rest, Ice, compression, Elevation_
21. DMARD _Disease-modifying antirheumatic drugs_
22. DEXA _Dual-energy x-ray absorptiometry_
23. NCV _Nerve Conduction Velocity._
24. CRP _C-reactive protein._
25. RF _Rheumatoid Factor._

SKILLS AND CONCEPTS

Answer the following questions. Write your answer on the line or in the space provided.

A. Anatomy of the Musculoskeletal System

1. What are the main functions of the musculoskeletal system? _• Body movement • Protection, support, and framework for organ systems of the body. • Storage for important minerals such as calcium and phosphorus._

B. Bones

1. The axial skeleton is made up of: _80 bones_

2. Name the three ossicles of the middle ear. _Incus, malleus, stapes_

3. The appendicular skeleton is made up of: _126 bones_

4. Label the following diagram of a long bone with the terms below.

- Carpals
- Femur
- Skull
- Metatarsals
- Sternum
- Ribs

- Ilium
- Metacarpals
- Sacrum
- Ulna
- Clavicle
- Tibia

- Phalanges
- Fibula
- Vertebral column
- Mandible
- Humerus

- Patella
- Tarsals
- Scapula
- Radius

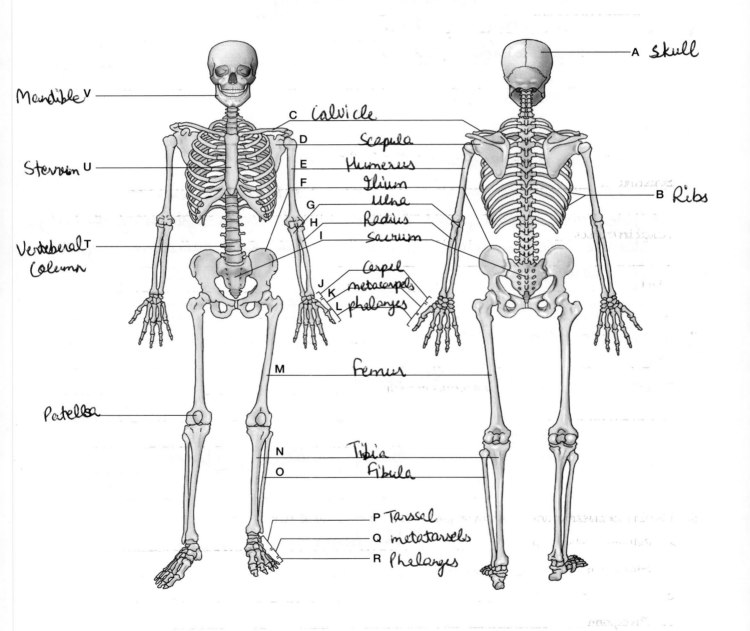

A Skull

Mandible V

C Calvicle

D Scapula

E Humerus

F Ilium

G Ulna

H Radius

I Sacrum

Sternum U

B Ribs

Verteberal T Column

J Carpel
K metacarpals
L phalanges

Patella

M Femur

N Tibia

O Fibula

P Tarsal
Q metatarsels
R Phalanges

5. What are the five categories of bone shape? Long, short, flat, sesamoid, Irregular

6. Describe the role of osteoblasts and osteoclasts in bone health. Both continuously remodel bones, making them strong, durable, and able to heal.

7. What is the function of red bone marrow? It produces red blood cells.

8. Compare compact bone and spongy bone. Spongy bone have some pores in it, and compact bone present in the outer layer of long bones.

C. Joints

1. In your own words, describe the range of motion for the three categories of joints.

   Synarthroses Immovable joints held together by fibrous cartilaginous tissue.

   Amphiarthroses limited range of motion joints, which are joined together by cartilage that is slightly movable.

   Diarthroses Full range of motion joints.

2. Describe a bursa and how it works in a joint. Bursae is a sacs of fluid located between joint and tendons. It help cushion and supports the joints.

3. Describe the meniscus and how it works in a joint. The meniscus consists of crescent-shaped cartilage in the knee joint that also cushions the joints.

4. Describe a ligament. It connects one bone with another bone.

5. List the six classifications of synovial joints. Give an example of each type of joint.

   a. Ball-and-socket joint Allows free movements. Ex. shoulder.

   b. Hinge joint Permits flexion and extension. Ex. elbow.

   c. Saddle joint Allow for flexion, extension, and other movements. ex. thum cross palm

   d. Pivot joint Permit rotation. Ex. cervical vertebral.

   e. Gliding joint Allow a bone to slide over another bone. Ex. wrist.

   f. Condyloid joint Permit flexion, extension, circular motion. Ex. movement of atlas.

D. Muscles

1. List the three types of muscles in the body. _____

    skeletal muscle, smooth muscle, cardiac muscle.

2. Label the following diagram of skeletal muscles with the terms below.

    - Deltoid
    - Iliopsoas
    - Biceps brachii
    - Gastrocnemius
    - Vastus medialis
    - Trapezius
    - External abdominal oblique

    - Sartorius
    - Soleus
    - Pectoralis major
    - Tibialis anterior
    - Serratus anterior

Trapezius A

Deltoid L

Biceps Brachii K

Serratus anterior J

Pectoralis major B

External abdominal Oblique C

Iliopsoas D

Sartorius I

Vastus medialis E

Gastrocnemius H

Soleus F

Tibialis Anterior G

3. Describe how the musculoskeletal system changes as we age. _____

People lose bone mass or density as they age, especially women after menopause. As we age, the structure of bone changes.

E. Physiology of the Musculoskeletal System

1. Describe the role of the synapse in muscle contraction. The synapse is a specialized structure that allows one neuron to communicate with another neuron.

2. Describe how a neurotransmitter works. _____

Neurotransmitter must travel across the synaptic cleft to continue the stimulus and generate a muscle contraction.

3. Briefly describe how ATP is used in a muscle. _____

Muscle need calcium and energy in the form of ATP to contract.

4. In your own words, define the terms *isotonic* and *isometric*, and give an example of each type of muscle contraction.

Isotonic muscle contraction that usually produces movement at a joint.

Isometric muscle contraction usually does not produce movement.

F. Disorders of the Musculoskeletal System

1. List common signs and symptoms of musculoskeletal diseases and disorders. _____

malaise, myalgia, inflammation, pain of the muscle, temporary loss of function.

2. List common etiology of musculoskeletal diseases and disorders. _____

Fracture, Trauma, deformity.

3. List three common CLIA-waived tests used to diagnose musculoskeletal conditions. _____

X-ray, CT scan, MRI

4. The following relate to osteoporosis.

   a. Describe osteoporosis. _A condition that causes bones to become brittle and weak._

   b. List at least five risks for developing osteoporosis. _Menopause, family history, small body frame, hormonal imbalance, cancer._

   c. List three signs and symptoms of osteoporosis. _Back pain, height loss, stooped posture._

   d. List one diagnostic procedure used for osteoporosis. _Bone density test_

   e. List four treatments commonly ordered by the provider for osteoporosis. _medication, weight-bearing exercise, Calcium and Vitamin D intake, modifying risk factors._

5. The following relate to rheumatoid arthritis (RA).

   a. Describe RA. _when immune system attacks the healthy cells, causing inflammation in the joints, eyes, lungs, and mouth._

   b. List the cause (etiology) of RA. _Genetics, cigarette use, obesity._

   c. List three signs or symptoms of RA. _Pain, achiness, stiffness._

   d. List two diagnostic procedures used for RA. _Blood test, MRI._

6. The following relate to muscular dystrophy.

   a. Describe muscular dystrophy. _A collection of over 30 inherited diseases that cause muscle weakness and muscle loss._

   b. List two causes (etiology) of muscular dystrophy. _Genetic mutation, muscle weakness_

c.   List three signs and symptoms of muscular dystrophy. _____

muscle pain, stiffness, learning disabilities.

_____

d.   List two diagnostic procedures used for muscular dystrophy. _____

CK Blood test, Muscle Biopsy

e.   List two treatments commonly ordered by the provider for muscular dystrophy. _____

stretching exercise, corticosteriods.

THE MEDICAL ASSISTANT'S ROLE IN ORTHOPEDICS AND RHEUMATOLOGY PROCEDURES

G. Assisting with the Examination

1.   Describe the 0-10 pain rating scale. Zero is no pain and 10 is the
worst pain ever.

2.   Briefly describe a gait assessment. _____
It is used to assess and treat individuals with
conditions affecting their ability to walk.

H. Assisting with Diagnostic Procedures
Refer to Tables 35.5 and 35.6 to complete the answers below.

1.   Describe the following diagnostic procedures;

a.   Computed tomography (CT) scan A CT scan is a diagnostic
imaging procedure that uses a combination of x-ray to produce image.

b.   Arthrogram It uses imaging equipment to evaluate a
joint like shoulder, elbow, wrist, hip, knee or ankle.

c.   Myelogram It uses a contrast dye to look for
problems in the spinal cord.

d.   Electromyography Recording of changes in skin voltage
produced by underlying skeletal muscle contraction.

e.   Rheumatoid factor (RF) A blood test that measures the
amount of RF antibody in the blood.

I. Range of Motion Measurement

1. Describe a goniometer and how it is used to assess range of motion. _A goniometer is used to measure the ROM of a joint. It have calibration markings to indicate the measurement._

J. Muscle Strength Evaluation

1. Describe how a dynamometer is used to evaluate hand grip strength. _Digital and nondigital dynamometer are available. A dynamometer provides an objective measurement of hand grip strength._

K. Assisting with Treatments

Fill in the blank with the medication classification described below.

1. Used to treat chronic inflammatory diseases (e.g., arthritis) _Sulfasaline_
2. Used to treat gout _allopurinol_
3. Used to treat neuromuscular disorders and epilepsy _Anticonvulsants_
4. Used to relieve pain _Analgesics_
5. Used to promote bone mineral density _osteoporosis agents_
6. Used to treat autoimmune disorders _Tumor necrosis factor inhibitors._

L. Casts and Splints

1. Describe splints, including their appearance and purpose. _A splint consists of a strip of rigid material that immobilizes an extremity. It provides partial protection while the site heels._

2. Describe three home care instructions that need to be given to a patient with a new cast. _The medical assistant needs to provide cast care instructions to patients. It is important to teach patients about check CSMT._

3. Describe CSMT, including what is normal and abnormal.

   a. Color _should be pink normal. abnormal — pale skin_

b. Sensation _normal — normal sensation_
Abnormal — Increased pain, Unable to feel light touch.

c. Motion _normal — movement of toes and fingers is normal_
abnormal — unable to move toes or fingers

d. Temperature _normal — should be warm_
abnormal — cooler than opposite extremity

M. Hot and Cold Therapies

1. When a patient must use a cold or hot application, what directions should be given to the patient?

The applications can be dry or moist. Dry means no moisture is left on skin, moist tend to increase tissue elasticity.

2. Describe three reasons why cold therapy is used. _It is used for sprains, strains, fractures, joint injuries_

3. List three conditions that can be helped with heat therapy. _acute pain, sinus congestion, Infection_

4. Describe the uses of paraffin bath therapy. _It is used to reduce pain. It has been found to maintain muscle strength and increase mobility._

5. Why are heat lamps with red-colored near-infrared bulbs used? _Red used to treat skin condition and other penetrates heal tissue._

6. Describe ultrasound therapy. _Ultrasound therapy used to treat pain and promote healing._

7. When is RICE therapy used? _During orthopedic injuries._

8. Describe what RICE stands for. _Rest, Ice, Compression, Elevation._

9. List the benefits of exercise therapy. • It helps to improve mobility
• Reduce or eliminate pain
• recover from a sport injury

10. Briefly describe how a TENS unit is used for pain relief. _____

It sends electrical pulses through the skin to start your body's own pain killers. TENS can reduce pain.

N. Assistive Devices

1. Axillary crutches are the most common types of assistive devices and are used when recovering from a lower extremity injury or surgery.

2. Describe how to fit axillary crutches. Put the crutches under your arms. There should be 2 inch space between your armpit and top of the crutch.

3. Describe the following limitations that are typically indicated by the provider.

   a. Weight bearing as tolerated Patients can place more than half of their body weight on their affected extremity if not painful.

   b. Partial weight bearing The provider will indicate how much weight can placed on the affected extremity.

   c. Toe-touch weight bearing Patients can touch ground with their toes on their affected side.

   d. Non-weight-bearing Patient cannot put weight on their affected extremity.

4. Describe how to fit walkers. _____

adjust your walker so that it fits your arm comfortably.

5. Describe how to fit a cane. Check your elbow bend. With the cane in your hand, your elbow should bend at a comfortable angle, about 15 degrees

CERTIFICATION PREPARATION

Circle the correct answer.

1. What bones are part of the shoulder girdle?
   a. Clavicle
   b. Scapula
   c. Femur
   d. Both a and b

2. What is the main function of the musculoskeletal system?
   a. Body movement
   b. pH balance
   c. Waste removal
   d. All of the above

3. Which is a CLIA-waived test?
   a. Erythrocyte sedimentation rate
   b. Rheumatoid factor
   c. Lyme disease blood antibodies
   d. All of the above

4. A ligament connects which two structures?
   a. Muscles to bone
   b. Muscles to muscles
   c. Bones to bones
   d. Muscles to tendons

5. RA is caused by
   a. a bacterial infection that destroys the joints.
   b. a fracture within a joint.
   c. a genetic condition that cannot be prevented.
   d. an autoimmune reaction that attacks the lining of the joints.

6. Which disease is caused by a buildup of uric acid in the blood?
   a. Gout
   b. Osteoporosis
   c. Degenerative joint disease
   d. Lyme disease

7. Which medication classification is used to treat neuromuscular disorders and epilepsy?
   a. Antigout
   b. Corticosteroids
   c. Anticonvulsants
   d. Antiinflammatories

8. Which is not a dry cold application?
   a. Chemical cold pack
   b. Ice bag
   c. Cold compress
   d. Bead pack

9. Fit axillary crutches so they are _____ below the armpit.
   a. ½ to 1 inch
   b. 1 to 1 ½ inches
   c. 2 fingerwidths
   d. Both b and c

10. When fitting a cane, which statement is correct?
    a. The cane should be held on the weak side.
    b. The top of the cane should be near the crease in the wrist.
    c. The elbow should be bent 30 degrees.
    d. All of the above

WORKPLACE APPLICATIONS

1. A young woman calls in and says that she is concerned about a rash she has on her leg. She is an avid hiker and spends most of her weekends hiking and camping. She frequently finds ticks on her clothing and is careful about using preventive measures to limit her exposure to tick bites. She has noticed a red rash on her leg today and for the last day or two has been feeling very tired and achy. She is afraid she might have Lyme disease.

   a. What type of testing can be done to help diagnose her condition? _____

   _____

   b. What organism causes Lyme disease? _____

   c. What type of preventive measure can be taken to guard against a tick bite? _____

   _____

   _____

2. Walter Biller is in to see Dr. James Martin at Walden-Martin Family Medical (WMFM) Clinic to go over some tests results. Walter's rheumatoid factor (RF) test is negative, and his C-reactive protein (CRP) and erythrocyte sedimentation rate (ESR) are elevated. What do these results mean?

_____

_____

3. Marcie Nguyen was playing softball last night and slid into second base, and in the process she twisted her ankle. She is afraid she may have a sprained ankle. What is the difference between and strain and a sprain?

_____

_____

How would the injury be treated if the diagnosis is a Grade I ankle sprain? _____

_____

_____

INTERNET ACTIVITIES

1. Using online resources, research a test used for diagnosing musculoskeletal disease. Create a poster presentation, a PowerPoint presentation, or a written paper summarizing your research. Include the following points in your project:
   a. Description of the test
   b. Any contraindications for the test
   c. Patient preparation for the test
   d. What occurs during the test

2. Using online resources, research a musculoskeletal disease. Create a poster presentation, a PowerPoint presentation, or an infographic summarizing your research. Include the following points in your project:
   a. Description of the disease
   b. Etiology
   c. Signs and symptoms
   d. Diagnostic procedures
   e. Treatments
   f. Prognosis
   g. Prevention

3. Using online resources, research the three abnormal curvatures of the spine presented in this chapter: lordosis, kyphosis, and scoliosis. In a one-page paper, describe each abnormal curve and describe how it is treated.

4. Using Table 35.7, Medication Classifications, select two generic medications from each of the following classifications: antigout and antiinflammatory. Using a reliable online drug resource, for each medication identify:
   a. Reasons for use
   b. Desired effects
   c. Side effects
   d. Adverse reactions

   Write a short paper addressing each of these four areas for each medication.

Procedure 35.1   Assist with the Application of a Cast

Name _____ **Date** _____ **Score** _____

Task: Assist the provider in applying a fiberglass cast. Document the procedure in the patient's health record.

Scenario: You are working with Dr. David Kahn as he applies a fiberglass cast on Johnny Parker's (DOB: 06/15/2010) left lower leg. You will assist the provider.

Equipment and Supplies:
- Patient's health record
- Rolls of fiberglass
- Basin for casting material
- Bandage
- Stockinette
- Gloves
- Sheet wadding and/or spongy padding
- Stand to support foot (lower extremity)
- Tape
- Scissors
- 2-3 towels
- Water
- Cast care instructions (optional)

Standard: Complete the procedure and all critical steps in _____ minutes with a minimum score of 85% within two attempts (*or as indicated by the instructor*).

Scoring: Divide the points earned by the total possible points. Failure to perform a critical step, indicated by an asterisk (*), results in grade no higher than an 84% (*or as indicated by the instructor*).

Time: Began_____ Ended_____ Total minutes: _____

Steps	Possible Points	Attempt 1	Attempt 2
1. Wash hands or use hand sanitizer. Assemble the necessary equipment.	5*		
2. Greet the patient. Identify yourself. Verify the patient's identity with full name and date of birth. Explain the procedure to be performed in a manner that the patient understands. Answer any questions the patient may have about the procedure.	10*		
3. Seat the patient comfortably, as directed by the provider. If the cast is being applied to the lower extremity, the toes must be supported by a stand.	5		
4. Clean the area that the cast will cover. Note any objective signs and ask about subjective symptoms (chart them at the end of the procedure).	10		
5. Cut the stockinette to fit the area the cast will cover. Apply the stockinette smoothly to the area the cast will cover. Leave 1 or 2 inches of excess stockinette above and below the cast area to finish the cast. Excess stockinette may be cut away where wrinkles form, such as at the front of the ankle.	5		

6.	Apply sheet wadding along the length of the cast using a spiral bandage turn. Extra padding may be used over bony prominences, such as the bones of the elbow or ankle.	**10**		
7.	Put on gloves. With lukewarm water in the basin, wet the fiberglass tape as directed by the provider.	10		
8.	Assist as directed as the provider applies the inner layer of fiberglass tape. A length of 1 to 2 inches of stockinette is rolled over the inner layer of the cast to form a smooth edge when the outer layer is applied.	10		
9.	As directed by the provider, help open and apply an outer layer of fiberglass tape.	10		
10.	Help shape the cast as directed. All contours must be smooth.	5		
11.	Discard the water and excess materials. Remove your gloves and wash your hands.	5*		
12.	Reassure the patient, review cast care verbally, and provide written instructions (optional).	5*		
13.	Document the procedure in the patient's health record. Include the provider's name, the procedure, what was taught, and how the patient responded.	10*		
	Total Score	100		

Documentation

Comments

CAAHEP Competencies	Step(s)
I.P.8. Instruct and prepare a patient for a procedure or a treatment	2
X.P.3. Document patient care accurately in the medical record	13
ABHES Competencies	**Step(s)**
4. Medical Law and Ethics a. Follow documentation guidelines	13
8. Clinical Procedures h. Teach self-examination, disease management and health promotion	12

Procedure 35.2   Assist with Cast Removal

Name _____ Date _____ Score _____

Task: Document the procedure in the patient's health record.

Scenario: You are working with Dr. David Kahn, and he orders removal of the lower left leg cast on Johnny Parker (DOB 06/15/2010).

Equipment and Supplies:
- Patient's health record
- Cast cutter
- Cast spreader
- Large bandage scissors
- Basin of warm water
- Mild soap
- Towel
- Skin lotion

Standard: Complete the procedure and all critical steps in _____ minutes with a minimum score of 85% within two attempts (*or as indicated by the instructor*).

Scoring: Divide the points earned by the total possible points. Failure to perform a critical step, indicated by an asterisk (*), results in grade no higher than an 84% (*or as indicated by the instructor*).

Time: Began_____ Ended_____ Total minutes: _____

Steps	Possible Points	Attempt 1	Attempt 2
1. Wash hands or use hand sanitizer. Assemble the necessary equipment.	15*		
2. Greet the patient. Identify yourself. Verify the patient's identity with full name and date of birth. Explain the procedure to be performed in a manner that the patient understands. Answer any questions the patient may have about the procedure.	15*		
3. Provide adequate support for the limb throughout the procedure. Using the cast cutter, make a cut on the medial and lateral sides of the long axis of the cast.	15		
4. Use the cast spreader to pry apart the two halves. Carefully remove the two parts of the cast. Use the large bandage scissors to cut away the stockinette and padding remaining.	15		
5. Gently wash the area that was covered by the cast with mild soap and warm water. Dry the area and apply a gentle skin lotion.	10		
6. Give the patient appropriate instructions about exercising and using the limb, as directed by the provider.	15		
7. Document the procedure in the patient's health record. Include the provider's name, the procedure, what was taught, and how the patient responded.	15*		
Total Score	**100**		

Documentation

Comments

CAAHEP Competencies	Step(s)
I.P.8. Instruct and prepare a patient for a procedure or a treatment	2
V.P.4.d. Coach patients regarding: treatment plan	6
X.P.3. Document patient care accurately in the medical record	7
ABHES Competencies	**Step(s)**
4. Medical Law and Ethics a. Follow documentation guidelines	7
8. Clinical Procedures h. Teach self-examination, disease management and health promotion	6

Procedure 35.3   Apply a Cold Pack

Name _____ **Date** _____ **Score** _____

Task: Apply a cold pack (chemical, gel, or bead) to a body area to reduce pain and prevent further swelling per treatment plan. Document the procedure in the patient's health record.

Scenario: You are working with Dr. David Kahn. Johnny Parker (DOB: 06/15/2010) arrives holding his arm and crying. Another medical assistant brings the patient and parent to the exam room. The medical assistant comes out and updates you on Johnny. His parent states that Johnny fell off his bike an hour ago and has since been complaining of pain in his right wrist. The department has a standing order to apply a cold pack to orthopedic injuries if the patient does not arrive with one in place. The medical assistant asks you to apply the cold pack as he completes the vital signs and medical history on Johnny.

Equipment and Supplies:
- Cold pack (chemical, gel, or bead)
- Towel or another type of protective covering for the cold pack
- Provider's order or standing order for orthopedic injuries
- Patient's health record

Standard: Complete the procedure and all critical steps in _____ minutes with a minimum score of 85% within two attempts (*or as indicated by the instructor*).

Scoring: Divide the points earned by the total possible points. Failure to perform a critical step, indicated by an asterisk (*), results in grade no higher than an 84% (*or as indicated by the instructor*).

Time: Began_____ Ended_____ Total minutes: _____

Steps	Possible Points	Attempt 1	Attempt 2
1. Wash hands or use hand sanitizer.	15*		
2. Read the standing order or the provider's order. Assemble the equipment. If using a chemical cold pack, activate the pack by squeezing it.	15		
3. Greet the patient. Identify yourself. Verify the patient's identity with full name and date of birth. Explain the procedure to be performed in a manner that the patient understands. Answer any questions the patient may have about the procedure.	15*		
4. Cover the cold pack with a towel or protective covering.	15		
5. Assist the patient to position the cold pack over the injured area.	10		
6. Coach patient on the use of a cold pack. Advise the patient to leave the cold pack in place for 15 to 20 minutes or until the area feels numb, whichever comes first.	15		
7. Document the procedure in the patient's health record. Include the provider's name, the order, what was taught, and how the patient responded.	15*		
Total Score	100		

Documentation

Comments

CAAHEP Competencies	Step(s)
I.P.8. Instruct and prepare a patient for a procedure or a treatment	3
V.P.4.d. Coach patients regarding: treatment plan	6
X.P.3. Document patient care accurately in the medical record	7
ABHES Competencies	**Step(s)**
4. Medical Law and Ethics a. Follow documentation guidelines	7
8. Clinical Procedures h. Teach self-examination, disease management and health promotion	6

Procedure 35.4   Apply a Hot Pack

Name _____ Date _____ Score _____

Task: Apply a hot pack (chemical, gel, or bead) to an infected wound. Document the procedure in the patient's health record.

Scenario: You are working with Dr. David Kahn. Jana Green (DOB 5/1/1936) has an infected wound on her arm. Dr. Kahn orders a hot pack to be applied to the wound for 15 minutes and coaching for the patient to continue the treatment at home four times a day for the next 3 days.

Equipment and Supplies:
- Hot pack (chemical, gel, or bead)
- Towel or another type of protective covering for the hot pack
- Provider's order
- Patient's health record

Standard: Complete the procedure and all critical steps in _____ minutes with a minimum score of 85% within two attempts (*or as indicated by the instructor*).

Scoring: Divide the points earned by the total possible points. Failure to perform a critical step, indicated by an asterisk (*), results in grade no higher than an 84% (*or as indicated by the instructor*).

Time: Began_____ Ended_____ Total minutes: _____

Steps	Possible Points	Attempt 1	Attempt 2
1. Wash hands or use hand sanitizer.	15*		
2. Read the provider's order. Assemble the equipment. If using a chemical hot pack, activate the pack by squeezing it. If pack needs to be warmed, follow the manufacturer's directions.	15		
3. Greet the patient. Identify yourself. Verify the patient's identity with full name and date of birth. Explain the procedure to be performed in a manner that the patient understands. Answer any questions the patient may have about the procedure.	15*		
4. Cover the hot pack with a towel or protective covering.	15		
5. Assist the patient to position the hot pack over the covered wound.	10		
6. Coach the patient on the use of a hot pack. Advise the patient to leave the hot pack in place for 15 minutes per the provider's order or until the area feels warm, whichever comes first.	15		
7. Document the procedure in the patient's health record. Include the provider's name, the order, what was taught, and how the patient responded.	15*		
Total Score	100		

Documentation

Comments

CAAHEP Competencies	Step(s)
I.P.8. Instruct and prepare a patient for a procedure or a treatment	3
V.P.4.d. Coach patients regarding: treatment plan	6
X.P.3. Document patient care accurately in the medical record	7
ABHES Competencies	**Step(s)**
4. Medical Law and Ethics a. Follow documentation guidelines	7
8. Clinical Procedures h. Teach self-examination, disease management and health promotion	6

Procedure 35.5   Coach a Patient in the Use of Axillary Crutches

Name _____ Date _____ Score _____

Task: Fit crutches to the patient. Coach the patient to use crutches properly, considering the patient's developmental life stage. Document your teaching in the patient's health record.

Scenario: You are working with Dr. David Kahn. He has ordered you to teach Daniel Miller (DOB: 3/21/2012) how to use axillary crutches. Daniel broke his left leg, and his treatment plan requires that he not bear weight on the left leg for 6 weeks. Daniel's bedroom is on the second floor, so he has to learn how to use crutches on the stairs also.

Equipment and Supplies:
- Axillary crutches
- Handout on crutch walking (optional)
- Provider's order
- Patient's health record

Standard: Complete the procedure and all critical steps in _____ minutes with a minimum score of 85% within two attempts (*or as indicated by the instructor*).

Scoring: Divide the points earned by the total possible points. Failure to perform a critical step, indicated by an asterisk (*), results in grade no higher than an 84% (*or as indicated by the instructor*).

Time: Began_____ Ended_____ Total minutes: _____

Steps	Possible Points	Attempt 1	Attempt 2
1. Wash hands or use hand sanitizer.	10*		
2. Read the provider's order. Assemble the equipment.	5		
3. Greet the patient. Identify yourself. Verify the patient's identity with full name and date of birth. Explain the procedure to be performed in a manner that the patient understands. Answer any questions the patient may have about the procedure.	10*		
4. Ensure the patient is wearing shoes and ask the patient to stand up straight. Assist as needed. Fit the crutches to the patient so they are 1 to 1 1/2 inches (about 2 finger-widths) below the armpit. The crutch should be about 4 to 6 inches to the side and front of each foot.	5		
5. Adjust the handgrips so they are near the patient's wrist and even with the top of the hip line. This should allow for a 15- to 30-degree bend in the elbow when the patient's hands are on the handgrip.	5		
6. Coach the patient using strategies appropriate for the patient's developmental stage. Encourage discussion and questions. Use concrete terms when explaining the procedure. Show simple pictures.	5*		
7. Using age-appropriate language, instruct the patient to keep the injured leg as relaxed as possible. The knee should be slightly bent, and the patient should look forward when walking. Instruct the patient not to bear weight on the axilla.	10		
8. Have the patient start in the tripod position and then move the crutches about 12 inches in front of his or her body (or less for a child).	5		

9. Have the patient put his weight on the crutches and move the body forward. Finish the step by having the patient swing the "good" or unaffected leg forward. Do not place weight on the "bad" or affected leg. Continue with these steps.	**5**		
10. To sit down: Instruct the patient to do the following: Back up to the chair, toilet, or bed until the seat touches the back of the legs. Move the "bad" or affected leg forward, balancing on the "good" or unaffected leg. Hold both crutches on the side with the "bad" or affected leg. Use the free hand to grab the seat or armrest. Slowly sit down.	**5**		
11. To stand up: Instruct the patient to do the following: Move toward the front of the seat and move the "bad" or affected leg forward. Hold both crutches on the side with the "bad" or affected leg. Use the free hand to push up from the seat to stand up. Balance on the "good" or unaffected leg while placing a crutch in each hand. Balance is needed before moving.	**5**		
12. To go up the stairs: Instruct the patient to do the following: Step up with the "good" or unaffected leg first. Then bring the crutches up, one in each arm. Finally place weight on the "good" or unaffected leg and bring the "bad" or affected leg up.	**5**		
13. To go down stairs: Instruct the patient to do the following: With a crutch in each hand, place the crutches on the first step. Then move the "bad" or affected leg forward and down. Lastly, follow with the "good" or unaffected leg.	**5**		
14. Instruct the patient and family on ways to prevent falls.	**10***		
15. Document the patient education in the patient's health record. Include the provider's name, the order, what was taught, how the patient responded, how the patient did the demonstration, and any handouts provided.	**10***		
Total Score	**100**		

Documentation

Comments

CAAHEP Competencies	Step(s)
I.P.8. Instruct and prepare a patient for a procedure or a treatment	3
V.P.4.d. Coach patients regarding: treatment plan	10-13
V.P.5.b. Coach patients appropriately considering: developmental life stage	6, 7
X.P.3. Document patient care accurately in the medical record	15
ABHES Competencies	**Step(s)**
4. Medical Law and Ethics a. Follow documentation guidelines	15
5. Human Relations d. Adapt care to address the developmental stages of life	6, 7
8. Clinical Procedures h. Teach self-examination, disease management and health promotion	10-13
8.k. Make adaptations to care for patients across their lifespan	6, 7

Procedure 35.6   Coach a Patient in the Use of a Walker

Name _____ **Date** _____ **Score** _____

Task: Fit a standard walker to the patient. Coach patient to use a standard walker properly, considering the patient's communication barrier and developmental life stage. Document teaching in the patient's health record.

Scenario: You are working with Dr. David Kahn. He has ordered you to teach Jana Green (DOB: 5/1/1936) how to use a standard walker. Jana needs the walker for extra stability. She has a hearing impairment. She can hear best with her right ear. She has no hearing in the left ear.

Equipment and Supplies:
- Standard walker
- Walker handout (optional)
- Provider's order
- Patient's health record

Standard: Complete the procedure and all critical steps in _____ minutes with a minimum score of 85% within two attempts (*or as indicated by the instructor*).

Scoring: Divide the points earned by the total possible points. Failure to perform a critical step, indicated by an asterisk (*), results in grade no higher than an 84% (*or as indicated by the instructor*).

Time: Began_____ Ended_____ Total minutes: _____

Steps	Possible Points	Attempt 1	Attempt 2
1. Wash hands or use hand sanitizer.	10*		
2. Read the provider's order. Assemble the equipment.	10		
3. Greet the patient. Identify yourself. Verify the patient's identity with full name and date of birth. Explain the procedure to be performed in a manner that the patient understands. Answer any questions the patient may have about the procedure.	10*		
4. Face the person when speaking. Position yourself so your voice is directed toward the patient's good ear. Use a low-pitched voice and speak clearly, slowly, and distinctly. Speak naturally. Limit medical terminology as you speak.	10		
5. Use simpler language when talking. Speak clearly. Communicate with dignity and respect. Allow time for the patient to respond. Listen to the patient's concerns.	10		
6. Ensure the patient is wearing shoes and ask the patient to step into the walker. The top of the walker grip should be even with the top of the hip line and near the crease in the wrist when the arms are at the side of the body. Adjust as needed. Keeping the shoulders relaxed and the hands on the grips will ensure the elbows are bent at a 15-degree angle.	10		

7.	Have the patient place the walker one step ahead of his or her body. Instruct the patient to use the "bad" or affected leg to step into the walker. The patient should not touch the front bar with the leg. Have the patient step forward with his or her other leg to complete the step. The patient will continue with this pattern while holding up the head and looking forward.	10		
8.	To sit down: Instruct the patient to back up to the chair, toilet, or bed until the seat touches the back of the legs. The patient can then use one hand to grab the seat or armrest and slowly sit down.	5		
9.	To stand up: Instruct the patient to move toward the front of the seat. Have the walker in front of the person. Have the patient use one hand to push up from the seat to stand up and then place hands on the walker. Remind patients to make sure they have their balance before moving.	5		
10.	Instruct the patient on ways to prevent falls. The walker should never be used on stairs or an escalator. If the patient will be using a bag on the front of the walker, instruct him or her to make sure not to overload it. Make sure to place all four legs of the walker on the ground before moving into the walker. Wash hands or use hand sanitizer.	10*		
11.	Document the patient education in the patient's health record. Include the provider's name, the order, what was taught, how the patient responded, how the patient did the demonstration, and any handouts provided.	10*		
	Total Score	100		

Documentation

Comments

CAAHEP Competencies	Step(s)
I.P.8. Instruct and prepare a patient for a procedure or a treatment	3
V.P.4.d. Coach patients regarding: treatment plan	8, 9
V.P.5.c. Coach patients appropriately considering: communication barriers	4, 5
X.P.3. Document patient care accurately in the medical record	11
ABHES Competencies	**Step(s)**
4. Medical Law and Ethics a. Follow documentation guidelines	11
8. Clinical Procedures h. Teach self-examination, disease management and health promotion	8, 9
8.j. Make adaptations for patients with special needs (psychological or physical limitations)	4, 5
8.k. Make adaptations to care for patients across their lifespan	4, 5

Procedure 35.7   Coach a Patient in the Use of a Cane

Name _____   Date _____   Score _____

Task: Fit a cane to a patient. Coach the patient to use a cane. Document teaching in the patient's health record.

Scenario: You are working with Dr. David Kahn. He has ordered you to teach Ella Rainwater (DOB: 7/11/1959) how to use a cane. Ella has left side weakness.

Equipment and Supplies:
- Cane
- Handout on cane walking (optional)
- Provider's order
- Patient's health record

Standard: Complete the procedure and all critical steps in _____ minutes with a minimum score of 85% within two attempts (*or as indicated by the instructor*).

Scoring: Divide the points earned by the total possible points. Failure to perform a critical step, indicated by an asterisk (*), results in grade no higher than an 84% (*or as indicated by the instructor*).

Time: Began_____ Ended_____ Total minutes: _____

Steps	Possible Points	Attempt 1	Attempt 2
1. Wash hands or use hand sanitizer.	**15***		
2. Read the provider's order. Assemble the equipment.	**10**		
3. Greet the patient. Identify yourself. Verify the patient's identity with full name and date of birth. Explain the procedure to be performed in a manner that the patient understands. Answer any questions the patient may have about the procedure.	**10***		
4. Ensure the patient is wearing shoes. The top of the cane should be near the crease in the wrist, when the arms are at the side of the body. Adjust as needed. With the patient's shoulders relaxed and hand on the cane, ensure the elbows are bent at a 15-degree angle.	**10**		
5. Instruct the patient to hold the cane on the "good" or unaffected side. The patient should take a step moving the "bad" or affected leg and the cane forward at the same time and then step forward with the "good" leg. Instruct the patient to lean on the cane as needed.	**10**		
6. To sit down: Instruct the patient to back up to the chair, toilet, or bed until the seat touches the back of the legs. The patient can then use a hand to grab the seat or armrest and slowly sit down.	**5**		
7. To stand up: Instruct the patient to move toward the front of the seat and move the "bad" or affected leg forward. The patient can then use a hand to push up from the seat to stand up. Remind patients to make sure to get their balance before moving.	**5**		
8. To go up the stairs: Instruct the patient to step up with the "good" or unaffected leg first while holding onto the rail. Then the patient should bring up the "bad" or affected leg to the same step. If there is no handrail, the cane and the "bad" leg should be placed on the stair at the same time.	**5**		

9.	To go down stairs: Instruct the patient to hold onto the rail and move the "bad" or affected leg down first. Then the patient should place the "good" or unaffected leg on the same step as the "bad" leg. When there is no handrail, instruct the patient to place the cane on the lower step, then place the "bad" or affected leg, and lastly place the "good" or unaffected leg next to the "bad" or affected leg.	**5**		
10.	Instruct the patient on ways to prevent falls.	**10***		
11.	Document the patient education in the patient's health record. Include the provider's name, the order, what was taught, how the patient responded, how the patient did the demonstration, and any handouts provided.	**15***		
	Total Score	**100**		

Documentation

Comments

CAAHEP Competencies	Step(s)
I.P.8. Instruct and prepare a patient for a procedure or a treatment	3
V.P.4.d. Coach patients regarding: treatment plan	5-9
X.P.3. Document patient care accurately in the medical record	11
ABHES Competencies	**Step(s)**
4. Medical Law and Ethics a. Follow documentation guidelines	11
8. Clinical Procedures h. Teach self-examination, disease management and health promotion	5-9
8.j. Make adaptations for patients with special needs (psychological or physical limitations)	4, 5

Neurology

CAAHEP Competencies	Assessment
I.C.4. List major organs in each body system	Skills and Concepts – A. 1-4, 6; Certification Preparation – 1
I.C.5. Identify the anatomical location of major organs in each body system	Skills and Concepts – A. 4, 7-10; Certification Preparation – 6
I.C.6. Compare structure and function of the human body across the life span	Skills and Concepts – A. 11; Certification Preparation – 8, 10
I.C.7. Describe the normal function of each body system	Skills and Concepts – A. 4, 5, 7, B. 1-9
I.C.8.a. Identify common pathology related to each body system including: signs	Skills and Concepts – C. 1, 7; Certification Preparation – 7; Workplace Application – 1-3
I.C.8.b. Identify common pathology related to each body system including: symptoms	Skills and Concepts – C. 1, 7; Certification Preparation – 7; Workplace Application – 1-3
I.C.8.c. Identify common pathology related to each body system including: etiology	Skills and Concepts – C. 4, 11, 12; Workplace Application – 2, 3
I.C.9.a. Analyze pathology for each body system including: diagnostic measures	Skills and Concepts – D. 3; Internet Activities – 1, 2
I.C.9.b. Analyze pathology for each body system including: treatment modalities	Skills and Concepts – C. 8 D. 4, 6; Workplace Application – 2-4
I.P.8. Instruct and prepare a patient for a procedure or a treatment	Procedure 36.2-36.4
V.C.10. Define medical terms and abbreviations related to all body systems	Vocabulary Review – 1-24; Abbreviations – 1-29
X.P.3. Document patient care accurately in the medical record	Procedure 36.1, 36.3, 36.4

ABHES Competencies	Assessment
2. Anatomy and Physiology a. List all body systems and their structures and functions	Skills and Concepts – A. 1-10, B. 1-9; Certification Preparation – 6
2.b. Describe common diseases, symptoms, and etiologies as they apply to each system	Skills and Concepts – C. 1, 4, 7, 11, 12; Certification Preparation – 7; Workplace Application – 1-3
2.c. Identify diagnostic and treatment modalities as they relate to each body system	Skills and Concepts – C. 8, D. 34, 36; Workplace Application – 2-4; Internet Activities – 1, 2
3. Medical Terminology c. Apply medical terminology for each specialty	Vocabulary Review – A. 1-10, B. 1-10, C. 1-9

ABHES Competencies	Assessment
3.d. Define and use medical abbreviations when appropriate and acceptable	Abbreviations – 1-24
4. Medical Law and Ethics a. Follow documentation guidelines	Procedure 36.1, 36.3, 36.4
8.e. Perform specialty procedures, including but not limited to minor surgery, cardiac, respiratory, OB-GYN, neurological, and gastroenterology	Procedure 36.2, 36.3

VOCABULARY REVIEW

Using the word pool on the right, find the correct word to match the definition. Write the word on the line after the definition.

Group A

1. Consists of several structures including the amygdala, hippocampus, and hypothalamus; plays an important role with behavior, memories, and emotions _____

2. Nerve tissue that lacks the insulation that causes a white appearance to other nerves; looks gray _____

3. Grooves or depressions on the surface of the brain between the gyri _____

4. A ridge in the floor of the lateral ventricle; composed of gray matter; involved with the limbic system and with creating and filing new memories _____

5. Folds or convolutions on the surface of the cerebral hemisphere, which increase the gray matter surface area

   _____

6. A system of tissues and/or organs that function together

   _____

7. Partial or complete loss of the ability to articulate ideas or understand written or spoken language _____

8. A small organ in the brain that secretes melatonin, a hormone that regulates the sleep/wake cycle _____

9. A groove that divides an organ into lobes or parts

   _____

10. A small mass of gray matter found in each temporal lobe of the cerebrum that is involved with memories, emotions, and activating the fight-or-flight response; part of the limbic system

    _____

Word Pool
- fissure
- aphasia
- amygdala
- limbic system
- gray matter
- gyri
- sulci
- pineal gland
- tract
- hippocampus

Group B

1. Pertaining to carrying away from a structure
   _____

2. A protective insulation that covers the axons and helps with the transmission of nerve impulses _____

3. Detectable cellular indicators used as a marker for a substance or disease process _____

4. The internal environment of the body that is compatible with life; a steady state that is created by all the body systems working together to provide a consistent and unvarying internal environment _____

5. A chemical that helps a nerve cell communicate with another nerve cell or muscle _____

6. An immune response against a person's own tissues, cells, or cell parts, leading to the deterioration of tissue
   _____

7. A long extension of a nerve fiber that conducts the impulse away from the nerve cell body _____

8. Pertaining to carrying toward a structure
   _____

9. The destination or intended tissue in the nervous impulse (e.g., a muscle) _____

10. A large opening in the base of the skull; forms a passageway for the spinal cord _____

Word Pool
- foramen magnum
- axons
- homeostasis
- afferent
- efferent
- neurotransmitters
- target tissue
- myelin sheath
- biomarkers
- autoimmune

Group C

1. A type of brain injury resulting from a blow to the head or body that causes the brain to move rapidly back and forth
   _____

2. Condition resulting from internal head injuries that occur when a baby or young child is violently shaken _____

3. An abnormal accumulation of cerebrospinal fluid that causes enlargement of the skull and compression of the brain
   _____

4. A scale used to measure the level of consciousness and severity of a head injury _____

5. An abnormal blood-filled sac formed from a localized dilation of the wall of a vein, artery, or heart _____

6. Sharp, spasm-like pain in a nerve or along the course of one or more nerves _____

7. A nerve response test that uses electrodes, which are placed on the scalp to measure brain reaction to a stimulus
   _____

8. A soft membranous gap between the incompletely formed cranial bones of an infant; also called a *soft spot* _____

9. Category of medication used to relieve pain
   _____

Word Pool
- evoked potential test
- analgesics
- shaken baby syndrome
- fontanel
- concussion
- Glasgow coma scale
- neuralgia
- hydrocephalus
- aneurysm

ABBREVIATIONS

Write out what each of the following abbreviations stands for.

1. CNS _____

2. PNS _____

3. ANS _____

4. CSF _____

5. BBB _____

6. ALS _____

7. AD _____

8. PET _____

9. HD _____

10. MS _____

11. PD _____

12. DHE _____

13. SPECT _____

14. TBI _____

15. NCV _____

16. EMG _____

17. CVA _____

18. TIA _____

19. A&Ox3 _____

20. LP _____

21. EEG _____

22. SBS _____

23. ICP _____

24. DBS _____

SKILLS AND CONCEPTS

Answer the following questions. Write your answer on the line or in the space provided.

A. Anatomy of the Nervous Systems

1. Describe the structures that make up the central nervous system (CNS). _____
   _____

2. Describe the structures that make up the peripheral nervous system (PNS). _____
   _____
   _____

3. The PNS is made up of two subsystems, the _____ and the
   _____.

4. Briefly describe the function of each lobe of the cerebrum. _____
   _____
   _____

5. Briefly describe the function of the cerebellum. _____
   _____

6. What structures make up the diencephalon? _____
   _____

7. Briefly describe the function of the brainstem. _____
   _____
   _____

8. Where does the spinal cord start and end? _____
   _____

9. List the three layers of the meninges that cover the spinal cord, from outer to inner. _____
   _____

10. The peripheral nervous system (PNS) is made up of the nerves that exit the _____ or
    _____. The peripheral nerves exiting the brain directly through the skull are called
    _____. The peripheral nerves that exit the spinal canal through spaces between the
    vertebrae are called _____.

11. Describe the changes in the neurologic system across the life span. _____
    _____
    _____
    _____

B. Physiology of the Nervous System

1. What are the three functions of the nervous system? _____

    _____

    _____

2. The nervous system is made up of two types of cells; _____ carry out the work of
    the nervous system and _____ provide a supportive function to the neurons.

3. A nerve impulse is also called a(n) _____.

4. A nerve impulse is an electrical impulse as it travels down an axon, but then becomes a chemical im-
    pulse as it moves across the _____. The chemical impulse moves across the synapse
    with the help of _____.

5. Define *target tissue* in your own words. _____

    _____

6. Give two examples of a neurotransmitter. _____

    _____

    _____

    _____

7. List the four types of neuroglia or glia cells in the nervous system. _____

    _____

8. Describe the myelin sheath in your own words. What structure does it cover in the nervous system?

    _____

    _____

9. The autonomic nervous system (ANS) is divided into two subsystems. Name the systems and their
    quick-phrase function.

    _____

    _____

C. Disorders of the Nervous System

1. List common signs and symptoms of nervous system diseases and disorders. _____

    _____

    _____

2. Briefly describe ALS. _____

    _____

    _____

3.   Name and describe the most common form of dementia. _____

_____

_____

_____

4.   Describe the cause of Huntington disease. _____

_____

_____

5.   Describe multiple sclerosis. _____

_____

_____

6.   List the four types of multiple sclerosis. _____

_____

_____

7.   Describe the signs and symptoms of Parkinson disease. _____

_____

_____

8.   List common medication used to treat headaches. _____

_____

9.   How are seizure disorders diagnosed? _____

_____

_____

10. Define *encephalitis.*_____

_____

_____

_____

11. What is meningitis and what causes the condition? _____

_____

_____

12. What is the cause of Guillain-Barré syndrome? _____

_____

_____

13. What is the mildest form of traumatic brain injury? _____

14. Define the following terms.

    a. Quadriplegia _____

    b. Paraplegia _____

    c. Peripheral neuropathy _____

    d. Shingles _____

    e. Spina bifida _____

    f. Meningocele _____

    g. Myelomeningocele _____

15. A cerebrovascular accident (CVA) is also called a(n) _____.

16. List the three types of strokes. _____

_____

_____

_____

D. The Medical Assistant's Role in Neurology Procedures

1. List assessments that may be included in a neurology examination for an adult or child. _____

_____

_____

2. List assessments that may be included in a neurology examination for a newborn or infant. _____

_____

_____

3. Briefly describe a lumbar puncture. _____

_____

_____

4. Which medications may increase the risk of bleeding during a lumbar puncture? _____

_____

5. What are some side effects that may be experienced after a lumbar puncture? _____

_____

_____

_____

6. Patients with neurologic disorders are prescribed a variety of medications. Briefly describe the following classifications of medications.

    a. Analgesics _____

    b. Anesthetics _____

    c. Anti-Alzheimer _____

    d. Anticonvulsants _____

    e. Antidepressants _____

    f. Antimigraines _____

    g. Corticosteroids _____

CERTIFICATION PREPARATION

Circle the correct answer.

1. The central nervous system contains which structure(s)?
    a. Cranial nerves
    b. Brain
    c. Spinal cord
    d. Both b and c

2. Which subsystem is part of the autonomic nervous system?
    a. Somatic nervous system
    b. Parasympathetic nervous system
    c. Central nervous system
    d. Peripheral nervous system

3. The nervous system works in partnership with which other system to help the body maintain homeostasis?
    a. Endocrine system
    b. Cardiovascular system
    c. Respiratory system
    d. None of the above

4. Which structure of a nerve cell carries impulses away from the cell body?
    a. Glia
    b. Dendrite
    c. Myelin sheath
    d. Axon

5. A chemical that helps a nerve cell communicate with another nerve cell or muscle is
    a. a synapse.
    b. the cerebrospinal fluid.
    c. a neurotransmitter.
    d. the myelin sheath.

6. The pons is located in the
    a. cerebrum.
    b. cerebellum.
    c. brainstem.
    d. spinal cord.

7. Which could be a sign or symptom of a cerebrovascular accident?
    a. Numbness or weakness of the face, leg, or arm
    b. Difficulty speaking
    c. Loss of balance or coordination
    d. All of the above

8. Alzheimer disease is most commonly diagnosed in which age group?
    a. 40-50
    b. 50-60
    c. After age 65
    d. None of the above

9. Which term is defined as a fold or convolution on the surface of the cerebral hemisphere?
    a. Gyri
    b. Sulci
    c. Fissure
    d. Tract

10. Which condition can be detected before birth?
    a. Spina bifida
    b. Cerebral palsy
    c. ADHD
    d. All of the above

WORKPLACE APPLICATIONS

1. Tia goes into the waiting room and starts to call back the next patient, Charlie Wayne-Thomas. Charlie is a regular patient at Walden-Martin Family Medical (WMFM) Clinic. He is 62 years old and in good health. When Tia calls him, he looks at her but only mumbles, he is pointing to his right leg and shaking his head back and forth as if to say "no." Tia tries to talk to Charlie, but she cannot understand his mumbling. Given this limited information, answer the questions below.

    a. What condition or conditions could be causing Charlie's signs and symptoms? _____

    _____

    b. Would this situation be considered a medical emergency? _____

    _____

    c. What should Tia do next?_____

    _____

    _____

    _____

2. Tia is reviewing nervous system diseases and disorders as part of a continuing education course. Briefly describe the nervous system conditions below, and include common signs and symptoms.

    a. Huntington disease or Huntington chorea _____

    _____

    b. Concussion _____

    _____

    c. Bell palsy_____

    _____

    _____

3. Sherman Potter was recently diagnosed with migraine headaches.

    a. What is the cause of migraine headaches?_____

    _____

    _____

    b. Briefly describe the signs and symptoms of a migraine headache. _____

    _____

    _____

    _____

    _____

INTERNET ACTIVITIES

1. Using online resources, research a test used for diagnosing a nervous system disease. Create a poster presentation, a PowerPoint presentation, or a written paper summarizing your research. Include the following points in your project:
   a. Description of the test
   b. Any contraindications for the test
   c. Patient preparation for the test
   d. What occurs during the test

2. Using online resources, research a nervous system disease or disorder. Create a poster presentation, a PowerPoint presentation, or a written paper summarizing your research. Include the following points in your project:
   a. Description of the disease
   b. Etiology
   c. Signs and symptoms
   d. Diagnostic procedures
   e. Treatments
   f. Prognosis
   g. Prevention

3. Using online resources, research the effect that diet can have on the management of multiple sclerosis. In a one-page paper, summarize the information that you found.

4. Using Table 36.7, Medication Classifications, select two medications from each of the following classifications: anticonvulsants and antimigraine. Using the information in Table 36.7, identify for each medication:
   a. Reasons for use
   b. Desired effects
   c. Side effects
   d. Adverse reactions

   Write a short paper addressing each of these four areas for each medication.

Procedure 36.1   Perform a Neurologic Status Exam

Name _____ Date _____ Score _____

Task: Administer and score a neurologic status exam.

Scenario: Dr. Arzt ordered a neurologic status exam form to be completed on Robert Caudill (date of birth [DOB] 10/31/1940). He is being accompanied by his caregiver. Role-play this scenario with two peers.

Equipment and Supplies:
- Patient's health record
- Order for the neurologic status exam
- Neurologic Status Exam Form (Work Product 36.1) or SimChart for the Medical Office (SCMO).

Standard: Complete the procedure and all critical steps in _____ minutes with a minimum score of 85% within two attempts (*or as indicated by the instructor*).

Scoring: Divide the points earned by the total possible points. Failure to perform a critical step, indicated by an asterisk (*), results in grade no higher than an 84% (*or as indicated by the instructor*).

Time: Began_____ Ended_____ Total minutes: _____

Steps:	Point Value	Attempt 1	Attempt 2
1. Wash hands or use hand sanitizer.	10		
2. SCMO: Click on the Form Repository and select the Neurologic Status Exam on the INFO PANEL. <u>For both forms:</u> Read the directions for the test.	10		
3. Greet the patient. Identify yourself. Verify the patient's identity with full name and date of birth. Explain the procedure to be performed in a manner that the patient understands. Answer any questions the patient may have about the procedure.	10		
4. SCMO: Click on Patient Search. Select the patient and verify the DOB. Click Select and the patient's name and DOB will autofill into the form field. Key in the information for the Performed By and Date fields. <u>Paper form:</u> Complete the following information on the exam form: patient name, date of birth, performed by, and date.	10		
5. Ask for the caregiver's name and clearly ask the caregiver-related questions from the form. Accurately document the information obtained.	15		
6. Perform the patient interview, following the directions on the form. Clearly provide the patient with the directions and the questions. Accurately document the information obtained from the patient.	30		
7. Accurately score the test as indicated by the directions. <u>SCMO:</u> Key the scores in the total fields. Save the form when completed. <u>Paper form:</u> Write the scores on the total line. Give the completed form to the provider.	15*		
Total Points	100		

Comments

CAAHEP Competencies	Step(s)
X.P.3. Document patient care accurately in the medical record	4-7
ABHES Competencies	**Step(s)**
4. Medical Law and Ethics a. Follow documentation guidelines	4-7

Work Product 36.1   Neurologic Status Exam

Name _____ Date _____ Score _____

WALDEN-MARTIN
FAMILY MEDICAL CLINIC
1234 ANYSTREET | ANYTOWN, ANYSTATE 12345
PHONE 123-123-1234 | FAX 123-123-5678

Neurological Status Exam

The Neurological Status Examination tests the individual's sense of cognitive functions and quickly allows the provider to screen for cognitive impairment and/or loss. In addition to testing language recall and motor skills, the NSE also allows you to test an individual's orientation to time, detail, and attention.

There are five sections. Each section of the test involves relating a series of questions or commands to a patient; the patient should receive one point for each correct answer. Conduct the test without interruptions in a well-lit, private exam room. Instruct the patient to listen carefully and to answer each question as accurately as possible. In the event that there is a caregiver accompanying the patient, ask the Caregiver Questions and record the responses (these are not part of the final score).

Read each question once and document the patient's response. Do not time the patient's answers or duration of the test overall; once completed, score the test immediately. To do so, add only the number of correct responses. The individual can receive a maximum score of 10 points; a score below 4 indicates cognitive impairment.

Patient Name: _____   **Date of Birth:** _____

Performed By: _____   **Date:** _____

Caregiver Questions (if available): (Yes, No, Not Aware)

Name of Caregiver: _____	Yes	No	Not Aware
• Does the patient have difficulty remembering recent events or conversions?	☐	☐	☐
• Does the patient have difficulty performing activities of daily living (bath, driving, cooking, etc.)	☐	☐	☐
• Have you noticed changes to speech patterns?	☐	☐	☐

Patient Interview

Sequencing:

Read the following statement to the patient three consecutive times: **"Drive the red car to Washington Street"**. Then ask the patient to restate the sentence; you will ask the patient to recall the statement later in the test.

	Yes	No
The patient was able to repeat the exact statement to you.	☐	☐

Total: _____

Time Orientation:

Ask the patient the following questions:

	Correct	Incorrect
• What is today's date?	☐	☐
• What season is it?	☐	☐

- What is the day of the week?

☐   ☐

Total: _____

Drawing:

Give the individual a piece of paper and ask him/her to copy a design of the two intersecting shapes. One point is awarded for correctly copying the shapes. All angles on both figures must be present, and the figures must have one overlapping angle.

Correct   **Incorrect**

☐   ☐

Total: _____

Information:

Ask the patient the following questions:

Correct   **Incorrect**

- Who is president of the United States?   ☐   ☐
- How many stars are on the American flag?   ☐   ☐

Total: _____

Recall:

Ask the patient to restate the sentence that you asked him/her at the beginning of the procedure. One point is given for repeating each of the following words.

Correct   **Incorrect**

- Drive   ☐   ☐
- Red Car   ☐   ☐
- Washington Street   ☐   ☐

Total: _____

Total Exam Score: _____

Procedure 36.2 Assist with the Neurologic Exam

Name _____ **Date** _____ **Score** _____

Tasks: Set up for a neuro exam and prepare a patient for the procedure. Assist the provider and the patient during the neuro exam.

Equipment and Supplies:
- Patient's health record
- Patient gown
- Drape
- Otoscope
- Ophthalmoscope
- Percussion hammer
- Disposable pinwheel
- Penlight
- Tuning fork
- Cotton ball
- Tongue depressor
- Small vials of warm, cold, sweet, and salty liquids
- Small vials of substances with distinct odors (e.g., spices, coffee, vanilla)
- Gloves
- Disinfecting wipes
- Biohazard sharps container
- Waste container

Standard: Complete the procedure and all critical steps in _____ minutes with a minimum score of 85% within two attempts (*or as indicated by the instructor*).

Scoring: Divide the points earned by the total possible points. Failure to perform a critical step, indicated by an asterisk (*), results in grade no higher than an 84% (*or as indicated by the instructor*).

Time: Began_____ Ended_____ Total minutes: _____

Steps:	Point Value	Attempt 1	Attempt 2
1. Wash hands or use hand sanitizer.	10		
2. Assemble supplies and equipment in the exam room.	25		
3. Greet the patient. Identify yourself. Verify the patient's identity with full name and date of birth. Explain the procedure to be performed in a manner that the patient understands. Answer any questions the patient may have about the procedure. Encourage the patient to use the restroom before the procedure.	15		
4. Instruct the patient to change into the gown. The opening should be in the back. Ask the patient if assistance is needed. If so, help. If not, leave the room and allow the patient time to change. When reentering the room, provide a courtesy knock on the door.	10		
5. During the examination, be prepared to assist the patient in changing positions as necessary. Have the necessary examination instruments ready for the provider at the appropriate time during the examination. Record all results from the examination as indicated by the provider.	20		

6.	After the exam, put on gloves and clean the exam room. Discard sharps in the biohazard sharps container. Discard other waste in the appropriate waste containers. Disinfect equipment and surfaces (e.g., exam table). Remove gloves and discard.	**10**		
7.	Wash hands or use hand sanitizer.	**10**		
	Total Points	**100**		

Comments

CAAHEP Competencies	**Step(s)**
I.P.8. Instruct and prepare a patient for a procedure or a treatment	3, 4, 5
ABHES Competencies	**Step(s)**
8.e. Perform specialty procedures, including but not limited to minor surgery, cardiac, respiratory, OB-GYN, neurological, and gastroenterology	Entire procedure

Procedure 36.3   Assist with a Lumbar Puncture

Name _____ Date _____ Score _____

Tasks: Set up for a lumbar puncture and prepare a patient for the procedure. Assist the provider during the lumbar puncture procedure. Document the procedure in the patient's health record.

Equipment and Supplies:
- Patient's health record
- Patient gown
- Drape
- Local anesthetic vial
- Syringe and needle
- Alcohol wipes
- Sterile, disposable lumbar puncture kit with specimen tubes
- Mayo stand
- Permanent marker or printed patient labels
- Laboratory requisition and specimen transport bag
- Gloves
- Biohazard waste container
- Waste container
- Consent form
- Lumbar puncture instructions (optional)

Standard: Complete the procedure and all critical steps in _____ minutes with a minimum score of 85% within two attempts (*or as indicated by the instructor*).

Scoring: Divide the points earned by the total possible points. Failure to perform a critical step, indicated by an asterisk (*), results in grade no higher than an 84% (*or as indicated by the instructor*).

Time: Began_____ Ended_____ Total minutes: _____

Steps:	Point Value	Attempt 1	Attempt 2
1. Wash hands or use hand sanitizer.	5		
2. Assemble supplies and equipment in the treatment room.	5		
3. Greet the patient. Identify yourself. Verify the patient's identity with full name and date of birth. Explain the procedure to be performed in a manner that the patient understands. Answer any questions the patient may have about the procedure. Encourage the patient to use the restroom before the procedure.	5		
4. Check if the consent form was signed. If the consent was not signed, ask the patient if he or she has any questions. If there are no questions, explain the consent form and have the patient sign the form. If the patient has questions, let the provider know.	5*		
5. Instruct the patient to change into the gown. The opening should be in the back. Ask the patient if assistance is needed. If so, help. If not, leave the room and allow the patient time to change. When reentering the room, provide a courtesy knock on the door.	5		

6. Assist the patient into a left side-lying position with the knees drawn up to the chest, or into a sitting position leaning forward on a stable surface. Support the patient's head with a pillow as necessary and provide a pillow for between the knees if needed.	5		
7. Prepare the skin preparation for the provider to use. Open the sterile disposable lumbar puncture kit on a Mayo stand. Without contaminating the supplies, add a sterile needle and sterile syringe to the sterile field.	10*		
8. If needed, help the patient remain in the proper position. Use the drape to cover the patient. Give verbal encouragement to the patient during the procedure.	5		
9. Assist the provider as needed during the procedure. When the provider is ready for the anesthetic, wipe the top of the vial with alcohol. Show the label to the provider and then hold the vial upside down as the provider withdraws the medication needed.	10		
10. Attach the printed labels to the specimen tubes or using the permanent marker label the specimens #1, #2, #3, and so on in the order in which they are collected.	5*		
11. Complete the laboratory requisition form and prepare the CSF specimens for transport to the laboratory.	5*		
12. Put on gloves. Discard the needle/syringe in a biohazard sharps container. Make sure to put the needle in first. Clean up the area. Discard the waste in the appropriate waste container. Remove gloves and discard.	5		
13. Wash hands or use hand sanitizer.	5		
14. Monitor the patient and give liquids as directed by the provider. When the patient is ready to leave, instruct the patient to get dressed. Ask the patient if assistance is needed. If so, help. If not, leave the room and allow the patient time to change.	5		
15. After the patient leaves, put on gloves and clean the room. Disinfect surfaces and discard waste. Remove gloves and discard.	5		
16. Wash hands or use hand sanitizer.	5		
17. Document the procedure in the patient's health record. Include the provider's name, the samples obtained, how the patient tolerated the procedure, and any instructions given.	10		
Total Points	100		

Documentation

Comments

CAAHEP Competencies	Step(s)
I.P.8. Instruct and prepare a patient for a procedure or a treatment	3, 5, 6, 8
X.P.3. Document patient care accurately in the medical record	15
ABHES Competencies	**Step(s)**
4. Medical Law and Ethics a. Follow documentation guidelines	15
8.e. Perform specialty procedures, including but not limited to minor surgery, cardiac, respiratory, OB-GYN, neurological, and gastroenterology	Entire procedure

Procedure 36.4 Coach a Patient for an Electroencephalogram

Name _____ Date _____ Score _____

Tasks: Coach a patient on the preparation needed for an electroencephalogram (EEG). Document in the patient's health record.

Order: Provide EEG instructions.

Equipment and Supplies:
- Patient's health record
- Instruction sheet for EEG (optional)

Standard: Complete the procedure and all critical steps in _____ minutes with a minimum score of 85% within two attempts (*or as indicated by the instructor*).

Scoring: Divide the points earned by the total possible points. Failure to perform a critical step, indicated by an asterisk (*), results in grade no higher than an 84% (*or as indicated by the instructor*).

Time: Began_____ Ended_____ Total minutes: _____

Steps:	Point Value	Attempt 1	Attempt 2
1. Wash hands or use hand sanitizer.	5		
2. Greet the patient. Identify yourself. Verify the patient's identity with full name and date of birth. Explain the procedure to be performed in a manner that the patient understands. Answer any questions the patient may have about the procedure.	10		
3. Explain the purpose of an EEG. An EEG is done to check for changes in the brain activity and can be helpful when diagnosing different disorders.	15		
4. Explain how the patient should prepare for the test. The patient should avoid caffeine on the day of the test. Take daily medications unless the provider indicates to hold medications until after the test. Wash hair the night before or the morning of the test, but do not use conditioners or any other hair care products. If the patient is to sleep during the EEG test, encourage the patient to stay up later the night before the test or to avoid sleeping.	20		
5. Explain what the patient should expect during the test. Electrodes (patches with wires) will be attached to the head either with adhesive or by using a special cap. There will be little to no discomfort during the test. The technician may ask the patient questions during the test.	15		
6. Explain what the patient should expect after the test. The technician will remove the electrodes. If sedation was given, the patient will need a ride home, must rest for the remaining part of the day, and must not drive.	15		
7. Let the patient know when to anticipate the results from the EEG. Also, give the patient the appointment information for the EEG, including the location and time.	10		
8. Document the teaching inthe patient's health record. Include the provider's name and the information given: the type of instructions, appointment information, and any materials.	10		
Total Points	**100**		

Documentation

Comments

CAAHEP Competencies	Step(s)
I.P.8. Instruct and prepare a patient for a procedure or a treatment	2-6
X.P.3. Document patient care accurately in the medical record	7
ABHES Competencies	**Step(s)**
4. Medical Law and Ethics a. Follow documentation guidelines	7

Behavioral Health

CAAHEP Competencies	Assessment
I.C.6. Compare structure and function of the human body across the life span	Skills and Concepts – C. 2
I.C.8.a. Identify common pathology related to each body system including: signs	Skills and Concepts – C. 6, 11, 12, 17, D. 2; Internet Activity – 2
I.C.8.b. Identify common pathology related to each body system including: symptoms	Skills and Concepts – C. 6, 11, 12, 17, D. 2; Certification Preparation – 7; Internet Activity – 2
I.C.8.c. Identify common pathology related to each body system including: etiology	Skills and Concepts – C. 4; Internet Activity – 2
I.C.9.a. Analyze pathology for each body system including: diagnostic measures	Skills and Concepts – C. 7, 13, E. 1; Internet Activity – 1, 2
I.C.9.b. Analyze pathology for each body system including: treatment modalities	Skills and Concepts – C. 8, 14, E. 2, 3; Certification Preparation – 8; Internet Activity – 2, 4
V.C.10. Define medical terms and abbreviations related to all body systems	Vocabulary Review – A. 1-7, B. 1-8; Abbreviations – 1-25

ABHES Competencies	Assessment
2. Anatomy and Physiology 2.b. Describe common diseases, symptoms, and etiologies as they apply to each system	Skills and Concepts – C. 4, 6, 11, 12, 17, D. 2; Certification Preparation – 7; Internet Activity – 2
2.c. Identify diagnostic and treatment modalities as they relate to each body system	Skills and Concepts – C. 7, 8, 13, 14, E. 1-3; Certification Preparation – 8; Internet Activity – 1, 2, 4
3. Medical Terminology c. Apply medical terminology for each specialty	Vocabulary Review – A. 1-7, B. 1-8
3.d. Define and use medical abbreviations when appropriate and acceptable	Abbreviations – 1-26

VOCABULARY REVIEW

Using the word pool on the right, find the correct word to match the definition. Write the word on the line after the definition.

Group A

1. A small mass of gray matter found in each temporal lobe of the cerebrum; involved with memories, emotions, and activating the fight-or-flight response _____

2. Abnormally elated mental state; the person may have feelings of euphoria, lack of inhibitions, sleeplessness, talkativeness, risk-taking behaviors, and irritability _____

3. Unshakable belief in something untrue; maybe accompanied by hallucinations and/or paranoia _____

4. The relative frequency of deaths in a specific population

   _____

5. A sensory experience (e.g., a smell, sound, sight, touch, or taste) involving something that is not present _____

6. A treatment of behavioral health disorders which encourage communication of conflicts and insights into the person's problems; goals include symptoms relief, changes in behavior, improved social and vocational function, and personality growth

   _____

7. The rate of the disease in a population _____

Word Pool
- psychotherapy
- morbidity
- mortality
- amygdala
- delusions
- hallucinations
- mania

Group B

1. Alternative perception of the self; a person's own reality is lost; people feel they are not in control of their own actions or speech

   _____

2. An unfounded or excessive suspicion of the motives of others

   _____

3. Patient-provider details from private, group, or family therapy, including what the patient stated and the provider's analysis of the statements and situation _____

4. Memory loss _____

5. Loss of sensation of the reality of one's surroundings

   _____

6. The external emotional expression _____

7. Awareness of one's environment, with reference to people, place, and time _____

8. An exaggerated sense of physical and mental well-being

   _____

Word Pool
- euphoria
- amnesia
- depersonalization
- derealization
- paranoia
- affect
- orientation
- psychotherapy notes

ABBREVIATIONS

Write out what each of the following abbreviations stands for.

1. LCSW _____

2. LICSW _____

3. LSW _____

4. DSM _____

5. ICD _____

6. GAD _____

7. CBT _____

8. OCD _____

9. HD _____

10. SSRI _____

11. SNRI _____

12. ASD _____

13. ADHD _____

14. ODD _____

15. CD _____

16. PTSD _____

17. EMDR _____

18. AUD _____

19. WAIS _____

20. IQ _____

21. DAP test _____

22. MMPI _____

23. TAT _____

24. IPT _____

25. DBT _____

26. SOB _____

SKILLS AND CONCEPTS

Answer the following questions. Write your answer on the line or in the space provided.

A. Behavioral Health Professionals

1. Describe the behavioral health professionals listed below.

    a. Psychiatrist _____

    _____

    b. Psychologist _____

    _____

    c. Social worker _____

    _____

    d. Cognitive behavioral therapist (CBT)_____

    _____

    e. Psychiatric nurse _____

    _____

    f. Substance abuse (or addiction) therapist or counselor _____

    _____

    g. Mental health therapist or counselor _____

    _____

B. Diagnostic and Statistical Manual of Mental Disorders

1. The DSM-5 contains the International Classification of Disease (ICD) codes required for insurance reimbursement and for monitoring the _____ and _____ statistics.

C. Mental Health Disorders

1. Mental health disorders are conditions that cause changes in the _____, _____, or _____ of an individual.

2. Describe behavioral health concerns across the life span. _____

    _____

    _____

    _____

    _____

3. Briefly describe generalized anxiety disorder (GAD). _____

   _____

   _____

4. What are the etiology and risk factors for OCD? _____

   _____

   _____

5. Define *panic disorder.* _____

   _____

   _____

6. What are the signs and symptoms of panic disorder? _____

   _____

7. How is panic disorder diagnosed? _____

   _____

   _____

   _____

8. How is panic disorder treated? _____

   _____

9. Define *phobia.* _____

   _____

   _____

10. There are many types of phobias. Using Table 37.1 in the textbook, name the following phobias.

    a. A fear of heights _____

    b. A fear of water _____

    c. A fear of spiders _____

    d. A fear of flying _____

    e. A fear of pain _____

    f. A fear of closed spaces _____

    g. A fear of needles _____

    h. A fear of speaking in front of people _____

    i. A fear of disease _____

11. List the signs and symptoms associated with social anxiety disorder. _____

_____

_____

_____

12. What are the signs and symptoms of autism spectrum disorder? _____

_____

_____

_____

_____

13. How is depression diagnosed? _____

_____

_____

_____

14. What medication may be used to treat depression? List the generic and brand names of the medications.

_____

15. Describe bipolar disorder. _____

_____

_____

_____

_____

16. Disruptive behavior disorder involves _____ or _____ action patterns of behavior. The person may have temper tantrums, _____, demonstrate _____ behaviors, and fight with others. People with disruptive behavioral disorder have problems controlling their _____ and _____, leading to is-sues at school and home.

17. List the signs and symptoms of ADHD. _____

_____

18. List three types of oppositional defiant disorder. _____

_____

19. Describe the following conditions.

a. Anorexia nervosa_____

b. Binge eating disorder _____

c. Bulimia nervosa _____

20. _____ is a condition that occurs after experiencing or witnessing a traumatic or terrifying event.

21. _____ causes disruptions in thought processes, perceptions, emotional responsiveness, and social interactions. Usually diagnosed in the _____ to the early thirties. It is more common in _____ than _____.

22. _____ is death caused by a self-inflicted injury with an intent to die as a result of the behavior.

23. List four warning signs of suicide. _____

_____

_____

D. Substance Use Disorders and Other Addictions

1. List five possible substances of abuse or dependence. _____

_____

_____

2. List three general signs and symptoms of substance abuse or dependence._____

_____

_____

3. List five other addictions that are not substance abuse. _____

_____

E. The Medical Assistant's Role in Mental and Behavioral Health Procedures

1. List four tests used by providers to assess mental status or cognitive functioning._____

_____

_____

_____

2. Fill in the use for each type of medication listed below.

   a. Antianxiety _____

   b. Anticonvulsants and mood stabilizers _____

   c. Antidepressants _____

   d. Antipsychotics _____

   e. Sedative-hypnotics _____

   f. Stimulants _____

3. List five types of psychotherapy that may be used by a behavioral health therapist. _____

_____

_____

_____

CERTIFICATION PREPARATION

Circle the correct answer.

1. Which term means an unreal sensory perception that occurs with no external cause?
    a. Hallucination
    b. Delusion
    c. Psychosis
    d. Dysphoria

2. Which term describes the rate of a disease in a population?
    a. Mortality
    b. Morbidity
    c. Orientation
    d. Affect

3. Which term means an unshakable belief in something untrue?
    a. Hallucination
    b. Mania
    c. Delusion
    d. Affect

4. Brontophobia is the fear of
    a. flying.
    b. computers.
    c. blood or injury.
    d. thunder.

5. Drugs of abuse include
    a. cocaine.
    b. heroin.
    c. prescription opioids.
    d. all of the above.

6. Which anxiety disorder is described as a persistent difficulty getting rid of personal possessions?
    a. GAD
    b. HD
    c. OCD
    d. None of the above

7. Which is *not* a symptom of depression?
    a. Feeling sad
    b. Loss of interest in hobbies
    c. Mania
    d. Thoughts of death or suicide

8. ADHD is often treated with what type of medication?
    a. Stimulants
    b. Antidepressants
    c. Mood stabilizers
    d. All of the above

9. Amnesia is defined as
    a. loss of hope for the future.
    b. memory loss.
    c. inability to cope.
    d. both a and c.

10. A trained medical doctor with four years of residency describes which behavioral health professional?
    a. Psychiatrist
    b. Psychologist
    c. Social worker
    d. Cognitive behavioral therapist

WORKPLACE APPLICATIONS

1. Mike is taking Celeste back to an examination room to see the provider. Celeste has been diagnosed with anorexia nervosa.

    a. Mike has Celeste step on the scale to take her weight. How might Mike ensure an accurate weight is obtained?

    _____

    _____

    b. Should Mike position Celeste at the scale any differently than any other patient? If yes, explain why.

    _____

    _____

    c. Should Mike tell Celeste her weight at the time of her weigh-in? Explain your answer._____

    _____

    _____

2. Mike is preparing Celeste's medical records to be sent to another provider. How should Celeste's psychotherapy notes be treated in this situation? Should they be included with all of her health records?

    _____

    _____

    _____

3. Susan is a medical assistant working in behavioral health. She often needs to coach patients on the use of medication for their conditions. Medication compliance is an important factor for a behavioral health patient. What types of information should Susan emphasize when coaching a patient on medication compliance?

    _____

    _____

    _____

    _____

INTERNET ACTIVITIES

1. Using online resources, research a test used for diagnosing mental and behavioral health disorders. Create a poster presentation, a PowerPoint presentation, or a written paper summarizing your research. Include the following points in your project:
    a. Description of the test
    b. Any contraindications for the test
    c. Patient preparation for the test
    d. What occurs during the test

2. Using online resources, research a mental or behavioral health disorder. Create a poster presentation, a PowerPoint presentation, or an infographic summarizing your research. Include the following points in your project:
   a. Description of the disease
   b. Etiology
   c. Signs and symptoms
   d. Diagnostic procedures
   e. Treatments
   f. Prognosis
   g. Prevention

3. Using online resources, research the three different types of eating disorders covered in this chapter: anorexia nervosa, binge eating disorder, bulimia nervosa. In a one-page paper, describe each eating disorder and describe how it is treated.

4. Using Table 37.6, Medication Classifications, select two medication from each of the following classifications: antianxiety and antipsychotic. Using the information in Table 37. 6, for each medication identify:
   a. Reasons for use
   b. Desired effects
   c. Side effects
   d. Adverse reactions

Write a short paper addressing each of these four areas for each medication.

Endocrinology

CAAHEP Competencies	Assessment
I.C.4. List major organs in each body system	Skills and Concepts – A. 2, 3
I.C.5. Identify the anatomical location of major organs in each body system	Skills and Concepts – A. 3, 16; Certification Preparation – 5, 6
I.C.6. Compare structure and function of the human body across the life span	Skills and Concepts – A. 21; Certification Preparation – 8, 10
I.C.7. Describe the normal function of each body system	Skills and Concepts – A. 5-15, 17-19, B. 1-5
I.C.8.a. Identify common pathology related to each body system including: signs	Skills and Concepts – C. 12, 14, 16c ,18, 19, 20 Certification Preparation – 7; Internet Activity – 2
I.C.8.b. Identify common pathology related to each body system including: symptoms	Skills and Concepts – C. 12, 14, 16d, 18, 19, 20 Certification Preparation – 7; Internet Activity – 2
I.C.8.c. Identify common pathology related to each body system including: etiology	Skills and Concepts – C. 16b; Workplace Application – 3; Internet Activity – 2
I.C.9.a. Analyze pathology for each body system including: diagnostic measures	Workplace Application – 1; Internet Activity – 1, 2
I.C.9.b. Analyze pathology for each body system including: treatment modalities	Internet Activity – 2, 4
I.C.10. Identify CLIA-waived tests associated with common diseases	Skills and Concepts – D. 3; Certification Preparation – 4
V.C.10. Define medical terms and abbreviations related to all body systems	Vocabulary Review – A. 1-9, B. 1-8; Abbreviations – 1-23
V.P.4.b. Coach patients regarding: health maintenance	Procedure 38.1
X.P.3. Document patient care accurately in the medical record	Procedure 38.1

ABHES Competencies	Assessment
2. Anatomy and Physiology a. List all body systems and their structures and functions	Skills and Concepts – A. 2, 3, 5-19, B. 1-5; Certification Preparation – 5, 6
b. Describe common diseases, symptoms, and etiologies as they apply to each system	Skills and Concepts – C. 12, 14, 16bcd, 18, 19, 20; Certification Preparation – 7; Workplace Application – 3; Internet Activity – 2
c. Identify diagnostic and treatment modalities as they relate to each body system	Workplace Application – 1; Internet Activity – 1, 2, 4

ABHES Competencies	Assessment
3. Medical Terminology c. Apply medical terminology for each specialty	Vocabulary Review – A. 1-9, B. 1-8
d. Define and use medical abbreviations when appropriate and acceptable	Abbreviations – 1-23
8. Clinical Procedures d. Assist provider with specialty examination, including cardiac, respiratory, OB-GYN, neurological, and gastroenterology procedures.	Procedure 38.1
8.e. Perform specialty procedures, including but not limited to minor surgery, cardiac, respiratory, OB-GYN, neurological, and gastroenterology.	Procedure 38.1

VOCABULARY REVIEW

Using the word pool on the right, find the correct word to match the definition. Write the word on the line after the definition.

Group A

1. Result when fats are broken down; used by the body for energy and tissue development _____

2. The space in the thoracic cavity that lies between the lungs; contains the heart, trachea, and esophagus

   _____

3. A naturally occurring element that is necessary for many body functions, including strong bones and teeth, proper blood clotting, nerve conduction, and muscle contractions

   _____

4. A test to measure the amount and concentration of urine produced when water is withheld from a patient for a period of time _____

5. An output or response that affects the input of a system

   _____

6. Structures or sites on or in a cell that bind with substances such as hormones, antigens, or drugs _____

7. A cell selectively affected by a specific agent such as a drug, hormone, or virus _____

8. An inorganic compound, usually a salt; a major factor in controlling fluid balance within the body

   _____

9. The internal environment of the body that is compatible with life; steady state that is created to provide a consistent and unvarying internal environment _____

Word Pool
- target cells
- homeostasis
- electrolyte
- calcium
- fatty acids
- mediastinum
- negative feedback
- receptors
- water deprivation test

Group B

1. Increase in the fluid pressure in the eye, can lead to blindness if not treated _____

2. Clouding of the lens, leading to decreased vision _____

3. Sexual drive or instinct _____

4. Diabetes mellitus damages the blood vessels in the retina leading to loss of vision and eventual blindness _____

5. A specialized organelle of a cell that is encased in a membrane and directs growth, metabolism, and reproduction of the cell _____

6. A structure within a cell that performs a specific function _____

7. To spread, scatter, disperse, or move _____

8. A form of toxemia during pregnancy characterized by high blood pressure, fluid retention, and protein in the urine _____

Word Pool
- nucleus
- organelle
- diffuse
- libido
- preeclampsia
- diabetic retinopathy
- glaucoma
- cataract

ABBREVIATIONS

Write out what each of the following abbreviations stands for.

1. ACTH _____

2. FSH _____

3. GH _____

4. LH _____

5. PRL _____

6. TSH _____

7. ADH _____

8. OT _____

9. T_3 _____

10. T_4 _____

11. PTH _____

12. GHRL _____

13. PG _____

14. DI _____

15. RAIU _____

16. DM _____

17. A1c _____

18. DKA _____

19. CKD_____

20. SIADH _____

21. FBG _____

22. OGTT _____

23. TFT _____

SKILLS AND CONCEPTS

Answer the following questions. Write your answer on the line or in the space provided.

A. Anatomy of the Endocrine System

1. Through the endocrine system, hormones regulate many body functions. List four functions that are regulated by hormones.

   _____

   _____

2. List the endocrine glands of the body._____

   _____

   _____

3. What structure in the brain is the major connection for the nervous and endocrine systems? _____

   _____

4. The _____ is called the *master gland*. It is made up of two lobes, the _____ and _____.

5. List the hormones made in the anterior pituitary gland. _____

   _____

6. List the hormones stored in the posterior pituitary gland._____

   _____

7. Where are the hormones stored in the posterior pituitary gland made? _____

   _____

8. List the three hormones made in the thyroid gland._____

   _____

9. Which hormone is made in the parathyroid gland? _____

10. Compare the actions of parathyroid hormone and calcitonin. _____

    _____

    _____

    _____

    _____

11. List and briefly describe the actions of the hormones produced by the adrenal cortex. _____

    _____

    _____

    _____

    _____

12. List and briefly describe the actions of the hormones produced by the adrenal medulla. _____

    _____

    _____

13. The pancreas is an endocrine gland and secretes _____, but it is also an exocrine
    gland and secretes _____.

14. List and briefly describe the actions of the hormones produced by the pancreas._____

    _____

    _____

15. What is the action of thymosin on T cells? _____

    _____

16. Describe the location of the mediastinum in the body._____

    _____

    _____

    _____

17. Describe the general function of the sex hormones, testosterone, estrogen, and progesterone._____

    _____

    _____

18. The pineal gland secretes the hormone _____.

19. Describe the function of melatonin. _____

    _____

    _____

20. Describe the changes in the endocrine system across a life span. _____

_____

_____

_____

B. Physiology of the Endocrine System

1. Briefly explain the three mechanisms that help regulate hormone secretions in the body. _____

_____

_____

_____

2. Define and describe *target cells*._____

_____

_____

_____

_____

3. Describe how nonsteroid hormones work._____

_____

_____

4. Describe how steroid hormones work. _____

_____

_____

_____

5. Describe the action of prostaglandins._____

_____

_____

_____

C. Disorders of the Endocrine System

Write out a definition in your own words for each term or condition listed below.

1. Exophthalmia _____

_____

2. Glucosuria _____

   _____

3. Ketoacidosis _____

   _____

4. Acromegaly _____

   _____

5. Pheochromocytoma _____

   _____

6. Gigantism _____

   _____

7. Panhypopituitarism _____

   _____

8. Prolactinoma _____

   _____

9. Polyphagia _____

   _____

10. Briefly describe diabetes insipidus. _____

    _____

    _____

11. Briefly describe hyperthyroidism _____

    _____

    _____

12. List the common signs and symptoms of hyperthyroidism. _____

    _____

    _____

13. Briefly describe hypothyroidism. _____

    _____

    _____

14. List the common signs and symptoms of hypothyroidism. _____

    _____

15. Circle the correct response below for each statement.

    a.   Hyperparathyroidism (increases or decreases) blood calcium levels

    b.   Hypoparathyroidism (increases or decreases) blood calcium levels.

    c.   Addison's disease is a (hypo- or hyper-) secretion of cortisol.

    d.   Cushing's disease is a (hypo- or hyper-) secretion of cortisol.

16. The following relate to type 1 diabetes mellitus.

    a.   Describe type 1 diabetes mellitus. _____

    _____

    _____

    b.   List the cause (etiology) of type 1 diabetes mellitus. _____

    _____

    c.   List three signs of type 1 diabetes mellitus. (Signs are objective and can be measured or observed by others.)

    _____

    _____

    d.   List two symptoms of type 1 diabetes mellitus. (Symptoms are subjective and can only be perceived by the patient.)

    _____

    _____

17. Briefly describe diabetic ketoacidosis. _____

    _____

    _____

18. List four signs and symptoms of DKA. _____

    _____

    _____

19. List the early signs and symptoms of hypoglycemia. _____

    _____

    _____

20. List the signs and symptoms of hypoglycemia as it worsens. _____

    _____

    _____

21. List four possible complications of diabetes mellitus._____

_____

_____

D. The Medical Assistant's Role in Endocrinology Procedures

1. What are two specific screening questions that a medical assistant may ask a diabetic patient concerning peripheral neuropathy?

_____

_____

2. What information should be part of a medical assistant's patient coaching regarding diagnostic procedures?

_____

_____

3. Looking at Tables 38.8 and 38.9 in the textbook, answer the following questions.

    a. Is a calcium blood test a CLIA-waived test?   Yes   No

    b. Is a glucose urine test a CLIA-waived test?   Yes   No

    c. Does a patient have to be fasting for a random blood glucose test?   Yes   No

    d. Does a thyroid function test measure calcitonin in the blood?   Yes   No

    e. Is an A1c result of 10 normal?   Yes   No

    f. Is an A1c result of 6.0 prediabetic?   Yes   No

4. Different types of insulins work differently, but the terminology used to describe insulin is consistent. Fill in the proper term for the sentences below.

    a. The _____ is the length of time before the insulin begins to work.

    b. The _____ is the period when the insulin is most effective.

    c. The _____ is the length of time the insulin exerts an effect on the body.

CERTIFICATION PREPARATION
Circle the correct answer.

1. Which is *not* an endocrine gland?
    a. Thymus
    b. Thyroid
    c. Spleen
    d. Pancreas

2. Which hormone is produced by the anterior pituitary gland?
    a. Testosterone
    b. Follicle-stimulating hormone
    c. Cortisol
    d. Melatonin

3. What specific cells of the pancreas produce insulin?
    a. Beta islet cells
    b. Alpha islet cells
    c. Adrenal cortex cells
    d. Both a and b

4. Which is a CLIA-waived test?
    a. A1c
    b. Fasting blood glucose
    c. Ketones urine test
    d. All of the above

5. Which gland is located in the brain?
    a. Adrenal gland
    b. Parathyroid gland
    c. Pineal gland
    d. Thymus

6. The pancreas is located in which body cavity?
    a. Thoracic cavity
    b. Pelvic cavity
    c. Abdominal cavity
    d. None of the above

7. Which could be a sign or symptom of a type II diabetes mellitus?
    a. Polydipsia
    b. Night sweats
    c. Polyuria
    d. Both a and c

8. Gestational diabetes is more common in women with
    a. existing prediabetes.
    b. being overweight.
    c. being younger than 25 years of age.
    d. both a and b.

9. Hyperparathyroidism causes blood calcium levels to
    a. increase.
    b. decrease.
    c. stay the same.
    d. parathyroid hormone does not affect blood calcium.

10. Which condition would most likely be diagnosed in an older adult patient?
    a. Type I diabetes
    b. Gigantism
    c. Type II diabetes
    d. Gestational diabetes

WORKPLACE APPLICATIONS

1. Lexie greets her patient, Mr. Ironsides, and takes him back to the exam room. Mr. Ironsides is coming in for a follow-up visit for his type II diabetes. Once vital signs are completed, Lexie checks his blood sugar. He has not eaten in about 4 hours and his blood sugar is 101 mg/dL. Lexie checks his electronic health record and his last recorded blood sugar was 155 mg/dL after 4 hours without food. Is Mr. Ironsides' 101 mg/dL blood sugar within the normal range? Explain your answer.

    _____

    _____

    What should Mr. Ironsides A1c result be? _____

2. Lexie is reviewing endocrine diseases and disorders as part of a continuing education course. Briefly define the following endocrine disorders.

    a. Gigantism _____

    _____

    b.   Growth hormone deficiency _____

          _____

    c.   Cretinism_____

          _____

    d.   Myxedema _____

          _____

    e.   Hashimoto thyroiditis_____

          _____

3.   Lisa Tenivoldi has been diagnosed with hyperthyroidism. What are the possible causes of hyperthyroidism?

          _____

          _____

INTERNET ACTIVITIES

1.   Using online resources, research a test used for diagnosing an endocrine system disease. Create a poster presentation, a PowerPoint presentation, or a written paper summarizing your research. Include the following points in your project:
    a.   Description of the test
    b.   Any contraindications for the test
    c.   Patient preparation for the test
    d.   What occurs during the test

2.   Using online resources, research an endocrine system disease or disorder. Create a poster presentation, a PowerPoint presentation, or a written paper summarizing your research. Include the following points in your project:
    a.   Description of the disease
    b.   Etiology
    c.   Signs and symptoms
    d.   Diagnostic procedures
    e.   Treatments
    f.   Prognosis
    g.   Prevention

3.   Using online resources, research the effect that diet can have on the management of type II diabetes mellitus. In a one-page paper, summarize the information that you found.

4.   Using Table 38.11, Medication Classifications, select one medication from each of the following classifications: antihyperglycemics, diuretics, and hormone replacement (noninsulin). Using the information in Table 38.11, identify for each medication:
    a.   Reasons for use
    b.   Desired effects
    c.   Side effects
    d.   Adverse reactions

Write a short paper addressing each of these four areas for each medication.

Procedure 38.1   Perform a Monofilament Foot Exam

Name _____ Date _____ Score _____

Tasks: Perform a monofilament foot exam to screen for peripheral neuropathy. Provide health maintenance coaching by providing foot care instructions. Document test results in the patient's health record.

Equipment and Supplies:
- 10 g monofilament tool
- Gloves
- Paper towel
- Provider's order or standing order
- Patient's health record

Standing Order:
For all patients with diabetes:
- Monofilament foot exam bilateral for all physical exam appointments.
- Coach patient on foot care.

Standard: Complete the procedure and all critical steps in _____ minutes with a minimum score of 85% within two attempts (*or as indicated by the instructor*).

Scoring: Divide the points earned by the total possible points. Failure to perform a critical step, indicated by an asterisk (*), results in grade no higher than an 84% (*or as indicated by the instructor*).

Time: Began_____ Ended_____ Total minutes: _____

Steps:	Point Value	Attempt 1	Attempt 2
1. Wash hands or use hand sanitizer.	5		
2. Read the provider's order. Assemble equipment.	5		
3. Greet the patient. Identify yourself. Verify the patient's identity with full name and date of birth. Explain the procedure to be performed in a manner that is understood by the patient. Answer any questions the patient may have on the procedure.	10		
4. Ask the patient to remove socks and shoes and rest the feet on the paper towel. The paper towel should be placed under the person's feet either on the floor or on the exam table step.	10		
5. Using your hand, demonstrate that the monofilament is flexible and not sharp. Also demonstrate the monofilament on the patient's hand.	10		
6. Instruct the patient to close his or her eyes. Tell the patient to say "yes" when he or she feels the monofilament on the foot.	10		
7. Start with the great toe and place the monofilament perpendicular to the skin. Press the monofilament until it bends, hold for one second and release. Pause to give the patient an opportunity to confirm it was felt. A confirmation is a positive or normal response. The test result is abnormal if the patient cannot feel in one area.	10		

8.	Do not cue the patient if no confirmation is given. Just move to the next location. Randomly test 9-12 locations on the anterior and posterior side of each foot or as the provider indicates. If a patient doesn't feel the site, check it three times randomly. Make sure to space out testing times (e.g., time between each check).	**15**		
9.	Discard supplies in waste container. Remove gloves and wash hands or use hand sanitizer.	**5**		
10.	Coach patient on proper foot care to prevent sores. Include when to check feet, what to look for, and how to care for feet daily. Suspicious areas need to be watched carefully and reported to the provider if they do not go away.	**10***		
11.	Document the test results in the patient health record. Include the provider's name, the order, and the results of the test. For the test, the first number indicates the total felt and the last number indicates the total times done.	**10***		
	Total Points	**100**		

Documentation

Comments

CAAHEP Competencies	Step(s)
V.P.4.b. Coach patients regarding: health maintenance	10
X.P.3. Document patient care accurately in the medical record	11
ABHES Competencies	**Step(s)**
8. Clinical Procedures d. Assist provider with specialty examination, including cardiac, respiratory, OB-GYN, neurological, and gastroenterology procedures.	Entire procedure
e. Perform specialty procedures, including but not limited to minor surgery, cardiac, respiratory, OB-GYN, neurological, and gastroenterology.	Entire procedure

Cardiology

CAAHEP Competencies	Assessment
I.C.4. List major organs in each body system	Skills and Concepts – A. 2-5; Certification Preparation – 1
I.C.5. Identify the anatomical location of major organs in each body system	Skills and Concepts – A. 7; Certification Preparation – 2
I.C.6. Compare structure and function of the human body across the life span	Skills and Concepts – A. 20a-e, 21-23; Certification Preparation – 6
I.C.7. Describe the normal function of each body system	Skills and Concepts – A. 1; Certification Preparation – 3-5, 7-8
I.C.8.a. Identify common pathology related to each body system including: signs	Skills and Concepts – C. 1, 3-5, 7-8, 9c, 10c, 11c, 12c, 13c; Online Activities – 2-3
I.C.8.b. Identify common pathology related to each body system including: symptoms	Skills and Concepts – C. 2, 6, 9d, 10d, 11d, 12d, 13d; Online Activities – 2-3
I.C.8.c. Identify common pathology related to each body system including: etiology	Skills and Concepts – C. 9b, 10b, 11b, 12b, 13b; Online Activity – 2
I.C.9.a. Analyze pathology for each body system including: diagnostic measures	Skills and Concepts – C. 9e, 10e, 11e, 12e, 13e, 15a-e, 16; Certification Preparation – 10; Online Activities – 1-2
I.C.9.b. Analyze pathology for each body system including: treatment modalities	Skills and Concepts – C. 9f, 10f, 11f, 12f, 13f, 17-21; Certification Preparation – 9; Workplace Applications – 1; Online Activities – 2-4
I.C.10. Identify CLIA-waived tests associated with common diseases	Skills and Concepts – C. 16; Certification Preparation – 10
I.P.1.a. Measure and record: blood pressure	Procedure 39.1
I.P.1.c. Measure and record: pulse	Procedure 39.1
V.C.10. Define medical terms and abbreviations related to all body systems	Abbreviations 1-28
X.P.3. Document patient care accurately in the medical record	Procedure 39.1

ABHES Competencies	Assessment
2. Anatomy and Physiology a. List all body systems and their structures and functions	Skills and Concepts – A. 1-20, 24-26; B. 1-5 Certification Preparation – 1, 3-5, 7-8

ABHES Competencies	Assessment
2b. Describe common diseases, symptoms, and etiologies as they apply to each system	Skills and Concepts – C. 1-8, 9a-d, 10a-d, 11a-d, 12a-d, 13a-d; Online Activities – 2-3
2c. Identify diagnostic and treatment modalities as they relate to each body system	Skills and Concepts – C. 9e-f, 10e-f, 11e-f, 12e-f, 13e-f, 15a-e, 16; Certification Preparation – 9-10 Workplace Applications – 1 Online Activities – 1-4
3. Medical Terminology c. Apply medical terminology for each specialty	Vocabulary Review – A. 7; B. 4-5, C. 1-3. 6; E. 4-5, 7-9; F. 1-5
3d. Define and use medical abbreviations when appropriate and acceptable	Abbreviations – 1-28
4. Medical Law and Ethics a. Follow documentation guidelines	Procedure 39.1
8. Clinical Procedures d. Assist provider with specialty examination, including cardiac, respiratory, OB-GYN, neurological, and gastroenterology procedures.	Procedure 39.1
8.e. Perform specialty procedures, including but not limited to minor surgery, cardiac, respiratory, OB-GYN, neurological, and gastroenterology.	Procedure 39.1

VOCABULARY REVIEW

Using the word pool on the right, find the correct word to match the definition. Write the word on the line after the definition.

Group A

1. Strong, stretchy, thick-walled vessels that carry blood from the heart _____

2. Thin-walled vessels that allow for exchange of substances _____

3. Collect blood from the venules and return blood to the heart _____

4. Smaller arteries that move blood to the capillaries _____

5. Pointed tip _____

6. Collect blood from capillaries _____

7. Area of the chest wall anterior to the heart and lower thorax _____

8. Two upper heart chambers _____

9. Two larger lower heart chambers _____

10. Another name for the cardiovascular system _____

Word Pool
- arterioles
- venules
- atria
- arteries
- capillaries
- veins
- apex
- ventricles
- circulatory system
- precordium

Group B

1. Inner thin endothelial layer that lines the chambers and valves
   _____

2. Tendon-like cords that attach the papillary muscle to the heart valve _____

3. Leaky valves _____

4. The middle and thickest layer of the heart
   _____

5. Outer layer of the heart _____

6. Deoxygenated blood is pumped from the right side of the heart to the lungs _____

7. Oxygen-deficient _____

8. A simple sugar that is absorbed by the intestines and found in the blood _____

9. A liquid that is able to dissolve other substances
   _____

10. Oxygenated blood is pumped from the left side of the heart and moves through the body _____

Word Pool
- epicardium
- chordae tendineae
- endocardium
- myocardium
- pulmonary circulation
- systemic circulation
- incompetent valves
- glucose
- deoxygenated
- solvent

Group C

1. Red blood cells (RBCs) _____

2. White blood cells (WBCs) _____

3. Platelets _____

4. Undifferentiated cells that can become specialized cells in the body _____

5. The process of changing a liquid to a solid
   _____

6. Controlling the blood flow _____

7. Clump together _____

8. A reddish pigment that results from the breakdown of RBCs in the liver _____

9. Curved inward on both sides _____

10. A hormone produced in the kidney that stimulates RBC production _____

Word Pool
- biconcave
- leukocytes
- stem cells
- coagulation
- erythropoietin
- bilirubin
- hemostatis
- agglutinate
- erythrocytes
- thrombocytes

Group D

1. Complete heartbeat _____

2. The _____ phase occurs when the heart is contracting

3. Phase when the heart is at rest and the atria fill with blood _____

4. State of a cell when the impulse moves through the cell causing action potential _____

5. The cells create and discharge the electrical impulse _____

6. Recovery phase of a cell _____

7. The cells respond to the electrical impulse _____

8. High blood pressure _____

9. The cells transmit electrical impulses to other cells _____

10. Waiting stage, no electrical activity occurring _____

Word Pool
- automaticity
- excitability
- polarized state
- conductivity
- diastole
- depolarized state
- repolarized state
- systole
- cardiac cycle
- hypertension

Group E

1. Amount of blood that is pushed out of the left ventricle compared to the total volume of blood that filled the ventricle _____

2. Thickness of a fluid _____

3. Inner opening of arteries _____

4. A condition caused by an abnormally large number of RBCs in the blood _____

5. Heart rate or rhythm is abnormal _____

6. An air bubble, blood clot, or foreign body that travels through the bloodstream and blocks a blood vessel _____

7. Bluish discoloration of the skin, lips, and nail beds _____

8. A blood clot that blocks the flow of the blood _____

9. A waxy lesion made up of cholesterol, fat, calcium, cells, and other substances that builds up on the inner wall of an artery _____

10. Excessive fluid in the intercellular spaces in the tissue; when external pressure (e.g., socks, finger pressure) is relieved, a depression is seen in the tissue _____

Word Pool
- embolus
- thrombus
- viscosity
- lumen
- cyanosis
- pitting edema
- polycythemia
- atheroma
- arrhythmia
- stroke volume

Group F

1. Tissue death _____

2. Inflammatory condition of a valve caused most commonly by rheumatic fever, bacterial endocarditis, or syphilis

   _____

3. A temporary fall in blood pressure that occurs when a person rapidly changes from a recumbent position to a standing position

   _____

4. Occurs when the heart valve flaps are stiff or fused together, thus narrowing the valve _____

5. The valve does not close completely and allows blood to leak backward across the valve into the prior chamber

   _____

Word Pool

- stenosis
- orthostatic hypotension
- infarction
- insufficiency
- valvulitis

ABBREVIATIONS

Write out what each of the following abbreviations stands for.

1. RBC _____

2. SA node _____

3. BP _____

4. SOB _____

5. CABG _____

6. CHF _____

7. CAD _____

8. DVT _____

9. PE _____

10. CBC _____

11. MI _____

12. CK-MB _____

13. CK _____

14. POTS _____

15. HDL _____

16. CTA _____

17. TEE _____

18. LDL _____

19. ICD _____

20. CHD _____

21. PAD _____

22. ASD _____

23. PFO _____

24. PDA _____

25. CLL _____

26. CML _____

27. CPK _____

SKILLS AND CONCEPTS
Answer the following questions. Write your answer on the line or in the space provided.

A. Anatomy of the Cardiovascular System

1. Describe the function of the cardiovascular system. What does it deliver and take away from the cells?

    _____

    _____

2. The cardiovascular system is a closed system that includes which three structures? _____

    _____

    _____

3. _____ include arteries, arteries, arterioles, capillaries, venules, and veins, which act as pipes to carry the blood around the body.

4. The _____ pumps the blood.

5. _____ contains the nutrients for the cells and the waste products to be excreted.

6. Describe the difference between arteries and veins. _____

    _____

    _____

7. Describe the anatomical location of the heart. _____

    _____

8. Describe the structure of the heart, including the chambers and the muscular wall. _____

    _____

    _____

    _____

9. Label the four chambers using RA, LA, RV, and LV. Using the word list, label the structures and write the words on the lines.

- Aorta
- AV node
- Bundle of His
- Inferior vena cava
- Internodal pathways

- Left bundle branch
- Mitral (bicuspid) valve
- Pulmonary artery

- Pulmonary veins
- Purkinje fibers
- Right bundle branch
- SA node

- Superior vena cava
- Tricuspid valve
- Coronary arteries

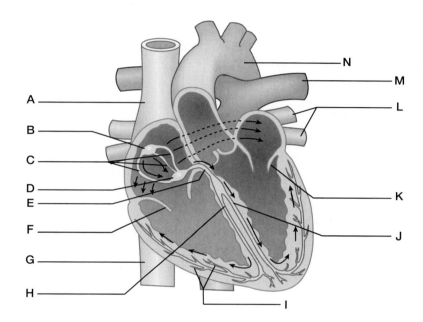

10. _____ is the AV valve located between the right atrium and ventricle.

11. _____ is the AV valve located between the left atrium and ventricle.

12. _____ is the SL valve located between the left ventricle and the aorta.

13. _____ is the SL valve located between the right ventricle and the pulmonary artery.

14. What occurs in the heart to create the "lub dup" sound? _____

_____

_____

15. Describe the two phases of the cardiac cycle. _____

_____

_____

16. Describe the flow of blood starting with the inferior vena cava and the superior vena cava and ending with the aorta. Include the names of the valves and chambers, along with the different types of vessels (e.g., capillaries) in your answer.

    _____

    _____

    _____

    _____

17. Deoxygenated blood is in the _____ atrium and oxygenated blood is in the _____ atrium.

18. The coronary arteries provide oxygen and nutrients to the _____ tissue. The right and left coronary arteries are the first to branch off the _____. Coronary veins drain into the _____, which empties into the _____ atrium.

19. In the hepatic portal circulation, veins from the spleen, gallbladder, pancreas, stomach, and intestines dump the blood into the _____, which takes the blood to the _____. After the blood is filtered in the liver, it drains into the hepatic vein before emptying into the _____.

20. The following relate to fetal circulation.

    a. The umbilical cord contains two _____ and one _____.

    b. The umbilical _____ carries oxygen and nutrients to the baby.

    c. The _____ helps most of the blood from the umbilical vein empty into the inferior vena cava. This allows the blood to bypass the immature _____.

    d. The _____ allows the blood to move from the right atrium to the left atrium, bypassing the immature _____.

    e. The _____, a short vessel, allows the blood from the pulmonary artery to be redirected to the aorta, bypassing the immature _____.

21. Describe two changes that occur in the cardiovascular system as a child grows and matures._____

    _____

    _____

22. Describe the changes that occur in the cardiovascular system with pregnancy. _____

    _____

    _____

23. Describe changes in the heart with age. _____

    _____

    _____

24. Describe the components of plasma. _____

_____

_____

25. List the three types of granulocytes and the two types of agranulocytes. _____

_____

_____

_____

26. What is the role of erythropoietin in the cardiovascular system? _____

_____

_____

27. List the four blood types using the ABO system and indicate which is the universal donor and universal recipient.

_____

_____

B. Physiology of the Cardiovascular System

1. List the five conduction system structures in order. _____

_____

_____

2. The _____ is considered the pacemaker of the heart.

3. The _____ take the impulse to the left atrium.

4. In the _____, the impulse moves very slowly through the node.

5. The _____ state is considered the "waiting" stage and no electrical activity occurs during this state.

6. Name the two states of a cardiac cell when electrical activity is created. _____

_____

_____

7. The _____ records the electrical activity of the heart and the _____ is used to assess the mechanical action of the heart.

8. The heart is controlled by the _____ nervous system and its own conduction system.

9. _____ is the resulting force of blood against the arterial walls.

10. List two things that increase blood volume and three things that decrease blood volume. _____

_____

_____

_____

11. Name three factors that influence the blood pressure. _____

_____

_____

12. _____ is the amount of blood that is pushed out of the left ventricle compared to the total volume of blood that filled the ventricle.

13. Name three factors that increase the resistance of blood flow. _____

_____

_____

14. Describe the process involved in forming a blood clot. _____

_____

_____

_____

_____

C. Diseases and Disorders of the Cardiovascular System

1. _____ means a slow heartbeat with ventricular contractions less than 60 bpm.

2. _____ means chest pain.

3. _____ is a bluish or grayish discoloration of skin, lips, and nail beds.

4. _____ means swelling.

5. _____ is profuse sweating.

6. _____ is breathlessness.

7. _____ is fainting.

8. _____ is a rapid heartbeat of more than 100 bpm.

9. The following relate to arrhythmias.

   a. Describe arrhythmias. _____

   _____

   _____

b. List four causes (etiology) of arrhythmias. _____

_____

_____

c. List three signs of arrhythmias. (Signs are objective and can be measured or observed by others.)

_____

_____

d. List three symptoms of arrhythmias. (Symptoms are subjective and can only be perceived by the patient.)

_____

_____

e. List four diagnostic procedures used for arrhythmias. _____

_____

_____

f. List three treatments for arrhythmias. _____

_____

_____

10. The following relate to cardiomyopathy.

a. Describe cardiomyopathy. _____

_____

_____

b. List the causes (etiology) of cardiomyopathy._____

_____

_____

c. List two signs of cardiomyopathy. (Signs are objective and can be measured or observed by others.)

_____

d. List one symptom of cardiomyopathy. (Symptoms are subjective and can only be perceived by the patient.)

_____

_____

e. List three diagnostic procedures used for cardiomyopathy. _____

_____

_____

f. List three treatments used for cardiomyopathy._____

_____

_____

11. The following relate to congestive heart failure.

a. Describe congestive heart failure. _____

_____

_____

b. List the five causes (etiology) of congestive heart failure._____

_____

_____

c. List three signs of congestive heart failure. (Signs are objective and can be measured or observed by others.)

_____

_____

d. List three symptoms of congestive heart failure. (Symptoms are subjective and can only be perceived by the patient.)

_____

_____

e. List one diagnostic procedure used for congestive heart failure._____

_____

_____

f. List three treatments for congestive heart failure. _____

_____

_____

12. The following relate to hypertension.

a. Describe hypertension. _____

_____

_____

b. List the three causes (etiology) of hypertension._____

_____

_____

c. List a sign of hypertension. (Signs are objective and can be measured or observed by others.)

_____

d. Discuss symptoms of hypertension. (Symptoms are subjective and can only be perceived by the patient.)

_____

e. List a diagnostic procedure used for hypertension. _____

_____

f. List two treatments used for hypertension. _____

_____

_____

13. The following relate myocardial infarction.

a. Describe a myocardial infarction. _____

_____

_____

b. List one cause (etiology) of a myocardial infarction. _____

_____

c. List two signs of a myocardial infarction. (Signs are objective and can be measured or observed by others.)

_____

_____

d. Discuss four symptoms of a myocardial infarction. (Symptoms are subjective and can only be perceived by the patient.)

_____

_____

_____

e. List two diagnostic procedures used for myocardial infarction. _____

_____

_____

f. List two immediate treatments used for myocardial infarction. _____

_____

_____

14. Describe the following types of shock.

    a. Anaphylactic_____

        _____

    b. Cardiogenic_____

        _____

    c. Hypovolemic _____

        _____

    d. Neurogenic _____

        _____

    e. Septic _____

        _____

15. Describe the following diagnostic procedures.

    a. Electrocardiography _____

        _____

    b. Exercise stress test _____

        _____

    c. Angiography _____

        _____

    d. Cardiac catheterization_____

        _____

    e. Echocardiography _____

        _____

16. What are two common CLIA-waived tests used to diagnose and monitor heart disease? _____

    _____

17. _____ medications are used to treat arrhythmias.

18. _____ medications are used to lower and control blood pressure.

19. _____ medications are used to prevent blood clots.

20. _____ medications increase urinary output and lower the blood pressure.

21. _____ medications are antihypertensives that reduce the heart rate, the workload, and the output of the heart.

CERTIFICATION PREPARATION

Circle the correct answer.

1. Which are components of the cardiovascular system?
   a. Blood
   b. Vessels
   c. Heart
   d. All of the above

2. What is the anatomic location of the heart?
   a. In the abdominal cavity, slightly left of the midline
   b. In the thoracic cavity, slightly left of the midline
   c. In the abdominal cavity, slightly right of the midline
   d. In the thoracic cavity, slightly right of the midline

3. What is the function of the cardiovascular system?
   a. Brings oxygen to the cells and carries carbon dioxide away from the cells
   b. Brings nutrients, water, and other substances (e.g., salts and hormones) to the cells
   c. Carries waste products (e.g., metabolic waste) away from the cells to be excreted
   d. All of the above

4. The pulmonary veins bring oxygenated blood back to the _____.
   a. left atrium
   b. left ventricle
   c. right atrium
   d. right ventricle

5. Which arteries bring oxygenated blood to the heart tissue?
   a. Pulmonary arteries
   b. Aorta
   c. Coronary arteries
   d. Carotid arteries

6. In unborn babies, which structure shifts most of the blood from the umbilical vein to the inferior vena cava, bypassing the immature liver?
   a. Foramen ovale
   b. Ductus arteriosus
   c. Ductus venosus
   d. Both b and c

7. Which conduction system structure is considered the pacemaker of the heart?
   a. Bundle of His (AV bundle)
   b. Right and left bundle branches
   c. Atrioventricular (AV) node
   d. Sinoatrial (SA) node

8. What factor influences blood pressure?
   a. Blood volume
   b. Ventricular contraction strength
   c. Resistance to blood flow
   d. All of the above

9. Which treatment procedure is used to destroy abnormal tissue that causes arrhythmias?
   a. Percutaneous transluminal coronary angioplasty
   b. Cardiac ablation
   c. Pericardiocentesis
   d. Left ventricular assist device

10. Which CLIA-waived test is used for anticoagulant therapy and heart disease?
    a. Cardiac enzymes test
    b. Cholesterol test
    c. Lipid profile
    d. Prothrombin test

WORKPLACE APPLICATIONS

1. Ken Thomas asked Lizzy how a low-sodium diet helps lower the blood pressure. How would you respond to this question?

   _____

   _____

2. You are working with a patient who was just diagnosed with tricuspid stenosis. The patient has a sibling with tricuspid insufficiency. She asks you to explain the difference between stenosis and insufficiency. Describe how you would explain the difference between these two conditions.

   _____

   _____

   _____

3. You are working with a patient who has a sibling that was just diagnosed with POTS. The patient asks you to explain this condition. Describe how you would explain POTS.

   _____

   _____

INTERNET ACTIVITIES

1. Using online resources, research a test used for diagnosing cardiovascular diseases. Create a poster presentation, a PowerPoint presentation, or write a paper summarizing your research. Include the following points in your project:
   a. Description of the test
   b. Any contraindications for the test
   c. Patient preparation for the test
   d. What occurs during the test

2. Using online resources, research a cardiovascular disease. Create a poster presentation, a PowerPoint presentation, or write a paper summarizing your research. Include the following points in your project:
   a. Description of the disease
   b. Etiology
   c. Signs and symptoms
   d. Diagnostic procedures
   e. Treatments

3. Using online resources, research right-sided heart failure and left-sided heart failure. In a one-page paper, describe each type of heart failure including the signs, symptoms, and possible treatments.

4. Using Table 39.12, Medication Classifications, select a generic medication from each of the following classifications: antiarrhythmic, anticoagulant, antihypertensive, antiplatelet, cholesterol-lowering agent, diuretic, hematopoietic, and hemostatic. Using a reliable online drug resource, identify for each medication:
   a. Reasons for use
   b. Desired effects
   c. Side effects
   d. Adverse reactions

   Write a short paper addressing each of these four areas for each medication.

Procedure 39.1   Measuring Orthostatic Vital Signs

Name _____ Date _____ Score _____

Tasks: Obtain orthostatic vital signs. Document results in the patient's health record.

Scenario: Dr. Walden ordered orthostatic vital signs to be completed on Erma Willis (date of birth [DOB] 12/09/1947). She has had episodes of dizziness and lightheadedness with standing up. Role-play this scenario with a peer.

Equipment and Supplies:
- Sphygmomanometer and stethoscope or digital blood pressure monitor
- Watch

Standard: Complete the procedure and all critical steps in _____ minutes with a minimum score of 85% within two attempts (*or as indicated by the instructor*).

Scoring: Divide the points earned by the total possible points. Failure to perform a critical step, indicated by an asterisk (*), results in grade no higher than an 84% (*or as indicated by the instructor*).

Time: Began_____ Ended_____ Total minutes: _____

Steps:	Point Value	Attempt 1	Attempt 2
1. Wash hands or use hand sanitizer.	5		
2. Greet the patient. Identify yourself. Verify the patient's identity with full name and date of birth. Explain the procedure to be performed in a manner that the patient understands. Answer any questions the patient may have about the procedure.	15		
3. Assist the patient onto the exam table and have patient lie down for 5 minutes.	5		
4. After 5 minutes, accurately obtain the patient's blood pressure and pulse rate. Keep the cuff on the patient. Write down the vital signs and indicate the patient's position and time.	15		
5. Assist the patient into a standing position and note the time. Ask the patient if he or she has any lightheadedness or dizziness. Continue to check with the patient throughout the procedure.	10		
6. After 1 minute of standing, accurately obtain the patient's blood pressure and pulse rate. Write down the vital signs and indicate the patient's position and time.	15		
7. After 3 minute of standing, accurately obtain the patient's blood pressure and pulse rate. Write down the vital signs and indicate the patient's position and time	15		
8. Assist the patient to the chair or exam table, if he or she is not dizzy. If the patient is dizzy, have the patient lie on the exam table.	5		
9. Wash hands or use hand sanitizer.	5		
10. Accurately document the vital signs in the patient's health record. Include the name of the provider ordering the test, the patient's position, and the length of time in the position. Specify the arm used to check the blood pressure.	10		
Total Points	100		

Documentation

Comments

CAAHEP Competencies	Step(s)
I.P.1.a. Measure and record: blood pressure	4, 6, 7
I.P.1.c. Measure and record: pulse	4, 6, 7
I.P.8. Instruct and prepare a patient for a procedure or a treatment	2
X.P.3. Document patient care accurately in the medical record	10
ABHES Competencies	**Step(s)**
4. Medical Law and Ethics a. Follow documentation guidelines	10
8. Clinical Procedures d. Assist provider with specialty examination, including cardiac, respiratory, OB-GYN, neurological, and gastroenterology procedures.	Entire procedure
8.e. Perform specialty procedures, including but not limited to minor surgery, cardiac, respiratory, OB-GYN, neurological, and gastroenterology.	Entire procedure

Pulmonology

chapter

40

CAAHEP Competencies	Assessment
I.C.4. List major organs in each body system	Skills and Concepts – A. 2, 6-14; Certification Preparation – 1
I.C.5. Identify the anatomical location of major organs in each body system	Skills and Concepts – A. 2, 10; Certification Preparation – 2
I.C.6. Compare structure and function of the human body across the life span	Skills and Concepts –A. 19-20; Certification Preparation – 8
I.C.7. Describe the normal function of each body system	Skills and Concepts – A. 1, 3, 18; B. 1; Certification Preparation – 3
I.C.8.a. Identify common pathology related to each body system including: signs	Skills and Concepts – C. 1-3, 5, 7-11, 12c, 17c, 18c, 19c, 20c; Workplace Applications – 2; Internet Activities – 2
I.C.8.b. Identify common pathology related to each body system including: symptoms	Skills and Concepts – C. 4, 6, 12d, 17d, 18d, 19d, 20d; Internet Activities – 2
I.C.8.c. Identify common pathology related to each body system including: etiology	Skills and Concepts – C. 12b, 17b, 18b, 19b, 20b; Certification Preparation – 7
I.C.9.a. Analyze pathology for each body system including: diagnostic measures	Skills and Concepts – C. 12e, 17e, 18e, 19e, 20e; D. 1, 2a-d, 3; Certification Preparation – 4, 9; Internet Activities – 1-2
I.C.9.b. Analyze pathology for each body system including: treatment modalities	Skills and Concepts – C. 12f, 17f, 18f, 19f, 20f; D. 4a-f, 5-7; Certification Preparation – 5-6, 10; Workplace Applications – 1; Internet Activities – 2, 4
I.C.10. Identify CLIA-waived tests associated with common diseases	Skills and Concepts – D. 1; Certification Preparation – 4
V.C.10. Define medical terms and abbreviations related to all body systems	Abbreviations – 1-34; Certification Preparation – 9
I.P.8. Instruct and prepare a patient for a procedure or a treatment	Procedure 40.1, 40.2, 40.3
I.P.2.d. Perform: pulmonary function testing	Procedure 40.1, 40.2
I.P.4.a. Verify the rules of medication administration: right patient	Procedure 40.3
I.P.4.b. Verify the rules of medication administration: right medication	Procedure 40.3

871

CAAHEP Competencies	Assessment
I.P.4.c. Verify the rules of medication administration: right dose	Procedure 40.3
I.P.4.d. Verify the rules of medication administration: right route	Procedure 40.3
I.P.4.e. Verify the rules of medication administration: right time	Procedure 40.3
I.P.4.f. Verify the rules of medication administration: right documentation	Procedure 40.3
X.P.3. Document patient care accurately in the medical record	Procedure 40.1, 40.2, 40.3, 40.4

ABHES Competencies	Assessment
2. Anatomy and Physiology a. List all body systems and their structures and functions	Skills and Concepts – A. 1-3, 6-14, 18; B. 1-9 Certification Preparation – 1, 3
2.b. Describe common diseases, symptoms, and etiologies as they apply to each system	Skills and Concepts – C. 1-11, 12a-d, 17a-d, 18a-d, 19a-d, 20a-d; Certification Preparation – 7; Workplace Applications – 2
2.c. Identify diagnostic and treatment modalities as they relate to each body system	Skills and Concepts – C. 12e-f, 17e-f, 18e-f, 19e-f, 20e-f, D. 1-7; Certification Preparation – 4, 7, 9; Internet Activities – 1-2, 4
3. Medical Terminology c. Apply medical terminology for each specialty	Vocabulary Review A. 7-8, 10; B. 1-5, 10-12
3.d. Define and use medical abbreviations when appropriate and acceptable	Abbreviations – 1-34; Certification Preparation – 9
4. Medical Law and Ethics a. Follow documentation guidelines	Procedure 40.1, 40.2, 40.3, 40.4
8. Clinical Procedures d. Assist provider with specialty examination, including cardiac, respiratory, OB-GYN, neurological, and gastroenterology procedures	Procedure 40.1, 40.2
8.e. Perform specialty procedures, including but not limited to minor surgery, cardiac, respiratory, OB-GYN, neurological, and gastroenterology	Procedure 40.1, 40.2, 40.3, 40.4

VOCABULARY REVIEW

Using the word pool on the right, find the correct word to match the definition. Write the word on the line after the definition.

Group A

1. A mixture of protein and fats that lines the alveoli and prevents the tissues from sticking together and collapsing during exhalation _____

2. A broad, dome-shaped muscle used for breathing; separates the thoracic and abdominopelvic cavities _____

3. Hollow, air-filled cavities in the skull and facial bones; lighten the weight of the skull and increase the tone, or resonance, of speech _____

4. Stoppage of breathing _____

5. Exhaling _____

6. Inhaling _____

7. Greater than normal level of carbon dioxide in the blood _____

8. Muscles located between the ribs that help with quiet respiration _____

9. Muscles in the neck, abdomen, and back that assist in breathing _____

10. Absence of breathing _____

Word Pool
- respiratory arrest
- intercostal muscles
- inspiration
- expiration
- hypercapnia
- apnea
- accessory muscle
- surfactant
- diaphragm
- paranasal sinuses

Group B

1. Low level of oxygen in the blood _____
2. Abnormally slow breathing _____
3. Nosebleed _____
4. The need to sit or stand to breathe comfortably _____
5. Deep, rapid, labored respiration that may occur because of exercise or pain and fever _____
6. High-pitched whistling sound related to labored breathing _____
7. A group of steroid hormones produced in the body or given as a medication _____
8. A cough that produces phlegm or mucus _____
9. A drug that relaxes smooth muscle contractions in the bronchioles to improve lung ventilation _____
10. A drug that is used to reduce a fever _____
11. A drug that reduces or eliminates pain _____
12. Aspiration of a fluid from the pleural cavity _____
13. A drug that is used for nasal congestion _____

Word Pool
- epistaxis
- analgesic
- wheezing
- productive cough
- decongestant
- antipyretic
- thoracentesis
- bradypnea
- orthopnea
- hyperpnea
- hypoxemia
- corticosteroids
- bronchodilator

ABBREVIATIONS
Write out what each of the following abbreviations stands for.

1. O_2 _____
2. CO_2 _____
3. COPD _____
4. CBC _____
5. MDI _____
6. AAT _____
7. SIDS _____
8. CF _____
9. CWP _____
10. OSA _____
11. CPAP _____
12. PE _____
13. ECG _____
14. TB _____
15. TST _____
16. PPD _____
17. QFT _____
18. RSV _____
19. AFB _____
20. SOB _____
21. ABG _____
22. CXR _____
23. VQ scan _____
24. TV _____
25. FVC _____
26. FEV_1 _____
27. ERV _____
28. IRV _____
29. VC _____

30. IC _____

31. FRC _____

32. RV _____

33. TLC _____

34. MVV _____

SKILLS AND CONCEPTS

Answer the following questions. Write your answer on the line or in the space provided.

A. Anatomy of the Respiratory System

1. Describe the purpose of the upper respiratory tract and the lower respiratory tract. _____

    _____

    _____

2. The upper respiratory tract structures start with the _____ and end with the _____, and they are all located outside of the _____ cavity.

3. List the three main functions of the upper respiratory tract. _____

    _____

    _____

4. The _____ separates the nares.

5. The _____ are small hairs in the nasal cavity that clean the air.

6. The _____ connects the middle ear to the nasopharynx and equalizes the pressure in the ear with the air pressure outside of the body.

7. The _____ or _____ are lymphatic tissue that help protect against pathogens.

8. Air enters the nasopharynx and then moves to the _____, then the _____, and then the _____ or voice box.

9. Describe the function of the epiglottis. _____

    _____

    _____

10. Label the following diagram.

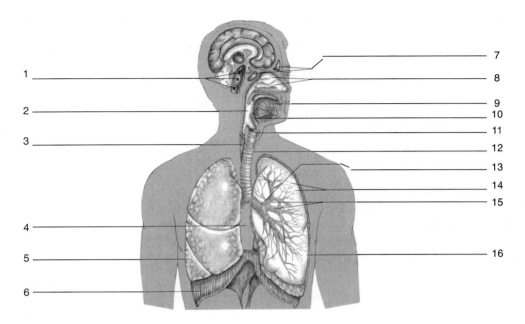

11. The lower respiratory tract consists of the _____, _____, and _____.

12. The lower respiratory tract structures are also lined with _____ and _____.

13. _____ is the space between the lungs.

14. The bronchi divide into smaller branches called the _____ that end in microscopic ducts capped by air sacs called _____.

15. Describe the role of surfactant. _____

_____

16. Each lung has a different number of lobes. Indicate the number of lobes for each lung and the names of each lobe.

_____

_____

17. The _____ is the double-folded, serous membrane that encases the lungs. The _____ lines the inner surface of the rib cage and the _____ is closest to the lungs.

18. Describe how the diaphragm and intercostal muscles work during normal, quiet respiration. (Include both inspiration and expiration in your answer.)

_____

_____

19. Describe how the respiratory system is different in infants compared to adults. _____

_____

_____

20. Describe how the respiratory system changes as a person ages._____

_____

_____

_____

B. Physiology of the Respiratory System

1. What are the two primary functions of the respiratory system?_____

_____

_____

2. Describe ventilation._____

_____

3. Describe external and internal respiration._____

_____

_____

_____

_____

4. Describe what triggers breathing for a healthy person and for a person with chronic obstructive pulmonary disease (COPD).

_____

_____

_____

5. When the breathing trigger is activated, it signals the medulla oblongata. Describe the process of inhaling starting with the respiratory center and ending with the expansion of the lungs.

_____

_____

_____

6. Explain why a person would use accessory muscles when breathing and describe four types of retractions.

_____

_____

_____

7. Describe the process of exhalation. _____

_____

_____

8. Describe the respiratory system's role in the acid-base balance in the body. _____

_____

9. Explain how the acid-base balance is changed when a person hyperventilates. _____

_____

_____

10. Explain how the acid-base balance is changed with hypoventilation. _____

_____

_____

C. Diseases and Disorders of the Respiratory System

1. _____ is an abnormal pattern of varying shallow and deep breathing.

2. _____ is an abnormal enlargement of the distal phalanges (fingers and toes) associated with cyanotic heart disease or advanced chronic pulmonary disease.

3. _____ is a bluish discoloration of the skin and mucous membrane.

4. _____ is a difficulty breathing.

5. _____ is excessive drainage from the nose.

6. _____ is breathlessness.

7. _____ or bubbling or popping sound heard on auscultation.

8. _____ is a continuous rumbling sound heard on auscultation.

9. _____ is a high-pitched, noisy breathing.

10. _____ is the expectoration of blood.

11. _____ is the abnormally rapid rate of breathing.

12. The following relate to COPD.

    a. Describe COPD, emphysema, and chronic bronchitis. _____

        _____

        _____

    b. List four causes (etiology) of COPD. _____

        _____

        _____

    c. List three signs of COPD. (Signs are objective and can be measured or observed by others.) _____

        _____

        _____

    d. List three symptoms of COPD. (Symptoms are subjective and can only be perceived by the patient.)

        _____

    e. List four diagnostic procedures used for COPD. _____

        _____

        _____

    f. List three treatments for COPD. _____

        _____

        _____

13. For the following body systems, list the effects of smoking.

    a. Respiratory system _____

        _____

    b. Nervous system _____

        _____

    c. Cardiovascular system _____

        _____

    d. Sensory system_____

        _____

    e. Digestive system _____

        _____

    f. Urinary system_____

        _____

14. List three conditions that can be caused by smokeless tobacco. _____

_____

15. List four substances found in e-cig aerosol. _____

_____

_____

16. Describe bronchiolitis obliterans or "popcorn lung" that can occur with e-cig use. _____

_____

_____

17. The following relate to cystic fibrosis (CF).

    a.   Describe CF. _____

          _____

    b.   List the cause (etiology) of CF._____

          _____

    c.   List four signs of CF. (Signs are objective and can be measured or observed by others.) _____

          _____

          _____

    d.   List two symptoms of CF. (Symptoms are subjective and can only be perceived by the patient.)

          _____

    e.   List two diagnostic procedures used for CF._____

          _____

    f.   List three treatments used for CF._____

          _____

          _____

18. The following relate to laryngeal cancer.

    a.   Describe laryngeal cancer. _____

          _____

    b.   List the one cause (etiology) of laryngeal cancer. _____

          _____

    c.   List three signs of laryngeal cancer. (Signs are objective and can be measured or observed by others.)

          _____

          _____

d. List three symptoms of laryngeal cancer. (Symptoms are subjective and can only be perceived by the patient.)

_____

_____

e. List one diagnostic procedure used for laryngeal cancer. _____

f. List three treatments for laryngeal cancer. _____

_____

19. The following relate to lung cancer.

a. Describe lung cancer. _____

_____

b. List the three causes (etiology) of lung cancer. _____

_____

c. List four signs of lung cancer. (Signs are objective and can be measured or observed by others.)

_____

_____

d. Discuss four symptoms of lung cancer. (Symptoms are subjective and can only be perceived by the patient.)

_____

_____

e. List a diagnostic procedure used for lung cancer. _____

f. List two treatments used for lung cancer. _____

_____

20. The following relate to pneumonia.

a. Describe pneumonia. _____

_____

b. List two causes (etiology) of pneumonia. _____

_____

c. List two signs of pneumonia. (Signs are objective and can be measured or observed by others.)

_____

d. Discuss four symptoms of pneumonia. (Symptoms are subjective and can only be perceived by the patient.)

_____

_____

e. List two diagnostic procedures used for pneumonia. _____

_____

f. List two treatments used for pneumonia. _____

_____

21. Describe the difference between latent tuberculosis (TB) infection and TB disease. _____

_____

_____

D. The Medical Assistant's Role in Pulmonary Procedures

1. List five CLIA-waived tests used to diagnose respiratory conditions._____

_____

_____

2. Describe the following pulmonary function tests.

a. Peak flow monitor _____

_____

b. Spirometry _____

_____

c. Arterial blood gas test_____

_____

d. Pulse oximetry _____

_____

3. Describe five important points to remember when doing a spirometry procedure. _____

_____

_____

4. Describe the following classifications of medications.

a. Antivirals _____

_____

b. Bronchodilators _____

_____

c. Corticosteroids (oral, nasal, and inhaled) _____

_____

d. Decongestants _____

_____

e. Expectorants _____

_____

f. Leukotriene receptor antagonists _____

_____

5. A(n) _____ is a long tube that is attached to the mouthpiece of the metered-dose inhaler (MDI) and slows the delivery of medication into the lungs.

6. Describe a nebulizer treatment. _____

_____

_____

7. Prior to a medical assistant applying oxygen to a patient, what must the medical assistant get from the provider?

_____

_____

CERTIFICATION PREPARATION

Circle the correct answer.

1. Which are components of the respiratory system?
   a. Nasal cavity
   b. Trachea
   c. Lungs
   d. All of the above

2. What is the anatomic location of the lungs and trachea?
   a. Cranial cavity
   b. Spinal cavity
   c. Thoracic cavity
   d. Abdominopelvic cavity

3. What is the function of the respiratory system?
   a. To maintain the acid-base balance in the body
   b. To carry waste products away from the cells to be excreted in the urine
   c. To exchange oxygen from the atmosphere for carbon dioxide waste
   d. Both a and c

4. Which test is a CLIA-waived test?
   a. VQ scan
   b. Arterial blood gas
   c. Sputum cytology
   d. Rapid strep A test

5. What medication is considered a quick-relief asthma medication?
   a. Fluticasone
   b. Montelukast
   c. Albuterol
   d. Budesonide

6. Which is surgical removal of the entire lung?
   a. Wedge resection
   b. Lobectomy
   c. Segmental resection
   d. Pneumonectomy

7. Which disease caused by a bacterial infection of the respiratory tract is also called *whooping cough*?
   a. Influenza
   b. Pertussis
   c. Croup
   d. Pleurisy

8. Which are characteristics of an infant's respiratory system?
   a. Airway collapses if the neck is overextended.
   b. Trachea is shorter and softer than in adults.
   c. Airway is narrow.
   d. All of the above

9. What is the maximum volume of air that can be as forcefully and rapidly exhaled as possible after taking in a full inhalation?
   a. TLC
   b. FVC
   c. RV
   d. FRC

10. What is true regarding oxygen delivery?
    a. A nasal cannula has a flow range between 1 and 6 L/min.
    b. The soft nasal cannula prongs must curve downwards when placed in the nose.
    c. A mask has a flow range of 5-10 L/min.
    d. All of the above are true.

WORKPLACE APPLICATIONS

1. Ken Thomas has COPD. He asks Renee why he needs to be on low levels of oxygen instead of higher levels. Describe how you would answer this question.

   _____

   _____

   _____

2. A mother calls and states her son is having difficulty breathing. Explain how you would ask her to check if he was using accessory muscles when breathing.

   _____

   _____

3. You are working with a patient who has a sibling who was just diagnosed with latent TB infection. The patient asks you to explain this condition. Describe how you would explain latent TB infection.

   _____

   _____

   _____

   _____

4. Read the peak flow meter measurements and label your answer.

A. _____

B. _____

C. _____

D. _____

E. _____

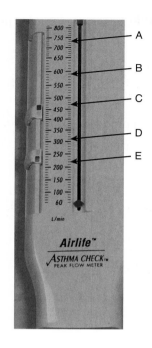

INTERNET ACTIVITIES

1. Using online resources, research a test used for diagnosing respiratory diseases. Create a poster presentation, a PowerPoint presentation, or write a paper summarizing your research. Include the following points in your project:
   a. Description of the test
   b. Any contraindications for the test
   c. Patient preparation for the test
   d. What occurs during the test

2. Using online resources, research a respiratory disease. Create a poster presentation, a PowerPoint presentation, or write a paper summarizing your research. Include the following points in your project:
   a. Description of the disease
   b. Etiology
   c. Signs and symptoms
   d. Diagnostic procedures
   e. Treatments

3. Using online resources, research the health risks attributed to smoking. Create a poster or a PowerPoint presentation summarizing the health risks associated with smoking and smokeless tobacco. Cite two online resources used.

4. Using Table 40.8, Medication Classifications, select a generic medication from each of the following classifications: antihistamines, antivirals, antitussives, bronchodilators, corticosteroids (oral), corticosteroids (nasal and inhaled), and decongestants. Using a reliable online drug resource, identify for each medication:
    a. Reasons for use
    b. Desired effects
    c. Side effects
    d. Adverse reactions

    Write a short paper addressing each of these four areas for each medication.

Procedure 40.1 Measure Peak Flow Rate

Name _____ Date _____ Score _____

Tasks: Perform a peak flow. Document the procedure in the patient's health record.

Equipment and Supplies:
- Peak flow meter
- Disposable mouthpiece
- Disinfection wipes
- Gloves
- Waste container
- Paper towel or denture cup (optional)
- Patient's health record

Standard: Complete the procedure and all critical steps in _____ minutes with a minimum score of 85% within two attempts (*or as indicated by the instructor*).

Scoring: Divide the points earned by the total possible points. Failure to perform a critical step, indicated by an asterisk (*), results in grade no higher than an 84% (*or as indicated by the instructor*).

Time: Began_____ Ended_____ Total minutes: _____

Steps:	Point Value	Attempt 1	Attempt 2
1. Wash hands or use hand sanitizer.	5		
2. Assemble equipment and supplies needed for the peak flow procedure. Place the mouthpiece on the peak flow meter. Move the indicator to the bottom of the calibration scale (if not using a digital meter).	5		
3. Greet the patient. Identify yourself. Verify the patient's identity with full name and date of birth. Explain the procedure to be performed in a manner that the patient understands. Answer any questions the patient may have on the procedure.	10		
4. Ask the patient to loosen any restrictive clothing. Have the patient remove any gum and loose dentures from his or her mouth. Make sure to provide a paper towel or denture cup if needed.	10		
5. With the patient in the seated position, ensure that his or her feet are flat on the floor and the legs uncrossed. The patient should sit straight up and against the back of the chair.	10		
6. Describe how the patient should do the test: "Take the deepest breath possible. Seal your lips around the mouthpiece. Blow as hard and as fast as you can." Encourage the patient to state when he or she is ready to start the test.	15*		
7. Coach the patient during the test. After the patient has blown through the meter, read the number next to the indicator. Write the number down. Reset the indicator to the bottom of the scale (if it's not a digital meter).	15		
8. Make any adjustments as needed. Repeat the test two additional times. Write down the last two numbers.	10		

9.	Put on gloves and remove the mouthpiece. Discard the mouthpiece in the waste container. Disinfect the peak flow meter. Remove gloves, and dispose of them in the waste container. Wash hands or use hand sanitizer.	10*		
10.	Notify the provider of the readings and document the readings in the patient's health record. Indicate the name of the provider who ordered the test, the name of the test, the results of the test, and how the patient tolerated the test.	10		
	Total Points	**100**		

Documentation

Comments

CAAHEP Competencies	**Step(s)**
I.P.2.d. Perform: pulmonary function testing	Entire procedure
I.P.8. Instruct and prepare a patient for a procedure or a treatment	4, 5, 6
X.P.3. Document patient care accurately in the medical record	10
ABHES Competencies	**Step(s)**
4. Medical Law and Ethics a. Follow documentation guidelines	10
8.d. Assist provider with specialty examination, including cardiac, respiratory, OB-GYN, neurological, and gastroenterology procedures	Entire procedure
8.e. Perform specialty procedures, including but not limited to minor surgery, cardiac, respiratory, OB-GYN, neurological, and gastroenterology	Entire procedure

Chapter 40 Pulmonology **889**

Procedure 40.2   Perform Spirometry Testing

Name _____ Date _____ Score _____

Tasks: Perform a spirometry test. Document the procedure in the patient's health record.

Equipment and Supplies:
- Spirometry machine with paper (and operator's manual if applicable)
- Disposable mouthpiece and tubing (if applicable)
- Nose clip
- Calibration equipment
- Disinfection wipes
- Gloves
- Waste container
- Paper towel or denture cup (optional)
- Patient's health record
- Scale (if no height and weight measurements were taken earlier that day)

Standard: Complete the procedure and all critical steps in _____ minutes with a minimum score of 85% within two attempts (*or as indicated by the instructor*).

Scoring: Divide the points earned by the total possible points. Failure to perform a critical step, indicated by an asterisk (*), results in grade no higher than an 84% (*or as indicated by the instructor*).

Time: Began_____ Ended_____ Total minutes: _____

Steps:	Point Value	Attempt 1	Attempt 2
1. Wash hands or use hand sanitizer.	5		
2. Assemble equipment and supplies needed for the spirometry procedure. Calibrate the machine according to the operator's manual and the facility's procedures.	5		
3. Greet the patient. Identify yourself. Verify the patient's identity with full name and date of birth. Explain the procedure to be performed in a manner that the patient understands. Answer any questions the patient may have on the procedure.	10		
4. Enter the patient's name, medical record number, age (or date of birth), race, gender, weight, and height into the machine. Enter any additional required information.	10		
5. Ask the patient to loosen any restrictive clothing. Have the patient remove any gum and loose dentures from his or her mouth. Make sure to provide a paper towel or denture cup if needed.	10		
6. With the patient in the seated position, ensure that his or her feet are flat on the floor and the legs uncrossed. The patient should sit straight up and against the back of the chair.	10*		
7. Describe how the patient should do the test: "Take the deepest breath possible. Seal your lips around the mouthpiece. Blow as hard and as fast as you can. Blow until you empty the air from your lungs."	10*		

Copyright © 2020, Elsevier Inc. All Rights Reserved.

8. Attach the mouthpiece to the machine. Explain the purpose of the nose clip to the patient. Apply the nose clip to the patient. Have the patient state when he or she is ready to start. Start the test as directed by the operator's manual.	**10**			
9. During the test, encourage the patient to empty the lungs. Repeat until three acceptable tests have been done. Allow the patient to rest between tests, if needed, and to indicate when he or she is ready for next test.	**10**			
10. Put on gloves and remove the mouthpiece. Discard the mouthpiece in the waste container. Disinfect the spirometer as indicated in the operator's manual. Remove gloves, and dispose of them in the waste container. Wash hands or use hand sanitizer.	**10**			
11. Document that the test was performed. Indicate the name of the provider who ordered the test, the name of the test, how the patient tolerated the test, and what you did with the test results. Any patient instructions regarding follow-up can also be documented.	**10**			
Total Points	**100**			

Documentation

Comments

CAAHEP Competencies	**Step(s)**
I.P.2.d. Perform: pulmonary function testing	Entire procedure
I.P.8. Instruct and prepare a patient for a procedure or a treatment	5, 6, 7
X.P.3. Document patient care accurately in the medical record	11
ABHES Competencies	**Step(s)**
4. Medical Law and Ethics a. Follow documentation guidelines	11
8.d. Assist provider with specialty examination, including cardiac, respiratory, OB-GYN, neurological, and gastroenterology procedures	Entire procedure
8.e. Perform specialty procedures, including but not limited to minor surgery, cardiac, respiratory, OB-GYN, neurological, and gastroenterology	Entire procedure

Procedure 40.3   Administer a Nebulizer Treatment

Name _____ Date _____ Score _____

Tasks: Perform a nebulizer treatment. Document the medication administration in the patient's health record.

Order: Levalbuterol 0.63 mg by nebulization.

Equipment and Supplies:
- Nebulizer machine
- Disposable nebulizer patient kit (tubing, medication cup, mouthpiece or mask, flexible tube, and tee)
- Medication as ordered
- Provider's order
- Normal saline (as ordered or according to the facility's protocol)
- Disinfection wipes
- Gloves
- Waste container
- Patient's health record

Standard: Complete the procedure and all critical steps in _____ minutes with a minimum score of 85% within two attempts (*or as indicated by the instructor*).

Scoring: Divide the points earned by the total possible points. Failure to perform a critical step, indicated by an asterisk (*), results in grade no higher than an 84% (*or as indicated by the instructor*).

Time: Began_____ Ended_____ Total minutes: _____

Steps:	Point Value	Attempt 1	Attempt 2
1. Wash hands or use hand sanitizer. Using the drug reference information and the order, review the information on the medication if needed. Clarify any questions you have with the provider.	5		
2. Select the right medication from the storage area. Check to see if the medication is concentrated and requires normal saline to dilute it. Check the medication label (and normal saline label, if used) against the order. Check for the right name, form, and route. Check the expiration date to make sure the drug has not expired. Verify that it is the right dose and time.	5*		
3. Assemble equipment and supplies needed for the nebulizer treatment.	5		
4. Perform the second medication check. Check the medication and normal saline label(s) against the order. Check for the right name, form, and route.	5*		
5. Add the medication, and if required, the normal saline to the medication cup. Secure the cover on the cup.	5		
6. Perform the third medication check. Check the medication label and normal saline label (if used) against the order. Check for the right name, form, and route. Verify that the amount of medication in the cup is correct with according to the order. Clean up the area.	5*		
7. Prior to entering the exam room, knock on the door and wait a moment. Greet the patient. Identify yourself. Verify the patient's identity with full name and date of birth. Make sure the patient's information matches the order and the record. Explain what you are going to do.	10*		

8.	Provide the right education to the patient. Explain the medication ordered, the desired effect, and common side effects; also identify the provider who ordered it. Answer any questions the patient may have. Use language the patient can understand. Ask the patient if he or she has any allergies. If the patient refuses the medication, notify the provider.	10*		
9.	Attach the mouthpiece (or mask). Attach the tubing to the medication cup and the machine.	5		
10.	Perform the right technique. The patient should be sitting upright on a chair to allow for total lung expansion. Instruct the patient to hold the mouthpiece between the teeth and seal the lips around the mouthpiece. Encourage the patient to take slow, deep breaths through the mouth. The patient should hold each breath 2-3 seconds before exhaling.	10*		
11.	Turn on the nebulizer and give the medicine cup and mouthpiece to the patient to start the treatment. Instruct the patient to put it into his or her mouth. If using a mask, position it securely and comfortably over the patient's nose and mouth.	10		
12.	Continue the treatment until the mist is no longer produced (approximately 10 minutes). Turn off the nebulizer. Encourage the patient to take several deep breaths and cough.	10		
13.	Put on gloves and dispose of the used supplies. Disinfect the nebulizer machine. Remove gloves, and dispose of them in the waste container. Wash hands or use hand sanitizer.	5		
14.	Document the procedure in the patient's health record. Include the name of the provider ordering the treatment, what was administered, how the patient tolerated the medication, and any follow-up assessments (e.g., vital signs).	10		
	Total Points	100		

Documentation

Comments

CAAHEP Competencies	Step(s)
I.P.4.a. Verify the rules of medication administration: right patient	7
I.P.4.b. Verify the rules of medication administration: right medication	2, 4, 6
I.P.4.c. Verify the rules of medication administration: right dose	2, 6
I.P.4.d. Verify the rules of medication administration: right route	2, 4, 6
I.P.4.e. Verify the rules of medication administration: right time	2
I.P.4.f. Verify the rules of medication administration: right documentation	14
I.P.8. Instruct and prepare a patient for a procedure or a treatment	8, 10
X.P.3. Document patient care accurately in the medical record	14
ABHES Competencies	**Step(s)**
4. Medical Law and Ethics a. Follow documentation guidelines	14
8.e. Perform specialty procedures, including but not limited to minor surgery, cardiac, respiratory, OB-GYN, neurological, and gastroenterology	Entire procedure

Procedure 40.4   Administer Oxygen per Nasal Cannula or Mask

Name _____ Date _____ Score _____

Tasks: Administer oxygen per nasal cannula or mask. Document the oxygen administration in the patient's health record.

Order 1: Administer 2 LPM of oxygen per nasal cannula.

Order 2: Administer 6 LPM of oxygen per simple mask.

Equipment and Supplies:
- Oxygen cylinder with oxygen regulator or oxygen flowmeter (wall unit)
- Adult nasal cannula or simple mask
- Provider's order
- Patient's health record

Standard: Complete the procedure and all critical steps in _____ minutes with a minimum score of 85% within two attempts (*or as indicated by the instructor*).

Scoring: Divide the points earned by the total possible points. Failure to perform a critical step, indicated by an asterisk (*), results in grade no higher than an 84% (*or as indicated by the instructor*).

Time: Began_____ Ended_____ Total minutes: _____

Steps:	Point Value	Attempt 1	Attempt 2
1. Wash hands or use hand sanitizer.	10		
2. Assemble equipment and supplies needed for the provider's order. If an oxygen cylinder is used, identify the amount of oxygen left in the cylinder.	10		
3. Verify the order if you have any questions.	10		
4. Greet the patient. Identify yourself. Verify the patient's identity with full name and date of birth. Make sure the patient's information matches the order and the record. Explain the procedure in a manner that the patient understands. Answer any questions the patient may have on the procedure.	10		
5. Connect the nasal cannula or mask to the regulator or flowmeter. Turn on the oxygen and adjust the flow rate to the correct amount per the provider's order. The ball should be centered on the number of liters ordered.	20		
6. Apply the mask or nasal cannula: a. Place the mask over the patient's nose, mouth, and chin. Place the elastic over the head. Adjust the elastic strap to tighten the mask on the face. Adjust the metal nasal bridge clamp, making sure it fits without obstructing the nose. Ensure that the mask fits tightly on the face. b. Insert the tips of the cannula into the nostrils. If the tips are curved, the curves face downward towards the bottom of the nose. Adjust the tubing around the back of the ears and then under the chin. Encourage the patient to breathe through the nose with the mouth closed.	20		
7. Make sure the patient is comfortable. Answer any questions he or she may have. Sanitize your hands.	10		

8.	Document the procedure. Include the name of the ordering provider, the number of liters of oxygen administered, the device used for administering the oxygen, and the patient's condition.	10		
	Total Points	100		

Documentation

Comments

CAAHEP Competencies	Step(s)
X.P.3. Document patient care accurately in the medical record	8
ABHES Competencies	**Step(s)**
4. Medical Law and Ethics a. Follow documentation guidelines	8
8.e. Perform specialty procedures, including but not limited to minor surgery, cardiac, respiratory, OB-GYN, neurological, and gastroenterology	Entire procedure

Urology and Male Reproduction

CAAHEP Competencies	Assessment
I.C.4. List major organs in each body system	Skills and Concepts – A. 1-7, 23
I.C.5. Identify the anatomical location of major organs in each body system	Skills and Concepts – A. 2, 8, 17, 21; Certification Preparation – 1
I.C.6. Compare structure and function of the human body across the life span	Skills and Concepts – B. 11-14; Certification Preparation – 4-5
I.C.7. Describe the normal function of each body system	Skills and Concepts – B. 1; Certification Preparation – 2, 6
I.C.8.a. Identify common pathology related to each body system including: signs	Skills and Concepts – C. 4-9, 10c, 11c, 12c, 13c; Internet Activities – 3
I.C.8.b. Identify common pathology related to each body system including: symptoms	Skills and Concepts – C. 1-3, 10d, 11d, 12d, 13d; Internet Activities – 3
I.C.8.c. Identify common pathology related to each body system including: etiology	Skills and Concepts – C. 10b, 11b, 11b, 12b; Internet Activities – 3
I.C.9.a. Analyze pathology for each body system including: diagnostic measures	Skills and Concepts – C. 10e, 11e, 12e, 13e, 14a-e, 15; Certification Preparation – 7, 8; Internet Activities – 1, 3
I.C.9.b. Analyze pathology for each body system including: treatment modalities	Skills and Concepts – C. 10f, 11f, 12f, 13f; Certification Preparation – 9, 10; Internet Activities – 2, 3
I.C.10. Identify CLIA-waived tests associated with common diseases	Skills and Concepts – C. 15; Certification Preparation – 8
V.C.10. Define medical terms and abbreviations related to all body systems	Abbreviations – 1-23
V.P.4.b. Coach patients regarding: health maintenance	Procedure 41.1
V.P.5.b. Coach patients appropriately considering: developmental life stage	Procedure 41.1
X.P.3. Document patient care accurately in the medical record	Procedure 41.1

ABHES Competencies	Assessment
2. Anatomy and Physiology a. List all body systems and their structures and functions	Skills and Concepts – A. 1-7, 23; B. 1; Certification Preparation – 1, 2, 6
2b. Describe common diseases, symptoms, and etiologies as they apply to each system	Skills and Concepts – C. 1-9, 10a-d, 11a-d, 12a-d, 13a-d; Internet Activities – 3
2c. Identify diagnostic and treatment modalities as they relate to each body system	Skills and Concepts – C. 10a-e, 11, 10e-f, 11e-f, 12e-f, 13e-f, 14a-e, 15; Certification Preparation – 7-8; Internet Activities – 1-3
3. Medical Terminology c. Apply medical terminology for each specialty	Vocabulary – C. 2-4, 6; D. 1, 3, 5, 7, 9-10; E. 3-4, 6-11; Skills and Concepts – C. 1-9; Certification Preparation – 8
3d. Define and use medical abbreviations when appropriate and acceptable	Abbreviations – 1-23 Certification Preparation – 8
8. k. Make adaptations to care for patients across their lifespan	Procedure 41.1

VOCABULARY REVIEW

Using the word pool on the right, find the correct word to match the definition. Write the word on the line after the definition.

Anandeep Kaur

Group A

1. Small arteries _____ arterioles _____
2. A very small vein _____ venule _____
3. Pertaining to carrying toward a structure _____ afferent _____
4. Fluid and substances that are filtered out of the blood in the Bowman capsule _____ filtrate _____
5. Pertaining to carrying away from a structure _____ efferent _____
6. A serous membrane lining of the abdominal cavity, which folds inward to enclose the viscera (internal organs) _____ Peritoneum _____
7. Folds in the wall of the organ _____ rugae _____
8. Sensory nerve ending that responds to a stretch stimulus _____ stretch receptor _____
9. Blood capillaries surrounding the proximal and distal convoluted tubules in the kidneys _____ peritubular capillaries _____
10. A type of cell found in the lining of hollow organs; it has ability to stretch with the contraction and distention of the organ _____ transitional epithelium _____

Word Pool

- filtrate
- peritoneum
- efferent
- transitional epithelium
- afferent
- arterioles
- rugae
- stretch receptor
- venule
- peritubular capillaries

Group B

1. A male gonad ___testis___

2. Tail of a sperm ___flagellum___

3. Tightly coiled tiny tubes in each testis ___seminiferous tubules___

4. Mature male reproductive cells ___spermatozoa___

5. Another name for the ductus deferens ___vas deferens___

6. Formation of sperm ___spermatogenesis___

7. Found below the bladder in males and surrounds the urethra
___prostate gland___

8. Coiled tube where the spermatozoa mature
___epididymis___

9. Part of the sperm; covered by the acrosome
___head___

10. Urine that remains in the bladder after micturition or urination
___residual urine___

Word Pool
- seminiferous tubules
- residual urine
- spermatogenesis
- epididymis
- head
- prostate gland
- testis
- vas deferens
- flagellum
- spermatozoa

Group C

1. A quality or characteristic of a material that allows another substance to pass through it ___permeability___

2. Scanty urination ___oliguria___

3. A hormone that is produced by the kidney cells and travels to the bone marrow to stimulate red blood cell formation
___erythropietin___

4. Bed wetting ___enuresis___

5. Need to urinate immediately ___urgency___

6. Between the cells ___interstitial___

7. Testosterone-secreting cells of testes that are found in the spaces between the seminiferous tubules ___interstitial cells___

8. Byproducts of drug metabolism ___metabolites___

9. Urinating more often than normal ___frequency___

10. A hormone secreted by the adrenal cortex; increases the movement of sodium out of the filtrate ___aldosterone___

Word Pool
- erythropoietin
- aldosterone
- frequency
- metabolites
- interstitial
- oliguria
- permeability
- enuresis
- urgency
- interstitial cells

Group D

1. A drug that reduces high blood pressure
   __antihypertensive__
2. Tissue taken from one area of the body and inserted into another area or person __graft__
3. An elevated level of lipids in the blood __hyperlipidemia__
4. A drug that increases the amount of urine produced
   __diuretic__
5. Pertains to the arteries and veins __arteriovenous__
6. A hollow, flexible tube that can be inserted into a vessel, organ, or cavity of the body to withdraw or instill fluid, monitor information, and visualize a vessel or cavity
   __catheter__
7. A decreased level of albumin (protein) in the blood
   __hypoalbuminemia__
8. A surgical procedure that creates a vein to remove and return blood during the hemodialysis procedure
   __vascular access__
9. An abnormal joining of an artery and vein
   __arteriovenous fistula__
10. Itching __pruritus__

Word Pool
- catheter
- antihypertensive
- pruritus
- hyperlipidemia
- graft
- diuretic
- arteriovenous fistula
- arteriovenous
- vascular access
- hypoalbuminemia

Group E

1. A group of steroid hormones produced in the body or given as a drug __corticosteroids__
2. A stiff ring inserted into the vagina that holds up the bladder
   ~~urostomy~~ __pessary__
3. A substance (i.e., medication or chemical) that prevents clotting of blood __anticoagulant__
4. A nervous system disorder of the peripheral nerves that causes discomfort, numbness, and weakness, especially in the extremities
   __neuropathy__
5. A temporary or permanent surgically created opening used for drainage (i.e., urine, stool) ~~urostomy~~ __stoma__
6. A drug that lowers the lipid levels in the blood
   __antihyperlipidemic__
7. A systemic infection involving pathologic microbes in the blood as a result of an infection that has spread from elsewhere in the body
   __septicemia__
8. Stones formed in the kidneys, gallbladder, and other parts of the body __calculi__
9. A surgically created opening on the abdominal wall used to drain urine __urostomy__
10. A backup of urine that causes dilation of the ureters and calyces; can increase pressure on the nephron units
    __hydronephrosis__
11. A decreased level of albumin (protein) in the blood
    __hypoalbuminemia__

Word Pool
- anticoagulant
- neuropathy
- hypoalbuminemia
- urostomy
- corticosteroids
- septicemia
- pessary
- hydronephrosis
- calculi
- antihyperlipidemic
- stoma

ABBREVIATIONS

Write out what each of the following abbreviations stands for.

1. ADH _Antidiuretic Hormone_
2. NH$_3$ _Ammonia_
3. K$^+$ _Potassium ion_
4. H$^+$ _Hydrogen ion_
5. RAAS _Renin – Angiotensin – Aldosterone System_
6. UTI _Urinary Tract Infection_
7. VCUG _Voiding Cystourethrogram_
8. ESRD _End-Stage Renal Disease_
9. BUN _Blood Urea Nitrogen_
10. ESR _Erythrocyte Sedimentation Rate_
11. RCC _Renal Cell Carcinoma_
12. PKD _Polycystic Kidney Disease_
13. IVP _Intravenous Pyelogram_
14. PSA _Prostate-Specific Antigen_
15. DRE _Digital Rectal Exam_
16. ESWL _Extracorporeal Shock Wave Lithotripsy_
17. UI _Urinary Incontinence_
18. UPJ _Ureteropelvic Junction_
19. VUR _Vesicoureteral Reflux_
20. BPH _Benign Prostatic Hyperplasia_
21. TURP _Transurethral Resection of the Prostate_
22. TSE _Testicular Self-Examination_
23. ED _Erectile Dysfunction_

SKILLS AND CONCEPTS

Answer the following questions. Write your answer on the line or in the space provided.

A. Anatomy of the Urinary System

1. List the four structures that make up the urinary system. _____

Two kidneys, two ureters, urinary bladder, urethra.

2. Label the structures of the urinary system using the figure below.

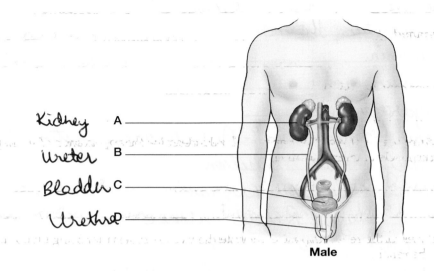

Kidney A

ureter B

Bladder C

Urethra

Male

3. The ___Kidney___ filter the blood and eliminate waste through the passage of urine.

4. The ___ureters___ move urine from the kidneys to the bladder.

5. The ___Bladder___ stores the urine until it is excreted.

6. The ___Urethra___ is the tube that conducts the urine out of the bladder.

7. The ___hilum___ is the indentation on the kidney.

8. Describe the anatomic location of the kidneys. The kidneys are loced posterior to the peritoneum, and between T12 and L3 vertebrae.

9. Describe the blood flow to, within, and from the kidney. Start with the abdominal aorta and end with the inferior vena cava.

The blood enters in aorta and moves to the renal artery. Then blood moves to interlobar artery via segmental artery. The blood enters in afferent glomerular arteriole. Glomerulus receive blood. Blood then enters in cortical radiate vein. Blood moves back to inferior vena cava.

10. Describe the following parts of the kidney.

   a. Capsule The fibrous outer covering of the kidney.

   b. Cortex The outer portion of the kidney.

   c. Renal column An extension of the cortex that dips down between medullary pyramids.

d. Medulla The inner portion that extends from ends of the cortex to the calyces.

e. Medullary pyramid Cone-shaped structure located in medulla and containing straight tubular structures and blood vessels.

f. Minor and major calyces and renal pelvis extensions of the ureter inside the kidney.

11. Describe the structure of a nephron. Your answer should describe the appearance of the nephron and include the renal corpuscle and renal tubule.

Each nephron is a very long tube, or tubule. One end of nephron is renal corpuscle and remaining section is renal tubule

12. Describe the structures of the renal corpuscle. Include the two arterioles that bring blood to and take blood away from the renal corpuscle.

End of the nephron is renal corpuscle. The afferent arteriole brings blood into glomerulus, and efferent arteriole take blood away from glomerulus.

13. Describe the sections of the renal tubule.

The renal tubule is made up of proximal tubule, Henle loop, Distal tubule, and collecting duct.

14. The ureter's muscular layer creates peristaltic waves that help move the urine through the ureter to the bladder.

15. transitional epithelium allows the ureters' walls to stretch to accommodate urine flow.

16. Explain the purpose of the ureterovesical junction. It is responsible for protection of the low pressure upper urinary tract from refluxing of urine from bladder.

17. Describe the anatomic location of the bladder. (Hint: What cavity contains the bladder?)

The urinary bladder is a hollow organ in pelvic cavity.

18. Explain the role of the rugae in the bladder. As the bladder starts to fill with urine, the rugae allow for greater bladder volume.

19. Describe what occurs when the detrusor muscle in the bladder relaxes and contracts.

It relax when bladder fills. It contract to push urine out.

20. The distal end of the urethra is called the urinary meatus and it is the final point before urine leaves the body.

21. Describe the location of the testes. _The testes are surrounded by a white, fibrous capsule and suspended together in a sac outside body called scrotum._

22. The _acrosome_ covers the head of the sperm and contains _enzymes_ to help penetrate the ovum.

23. Describe spermatogenesis, including where sperm are formed and where they mature. _The Spermatozoa are formed in series of tightly coiled tiny tubes in each testes. From seminiferous tubules, spermatoze travel to epididymis, where they mature._

24. Describe the pathway taken by sperm through the male reproductive system. _The ejaculatory duct begins where seminal vesicles join the vas deferens, and this "tube" joins the urethra. The urethra found within penis and transport semen outside the body._

B. Physiology of the Urinary System

1. Describe the normal function (the five roles) of the urinary system. _maintains fluid volume, maintains normal composition of body fluids, maintain an adequate blood pressure, activate vitamin D, control red blood production_

2. _Erithropoietin_ is secreted by the urinary system and is involved with red blood cell production.

3. Explain the importance of the afferent arteriole's larger diameter and the efferent arteriole's smaller diameter.

   It means blood moves into glomerulus faster that it leaves. The pressure inside glomerulus is high.

4. _filtrate_ is the substance in the Bowman capsule.

5. List three dissolved substances that move through the capillary wall in the glomerulus. _Electrolytes, waste products, aminoacids & glucose_

6. List three substances that are too large to pass through the capillary wall. _WBC, RBC and plasma protein._

7. Explain what happens to the amount of filtrate if a person's blood pressure falls due to a hemorrhage.

   The pressure in the glomerulus is not high enough to cause movement of the fluids, so little to no filterate is evacted.

8. List seven substances that move from the blood to the filtrate during the filtration process in the renal corpuscle.

   Water, Ammonia, Phosphorus, sodium, chloride, Urea, glucose

9. The _reabsorption_ process starts as the filtrate moves into the proximal tubule.

10. During the reabsorption process, substances move from the filtrate back to the blood. For each of the following structures, list the substances that move back into the blood.

    a. Proximal tubule _Water and solutes (sodium ions and glucose) move back into the blood._

    b. Henle loop _chloride and sodium, and water move back into blood._

    c. Distal tubule _Water move back into blood._

    d. Collecting duct _~~Ammonia, pot~~ Urea, water move back into blood._

11. Describe the structure and function of the urinary system in a baby and young child. _____

    when babies born they have same number of nephrons. A baby's kidney do not retain water like adult kidney do.

12. Describe the structure and function changes of the urinary system during adult years for both men and women.

    During childhood, the bladder continues to grow. Bladder control is learned usually between age 2 and 3.

13. Describe the structure and function changes of the urinary system during pregnancy. _During_ pregnancy, the filtration rate increase, but the number of nephrons remains the same.

14. Describe the structure and function changes of the urinary system with older adults. _____

    Bladder become less stretchy. The kidneys become less able to regulate water balance. Bladder muscle get weaker.

15. During the secretion process, substances move from the blood to the filtrate. For each of the following structures, list the substances that move to the filtrate.

    a. Henle loop_____ Urea _____

b. Distal tubule _Ammonia, certain drugs, hydrogen, potassium,_

c. Collecting duct _Potassium._

16. When renin is secreted, it raises the blood pressure. Describe the two ways renin increases the blood pressure.

- By creating more blood plasma volume.
- By constricting of blood vessels.

17. Explain when erythropoietin is released and its role in the body. _When kidney cell detect low oxygen level in blood, erythropoietin is released. It stimulate bone marrow to make more RBC._

18. Where is testosterone produced? _At puberty, interstitial cells in the testicles begins to produce testosterone._

19. What is the role of testosterone? _It is responsible for maintaing reproductive structures and for the development of sperm cells._

C. Diseases and Disorders of the Urinary System

1. _dysuria_ is a condition of painful urination.
2. _polyuria_ is a condition of excessive thirst.
3. _urgency_ is the intense sensation of the need to urinate immediately.
4. _Urinary incontinence_ means the inability to hold urine.
5. _albuminuria_ means albumin in the urine.
6. _bacteriuria_ is bacteria in the urine.
7. _glycouria_ is sugar in the urine.
8. _hematuria_ is blood in the urine.
9. _pyuria_ is pus in the urine.
10. The following relate to acute cystitis.

a. Describe acute cystitis. _Inflammation of the bladder._

b. List five causes (etiology) of acute cystitis. _Catheter, Bowel intontience, diabetes, Menopause, urinary tract procedure._

c. List three signs of acute cystitis. (Signs are objective and can be measured or observed by others.)

low grade fever, cramping, mental changes.

d. List three symptoms of acute cystitis. (Symptoms are subjective and can only be perceived by the patient.)

Foul-smell urine, Nocturia, Dysuria

e. List two diagnostic procedures used for acute cystitis. _____

Urinalysis, Urine Culture and Sensitivity test.

f. List one treatment commonly ordered by the provider and two home care treatments that can be done for acute cystitis.

Antibiotic therapy.
Home care :- avoid coffee, alcohol.

11. The following relate to polycystic kidney disease.

a. Describe polycystic kidney disease. An inherited condition in which cysts formed in the kidneys.

b. List the cause (etiology) of polycystic kidney disease. Genetic

c. List three signs of polycystic kidney disease. (Signs are objective and can be measured or observed by others.)

Pain in the flank, nocturia, drowsiness.

d. List one symptom of polycystic kidney disease. (Symptoms are subjective and can only be perceived by the patient.)

hematuria

e. List three diagnostic procedures used for polycystic kidney disease. _____

CBC, liver Blood test, Urinalysis.

f. List three treatments commonly used for polycystic kidney disease. _____

Anti hypertensive, diuretic, low-salt diet.

12. The following relate pyelonephritis.

a. Describe pyelonephritis. A Urinary tract Infection of one or both of the kidneys.

b.   List the two causes (etiology) of pyelonephritis. _Bacteria or ~~this~~ Virus._

c.   List four signs of pyelonephritis. (Signs are objective and can be measured or observed by others.)

fever, chills, vomiting, nausea,

d.   List three symptoms of pyelonephritis. (Symptoms are subjective and can only be perceived by the patient.)

low back pain, bad-smell urine, hematuria.

e.   List five diagnostic procedures used for pyelonephritis. _Urine culture, urinalysis, Physical exam, blood culture, blood work._

f.   List one treatment used for pyelonephritis._____

Antibiotic treatment.

13.   The following relate prostate cancer.

a.   Describe prostate cancer. _With prostate cancer, the gland can increase in size, obstructing urethra._

b.   List the etiology (cause) and five risk factors for prostate cancer. _Cells in prostate mutate, causing the cancer. Risk factors :- family history, lack exercise, Obese, tall, high intake of calcium_

c.   List three signs of prostate cancer. (Signs are objective and can be measured or observed by others.)

~~Back pain~~ loss of bladder, nocturia, Hematuria

d.   List one symptom of prostate cancer. (Symptoms are subjective and can only be perceived by the patient.)

Back pain, hip pain.

e.   List two diagnostic procedures used for prostate cancer. _____

DRE, PSA blood test.

f.   List two treatments used for prostate cancer. _____

Prostatectomy, Radiation.

14.   Describe the following diagnostic procedures.

a.   Cystoscopy and ureteroscopy _used to examine urethra, ureter and bladder._

b.   DMSA scan _Use to evaluate kidneys._

c. BUN test _to determine kidneys are working normally._

d. UA _To detect UTI, kidney disease and diabetes._

e. Urine culture _lab test to check for bacteria in a urine sample._

15. What is a common CLIA-waived test ordered for urinary symptoms? _Urine Culture_

CERTIFICATION PREPARATION

Circle the correct answer.

1. What statement is correct?
   a. The body has two urethras and one ureter.
   b. The kidneys are between T12 and L3 vertebrae.
   c. Urine moves from the bladder to the ureter and out of the body.
   d. The kidneys are anterior to the peritoneum.

2. The liquid in the renal tubule is called _____.
   a. electrolytes
   b. urine
   c. water
   d. filtrate

3. The point where the ureter enters the bladder is called _____.
   a. ureteral junction
   b. trigone
   c. ureterovesical junction
   d. rugae

4. During pregnancy, the filtration rate _____ and the number of nephrons _____.
   a. decreases; decreases
   b. increases; remains the same
   c. remains the same; increases
   d. increases; increases

5. The urinary system changes as a person ages. Which statement is *not* correct regarding older adults?
   a. Kidney tissue and the number of nephrons decrease.
   b. Renal arteries become hardened.
   c. Kidneys filter the blood faster.
   d. The bladder wall becomes less stretchy.

6. What is the normal role of the urinary system?
   a. Maintains fluid volume
   b. Controls red blood cell production
   c. Maintains an adequate blood pressure
   d. All of the above are normal roles of the urinary system

7. Which test measures the amount of urine left in the bladder after urination?
   a. Voiding cystourethrogram
   b. Ultrasound
   c. Postvoid residual urine test
   d. Intravenous pyelogram

8. What is a commonly used CLIA-waived test used to identify abnormal substances in the urine?
   a. Urinalysis
   b. Urine culture
   c. Cystoscopy
   d. Both a and c

9. Which medication is *not* an oral erectile dysfunction agent?
   a. Avanafil
   b. Sildenafil
   c. Warfarin
   d. Vardenafil

10. Which medication relaxes bladder muscles and decreases bladder contractions?
    a. Anticholinergic
    b. Antimuscarinic
    c. Alpha blockers
    d. Beta-3 adrenergic agonist

WORKPLACE APPLICATION

1. When Mrs. Williams was diagnosed with a urinary tract infection (UTI), she asked Hannah how females can decrease their risk for UTIs. How would you respond to this question?

    _____

    _____

2. You are working with a pediatric patient who was just diagnosed with diabetes insipidus. The child's mother asks you if it is "sugar diabetes." Describe how you would explain diabetes insipidus.

    _____

    _____

3. You are working with a patient who is confused about peritoneal dialysis and hemodialysis. Briefly explain both types of dialysis using words that a patient could understand.

    _____

    _____

    _____

INTERNET ACTIVITIES

1. Using online resources, research a test used for diagnosing urinary diseases. Create a poster presentation, a PowerPoint presentation, or write a paper summarizing your research. Include the following points in your project:
    a. Description of the test
    b. Any contraindications for the test
    c. Patient preparation for the test
    d. What occurs during the test

2. Using online resources, research a disorder of the urinary or male reproductive system. Create a poster presentation, a PowerPoint presentation, or write a paper summarizing your research. Include the following points in your project:
    a. Description of the disease
    b. Etiology
    c. Signs and symptoms
    d. Diagnostic procedures
    e. Treatments

3. Using online resources, research the different types of incontinence. In a one-page paper, describe each type of incontinence and how it is treated.

4. Using Table 41.7, Medication Classifications, select a generic medication from each of the following classifications: antibiotics, anticholinergics, antimuscarinics, diuretics, electrolytes, and erectile dysfunction agents. Using a reliable online drug resource, identify for each medication:
    a. Reasons for use
    b. Desired effects
    c. Side effects
    d. Adverse reactions

    Write a short paper addressing each of these four areas for each medication.

Procedure 41.1 Coach a Patient on Testicular Self-Exam

Name _____ **Date** _____ **Score** _____

Tasks: Coach a patient to do a testicular self-exam (TSE) while considering the patient's developmental life stage. Document your teaching in the patient's health record.

Equipment and Supplies:
- Testicular self-examination brochure (optional)
- Testicular model
- Provider's order
- Patient's health record

Scenario: You are working with Dr. David Kahn. He has ordered you to provide Truong Tran (date of birth [DOB] 05/30/1991) with TSE coaching.

Directions: Role-play this scenario with a peer.

Standard: Complete the procedure and all critical steps in _____ minutes with a minimum score of 85% within two attempts (*or as indicated by the instructor*).

Scoring: Divide the points earned by the total possible points. Failure to perform a critical step, indicated by an asterisk (*), results in grade no higher than an 84% (*or as indicated by the instructor*).

Time: Began_____ Ended_____ Total minutes: _____

Steps:	Point Value	Attempt 1	Attempt 2
1. Wash hands or use hand sanitizer.	**10**		
2. Read the provider's order. Assemble the equipment.	**10**		
3. Greet the patient. Identify yourself. Verify the patient's identity with full name and date of birth. Explain the procedure to be performed in a manner that the patient understands. Answer any questions the patient may have about the procedure.	**10**		
4. Ask the patient what he knows about the self-exam. Clarify any inaccuracies. Build on the patient's prior knowledge of the topic during the session. Identify the patient's motivating factor for learning about the self-exam. Listen to the patient's concerns.	**10**		
5. Explain to the patient that the best time to do the self-exam is after a warm shower or bath.	**10**		
6. Demonstrate on the model while discussing the technique. Instruct the patient to examine each testicle gently with both hands. a. Roll the testicle between the thumb and fingers. b. Show the patient the epididymis, the soft curved structure behind and on top of the testicle. c. Then show the patient how to examine the vas deferens, which is the tube that runs up the epididymis.	**10**		
7. Instruct the patient to feel for any abnormalities and lumps. These could be painless or painful. Instruct the person to look for changes in the size, texture, or shape.	**10**		

8.	Have the patient demonstrate the technique on the model. Coach the patient on ways to improve the exam if needed.	**10**		
9.	Answer any questions the patient may have. Provide the patient with a brochure to take home (optional).	**10**		
10.	Document the patient education in the patient's health record. Include the provider's name, the order, what was taught, how the patient responded, how the patient did the demonstration, and any handouts provided.	**10**		
	Total Points	**100**		

Documentation

Comments

CAAHEP Competencies	Step(s)
V.P.4.b. Coach patients regarding: health maintenance	Entire procedure
V.P.5.b. Coach patients appropriately considering: developmental life stage	4
X.P.3. Document patient care accurately in the medical record	10
ABHES Competencies	**Step(s)**
8.k. Make adaptations to care for patients across their lifespan	4

Obstetrics and Gynecology

CAAHEP Competencies	Assessment
I.C.4. List major organs in each body system	Skills and Concepts – A. 1, 2
I.C.5. Identify the anatomical location of major organs in each body system	Skills and Concepts – A. 1, 2
I.C.6. Compare structure and function of the human body across the life span	Skills and Concepts – B. 1, 2, 3; C. 8
I.C.7. Describe the normal function of each body system	Skills and Concepts – A. 5
I.C.8.a. Identify common pathology related to each body system including: signs	Skills and Concepts – C. 8
I.C.8.b. Identify common pathology related to each body system including: symptoms	Skills and Concepts – C. 8
I.C.8.c. Identify common pathology related to each body system including: etiology	Skills and Concepts – C. 7
I.C.9.a. Analyze pathology for each body system including: diagnostic measures	Skills and Concepts – C. 4, 5
I.C.9.b. Analyze pathology for each body system including: treatment modalities	Workplace Applications – 1
I.C.10. Identify CLIA-waived tests associated with common diseases	Skills and Concepts – D. 3
I.P.8. Instruct and prepare a patient for a procedure or a treatment	Procedure 42.1, 42.2
I.P.9. Assist provider with a patient exam	Procedure 42.1
V.C.10. Define medical terms and abbreviations related to all body systems	Vocabulary Review, Abbreviations
V.P.4.b. Coach patients regarding: health maintenance	Procedure 42.2
V.P.5.a. Coach patients appropriately considering: cultural diversity	Procedure 42.2
V.P.5.b. Coach patients appropriately considering: developmental life stage	Procedure 42.2
X.P.3. Document patient care accurately in the medical record	Procedure 42.2

ABHES Competencies	Assessment
2. Anatomy and Physiology a. List all body systems and their structures and functions	Skills and Concepts – B. 1, 2, 3; C. 8
2. Anatomy and Physiology b. Describe common diseases, symptoms, and etiologies as they apply to each system	Skills and Concepts – C. 4, 7, 8
2. Anatomy and Physiology c. Identify diagnostic and treatment modalities as they relate to each body system	Skills and Concepts – C. 5
3. Medical Terminology c. Apply medical terminology for each specialty	Vocabulary Review
3. Medical Terminology d. Define and use medical abbreviations when appropriate and acceptable	Vocabulary Review, Abbreviations
8. Clinical Procedures d. Assist provider with specialty examination, including cardiac, respiratory, OB-GYN, neurological, and gastroenterology procedures	All procedures
8. Clinical Procedures e. Perform specialty procedures, including but not limited to minor surgery, cardiac, respiratory, OB-GYN, neurological, and gastroenterology	All procedures

VOCABULARY REVIEW

Using the word pool on the right, find the correct word to match the definition. Write the word on the line after the definition.

Group A

1. The area between the opening of the vagina and the anus
   _____

2. The larger external folds of skin surrounding the opening of the vagina _____

3. Sensitive erectile tissue _____

4. Removal of the breast tumor and a small amount of the surrounding tissue _____

5. A mature sexual reproductive cell; spermatozoa or ovum
   _____

6. A fold of mucous membrane partly closing the external orifice of the vagina _____

7. The release of the ovum from the ovarian follicle
   _____

8. Organs that produce sex cells in both males and females
   _____

9. The smaller inner folds of skin surrounding the opening of the vagina _____

10. The vaginal opening _____

Word Pool
- gonads
- gamete
- orifice
- hymen
- labia majora
- labia minora
- clitoris
- perineum
- ovulation
- lumpectomy

Group B

1. Painful menstrual flow, cramps _____

2. A high-frequency electrical current running through a wire is used to remove abnormal tissue from both the cervix and the endocervical canal _____

3. Bands of scar tissue that can bind anatomic structures together

   _____

4. Removal of a limited number of lymph nodes to determine if the cancer has spread to the lymph nodes _____

5. Surgical removal of the fallopian tube and ovary

   _____

6. A sample of abnormal tissue from the cervix using a small spoon-shaped instrument called a *curette* _____

7. Surgical removal of the uterus and cervix

   _____

8. Removal of the entire breast _____

9. An extensive cervical biopsy during which a wedge of tissue is removed from the cervix and examined under a microscope

   _____

10. Using a microscope with a light source, the vagina and cervix are visually examined to locate and evaluate abnormal cells

    _____

Word Pool
- mastectomy
- sentinel node biopsy
- endocervical curettage
- colposcopy
- loop electrosurgical excision procedure
- cone biopsy
- hysterectomy
- salpingo-oophorectomy
- adhesions
- dysmenorrhea

Group C

1. A fluid-filled cyst in one of the vestibular glands located on either side of the vaginal orifice _____

2. Excessive menstrual flow and uterine bleeding other than that caused by menstruation _____

3. Lack of menstrual flow _____

4. Painful or difficult intercourse _____

5. Failure of the ovaries to release an ovum at the time of ovulation

   _____

6. A procedure used to visually examine the abdomen

   _____

7. Abnormal thinning of the bone structure, causing bones to become brittle and weak _____

8. Abnormally heavy menstrual flow or prolonged menstrual periods _____

9. Similarity in size, form, and arrangement of parts on opposite sides of the body _____

10. Pus-like _____

Word Pool
- dyspareunia
- menorrhagia
- menometrorrhagia
- laparoscopy
- purulent
- amenorrhea
- osteoporosis
- symmetry
- Bartholin cysts
- anovulation

Group D

1. A condition in which the spinal column has an abnormal opening that allows protrusion of the meninges and/or the spinal column _____

2. A deficiency in the enzyme phenylalanine hydroxylase, which is responsible for converting phenylalanine into tyrosine _____

3. Tissue death _____

4. An abnormal condition of pregnancy of unknown cause, marked by hypertension, edema, and proteinuria _____

5. Congenital absence of part or all of the brain _____

6. Implantation of the embryo in any location other than the uterus _____

7. A disorder that affects all the exocrine cells but affects the respiratory system the most; mucus is abnormally thick and blocks the alveoli, causing dyspnea _____

8. A genetic disorder in which abnormal cell division results in an extra chromosome 21 _____

9. An inherited anemia characterized by crescent-shaped red blood cells _____

10. Ability to live _____

11. A group of inherited blood disorders characterized by a deficiency of one of the factors necessary for the coagulation of blood _____

12. The protrusion of the meninges through an opening in the spinal column or skull _____

Word Pool

- necrosis
- viability
- ectopic pregnancy
- preeclampsia
- Down syndrome
- spina bifida
- meningocele
- anencephaly
- hemophilia
- sickle cell anemia
- cystic fibrosis
- phenylketonuria

ABBREVIATIONS

Write out what each of the following abbreviations stands for.

1. OB/GYN _____

2. hCG _____

3. MRI _____

4. HPV _____

5. LEEP _____

6. GN-RH _____

7. PID _____

8. DUB _____

9. PMDD _____

10. PMS _____

11. HDN _____

12. HRT _____

13. KOH _____

14. OCP _____

15. IUD _____

16. OSHA _____

17. PKU _____

18. IUFD _____

19. PPD _____

20. EPDS _____

21. AFP _____

22. CVS _____

SKILLS AND CONCEPTS

Answer the following questions. Write your answer on the line or in the space provided.

A. Anatomy of the Female Reproductive System

1. Label the structures in the following figures.

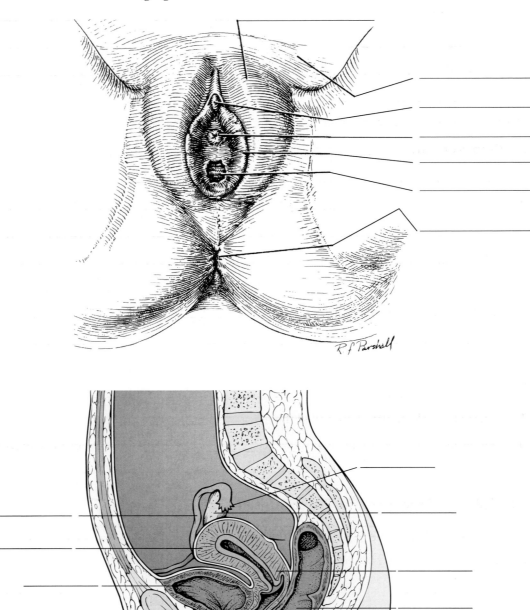

2. Which body cavity contains the ovaries, fallopian tubes, and uterus?_____

3. Describe each of the three layers of the uterus.

   a. Perimetrium _____

   _____

   b. Myometrium_____

   _____

   c. Endometrium _____

   _____

4. Describe the three areas of the uterus.

   a. Corpus or body _____

   _____

   b. Fundus_____

   _____

   c. Cervix _____

   _____

5. List the purposes of the vagina. _____

   _____

   _____

   _____

6. The external female genitalia are called the _____.

7. In addition to the pelvic organs, the _____ are also part of the female reproductive system.

B. Physiology of the Female Reproductive System

1. The term for the beginning of the menstrual cycle is _____.

2. Describe the three phases of the menstrual cycle. _____

   _____

   _____

   _____

   _____

   _____

   _____

3. Describe the journey that a zygote takes and what occurs as it develops. _____

_____

_____

_____

_____

_____

_____

_____

_____

4. From weeks 3 through 8 of development, the organism is called a(n) _____; from the week 9 through 38, it is called a(n) _____.

C. Disorders of the Female Reproductive System

1. _____ or _____ are the most often causes of PID.

2. Almost all cervical cancers are caused by _____.

3. List five risk factors for breast cancer.

   a. _____

   b. _____

   c. _____

   d. _____

   e. _____

4. Describe the screening test for cervical cancer. _____

   _____

   _____

   _____

5. List the diagnostic procedures for ovarian cancer. _____

   _____

   _____

   _____

   _____

   _____

6. The condition where functional endometrial tissue is located outside of the uterus is called
_____.

7. The vaginal infection commonly called a *yeast infection* is caused by what organism? _____
_____

8. List five symptoms of menopause.

    a. _____

    b. _____

    c. _____

    d. _____

    e. _____

D. The Medical Assistant's Role in Obstetrics and Gynecology Procedures

1. Describe the elements of a gynecologic history._____
_____
_____
_____
_____
_____
_____
_____
_____
_____
_____
_____
_____
_____

2. How can a medical assistant help prevent embarrassment for the patient when assisting with a gynecologic examination?
_____
_____
_____
_____
_____

3. Describe the CLIA-waived testing that can be done for pregnancy. _____

    _____

    _____

    _____

CERTIFICATION PREPARATION

1. The _____ starts the follicular phase of the menstrual cycle.
    a. hypothalamus
    b. pituitary gland
    c. ovary
    d. medulla

2. During implantation, the zygote functions as an endocrine gland by secreting which hormone?
    a. FSH
    b. hCG
    c. LSH
    d. GnRH

3. According to the American Cancer Society, what is the risk of a woman developing breast cancer?
    a. 1 in 2
    b. 1 in 8
    c. 1 in 20
    d. 1 in 100

4. What position is used for a pelvic examination?
    a. Supine
    b. Prone
    c. Sims
    d. Lithotomy

5. When testing for candidiasis, a drop of what solution is added to the slide?
    a. Sterile water
    b. Potassium hydroxide
    c. Saline
    d. Nothing is added to the slide

6. During a pelvic examination, what occurs after the provider has collected the specimen for a Pap test?
    a. Breast examination
    b. Bimanual examination
    c. Digital rectal examination
    d. Abdominal examination

7. A maturation index can assist in the diagnosis and treatment of which condition?
    a. Infertility issues
    b. Amenorrhea
    c. Menopause
    d. All of the above

8. What method of contraception either kills sperm or prevents them from entering the cervical os?
    a. Barrier methods
    b. Hormonal contraceptives
    c. Intrauterine devices
    d. None of the above

9. What procedure uses a microscope with a light source and magnifying lens?
    a. Cryotherapy
    b. Pap test
    c. LEEP
    d. Colposcopy

10. What term refers to the number of pregnancies that have gone to the age of viability?
    a. Gravida
    b. Multigravida
    c. Para
    d. Primipara

WORKPLACE APPLICATIONS

1. Anna Richardson is scheduled for a loop electrosurgical excision procedure (LEEP) today because of an abnormal Pap test. Explain to Anna how the procedure is performed and why Dr. Walden has ordered it.

   _____

   _____

   _____

   _____

2. Julia Berkley is in for her first prenatal visit. When taking her history, she tells you that she has a 2-year-old, four-year-old twins, and had a miscarriage last year. What is her gravida, para, and abortion information?

   _____

   _____

3. Dr. Walden has asked you to prepare a patient for a bimanual examination. How should the patient be gowned and draped? How should you position the patient? What type of supplies will Dr. Walden need to complete the examination? What is assessed during this examination?

   _____

   _____

   _____

   _____

   _____

   _____

INTERNET ACTIVITIES

1. IUDs are a highly recommended form of birth control. Research the types of IUDs online. Create a poster presentation, a PowerPoint presentation, or write a paper summarizing your research. Include the following points in your project:
   a. Describe the different types of IUDs and how they work.
   b. How are they inserted and removed?
   c. What are their potential complications?

2. Search the Internet for resources for pregnant and breastfeeding women. Develop a resource guide for these patients in an obstetric practice.

Procedure 42.1   Setting Up for and Assisting the Provider with a Gynecologic Examination

Name _____ **Date** _____ **Score** _____

Task: Prepare equipment for a gynecologic examination and assist the provider by placing the patient in the appropriate positions.

Equipment and Supplies:
- Gloves
- Fecal occult blood test kit
- Water-soluble lubricant
- Vaginal speculum
- Slide and fixative or liquid preparation container
- Cervical spatula or plastic-fronded broom
- Laboratory requisition form
- Cotton-tipped applicator
- Patient gown
- Patient drape sheet
- Tray or Mayo stand

Standard: Complete the procedure and all critical steps in _____ minutes with a minimum score of 85% within two attempts (*or as indicated by the instructor*).

Scoring: Divide the points earned by the total possible points. Failure to perform a critical step, indicated by an asterisk (*), results in grade no higher than an 84% (*or as indicated by the instructor*).

Time: Began_____ Ended_____ Total minutes: _____

Steps:	Point Value	Attempt 1	Attempt 2
1. Wash hands or use hand sanitizer.	5		
2. Assemble equipment needed for the gynecologic examination. Place on a tray or Mayo stand in a logical order.	5		
3. Change the table paper if needed.	5		
4. Greet the patient. Identify yourself. Verify the patient's identity with full name and date of birth. Explain the procedure to be performed in a manner that is understood by the patient. Answer any questions the patient may have about the procedure.	10		
5. Ask if the patient needs to empty her bladder and collect a urine specimen if needed.	10		
6. Instruct the patient to undress and put on the gown.	10		
7. Assist the patient onto the examination table and she should remain in the sitting position. Place the drape across her lap.	10		
8. Assist the patient into the supine position, providing a pillow for under her head for comfort. Pull out the leg extension on the examination table.	10		
9. With the stirrups in place on the examination table, assist the patient into the lithotomy position. The leg extension should then be pushed in.	15*		
10. When the examination is complete, assist the patient into the sitting position. Instruct the patient that she can get dressed.	10		

11. After the patient has dressed and left the exam room, clean the room and prepare specimens for transport to the laboratory.	**10**		
Total Points	**100**		

Comments

CAAHEP Competencies	**Step(s)**
I.P.9. Assist provider with a patient exam	Entire procedure
I.P.8. Instruct and prepare a patient for a procedure or a treatment	4-6
ABHES Competencies	**Step(s)**
8.d. Assist provider with specialty examination, including cardiac, respiratory, OB-GYN, neurological, and gastroenterology procedures	Entire procedure
8.e. Perform specialty procedures, including but not limited to minor surgery, cardiac, respiratory, OB-GYN, neurological, and gastroenterology	Entire procedure

Procedure 42.2   Coach a Patient on Breast Self-Exam

Name _____   Date _____   Score _____

Tasks: Coach a patient to do BSE while considering the patient's cultural beliefs and developmental life stage. Document teaching in the patient's health record.

Equipment and Supplies:
- Breast self-examination brochure (optional)
- Breast model
- Provider's order
- Patient's health record

Scenario: You are working with Dr. David Kahn. He has ordered you to show Binh, a 17-year-old Vietnamese patient, how to do a breast self-exam. She has a strong family history of breast cancer. The patient can fluently speak and understand English.

Directions: Role-play this scenario with another peer.

Standard: Complete the procedure and all critical steps in _____ minutes with a minimum score of 85% within two attempts (*or as indicated by the instructor*).

Scoring: Divide the points earned by the total possible points. Failure to perform a critical step, indicated by an asterisk (*), results in grade no higher than an 84% (*or as indicated by the instructor*).

Time: Began_____ Ended_____ Total minutes: _____

Steps:	Point Value	Attempt 1	Attempt 2
1. Wash hands or use hand sanitizer.	5		
2. Read the provider's order. Assemble equipment.	5		
3. Greet the patient. Identify yourself. Verify the patient's identity with full name and date of birth. Explain the procedure to be performed in a manner that the patient understands. Answer any questions the patient may have about the procedure.	10		
4. Provide privacy and independence during the session. Encourage the patient to ask questions and discuss her concerns.	5*		
5. Ask the patient if she is familiar with breast self-examinations. Ask about her thoughts on illness and if she does alternative therapies. Explain the importance of doing a self-exam.	5*		

6.   Explain to the patient that she will need to undress and look at her breast in the mirror to identify any changes.
  a. Let her know that she will need to check to see if they are the usual size, shape, and color.
  b. She should also look for swelling, redness, rash, dimpling, puckering, or bulging of the skin.
  c. She should check to see if the nipple position or appearance has changed.
  d. Finally, she should check to see if any fluid is coming from the nipple by placing her thumb and index finger on the tissue by the nipple and pulling outward towards the end of the nipple.
	10		

7.	Instruct the patient that she needs to change positions and continue to check the appearance of the breasts. She needs to place her hands on her hips and press down. This tightens the chest muscle under the breasts. While in this position, she should turn from side to side to see the outer part of the breasts. Instruct her to clasp her hands behind her head or raise her arms and look at the outer part of the breasts again.	**10**		
8.	Instruct the patient to bend forward and roll her shoulders and elbows forward while tightening her chest muscles. While in this position, she can check for changes in the shape of the breasts.	**10**		
9.	Instruct the patient to palpate the breast using one of the two techniques. Use the model as you explain the technique. • *Lying-down technique*: Instruct the patient to check the breast while lying down. Have her do the following: Tuck a small pillow under the side being checked. Tuck one arm under the head and with the other hand check the opposite breast (e.g., right hand checks the left breast). Use the first two or three finger pads. With fingers together, use a circular motion and a firm, smooth touch to check the entire breast. Start at the top outer breast tissue and move around the breast in a circular pattern. When the top of the breast is reached again, move in 1 inch towards the nipple and complete another circle around the breast. Repeat until the entire breast from the armpit to the cleavage is checked. Then place fingers flat on the nipple and feel for any changes beneath the nipple. Repeat these steps on the other breast. • *Shower technique*: Place the right hand on the right hip. With a soapy left hand, feel for changes in the right axilla area. Use two or three finger pads to press on the breast. Move in an up and down pattern over the breast tissue. Make sure to cover from the bra line to the collarbone. Repeat on the opposite side.	**10**		
10.	Have the patient select a technique that she will use. Encourage the patient to demonstrate the technique on the breast model. Coach the patient on ways to improve the exam if needed.	**10**		
11.	Answer any questions the patient may have. Provide the patient with a brochure to take home (optional).	**10**		
12.	Document the patient education in the patient's health record. Include the provider's name, the order, what was taught, how the patient responded, how the patient did the demonstration, and any handouts provided.	**10**		
	Total Points	**100**		

Documentation

Comments

CAAHEP Competencies	Step(s)
V.P.4.b. Coach patients regarding: health maintenance	Entire procedure
V.P.5.b. Coach patients appropriately considering: developmental life stage	4
V.P.5.a. Coach patients appropriately considering: cultural diversity	4, 5
X.P.3. Document patient care accurately in the medical record	12
ABHES Competencies	**Step(s)**
8.k. Make adaptations to care for patients across their lifespan	4

Pediatrics

CAAHEP Competencies	Assessment
I.P.1.g. Measure and record: length (infant)	Procedure 43.2
I.P.1.h. Measure and record: head circumference (infant)	Procedure 43.1
I.P.1.f. Measure and record: weight	Procedure 43.2
II.C.6.b. Analyze healthcare results as reported in: tables	Skills and Concepts – C. 1
II.C.6.a. Analyze healthcare results as reported in: graphs	Skills and Concepts – C. 1
II.P.4. Document on a growth chart	Procedure 43.1, 43.2
V.C.17.b. Discuss the theories of: Erikson	Skills and Concepts – A. 3
I.C.6. Compare structure and function of the human body across the life span	Skills and Concepts – A. 2
I.P.9. Assist provider with a patient exam	Procedure 43.1, 43.2
X.P.3. Document patient care accurately in the medical record	Procedure 43.1, 43.2

ABHES Competencies	Assessment
5. Human Relations d. Adapt care to address the developmental stages of life	Workplace Applications – 1-3

VOCABULARY REVIEW

Using the word pool on the right, find the correct word to match the definition. Write the word on the line after the definition.

1. A thin, watery serum-like drainage ___serous___

2. The state of being drowsy and dull, listless and unenergetic ___lethargy___

3. A space covered by thick membranes between the sutures of an infant's skull ___fontanelle___

4. The ability to function independently ___autonomy___

5. Abnormally small head associated with incomplete brain development ___microcephaly___

6. A disorder that does not have a cause that can be found in the body ___non-organic___

7. A thin layer of cartilage located at the ends of a long bone where new bone forms ___epiphyseal plates___

8. Weakened or changed ___attenuated___

9. Inflammation and irritation of the skin ___excoriation___

10. Hives ___urticaria___

11. Characterized by the formation and/or discharge of pus ___suppurative___

12. Enlargement of the cranium caused by abnormal accumulation of cerebrospinal fluid in the cerebral system ___hydrocephaly___

Word Pool
- epiphyseal plates
- autonomy
- excoriation
- lethargy
- nonorganic
- serous
- suppurative
- fontanelle
- hydrocephaly
- microcephaly
- attenuated
- urticaria

ABBREVIATIONS

Write out what each of the following abbreviations stands for.

1. CDC ___Centers For Disease Control and Prevention___

2. VIS ___Vaccine Information Statement___

3. BMI ___Body Mass Index___

4. AAP ___The American Academy of Pediatrics___

5. AAFP ___American Academy of Family Physicians___

6. ASD ___Autism Spectrum Disorder___

7. PDD ___Pervasive Developmental Disorders___

8. NCVIA ___National Childhood Vaccine Injury Act___

9. HPV ___Human Papilloma Virus___

SKILLS AND CONCEPTS

Answer the following questions. Write your answer on the line or in the space provided.

A. Normal Growth and Development

1. Explain the difference between growth and development. Growth refers to measurable changes, such as height and weight. Development refers to the stages of physical, cognitive and social growth.

2. What would be the expected growth pattern for the following age groups?

    a. 6 months birth weight doubles

    b. 1 year birth weight triples, length increased by 50%.

    c. 2 years gain 4 pounds in 1 year

    d. 3 years Gains 3-5 pounds in 1 year and grows 2 - 2½ inches

    e. 3-6 years Gains 3-5 pounds per year, grows 1/1, 2-2/2.1 inches per year

3. In your own words, describe each of Erikson's stages of development.

    a. Trust vs. mistrust Infants learn to rely on caregivers; mistrust occurs if needs are not met.

    b. Autonomy vs. shame and doubt Toddlers learn language skills and gain independence; they may feel shame and doubt if they cannot meet parental expectations.

c. Initiative vs. guilt Preschoolers actively seek out new experiences; children become hesitant if restrictions or reprimands make them feel guilty or afraid to try more challenging skills

d. Industry vs. inferiority school-aged children enjoy finishing projects and receiving recognition; they develop feeling of inferiority if they are not accepted by peers or if they cannot please their parents.

e. Identity vs. role confusion Adolescents face many physical and hormonal changes in this age. Teenagers work at figuring out who they are and where they fit; they are seeking a direction of their lives.

B. Pediatric Diseases and Disorders

1. Colic is a condition that is usually seen in infants between __2__ weeks and __4__ months of age. It involves crying episodes that occur at least __3__ times a week and last for longer than __3__ hours a day and lasting at least __3__ weeks.

2. List the symptoms of failure to thrive. Failure to thrive refers to children whose current weight or rate of weight gain is much lower than that of other children of similar age and gender. It is a symptom more than a disease.

3. Describe the possible signs of otitis media. Signs of the otitis media is inflammation of the middle ear, with fluid building up behind the tympanic membrane.

4. What are the possible causes of otitis media? It is caused by bacteria or a virus.

5. When and how should children be screened for autism spectrum disorder (ASD)? All children be screened for autism at their 18 and 24 month well-child checkup. Children with autism show wide range of neurologic and developmental behaviors.

6. What are three common characteristics of children with ASD? _____

   ✻ Poorly developed social skills

   ✻ difficulty with expressive and receptive communication

   ✻ The presence of restrictive and repetitive behaviors

   _____

   _____

   _____

7. Nearly _____20%_____ of all children and adolescents in the United States are obese.

8. List three possible reasons for childhood obesity. _____

   ✻ A family history of obesity

   ✻ high-calorie diets

   ✻ stress

C. Role of the Medical Assistant in Pediatric Procedures

1. Using the growth charts in the textbook (Figures 43.7 and 43.8), plot the measurements and answer the following questions.

   a. Simon Blackstone, 18 months: head circumference, 14.25 inches; 85 cm long; 14 kg.

      What is his height percentile? _____90_____

      What is his weight percentile?_____below 5_____

   b. Carla Toomis, 9 years old: 50 inches tall and weighs 88 pounds.

      What is her height percentile? _____25_____

      What is her weight percentile? _____95_____

2. All healthcare workers should be aware of the signs of children who are being abused, neglected, or exploited. Summarize what you have learned about the signs of child abuse.

   The Child Abuse and Prevention and Treatment Act states that all threats to child's physical or mental welfare must be reported. This means that every teacher, healthcare worker, and social workers, – in fact, every citizen – who suspects that a child is being neglected.

3. List eight details that must be documented when a vaccination is given.

   a. *date vaccine was administered* Write vaccine's manufacturer

   b. Type of vaccine and the dose

   c. Exact site injection was given

   d. Any reported observed side effect

   e. Publication date of the VIS form given the parent

   f. Parent education about possible side effect's

   g. Name and title of person who administered the vaccine

   h. _____

4. List the route of administration for the following vaccines.

   a. Dtap __Diphtheria tetanus pertusis__

   b. HAV __Hepatitis A__

   c. HBV __Hepatitis B__

   d. HPV __Human papillomavirus__

   e. Hib __Hemophilus Influenzae__

   f. Influenza __Trivalent Inactivated vaccine__

   g. IPV __Inactive poliovirus for polio__

   h. MMR __Measles mumps rubella__

   i. PCV __Pneumococcal pneumonia__

   j. Varicella __Varimax__

CERTIFICATION PREPARATION

Circle the correct answer.

1. During which period in a child's life does he or she gain weight the fastest?
   a. First 6 months
   b. Age 6 months to 1 year
   c. Preschool
   d. Adolescence

2. In which illness or condition are dehydration and electrolyte imbalance of particular concern when the disorder occurs in children?
   a. Colic
   b. Influenza
   c. Hepatitis B
   d. Diarrhea

3. The first dose of MMR vaccine should be administered at what age?
   a. 2 months
   b. 4 months
   c. 12 months
   d. 4 years

4. What method of evaluation is used to detect microcephaly?
   a. Culture of infectious material
   b. Developmental screening tests
   c. Laryngoscopy
   d. Measurement of the head circumference

5. Tetanus is part of which immunization?
   a. HBV
   b. Hib
   c. DTaP
   d. MMR

6. Which is a helpful approach to adolescent patients?
   a. The parents should be present for discussions about health problems.
   b. The medical assistant should recognize the importance of personal appearance to adolescents.
   c. The medical assistant should use distraction if painful procedures are performed.
   d. The medical assistant should give the adolescent advice on handling personal problems.

7. The varicella vaccine is usually administered to children in which age group?
   a. Newborns (first dose)
   b. 6 months
   c. 12-18 months
   d. Preschool age

8. Studies have shown that a child who is obese between the ages of _____ has an 80% chance of becoming an obese adult.
   a. 2 and 4
   b. 4 and 8
   c. 8 and 12
   d. 10 and 13

9. The Hib vaccine prevents _____.
   a. measles
   b. varicella
   c. meningitis
   d. hepatitis B

10. One of the primary causes of childhood injuries is _____.
    a. motor vehicle accidents
    b. drowning
    c. burns
    d. all of the above

WORKPLACE APPLICATIONS

1. Based on what you have learned about therapeutic approaches for the pediatric patient, what would be the best way to deal with the following patient situations?

   a. A crying 2-month-old scheduled for the first round of vaccinations _____

   _____

   _____

   b. A 3-year-old who is diagnosed with croup _____

   _____

   _____

   c. An 8-year-old who needs his blood glucose checked with a glucometer _____

   _____

   _____

   d. A 13-year-old who has to receive a penicillin injection in the ventrogluteal site _____

   _____

   _____

2. The grandmother of a 3-year-old patient calls today with concerns about her granddaughter, who has had diarrhea for 2 days. What types of questions should the medical assistant ask about the child's condition? What types of fluids and diet might the provider recommend?

    _____

    _____

    _____

    _____

3. Allison is trying to obtain vital signs on a 4-year-old child who refuses to stand on the scale or cooperate while her temperature is taken. What can Allison do to try to obtain the child's cooperation? What is the best way to take this patient's temperature?

    _____

    _____

    _____

    _____

INTERNET ACTIVITIES

1. Using internet resources, research childhood obesity. Create a poster presentation, a PowerPoint presentation, or write a paper summarizing your research. Include the following points in your project:
    a. Possible reasons for the increase in childhood obesity
    b. Possible solutions
    c. Describe how BMI is determined and used with pediatric patients

2. Using internet resources, research ADHD. Create a poster presentation, a PowerPoint presentation, or write a paper summarizing your research. Include the following points in your project:
    a. Possible causes of ADHD
    b. Treatment options for ADHD including nontraditional options
    c. Techniques a medical assistant can use when working with a patient with ADHD

Procedure 43.1   Measure the Circumference of an Infant's Head

Name _____   Date _____   Score _____

Task: To obtain an accurate measurement of the circumference of an infant's head and plot the result on the patient's growth chart.

Equipment and Supplies:
- Patient's record, with appropriate growth chart
- Flexible disposable tape measure
- Age- and gender-specific growth chart
- Pen

Standard: Complete the procedure and all critical steps in _____ minutes with a minimum score of 85% within two attempts (*or as indicated by the instructor*).

Scoring: Divide the points earned by the total possible points. Failure to perform a critical step, indicated by an asterisk (*), results in grade no higher than an 84% (*or as indicated by the instructor*).

Time: Began_____ Ended_____ Total minutes: _____

Steps:	Point Value	Attempt 1	Attempt 2
1. Wash hands or use hand sanitizer.	10		
2. Greet the patient and the parents or caregivers. Identify yourself. Verify the patient's identity with full name and date of birth. Explain the procedure to be performed in a manner that is understood by the patient. Answer any questions the patient may have on the procedure. If he or she is old enough, gain the child's cooperation through conversation.	10		
3. Place an infant in the supine position, or the infant may be held by the parent. An older child may sit on the examination table.	10		
4. Hold the tape measure with the zero mark against the infant's forehead, slightly above the eyebrows and the top of the ears. Ask the parent for assistance if necessary.	15*		
5. Bring the tape measure around the head, just above the ears, until it meets.	15*		
6. Read to the nearest 0.5 cm or 1/4 inch.	10		
7. Record the measurement on the growth chart and in the patient's health record.	10		
8. Dispose of the tape measure.	10		
9. Wash hands or use hand sanitizer.	10		
Total Points	100		

Documentation

Comments

CAAHEP Competencies	Step(s)
I.P.1.h. Measure and record: head circumference (infant)	Entire procedure
II.P.4. Document on a growth chart	7
ABHES Competencies	**Step(s)**
5.d. Adapt care to address the developmental stages of life	Entire procedure

Procedure 43.2 Measure an Infant's Length and Weight

Name _____ Date _____ Score _____

Task: To measure an infant's length and weight accurately so that growth patterns can be monitored and recorded.

Equipment and Supplies:
- Patient's record
- Infant scale with paper cover
- Flexible measuring tape
- Examination table paper
- Pen
- Pediatric length board, if available
- Gender-specific infant growth chart
- Waste container

Standard: Complete the procedure and all critical steps in _____ minutes with a minimum score of 85% within two attempts (*or as indicated by the instructor*).

Scoring: Divide the points earned by the total possible points. Failure to perform a critical step, indicated by an asterisk (*), results in grade no higher than an 84% (*or as indicated by the instructor*).

Time: Began _____ Ended _____ Total minutes: _____

Steps for measuring infant length:	Point Value	Attempt 1	Attempt 2
1. Wash hands or use hand sanitizer, assemble the necessary equipment.	5		
2. Greet the patient and parents or caregivers. Identify yourself. Verify the patient's identity with full name and date of birth. Explain the procedure to be performed in a manner that is understood by the patient. Answer any questions the parents or caregivers may have on the procedure.	5		
3. Undress the infant. The diaper may be left on.	5		
4. Cover the examination table with smooth, flat paper. Ask the caregiver to place the infant on his or her back on the examination table. If the table is a pediatric table with a headboard, ask the caregiver to hold the infant's head gently against the headboard while you straighten the infant's leg and note the location of the heel on the measurement area. If there is no headboard, ask the caregiver to gently hold the infant's head still while you draw a line on the paper at the top of the baby's head and at the heel after extending the leg.	10*		
5. Measure the infant's length with the tape measure and record it.	10		
6. Document the results in either inches or centimeters, depending on office policy, on the infant's growth chart, in the progress notes, and in the caregiver's record if requested.	5		
Steps for measuring infant weight:			
7. Wash hands or use hand sanitizer, assemble the necessary equipment, and explain the procedure to the infant's caregiver.	5		
8. Greet the patient and parents or caregivers. Identify yourself. Verify the patient's identity with full name and date of birth. Explain the procedure to be performed in a manner that is understood by the patient. Answer any questions the parents or caregivers may have on the procedure.	5		

9. If the scale is not a digital model, prepare the scale by sliding weights to the left; line the scale with disposable paper to reduce the risk of pathogen transmission.	5		
10. Completely undress the infant. If the diaper is clean and dry it can remain on.	5		
11. Place the infant gently on the center of the scale, keeping your hand directly above the infant's trunk for safety.	10		
12. If the scale is not a digital model, slide the weights across the scale until balance is achieved. Read the infant's weight while he or she is still.	10*		
13. If the scale is not a digital model, return the weights to the far left of the scale and remove the baby. Discard the paper lining the scale. If the scale became contaminated during the procedure, follow Occupational Safety and Health Administration (OSHA) guidelines for use of gloves and disposal of contaminated waste. Disinfect the equipment according to the manufacturer's guidelines.	10		
14. Wash hands or use hand sanitizer.	5		
15. Document the results in either pounds or kilograms, depending on office policy, on the infant's growth chart, in the progress notes, and in the caregiver's record if requested.	5		
Total Points	100		

Documentation

Comments

CAAHEP Competencies	**Step(s)**
I.P.1.g. Measure and record: length (infant)	1-6
II.P.4. Document on a growth chart	6, 13
ABHES Competencies	**Step(s)**
5.d. Adapt care to address the developmental stages of life	Entire procedure

Procedure 43.3   Document Immunizations

Name _____ Date _____ Score _____

Task: To document accurately the administration of a pediatric immunization.

Equipment and Supplies:
- Patient's record
- Vaccine administration record (VAR) (Work Product 43-3)
- Parent's immunization record (if used in the medical practice)
- Vaccine Information Sheet (VIS) for hepatitis B (a link to the current VIS forms can be accessed at www. cdc.gov/vaccines/hcp/vis/current-vis.html)

Scenario: Samantha Anderson, a 5-week-old infant, has just received her second dose of the hepatitis B (HBV) vaccine. Document the administration of the vaccine.

Standard: Complete the procedure and all critical steps in _____ minutes with a minimum score of 85% within two attempts (*or as indicated by the instructor*).

Scoring: Divide the points earned by the total possible points. Failure to perform a critical step, indicated by an asterisk (*), results in grade no higher than an 84% (*or as indicated by the instructor*).

Time: Began_____ Ended_____ Total minutes: _____

Steps:	Point Value	Attempt 1	Attempt 2
1. Gather the necessary forms.	20		
2. Make sure that the hepatitis B VIS form was given, and that all the parent's questions were answered before the vaccine is dispensed and administered.	20*		
Scenario update: The parent signed the required paperwork and you have the vaccine in the left vastus lateralis and now you need to document. 3. After the vaccine has been given, complete the information required on the VAR, including the name of the vaccine, the date given, the route of administration and site, the vaccine lot number and manufacturer, the date on the VIS form, the date it was given to the parent, and your signature or initials.	20		
4. In the parent's immunization record, record the date of administration, the name and address of the provider's practice, and the type of vaccine administered.	20		
5. After administering the HBV vaccine, record the following details in the child's health record: • Date the vaccine was administered • Vaccine's manufacturer, batch and lot numbers, and expiration date • Type of vaccine administered and dose • Route of administration and exact site if an injection was given • Any reported or observed side effects • Publication date of the VIS form given to the parent (on the bottom of the form) • Parent education about possible side effects of the vaccine • Name and title of the person who administered the vaccine	20*		
Total Points	**100**		

Documentation

Comments

ABHES Competencies	Step(s)
5.d. Adapt care to address the developmental stages of life	Entire procedure

Work Product 43.1 Vaccine Administration Record

Name _____ Date _____ Score _____

Vaccine Administration Record for Children and Teens

Patient name: _____

Birthdate: _____ Chart number: _____

Clinic name and address

Before administering any vaccines, give copies of all pertinent Vaccine Information Statements (VISs) to the child's parent or legal representative and make sure he/she understands the risks and benefits of the vaccine(s). Always provide or update the patient's personal record card.

Vaccine	Type of Vaccine[1]	Date given (mo/day/yr)	Funding Source (F,S,P)[2]	Route & Site[3]	Vaccine		Vaccine Information Statement (VIS)		Vaccinator[5] (signature or initials & title)
					Lot #	Mfr.	Date on VIS[4]	Date given[4]	
Hepatitis B[6] (e.g., HepB, Hib-HepB, DTaP-HepB-IPV) Give IM.[3]									
Diphtheria, Tetanus, Pertussis[6] (e.g., DTaP, DTaP/Hib, DTaP-HepB-IPV, DT, DTaP-IPV/Hib, Tdap, DTaP-IPV, Td) Give IM.[3]									
Haemophilus influenzae type b[6] (e.g., Hib, Hib-HepB, DTaP-IPV/Hib, DTaP/Hib, Hib-MenCY) Give IM.[3]									
Polio[6] (e.g., IPV, DTaP-HepB-DTaP-IPV/Hib, DTaP-IPV) Give IPV SC or IM.[3] Give all others IM.[3]									
Pneumococcal (e.g., PCV7, PCV13, conjugate; PPSV23, polysaccharide) Give PCV IM.[3] Give PPSV SC or IM.[3]									
Rotavirus (RV1, RV5) Give orally (po).[3]									

See page 2 to record measles-mumps-rubella, varicella, hepatitis A, meningococcal, HPV, influenza, and other vaccines (e.g., travel vaccines).

How to Complete This Record

1. Record the generic abbreviation (e.g., Tdap) or the trade name for each vaccine (see table at right).

2. Record the funding source of the vaccine given as either F (federal), S (state), or P (private).

3. Record the route by which the vaccine was given as either intramuscular (IM), subcutaneous (SC), intradermal (ID), intranasal (IN), or oral (PO) and also the site where it was administered as either RA (right arm), LA (left arm), RT (right thigh), or LT (left thigh).

4. Record the publication date of each VIS as well as the date the VIS is given to the patient.

5. To meet the space constraints of this form and federal requirements for documentation, a healthcare setting may want to keep a reference list of vaccinators that includes their initials and titles.

6. For combination vaccines, fill in a row for each antigen in the combination.

Abbreviation	Trade Name and Manufacturer
DTaP	Daptacel (sanofi); Infanrix (GlaxoSmithKline [GSK]); Tripedia (sanofi pasteur)
DT (pediatric)	Generic DT (sanofi pasteur)
DTaP-HepB-IPV	Pediarix (GSK)
DTaP/Hib	TriHIBit (sanofi pasteur)
DTaP-IPV/Hib	Pentacel (sanofi pasteur)
DTaP-IPV	Kinrix (GSK)
HepB	Engerix-B (GSK); Recombivax HB (Merck)
HepA-HepB	Twinrix (GSK), can be given to teens age 18 and older
Hib	ActHIB (sanofi pasteur); Hiberix (GSK); PedvaxHIB (Merck)
Hib-HepB	Comvax (Merck)
Hib-MenCY	MenHibrix (GSK)
IPV	Ipol (sanofi pasteur)
PCV13	Prevnar 13 (Pfizer)
PPSV23	Pneumovax 23 (Merck)
RV1	Rotarix (GSK)
RV5	RotaTeq (Merck)
Tdap	Adacel (sanofi pasteur); Boostrix (GSK)
Td	Decavac (sanofi pasteur); Generic Td (MA Biological Labs)

Technical content reviewed by the Centers for Disease Control and Prevention

This form was created by the Immunization Action Coalition • www.immunize.org • www.vaccineinformation.org

For additional copies, visit www.immunize.org/catg.d/p2022.pdf • Item #P2022 (4/14)

Geriatrics

CAAHEP Competencies	Assessment
I.P.9. Assist provider with a patient exam	Procedure 44.1
V.A.1.a. Demonstrate: empathy	Procedure 44.1
I.C.6. Compare structure and function of the human body across the life span	Skills and Concepts – A. 1, 2, 3, 5, 7, 9, 11, 12, 15, 18, 22, 25-28, 30; Workplace Application – 2; Internet Activities 2, 3
ABHES Competencies	**Assessment**
5. Human Relations d. Adapt care to address the developmental stages of life	Procedure 44.1

VOCABULARY REVIEW

Using the word pool, find the correct word to match the definition. Write the word on the line after the definition.

Group A

1. Rhythmic contraction of involuntary muscles lining the gastrointestinal tract _____

2. Fully and clearly expressed or demonstrated; leaving nothing merely implied _____

3. The most abundant structural protein found in skin and other connective tissues; provides strength and cushioning to many parts of the body _____

4. Nerve pain that occurs after a shingles outbreak and may become chronic _____

5. A temporary fall in blood pressure when a person rapidly changes from a recumbent position to a standing position

    _____

6. Skin surface areas supplied by a single afferent spinal nerve

    _____

7. The relative frequency of deaths in a specific population

    _____

8. Proceeding in a gradual, subtle way, but with harmful effects

    _____

Word Pool
- mortality
- orthostatic hypotension
- insidious
- explicit
- peristalsis
- collagen
- dermatome
- postherpetic neuralgia

Group B

1. A medicine or substance capable of damaging cranial nerve VIII or the organs of hearing and balance _____

2. A highly elastic protein in connective tissue that allows tissues to resume their shape after stretching or contracting; found abundantly in the dermis of the skin _____

3. Frequent urination at night _____

4. Chronic disease of the inner ear causing recurrent episodes of vertigo, progressive sensorineural hearing loss, and tinnitus

   _____

5. The secretion or discharge of tears _____

6. Surgical removal of the ovaries _____

7. Sores that develop over a bony prominence as the result of ischemia from prolonged pressure _____

8. Abnormal thinning of the bone structure causing bones to become brittle and weak _____

Word Pool
- osteoporosis
- oophorectomy
- decubitus ulcer
- nocturia
- elastin
- lacrimation
- Ménière's disease
- ototoxic

ABBREVIATIONS

Write out what each of the following abbreviations stands for.

1. CHF _____

2. DM _____

3. GERD _____

4. CVA _____

5. OTC _____

6. AD _____

7. CNS _____

8. REM _____

9. PLMD _____

10. COPD _____

SKILLS AND CONCEPTS

A. Changes in Anatomy, Physiology, and Diseases

1. The most common reason for hospitalization among older adults is _____.

2. Describe the changes in the cardiovascular system as a person ages. _____

   _____

   _____

   _____

3. Aging may bring on hypertension. How does hypertension affect the heart? _____

   _____

   _____

   _____

4. List the signs and symptoms of orthostatic hypotension. _____

   _____

   _____

5. The most common endocrine system disorder seen in aging patients is _____ .

6. What are the classic symptoms of diabetes mellitus? _____

   _____

7. When an older patient has diabetes mellitus, he or she needs to be aware of sensory abnormalities. List two sensory symptoms that may be seen in older patients.

   _____

8. Write a brief definition of the following terms.

   a. Dysphagia_____

      _____

   b. Peristalsis _____

      _____

   c. GERD_____

      _____

9. Exposure to UV light from the sun may frequently cause what skin conditions with aging? _____

   _____

   _____

10. List the three layers of the skin. _____

    _____

11. Loss of what substance in the skin causes it to sag and wrinkle? _____

12. Aging patients may not be able to regulate body temperature as efficiently as younger patients. How can the medical assistant make an older patient comfortable?

    _____

    _____

13. What are some suggestions that might help older patients prevent and treat dry skin? _____

    _____

14. The term for hair loss is _____.

15. Another term for age spots is _____.

16. Shingles is caused by the same virus that causes _____.

17. Briefly describe osteoarthritis. _____

_____

18. Muscular changes in the aging patient are directly related to the individual's _____.

19. List five risk factors for osteoporosis. _____

_____

_____

20. What are possible complications of a fall? _____

_____

_____

21. List five measures that can be taken to prevent falls. _____

_____

_____

_____

_____

22. Briefly describe how to ensure mental functioning in later life. _____

_____

_____

_____

23. Briefly define *Alzheimer's disease.* _____

_____

_____

24. List five conditions that can interfere with sleep. _____

_____

_____

25. Briefly describe how the respiratory system changes as a person ages._____

_____

_____

_____

26. List eye diseases and disorders that occur frequently in older patients. _____

    _____

    _____

27. Briefly describe presbycusis. _____

    _____

    _____

    _____

28. During the aging process, the abilities to _____ and _____ decline subtly. The ability to taste _____ and _____ flavors is reduced, but the ability to detect _____ and _____ flavors remains the same.

29. What term is defined as the involuntary loss of urine? _____

30. Aging decreases the female hormones _____ and _____, and increases _____. Aging men can experience a change in _____ levels, which can affect the _____.

B. The Medical Assistant's Role in Caring for the Older Patient

1. To be sensitive to the needs of older patients, what accommodations should an ambulatory care clinic make?

    _____

    _____

    _____

    _____

2. What are general guidelines for effective patient education with older adults? _____

    _____

    _____

    _____

    _____

    _____

    _____

    _____

CERTIFICATION PREPARATION

Circle the correct answer.

1. The most common disorder of the endocrine system is
   a. hyperthyroidism.
   b. diabetes mellitus.
   c. Alzheimer's disease.
   d. Meniere's disease.

2. The relative frequency of deaths in a specific population is the definition for
   a. insidious.
   b. explicit.
   c. mortality.
   d. exploitation.

3. Indications that a patient may be a victim of elder abuse may include
   a. recurrent injuries caused by accident.
   b. poor general appearance and hygiene.
   c. bruising, dehydration, and pressure injuries.
   d. all of the above.

4. Which taste buds decline as a person ages?
   a. Sweet
   b. Salty
   c. Bitter
   d. Both a and b

5. Hearing loss associated with normal aging is
   a. Meniere's disease.
   b. presbycusis.
   c. otosclerosis.
   d. ototoxic.

6. A condition that makes it difficult to focus in detail on objects close at hand is
   a. glaucoma.
   b. cataracts.
   c. macular degeneration.
   d. presbyopia.

7. Which medical condition does not interfere with sleep?
   a. Congestive heart failure
   b. Otosclerosis
   c. Parkinson's disease
   d. Joint and bone pain

8. The formation of amyloid plaques in the brain would be found in a patient with which disease or disorder?
   a. Congestive heart failure
   b. Macular degeneration
   c. Alzheimer's disease
   d. Depression

9. Risk factors for cognitive decline include
   a. hypertension.
   b. diabetes mellitus.
   c. sedentary lifestyle.
   d. all of the above.

10. The primary cause of hip fractures is
    a. osteoporosis.
    b. dementia.
    c. stroke.
    d. Parkinson's disease.

WORKPLACE APPLICATIONS

1. Patricia is a 75-year-old patient who has a cataract in her right eye. Patricia is going to have a phaco-emulsification of her right eye. How would you explain this procedure to Patricia in language that would help her understand the procedure? Write your answer below.

   _____

   _____

   _____

   _____

2. Gracie, a 68-year-old patient, has an appointment for a physical today. As the medical assistant talks to her, she mentions that her skin has become very dry over the last few years. How could the medical assistant coach her about maintaining the health of her skin as she ages?

_____

_____

_____

_____

3. Juan is reviewing the medications used to treat osteoporosis for a continuing education course he is taking. List the medications used below. List the generic, brand names, and brief action of the medication.

_____

_____

_____

_____

INTERNET ACTIVITIES

1. Using online resources, research an imaging test used for diagnosing Alzheimer's disease. Create a poster presentation, a PowerPoint presentation, or a written paper summarizing your research. Include the following points in your project:
    a. Description of the test
    b. Any contraindications for the test
    c. Patient preparation for the test
    d. What occurs during the test

2. Using online resources, research a disease or disorder that occurs in older patient populations. Create a poster presentation, a PowerPoint presentation, or a written paper summarizing your research. Include the following points in your project:
    a. Description of the disease
    b. Etiology
    c. Signs and symptoms
    d. Diagnostic procedures
    e. Treatments
    f. Prognosis
    g. Prevention

3. Using online resources, research the effect that diet can have on the aging process. In a one-page paper, summarize the information that you found.

Procedure 44.1 Understand the Sensorimotor Changes of Aging

Name _____ Date _____ Score _____

Task: To role-play an older adult to better understand the needs of aging people.

Equipment and Supplies:
- Yellow-tinted glasses, ski goggles, or laboratory goggles
- Pink, white, yellow "pills" (e.g., various colors of Tic Tacs)
- Petroleum jelly (e.g., Vaseline)
- Cotton balls
- Eye patches
- Tape
- Utility gloves
- Tongue depressors
- Elastic bandages
- Medical forms in small print
- Pennies
- Button shirts
- Walker

Standard: Complete the procedure and all critical steps in _____ minutes with a minimum score of 85% within two attempts (*or as indicated by the instructor*).

Scoring: Divide the points earned by the total possible points. Failure to perform a critical step, indicated by an asterisk (*), results in grade no higher than an 84% (*or as indicated by the instructor*).

Time: Began_____ Ended_____ Total minutes: _____

Steps:	Point Value	Attempt 1	Attempt 2
1. Role-play vision and hearing loss. • Put two cotton balls in each ear and an eye patch over one eye. Follow your partner's instructions. • *Partner:* Stand out of the line of vision (to prevent lip-reading). Without using gestures or changing your voice volume, tell your partner to cross the room and pick up a book.	10		
2. Role-play yellowing of the lens of the eye. • Line up "pills" of different pastel colors. • *Partner:* Pick out the different colors while wearing the yellow-tinted glasses.	10		
3. Role-play difficulty focusing. • Put on goggles smeared with petroleum jelly and follow your partner's directions. • *Partner:* Stand at least 3 feet in front of your partner and motion for him or her to come to you (your partner is deaf, so talking will not help).	10		
4. Role-play loss of peripheral vision. • Put on goggles with black paper taped to the sides. • *Partner:* Stand to the side, out of the field of vision, and motion for your patient to follow you.	10		

5. Role-play aphasia and partial paralysis. • You are unable to use your right arm or leg. Place tape over your mouth. Let your partner know you need to go to the bathroom. • *Partner:* Stand at least 3 feet away with your back to your partner and wait for instructions.	**10**		
6. Role-play problems with dexterity. • Put thick gloves on your hands and try to sign your name, button a shirt, tie your shoes, and pick up pennies.	**10**		
7. Role-play problems with mobility. • Use the walker to cross the room. • *Partner:* After your partner starts to use the walker, hand him or her a book to carry.	**10**		
8. Role-play changes in sensation. • Put a rubber utility glove on; turn on very warm water; test the difference in temperature between the gloved hand and the ungloved hand.	**10**		
9. Summarize and share with the group your impressions of the effect of age-related sensorimotor changes. *(Refer to the Checklist for Affective Behaviors)*	**20***		
Total Points	**100**		

Checklist for Affective Behaviors

Affective Behavior	*Directions:* Check behaviors observed during the role-play.					
	Negative, Unprofessional Behaviors	**Attempt**		**Positive, Professional Behaviors**	**Attempt**	
Empathy		**1**	**2**		**1**	**2**
	Did not acknowledge the age-related sensorimotor changes in the older population			Acknowledged the age-related sensorimotor changes in the older population		
	Failed to reassure patient; did not respond to the patient's concerns			Discussed the difficulty of doing the tasks; how it felt not being able to do what was asked when being the "older person"		
	Failed to identify ways to adapt interactions when working with older people that could accommodate the age-related sensorimotor changes			Verbalized ways to adapt interactions when working with older people while considering age-related sensorimotor changes		
	Other:			Other:		

Grading		Point Value	Attempt 1	Attempt 2
Does not meet Expectation	• Response lacks empathy. • Student demonstrated more than 2 negative, unprofessional behaviors during the interaction.	0		
Needs Improvement	• Response lacks empathy. • Student demonstrated 1 or 2 negative, unprofessional behaviors during the interaction.	0		
Meets Expectation	• Response was empathetic; no negative, unprofessional behaviors observed. • Responses where limited, more thought/consideration is needed.	20		
Occasionally Exceeds Expectation	• Response was empathetic; no negative, unprofessional behaviors observed. • Response provided more insights, more thought/consideration is needed.	20		
Always Exceeds Expectation	• Response empathetic; no negative, unprofessional behaviors observed. • Student's response showed a depth understanding that is consistent with a professional medical assistant.	20		

Comments

CAAHEP Competencies	Step(s)
V.A.1.a. Demonstrate: empathy	9
I.P.9. Assist provider with a patient exam	Entire procedure
ABHES Competencies	**Step(s)**
5. Human Relations d. Adapt care to address the developmental stages of life	Entire procedure

hemolyzed
stability
aliquot

Introduction to the Clinical Laboratory

CAAHEP Competencies	Assessment
I.C.12. Identify quality assurance practices in healthcare	Skills and Concepts – C. 1-5
II.C.6.a. Analyze healthcare results as reported in: graphs	Procedure 45.1
II.C.6.b. Analyze healthcare results as reported in: tables	Procedure 45.1
XII.C.1.a. Identify: safety signs	Skills and Concepts – E. 1
XII.C.1.b. Identify: symbols	Skills and Concepts – E. 1
XII.C.1.c. Identify: labels	Skills and Concepts – E. 6, 7
XII.C.2.a. Identify safety techniques that can be used in responding to accidental exposure to: blood	Skills and Concepts – E. 10-13
XII.C.2.b. Identify safety techniques that can be used in responding to accidental exposure to: other body fluids	Skills and Concepts – E. 10-13
XII.C.2.c. Identify safety techniques that can be used in responding to accidental exposure to: needlesticks	Skills and Concepts – E. 10-12
XII.C.2.d. Identify safety techniques that can be used in responding to accidental exposure to: chemicals	Skills and Concepts – E. 4-7, 10, 11
XII.C.5. Describe the purpose of Safety Data Sheets (SDS) in a healthcare setting	Skills and Concepts – E. 5; Workplace Applications – 3
XII.C.6. Discuss protocols for disposal of biological chemical materials	Online Activity – 4, Procedure 45.1
I.P.10. Perform a quality control measure	Procedure 45.1
II.P.3. Maintain lab test results using flow sheets	Procedure 45.1
VI.P.8. Perform routine maintenance of administrative or clinical equipment	Procedure 45.4
XII.P.1.a. Comply with: safety signs	Procedure 45.3
XII.P.1.b. Comply with: symbols	Procedure 45.3
XII.P.1.c. Comply with: labels	Procedure 45.3

CAAHEP Competencies		Assessment
XII.P.2.a. Demonstrate proper use of: eyewash equipment	Procedure 45.2	
XII.P.5. Evaluate the work environment to identify unsafe working conditions	Procedure 45.3	
ABHES Competencies		**Assessment**
9. Medical Laboratory Procedures a. Practice quality control	Procedure 45.1	
b. Perform selected CLIA-waived tests that assist with diagnosis and treatment	Procedure 45.1	
c. Dispose of biohazardous materials	Procedure 45.1	

VOCABULARY REVIEW

Using the word pool, find the correct word to match the definition. Write the word on the line after the definition.

Group A

1. A biological sample such as blood, urine, body fluids, feces, or tissue collected for analysis and evaluation ___Specimen___

2. A physician specially trained in the nature and cause of disease ___pathologist___

3. The substance or chemical being analyzed or detected in a specimen ___Analyte___

4. A laboratory that performs testing for another laboratory; testing varies from high-volume routine testing to low-volume unique or unusual testing ___Referral laboratory___

5. A series of laboratory tests associated with a particular organ or disease; also referred to as a *panel* of tests ___profile testing___

6. Tests are not necessarily diagnostic for one particular disease, but rather indicate that the disease state may exist ___screening test___

7. The study and science dealing with the effects, antidotes, and detection of poisons or drugs ___toxicology___

8. A test result is expressed as a number, usually with units of measure attached to numeric values ___quantitative___

9. The study of cells using microscopic testing methods ___cytology___

10. Tests that are reported as positive or negative, with no numeric value attached to the result ___qualitative___

Word Pool
- specimen
- referral laboratory
- pathologist
- analyte
- profile testing
- screening test
- toxicology
- qualitative
- quantitative
- cytology

Group B

1. Testing performed on organisms to establish an appropriate antibiotic therapy for that specific bacteria or fungus *sensitivity testing*
2. The study of tissues *histology*
3. Free from living pathogenic organisms *aseptically*
4. A solid, liquid, or semi-solid medium designed to support the growth of microorganisms, especially bacteria and fungus *culture media*
5. Free from all living organisms *sterile*
6. The growth of only one microorganism in a culture, or on a nutrient medium *pure culture*
7. Latin term meaning "in glass" and is commonly known as *in the laboratory* *in vitro*
8. International Normalized Ratio, also called *prothrombin time*; used to test the effectiveness of blood-thinning medication *INR*
9. A set of step-by-step instructions to help employees carry out routine operations efficiently, with high quality, and uniformity of performance *standard operating procedures*
10. Tests designed to have straightforward directions and procedures so that they have a minimal risk of incorrect results *waived*

Word Pool
- histology
- INR
- aseptically
- sterile
- sensitivity testing
- culture media
- pure culture
- in vitro
- standard operating procedures
- waived

Group C

1. Causing the gradual destruction of a substance by chemical action *corrosive*
2. Data results on a graph that make an abrupt change in value *trend*
3. Manufacturer-prepared samples that have a known quantity of a specific analyte used for quality-control purposes; also called *controls* or *quality controls* *control materials*
4. Any substance that can be breathed into the lungs *inhalant*
5. Data results on a graph that are obtained over time, which continue to go upward or downward in value *shift*
6. Capable of burning, corroding, or damaging tissue by chemical action *caustic*
7. Determining the accuracy of an instrument by comparing its output with that of a known standard or another instrument known to be accurate *calibration*
8. A substance for use in a chemical reaction *reagent*
9. The ability to consistently reproduce a test result *precision*
10. A measure of how close a test result is to the true value of the control material, as established by the manufacturer *accuracy*

Word Pool
- calibration
- control materials
- accuracy
- precision
- reagent
- trend
- shift
- caustic
- inhalant
- corrosive

Group D

1. A blood sample in which the red blood cells have ruptured
   hemolyzed

2. A portion of a well-mixed sample removed for testing
   aliquot

3. Medical term for devices with sharp points or edges that can puncture or cut skin; examples include needles, scalpels, or broken glass _sharps_

4. Scientific tests or techniques used regarding the detection or evidence of a crime _forensic_

5. Fluids that have escaped from blood vessels and are deposited in tissues or on tissue surfaces; examples would be a seeping cut, oozing sore, or leaking site of infection _exudates_

6. To withdraw fluid using suction _aspirate_

7. A substance (i.e., medication or chemical) that prevents clotting of blood _anticoagulant_

Word Pool
- exudate
- sharps
- aspirate
- anticoagulant
- hemolyzed
- aliquot
- forensic

ABBREVIATIONS

Write out what each of the following abbreviations stands for.

1. AAMA _____

2. POL _____

3. UTI _____

4. CMA _____

5. RMA _____

6. MT _____

7. MLT _____

8. AMT _____

9. ASCP _____

10. CCMA _____

11. CLS _____

12. CLT _____

13. MLA _____

14. ISCLT _____

15. CMLA _____

16. NHA _____

17. RMT _____

18. CPT _____

19. NCA _____

20. FOBT _____

21. RBC _____

22. WBC _____

23. INR _____

24. LDL _____

25. HDL _____

26. CSF _____

27. CLIA _____

28. CMS _____

29. FDA _____

30. CDC _____

31. HIV _____

32. SOP _____

33. QA _____

34. QC _____

35. OSHA _____

36. HCS _____

37. SDS _____

38. PPE _____

39. BBPS _____

40. OPIM _____

41. HMIS _____

42. HBV _____

43. HCV _____

44. PEP _____

45. STAT _____

46. EHR _____

47. PHI _____

48. C _____

49. F _____

50. SI _____

51. WHO _____

52. PPM(P) _____

53. KOH _____

54. CAP _____

55. HIPAA _____

56. CoW _____

57. (D)HHS _____

58. RPM _____

59. TSH _____

SKILLS AND CONCEPTS

Answer the following questions. Write your answer on the line or in the space provided.

A. Introduction—The Clinical Laboratory and Patient Care

1. A laboratory director is either a(n) _____pathologist_____ or clinical laboratory scientist with a(n) _____doctorate degree_____.

2. In an ambulatory care facility, the lab director may be a(n) _____physician_____; this type of laboratory is referred to as a(n) _____POL_____.

3. List the four main purposes of laboratory testing. ✱ To document the good health of a patient.
   ✱ To screen patients for diseases and conditions such as diabetes, etc.
   ✱ To help the provider diagnose a medical disease, disorders.
   ✱ To help the provider decide the most appropriate treatment.

4. List three laboratory-related activities a medical assistant may participate in. _____
   ✱ Proper patient preparation.
   ✱ Testing procedures common to the provider's practice.
   ✱ Normal range of results for common testing.

5. A change in the internal environment of the body often results in _____abnormal tests_____ that are outside the population's _____reference range_____.

6. Screening test results are often _____qualitative_____ and are reported as _____positive_____ or _____negative_____.

7. Quantitative test results are usually expressed as a(n) _____number_____, with units of measure attached to the value.

8. List the 12 laboratory departments. Urinalysis, hematology, chemistry, microbiology, specimen collection and processing, blood bank, coagulation, immunology/serology, histology, cytology, toxicology, and special chemistry.

9. What are the four types of testing most commonly done in a POL? _____
   Urinary, hematology, Chemistry, Microbiology

10. To perform a urinalysis, the specimen is tested with a multiple test strip called a(n) _____dipstick_____.

11. POL hematology testing is most frequently the following three screening tests: _____hemoglobin_____, _____hematocrit_____, and _____the INR_____.

12. Define *single analyte test* and *profile test* in your own words and give an example of each._____
   Single analyte is one test and profile test is more than one analyte is tested from a single sample.

13. Define the term *aseptically*._____
   Free from living germs or diseases

14. Free from all living organisms is the definition for _____sterile_____.

15. In microbiology, specimens may be grown on _____culture media_____.

16. Define *sensitivity testing* in your own words. _____
   It is a test that is done on organisms to see what antibiotics therpy would work best to kill it weather its bacteria or fungi.

17. List one microbiology test that is frequently performed in a POL._____
   A rapid strep tests

B. Government Legislation Affecting Clinical Laboratory Testing

1. Briefly describe CLIA. _It is designed to ensure that accuracy, precision, reliability, and timeliness of patient test results regardless of which laboratory performed the testing_

2. The U.S. Food and Drug Administration (FDA) is responsible for categorizing commercially marketed tests performed _____ in vitro _____, based on the CLIA guidelines.

3. List the three FDA complexity categories for laboratory tests. _waived tests, moderate complexity tests, and high complexity tests._

4. Define *waived testing*. _Laboratory tests and procedures that have been approved by the FDA for home use or that are simple laboratory tests and procedures to perform._

5. Describe *proficiency testing* in the laboratory. _They are testing that is done the same way as patient samples, the results are then reported to the proficiency testing agency, and the accuracy of the testing is verified._

C. Quality Assurance Guideline

1. Describe quality assurance (QA) in the laboratory. _____

2. List the three stages of laboratory QA. _____

3. Define *calibration* in your own words. _____

4. Define *quality control* or *control materials*. _____

_____

_____

5. Why is preventive maintenance so important in the laboratory? _____

_____

_____

D. Quality Control Guideline

1. What is the purpose of running quality control (QC) samples in the laboratory? _____

_____

_____

2. _____ is a measure of how close a test result is to the true value of the control material as established by the manufacturer.

3. The term for the ability to consistently reproduce a test result is _____.

4. When should QC samples be run in the clinical laboratory? _____

_____

_____

5. Define these graphing terms.

   a. Trend _____

   _____

   b. Shift _____

   _____

E. Laboratory Safety

1. Write the definition for each warning symbol in the spaces provided.

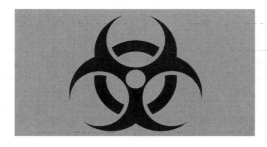 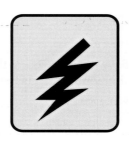 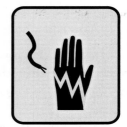

   A. _____   B. _____

2. The U.S. government created a system of safeguards and regulations under the

   _____.

3. What two programs are mandated by OSHA to ensure safety for laboratory personnel? _____

   _____

   _____

4. Briefly describe OSHA's Hazard Communication Standard (HCS). _____

   _____

   _____

   _____

   _____

   _____

   _____

5. Briefly describe a safety data sheet (SDS) and list the information included on each SDS. _____

   _____

   _____

   _____

   _____

   _____

   _____

6. Refer to textbook Figure 45.3 when answering this question. Describe the hazard each diamond represents.

   Top (red) diamond: _____

   Left (blue) diamond: _____

   Bottom (white) diamond: _____

   Right (yellow) diamond: _____

7. Refer to textbook Figure 45.3 when answering this question. The four-color chemical label can also have numbers from 0-4 in each diamond. What is the significance of the number?

   _____

   _____

   _____

8. Describe what a biohazard is in your own words. _____

_____

_____

9. List the types of specimens that have the potential to be infectious. _____

_____

_____

10. What are the five elements of Standard Precautions?_____

_____

_____

11. According to the CDC, the most effective means of preventing infection is _____.

12. The Bloodborne Pathogens Standard requires documentation of employee protection in an exposure control plan. List the information that must be included in an employer's exposure control plan.

_____

_____

_____

13. List three safety guidelines for Other Potentially Infectious Materials (OPIM)._____

_____

_____

_____

F. Specimen Collection, Processing, and Storage

1. What are the three most common specimens collected for the clinical laboratory?_____

   Blood, Urine, and wound or mucous membrane

2. If the patient is not _____identified_____ properly, the laboratory results that are generated will be useless.

3. When labeling a sample container, what information should always be included? _____

   Patient's full name, date of birth, medical record number, time and date collected, address, phone number,

4. If a specimen will be tested for the presence of microorganisms, a(n) _____*sterile*_____ container must be used.

5. Forensic specimens are also called _____*midstream*_____ specimens.

6. Describe the phrase *chain of custody*. Give one example of a specimen that would follow chain of custody rules.

   It refers to the stepwise method used to collect, process, and test a specimen. Blood is the one of example.

G. Laboratory Mathematics and Measurement

Express the following Greenwich times as military times. Use Table 45.5 for reference.

1. 8:10 AM = _____

2. 2:15 PM = _____

3. 6:30 PM = _____

4. 5:50 AM = _____

Express the following temperatures in Celsius.

5. 98.6° F = _____

6. 32° F = _____

7. 212° F = _____

8. 72° F = _____

9. What systems of measurement are used in the clinical laboratory? _____

_____

Use Table 45.9 for reference. Determine the type of specimen by which metric units of measure are used for the following.

10. 20 mL of reagent   volume   weight   length

11. 9.45 kg of tissue   volume   weight   length

12. 327 mcg of reagent   volume   weight   length

13. 41.5 cm of tubing   volume   weight   length

14. 7.25 cc of reagent   volume   weight   length

15. 10.5 mm of specimen   volume   weight   length

16. When liquids are measured into test tubes, the most common piece of glassware used is the
_____.

H. Laboratory Equipment

1. Which instrument is used to view objects too small to be seen with the naked eye?_____
_____

2. List the medical personnel who can make a final analysis of a microscope slide. _____
_____
_____
_____

3. An instrument used to separate blood cells from serum or plasma is called a(n)
_____.

4. Briefly explain how a centrifuge separates solid from liquid. _____
_____
_____

5. Cabinets that maintain constant temperatures are called _____, and are used most
frequently in the _____ department of a clinical laboratory.

CERTIFICATION PREPARATION

Circle the correct answer.

1. Which term is defined as the substance or chemical being analyzed or detected in a specimen?
   a. Electrolyte
   b. Reagent
   c. Analyte
   d. Identifiers

2. Which laboratory department studies tissues?
   a. Cytology
   b. Histology
   c. Toxicology
   d. Chemistry

3. Which laboratory department does sensitivity testing?
   a. Microbiology
   b. Chemistry
   c. Urinalysis
   d. Hematology

4. Which is a CLIA-waived test?
   a. Fasting blood glucose
   b. Dipstick urinalysis
   c. Rapid strep testing
   d. All of the above

5. Which government agency is responsible for determining the CLIA complexity of all laboratory tests?
   a. CMS
   b. HHS
   c. FDA
   d. OSHA

6. Which CLIA complexity tests can a medical assistant always perform?
   a. Waived tests
   b. Moderate-complexity tests
   c. High-complexity tests
   d. All of the above

7. Which term is defined as the ability to consistently reproduce a test result?
   a. Accuracy
   b. Reliability
   c. Trend
   d. Precision

8. According to the CDC, the single most effective means of preventing infection is
   a. wearing proper PPE during patient contact.
   b. always wearing gloves when working with blood specimens.
   c. proper and frequent hand sanitation.
   d. all of the above.

9. An example of a bloodborne pathogen is
   a. HIV.
   b. influenza.
   c. HBV.
   d. a and c.

10. Which piece of laboratory equipment is defined as a cabinet that maintains a constant temperature?
   a. Microscope
   b. Centrifuge
   c. Incubator
   d. Rotor

WORKPLACE APPLICATIONS

1. Greg is helping train a student medical assistant today and he is responsible for going through the following competency: Evaluate the work environment to identify unsafe working conditions. He has set up a number of items on a benchtop and is asking the student to review each environment.

   Evaluate each statement below and determine if the work environment described would be safe or unsafe. Circle your answer for each environment.

   • Two unopened rapid strep kits enclosed in their boxes sitting on a countertop at room temperature

      SAFE   UNSAFE

   • Two pipets containing an unknown yellow liquid, laying on absorbent laboratory paper

      SAFE   UNSAFE

   • A disinfectant wipes container that is open, and two wipes look like they have been used to clean up a pinkish-red spill, and are now laying on the counter

      SAFE   UNSAFE

   • A bottle of urinalysis dipsticks that are properly closed, sitting on the counter

      SAFE   UNSAFE

   • A countertop sharps container that has a few used pipets in it

      SAFE   UNSAFE

   • A pipet and bulb sitting on the counter, with a few small pieces of broken glass nearby

      SAFE   UNSAFE

   • An unlabeled beaker with a blue liquid inside of it

      SAFE   UNSAFE

2. Greg is giving a laboratory tour to a small group of new clinic employees. Greg meets them in the waiting area of the laboratory. A few people have water bottles with them and one person is checking their phone in the waiting room until the tour starts.

   Read each scenario below and answer each question at the end of the statement by circling YES or NO.

   - There is a sign on the door leading into the laboratory that states, "No food or drink beyond this point." To comply with the sign, should people bring their water bottles into the lab?

     YES   NO

   - Once inside the lab, there is a symbol showing a cell phone with a big red X over it. To comply with the symbol, should people bring their cell phones into the lab?

     YES   NO

   - Once inside the lab, there are lab coats with safety glasses in the pockets hanging on a coat rack. Each lab coat has a label on the sleeve that reads "guest." Above the coat rack a sign reads "Lab coats and safety glasses must be worn beyond this point." To comply with the wall sign and coat label, should each person put on a lab coat and safety glasses?

     YES   NO

   - As they finish their tour of the lab, there are two boxes—one labeled "lab coats here" the other labeled "safety glasses here." To comply with the labels on the boxes, can the people take the lab coats and safety glasses out of the laboratory?

     YES   NO

3. Greg is unpacking supplies that he ordered for the laboratory. One box contains a chemical reagent and the accompanying SDS. Briefly explain the purpose of SDS in a healthcare setting.

   _____

   _____

   _____

   _____

INTERNET ACTIVITIES

1. Using online resources, research one department of the laboratory. Create a poster presentation, a PowerPoint presentation, or a written paper summarizing your research. Include the following points in your project:
   a. Name of the department
   b. General overview of the testing performed in the department
   c. Common specimens tested
   d. Common disease states tested for in the department
   e. Common CLIA-waived tests performed in the department

2. Go to the website for the CDC (www.cdc.gov) and research a bloodborne pathogen of your choice. Create a poster presentation, a PowerPoint presentation, or a written paper summarizing your research. Include the following points in your project:
   a. Description of the pathogen
   b. Testing used to identify the blood-borne pathogen
   c. CLIA-waived testing available for the blood-borne pathogen
   d. Personal protective equipment (PPE) needed during testing procedures

3. Using online resources, research the preventive maintenance routinely performed on a microscope, centrifuge, or incubator. In a one-page paper, summarize the information that you found.

4. Go to www.cdc.gov or www.fda.gov and research protocols or guidelines for laboratory waste disposal. In a one-page paper, summarize the information that you found.

Procedure 45.1   Perform a Quality Control Measure on a Glucometer and Record the Results on a Flow Sheet

Name _____ **Date** _____ **Score** _____

Task: To test and analyze the results of glucometer controls to see whether a glucometer is producing reliable test results, and to record the results on the laboratory flow sheet.

Equipment and Supplies:
- Fluid-impermeable lab coat, gloves, and eye protection
- Glucometer
- Coded test strips designed for the glucometer used
- Control solution provided by the manufacturer
- Package insert showing directions on how to run the glucometer
- Biohazard waste container
- Glucose test control flow sheet

NOTE: Not all glucometers need to include the code strip step in the procedure. This is one example of one type of system used. Please disregard any unnecessary steps.

Standard: Complete the procedure and all critical steps in _____ minutes with a minimum score of 85% within two attempts (*or as indicated by the instructor*).

Scoring: Divide the points earned by the total possible points. Failure to perform a critical step, indicated by an asterisk (*), results in grade no higher than an 84% (*or as indicated by the instructor*).

Time: Began _____ Ended _____ Total minutes: _____

Steps:	Point Value	Attempt 1	Attempt 2
1. Wash hands or use hand sanitizer. Put on lab coat, gloves, and eye protection.	15*		
2. Take a coded strip out of the bottle and note the control level and range listed on the control bottle or the strip container. Close the coded strip bottle.	10		
3. Review the directions on the glucometer package insert and calibrate the meter by inserting the precoded test strip into the monitor or by manually inserting the code number into the monitor.	10		
4. Check the expiration date on the liquid control bottle and mix well by inverting and rolling the bottle between the palms of your hands.	10*		
5. Complete the top portion of the control log sheet with the test name, control lot number, and expiration date, and the control's reference range based on whether it is a low-, normal-, or high-level control.	10*		
6. Insert the strip into the glucometer and apply a drop of the liquid control to the strip according to the directions.	10		
7. Record the result on the glucose test control flow sheet or the glucose test control QC graph (whichever method is used in the laboratory). Note whether it falls within the manufacturer's reference range. If not, the test should be repeated with a new test strip.	10*		
8. When you have finished running the controls, properly dispose of the strips as recommended by the manufacturer.	10*		

9.	Remove gloves and eyewear. Wash hands or use hand sanitizer.	**15***		
	Total Points	**100**		

GLUCOSE TEST CONTROL FLOW SHEET

Control Lot #: _____			Expiration Date: _____		
Control Range: _____			Level: Low/Normal/High		
Date	**Student/MA Initials**	**Result**	**Accept**	**Reject**	**Corrective Action**

Comments

CAAHEP Competencies	**Step(s)**
I.P.10. Perform a quality control measure	Entire procedure
II.P.3. Maintain lab test results using flow sheets	7
II.C.6.a. Analyze healthcare results as reported in: graphs	7
II.C.6.b. Analyze healthcare results as reported in: tables	7
ABHES Competencies	**Step(s)**
9. Medical Laboratory Procedures a. Practice quality control	Entire procedure
b. Perform selected CLIA-waived tests that assist with diagnosis and treatment	Entire procedure
c. Dispose of biohazardous materials	8

Procedure 45.2 Use of the Eyewash Equipment: Perform an Emergency Eye Wash

Name _____ **Date** _____ **Score** _____

Task: To minimize the risk of occupational exposure to pathogens if body fluids contact the eyes.

Equipment and Supplies:
- Gloves
- Plumbed or self-contained eye wash unit

Standard: Complete the procedure and all critical steps in _____ minutes with a minimum score of 85% within two attempts (*or as indicated by the instructor*).

Scoring: Divide the points earned by the total possible points. Failure to perform a critical step, indicated by an asterisk (*), results in grade no higher than an 84% (*or as indicated by the instructor*).

Time: Began_____ Ended_____ Total minutes: _____

Steps:	Point Value	Attempt 1	Attempt 2
1. Wash hands or use hand sanitizer.	15*		
2. Remove contact lenses or glasses. Put on gloves.	10*		
3. Following the manufacturer's directions, turn on the eye wash unit. If it is a plumbed unit, the control valve should remain on until the unit is manually shut off.	10		
4. Hold the eyelids open with the thumb and index finger to ensure adequate rinsing of the entire eye and eyelid surface.	10*		
5. Avoid aiming the water stream directly onto the eyeball.	10		
6. Flush the eyes and eyelids for a minimum of 15 minutes, rolling the eyes periodically to ensure complete removal of the foreign material.	10		
7. Properly remove gloves, dispose of them in a labeled biohazard waste container.	10*		
8. Wash hands or use hand sanitizer.	15*		
9. After completion of the eye wash, follow postexposure follow-up procedures.	10		
Total Points	100		

Comments

CAAHEP Competencies	Step(s)
XII.P.2.a. Demonstrate proper use of: eyewash equipment	Entire procedure

Procedure 45.3 Evaluate the Laboratory Environment

Name _____ Date _____ Score _____

Task: Evaluate the laboratory environment and identify unsafe working conditions. Identify compliance with safety signs, symbols, and labels.

Equipment and Supplies:
- Laboratory environment evaluation form (Work Product 45.1)
- Pen

Standard: Complete the procedure and all critical steps with a minimum score of 85% within two attempts (*or as indicated by the instructor*).

Scoring: Divide the points earned by the total possible points. Failure to perform a critical step, indicated by an asterisk (*), results in grade no higher than an 84% (*or as indicated by the instructor*).

Steps:	Point Value	Attempt 1	Attempt 2
1. Observe use of safety signs, symbols, and labels in the laboratory setting. Document your findings on the work environment evaluation form (Work Product 45.1).	25*		
2. Explain if the laboratory personnel are complying with the safety signs, symbols, and labels.	25*		
3. Observe the environment for safety risks. Document your findings.	25*		
4. Based on your observations, summarize your findings. If risks are present, create a list of issues that need to be addressed. Describe what needs to be done for each risk.	25*		
Total Points	100		

Comments

CAAHEP Competencies	Step(s)
XII.P.1.a. Comply with: safety signs	1, 2
XII.P.1.b. Comply with: symbols	1, 2
XII.P.1.c. Comply with: labels	1, 2
XII.P.5. Evaluate the work environment to identify unsafe working conditions	Entire procedure

Work Product 45.1   Work Environment Evaluation Form

Name _____ **Date** _____ **Score** _____

To be used with Procedure 45.3.

Directions: Check either in the "Yes" or "No" column for each question. Check "NA" if it is not applicable. Include any issues in the comment column. Summarize your findings for each area, using the space indicated.

Complying with Safety Signs, Symbols, and Labels	Yes	No	NA	Comments
• Refrigerator displays a biohazard symbol.				
• Refrigerator displays a sign indicating "not for storage of food or medication."				
• Biohazard waste containers display a biohazard symbol .				
• Biohazard waste containers use a red biohazard bag.				
• Chemicals and reagents labeled with original manufacturer's label and a hazard identification system label (by the National Fire Protection Association).				
• Sign on the door indicating "No food or drink beyond this point."				
• A sign in the lab indicates no cell phones are allowed.				
• A sign at the entrance of the lab indicates that lab coats and safety glasses must be worn.				
Safety of the Laboratory Environment	**Yes**	**No**	**NA**	**Comments**
• Chemicals and reagents are sealed.				
• Safety Data Sheets are available for all chemicals used in the laboratory.				
• If using a chemical that produces toxic or flammable vapors, the person works under a fume hood that exhausts air to the outside.				
• Disinfection wipes available in work area				
• A fire extinguisher is available in the laboratory.				
• Ceiling sprinkler system is present.				
• A sink with running water is available for emergencies.				
• Eye wash station is present.				
• Are electrical cords and plugs free from cracks, fraying, or other damage?				
• Are power strips overloaded?				
• Are flammable chemicals and supplies stored according to manufacturers' guidelines?				
• Are combustibles (e.g., paper, cardboard, cloth, flammable chemicals) away from heat sources?				
Observations of unsafe practices:				

Are the laboratory personnel complying with the safety signs, symbols, and labels? Explain why or why not based on your observations.

If risks are present, create a list of issues that need to be addressed. Describe what needs to be done for each risk.

Procedure 45.4 Perform Routine Maintenance on Clinical Equipment (Microscope)

Name _____ Date _____ Score _____

Task: Focus the microscope properly using a prepared slide under low power, high power, and oil immersion, then perform routine maintenance on the microscope before storing it.

Equipment and Supplies:
- Microscope
- Lens cleaner
- Lens tissue
- Slide containing specimen
- Immersion oil

Standard: Complete the procedure and all critical steps in _____ minutes with a minimum score of 85% within two attempts (*or as indicated by the instructor*).

Scoring: Divide the points earned by the total possible points. Failure to perform a critical step, indicated by an asterisk (*), results in grade no higher than an 84% (*or as indicated by the instructor*).

Time: Began_____ Ended_____ Total minutes: _____

Steps:	Point Value	Attempt 1	Attempt 2
1. Wash hands or use hand sanitizer.	5*		
2. Gather the needed materials.	3		
3. Clean the lenses with lens tissue and lens cleaner.	5*		
4. Adjust the seating to a comfortable height.	3		
5. Plug the microscope into an electrical outlet and turn on the light switch.	3		
6. Place the slide specimen on the stage and secure it.	3		
7. Turn the revolving nosepiece to engage the 4× or 10× lens.	4*		
8. Carefully raise the stage while observing with the naked eye from the side.	3		
9. Focus the specimen using the coarse adjustment knob.	5*		
10. Adjust the amount of light by closing the iris diaphragm, by bringing the condenser up or down, or by adjusting the light from the source.	3		
11. Switch to the 40× lens. Use the fine adjustment knob to focus the specimen in detail.	5*		
12. Turn the revolving nosepiece to the area between the high-power objective and oil immersion.	3		
13. Place a small drop of oil on the slide.	4*		
14. Carefully rotate the oil immersion objective into place. The objective will be immersed in the oil.	3		
15. Adjust the focus with the fine adjustment knob.	5*		
16. Increase the light by opening the iris diaphragm and raising the condenser.	3		
17. Identify the specimen.	3		
18. Return to low power but do not drag the 40× lens through the oil.	4*		

19. Remove the slide and dispose of it in a biohazard sharps container.	5*		
20. Lower the stage.	3		
21. Center the stage.	3		
22. Switch off the light and unplug the microscope.	3		
23. Clean the lenses with lens tissue and remove oil with lens cleaner.	5*		
24. Wipe the microscope with a cloth.	3		
25. Cover the microscope.	3		
26. Sanitize the work area.	3		
27. Wash hands or use hand sanitizer.	5*		
Total Points	100		

Comments

CAAHEP Competencies	Step(s)
VI.P.8. Perform routine maintenance of administrative or clinical equipment	Entire procedure

Urinalysis

CAAHEP Competencies	Assessment
I.P.10. Perform a quality control measure	Procedure 46.4
I.P.11.c. Obtain specimens and perform: CLIA-waived urinalysis	Procedure 46.1, 46.2, 46.3, 46.5, 46.7, 46.8
II.P.2. Differentiate between normal and abnormal test results	Procedure 46.4, 46.5
II.A.1. Reassure a patient of the accuracy of the test results	Procedure 46.9

ABHES Competencies	Assessment
3.c. Apply medical terminology for each specialty	Vocabulary Review – A. 1-10, B. 1-9, C. 1-10, D. 1-6
3.d. Define and use medical abbreviations when appropriate and acceptable	Abbreviations 1-26
9.a. Practice quality control	Procedure 46.4
9.b. Perform selected CLIA-waived tests that assist with diagnosis and treatment 1) Urinalysis	Procedure 46.3, 46.5, 46.7, 46.8
9.c. Dispose of biohazardous materials	Procedure 46.3, 46.5, 46.8
9.d. Collect, label, and process a specimen	Procedure 46.1, 46.2
9.e. Instruct patients in the collection of 1) clean-catch midstream urine specimens	Procedure 46.2

VOCABULARY REVIEW

Using the word pool, find the correct word to match the definition. Write the word on the line after the definition

Group A

1. Microorganisms (mostly bacteria and yeast) that live on or in the body _____
2. A procedure for evaluating the glomerular filtration rate of the kidneys _____
3. Hollow, flexible tube that can be inserted into a vessel, organ, or cavity of the body to withdraw or instill fluid, monitor information, and visualize a vessel or cavity

    _____
4. To separate a solid substance from a solution

    _____
5. A body opening or passage, especially the external opening of a structure _____
6. A cloudy appearance; not clear _____
7. The functional unit of the kidney _____
8. A test result is expressed as a number, usually with units of measure attached to numeric values _____
9. The internal environment of the body that is compatible with life; steady state that is created by all the body systems working together _____
10. Fluid and substances that are filtered out of the blood in the Bowman capsule _____

Word Pool
- homeostasis
- nephron
- filtrate
- quantitative
- creatinine clearance rates
- catheter
- turbidity
- meatus
- normal flora
- precipitate

Group B

1. An electrically charged atom or the smallest component of an element (cation has a positive charge, anion has a negative charge)

    _____
2. Insoluble material that settles to the bottom of a urine specimen and to the bottom of centrifuged urine

    _____
3. An essential amino acid found in milk, eggs, and other foods

    _____
4. A narrow, tube-shaped container marked with horizontal lines to represent units of measurement; used to precisely measure the volume of liquids _____
5. A kidney disease affecting the glomeruli of the nephron; characterized by albumin in the urine, edema, and high blood pressure _____
6. A type of hemoglobin found in the muscle _____
7. A solid substance with a regular shape that is due to the structure of molecules _____
8. Complete or whole; not broken or altered

    _____
9. The yellow pigment normally found in urine; it is described as straw, yellow, or amber, based on its concentration

    _____

Word Pool
- urochrome
- crystals
- graduated cylinder
- phenylalanine
- glomerulonephritis
- ions
- sediment
- intact
- myoglobin

Group C

1. Any enzyme that breaks down esters (a type of organic molecule) into alcohols and acids _____

2. Yellow discoloration of the skin, whites of the eyes, and mucous membranes, due to an increase of bilirubin in the blood

    _____

3. To pour a liquid gently so that it does not disturb the remaining sediment _____

4. A dilute urine concentration _____

5. The continued breakdown of bilirubin in the liver produces this substance _____

6. A blood flow deficiency to the kidney(s) _____

7. A concentrated urine _____

8. Damaging or destructive to the kidneys

    _____

9. Old red blood cells are broken down in the liver and gradually converted into this substance _____

10. The clear liquid above the sediment in a centrifuged urine specimen _____

Word Pool
- bilirubin
- urobilinogen
- jaundice
- esterase
- decanting
- supernatant
- renal ischemia
- nephrotoxic
- hypertonic
- hypotonic

Group D

1. A hormone secreted by the anterior pituitary gland; it stimulates the growth of ovum (eggs) in the ovary and induces the formation of sperm in the testis _____

2. The injection of semen into the vagina or uterus using a catheter or syringe; nonsexual _____

3. A hormone produced by the anterior pituitary gland; stimulates ovulation and the development of the corpus luteum in females and the production of testosterone in males

    _____

4. A laboratory technique that uses the specific binding between an antigen and antibody to identify and quantify a substance in a sample; the sample in this technique moves in a sideways motion, usually on an absorbent paper _____

5. Single-celled organisms that are the most primitive form of animal life; most are microscopic _____

6. The intentional manipulation of a urine sample that allows someone to falsely pass a drug screening test

    _____

Word Pool
- protozoa
- lateral flow immunoassay
- artificial insemination
- luteinizing hormone
- follicle-stimulating hormone
- adulterated

ABBREVIATIONS

Write out what each of the following abbreviations stands for.

1. POL _____

2. CMA _____

3. AAMA _____

4. CLIA _____

5. C&S _____

6. FSH _____

7. LH _____

8. PKU _____

9. UTI _____

10. UA _____

11. PPP _____

12. CCMS _____

13. CPT _____

14. PPE _____

15. Na _____

16. K _____

17. RBC _____

18. WBC _____

19. FDA _____

20. PPM(P) _____

21. CLSI _____

22. hCG _____

23. OTC _____

24. SAMHSA _____

25. NIDA _____

26. (D)HHS _____

SKILLS AND CONCEPTS

Answer the following questions. Write your answer on the line or in the space provided.

A. Introduction and Urine Formation

1. Give two reasons why urine is the second most common specimen tested in the laboratory. _____

   _____

   _____

   _____

2. Blood passes through microscopic structures in the kidneys called _____, where blood is filtered to form a(n) _____. The composition of the filtrate is adjusted in the renal tubules by two processes, _____ and _____, until it reaches the final makeup and is called _____.

3. The average person voids about how much urine in a normal day? _____

4. What is the largest component of urine? _____

5. What are normal waste products found in urine? _____

   _____

   _____

6. What are abnormal waste products found in urine? _____

   _____

   _____

   _____

B. Collecting a Urine Specimen

1. If you think that the patient does not understand directions for a urine specimen collection, what can you do to ensure that he or she understands?

   _____

   _____

   _____

   _____

2. Is it okay if patients use a jar or container from home for urine sample collection? _____

   _____

3. What type of container should be used for collection if the patient may have a UTI? _____

   _____

4. What information, at a minimum, should be written or printed on the urine specimen label?_____

_____

_____

_____

5. Why should a patient not void directly into a 24-hour urine container, but rather collect the sample and then pour it into the 24-hour container?

_____

_____

6. What additional information should a medical assistant remind patients of if they are going to collect the 24-hour urine at home?

_____

_____

_____

7. Why is a clean-catch midstream urine collection ordered when the provider suspects the patient has a UTI?

_____

_____

_____

8. Explain what a culture and sensitivity test is, and why it is done. _____

_____

_____

9. How soon after the collection of a urine sample should it be tested in the laboratory? _____

_____

10. How should a urine specimen be stored until it is tested?_____

_____

_____

_____

11. Why are evacuated urine transport tubes used when sending a urine specimen to another laboratory?

_____

_____

C. Routine Urinalysis

1. What is the minimum sample volume of urine needed for a routine urinalysis (UA)?_____

_____

2. What three aspects of the urine are being tested with a complete UA? _____

_____

_____

3. What observations of urine should be made during a UA?_____

_____

_____

4. Should urine normally be any color other than yellow?_____

_____

5. A light yellow color is referred to as _____, a dark yellow color is referred to as
_____.

6. What are possible causes of urine turbidity? _____

_____

7. Define the term *aliquot*._____

_____

8. What is another term for specific gravity? _____

9. If a person has a change in urine specific gravity, what does that tell the provider?_____

_____

_____

10. Why are urine dipstick testing results so valuable to providers? _____

_____

_____

_____

11. Can a urine dipstick test be performed on a sterile specimen?   Yes   No

Can a urine dipstick test be performed on a nonsterile specimen?   Yes   No

12. What tests are included in a urine dipstick test? _____

_____

_____

13. What is the normal pH range for urine? _____

14. What other sugars are detected with a urine strip glucose reaction? _____

_____

15. Using glucose as an example, what is a renal threshold and why is it important? _____

_____

_____

_____

_____

16. What diseases or conditions could cause a positive ketone test on a urine reagent strip? _____

_____

_____

17. Is it normal to have protein in the urine?   Yes   No

18. Define the term *intact*. _____

_____

19. Define *myoglobinuria*. _____

_____

_____

20. List the causes of bilirubinuria._____

_____

_____

21. List the causes of urobilinogen in the urine._____

_____

_____

22. What common bacteria does not break down nitrate to nitrite? _____

_____

23. What are the limitations of a urine dipstick or reagent strip test? _____

_____

_____

_____

24. The FDA has categorized a reagent strip test for urine as a CLIA _____ test.

25. Briefly explain how a Chek-Stix works for UA quality control. _____

_____

_____

_____

_____

D. Microscopic Preparation and Examination of Urine Sediment

1. A microscopic examination of urine is categorized as a CLIA _____ test. Because of this, a POL must be certified to perform CLIA _____.

2. Can a medical assistant prepare and complete the microscopy of a UA? _____

_____

_____

_____

3. What are the three main categories of microscopic findings in a UA sample? _____

_____

4. List some of the cells that can be seen in a microscopic UA preparation. _____

_____

_____

E. Additional CLIA-Waived Tests Performed on Urine

1. Describe the Clinitest. _____

_____

_____

_____

_____

2. What hormone is being detected with a urine pregnancy test? _____

_____

3. What hormone is being detected with a lateral flow ovulation test? _____

_____

4. What hormone is being detected with a lateral flow menopause test? _____

_____

5. What substances are being detected with a urine test for drugs of abuse? _____

_____

6. Describe specimen adulteration. _____

_____

_____

_____

CERTIFICATION PREPARATION
Circle the correct answer.

1. Which structure is the functional unit of the urinary system?
   a. Renal tubules
   b. Glomerulus
   c. Kidney
   d. Nephron

2. Which substance is a normal constituent of urine?
   a. Protein
   b. Urea
   c. Glucose
   d. Red blood cells

3. What type of urine specimen should be collected for culture and sensitivity testing?
   a. Random specimen
   b. 2-hour postprandial specimen
   c. Clean-catch midstream specimen
   d. 24-hour specimen

4. Which is a CLIA-waived test?
   a. Ovulation test
   b. Dipstick urinalysis
   c. Urine microscopy
   d. Both a and b

5. Sensitivity limits for drug screening tests are set by which agency?
   a. SAMHSA
   b. NIDA
   c. (D)HHS
   d. All of the above

6. What hormone is being detected in a CLIA-waived urine pregnancy test?
   a. hCG
   b. FSH
   c. LH
   d. Both b and c

7. Which term is defined as pouring a liquid gently so that it does not disturb the remaining sediment?
   a. Supernatant
   b. Turbidity
   c. Decant
   d. Precipitate

8. A positive urine dipstick nitrite test is seen in which condition?
   a. Diabetes mellitus
   b. Glomerulonephritis
   c. Urinary tract infection
   d. All of the above

9. Which medical terminology root below means bend or deflect?
   a. orth/o
   b. morph/o
   c. prot/o
   d. refract/o

10. The definition of the term *cystitis* is
    a. inflammation of the kidney.
    b. infection of the kidney.
    c. inflammation of the bladder.
    d. infection of the bladder.

WORKPLACE APPLICATIONS

1. Becca is looking at the results of a patient dipstick urinalysis. Using the table of results below, indicate if the result is normal or abnormal by checking the appropriate box. *Use Table 46.4 as a reference for UA test normal values.*

Analyte	Patient Result	Normal	Abnormal
Specific gravity	1.020		
pH	6.0		
Protein (mg/dL)	NEG		
Glucose (mg/dL)	250 mg/dL		
Ketone (mg/dL)	40 mg/dL		
Bilirubin (mg/dL)	NEG		
Blood (mg/dL)	NEG		
Nitrite (mg/dL)	NEG		
Urobilinogen (Ehrlich units)	0.5 Ehrlich units		
White blood cells	NEG		

2. Julie is giving Ethel instructions about how to collect a random urine sample. Ethel is elderly and a little hard of hearing, but Julie is patient and goes through the written instructions with her. Julie then asks Ethel to repeat back some key information so that she is sure Ethel understands the directions. She asks Ethel if she has any questions and Ethel replies "Yes, I do. How do I know this urine test is accurate? I will collect the sample here, and then it goes to the lab. How do I know the results are correct? How do I know they are testing my urine sample?"

   How would you assure Ethel that the testing done in the laboratory is correct? _____

   _____

   _____

   _____

   _____

   _____

   _____

   _____

   _____

INTERNET ACTIVITIES

1. Using online resources, find the list of CLIA-approved provider-performed microscopy procedures (PPMP). (HINT: the www.fda.gov or www.cms.gov sites are a great place to start.) What tests in the urinalysis department are CLIA-PPMP tests? Write a one-page paper summarizing your research. Include the following points in your paper:
   a. Name and give a brief description of the tests
   b. List the CPT codes for each test

2. Using online resources, research one drug of abuse. Create a poster presentation, a PowerPoint presentation, or a written paper summarizing your research. Include the following points in your project:
   a. Description of the drug and its effects on the body
   b. Tests available that are used to identify the drug or its metabolites
   c. CLIA-waived testing available for the detection of the drug
   d. How long does the drug remain detectable in the body after use?

3. Using online resources, write a short paper that describes a lateral flow immunoassay procedure. Summarize your research and include the following points in your project.
   a. What substance does the test detect?
   b. What is the antigen and antibody in the test?
   c. What is the CLIA category for the test?
   d. Briefly describe the principle of the test.

Procedure 46.1 Instruct a Patient in the Collection of a 24-Hour Urine Specimen

Name _____ Date _____ Score _____

Task: Instruct a patient how to collect a urine specimen. Collect a 24-hour urine sample to test for creatinine clearance.

Equipment and Supplies:
- Patient's health record
- 2-4 L urine collection container
- Plastic cup or specimen collection pan for collecting urine (which is then poured into the collection container)
- Printed patient instructions
- Laboratory requisition
- Fluid-impermeable lab coat, protective eyewear, and gloves

Standard: Complete the procedure and all critical steps in _____ minutes with a minimum score of 85% within two attempts (*or as indicated by the instructor*).

Scoring: Divide the points earned by the total possible points. Failure to perform a critical step, indicated by an asterisk (*), results in grade no higher than an 84% (*or as indicated by the instructor*).

Time: Began_____ Ended_____ Total minutes: _____

Steps:	Point Value	Attempt 1	Attempt 2
1. Greet the patient. Identify yourself. Verify the patient's identity with full name, ask the patient to spell the first and last name, and give their date of birth. Explain the procedure to be performed in a manner that is understood by the patient. Answer any questions the patient may have on the procedure.	10*		
2. Label the container with the patient's name and the current date; identify the specimen as a 24-hour urine specimen; and include your initials. Check for preservative if needed.	5		
3. Explain the following instructions to adult patients or to the guardians of pediatric patients. **Patient Instructions: Obtaining a 24-Hour Urine Specimen** a. Empty your bladder into the toilet in the morning without saving any of the specimen. Record the time you first emptied your bladder on the label. b. For the next 24 hours, each time you empty your bladder, all the urine should be collected into the plastic cup or collection pan that is placed on the toilet. Then pour all the collected urine directly into the large specimen container. c. Put the lid back on the container after each urination and rinse out the plastic cup or collection pan and store the container in the refrigerator or at room temperature, as directed, throughout the 24 hours of the study. d. If at any time you forget to collect your specimen or if some urine is accidentally spilled, the test must be started over again with a new container and a newly recorded start time.	10		

	e. Collect the final urine specimen at the same time you started the collection process on the previous day. This last collected specimen is placed in the large container. Collection ends with the voided morning specimen on the second day, which completes the 24-hour period. f. As soon as possible after completing collection, return the specimen container to the provider's office or the designated laboratory.			
4.	Give the patient the specimen container and supplies with written instructions to confirm understanding.	**10**		
5.	Document details of the patient education session in the patient's record.	**10**		
Processing a 24-Hour Urine Specimen				
6.	Ask the patient whether he or she collected all voided urine throughout the 24-hour period or whether any problems occurred during the collection process.	**10**		
7.	Complete the laboratory request form. Make sure that all the information is filled out on the container label.	**10**		
8.	Wash hands or use hand sanitizer. Put on a fluid-impermeable lab coat, protective eyewear, and gloves before preparing the specimen for transport.	**10***		
9.	Store the specimen in the refrigerator until it is picked up by the laboratory.	**5**		
10.	Remove gloves and discard appropriately. Remove protective eyewear and lab coat. Wash hands or use hand sanitizer.	**10***		
11.	Document that the specimen was sent to the laboratory, including the type of test ordered, the date and time, the type of specimen, and your initials.	**10***		
	Total Points	**100**		

Documentation

Comments

CAAHEP Competencies	Step(s)
I.P.11.c. Obtain specimens and perform: CLIA-waived urinalysis	Entire procedure
ABHES Competencies	**Step(s)**
9.d. Collect, label, and process a specimen	Entire procedure

Procedure 46.2   Collect a Clean-Catch Midstream Urine Specimen

Name _____   Date _____   Score _____

Task: To instruct a patient on how to collect a contaminant-free urine sample for culture or analysis using the clean-catch midstream specimen (CCMS) technique.

Equipment and Supplies:
- Patient's record
- Form with written patient instructions
- Sterile container with lid and label
- Specimen bag
- Antiseptic towelettes
- Fluid-impermeable lab coat, protective eyewear, and gloves

Standard: Complete the procedure and all critical steps in _____ minutes with a minimum score of 85% within two attempts (*or as indicated by the instructor*).

Scoring: Divide the points earned by the total possible points. Failure to perform a critical step, indicated by an asterisk (*), results in grade no higher than an 84% (*or as indicated by the instructor*).

Time: Began_____ Ended_____ Total minutes: _____

Steps:	Point Value	Attempt 1	Attempt 2
1. Greet the patient. Identify yourself. Verify the patient's identity with full name, ask the patient to spell the first and last name, and give their date of birth. Explain the procedure to be performed in a manner that is understood by the patient. Answer any questions the patient may have on the procedure.	15*		
2. Label the sterile sealed container (not the lid) and give the patient the towelette supplies and written patient instructions form, if needed.	10		
3. Explain the following instructions to adult patients or to the guardians of pediatric patients, making sure you show sensitivity to privacy issues. **Patient Instructions:** *Obtaining a Clean-Catch Midstream Specimen (Female Patient)* 1. Wash your hands and open the towelette packages for easy access. 2. Remove the lid from the specimen container, being careful not to touch the inside of the lid or the inside of the container. Place the lid, facing up, on a paper towel. 3. Lower your underclothing and sit on the toilet. 4. Expose the urinary meatus by spreading apart the labia with one hand 5. Cleanse each side of the urinary meatus with a front-to-back motion, from the pubis toward the anus. Use a separate antiseptic wipe to cleanse each side of the meatus. 6. Cleanse directly across the meatus, front to back, using a third antiseptic wipe 7. Hold the labia apart throughout this procedure. 8. Void a small amount of urine into the toilet. 9. Move the specimen container into position and void the next portion of urine into it. Fill the container halfway. Remember, this is a sterile container. Do not put your fingers on the inside of the container.	25*		

10. Remove the cup and void the last amount of urine into the toilet. (This means that the first part and the last part of the urinary flow have been excluded from the specimen. Only the middle portion of the flow is included.) 11. Place the lid on the container, taking care not to touch the interior surface of the lid. Wipe in your usual manner, redress. Wash your hands and return the sterile specimen to the place designated by the medical facility. **Patient Instructions:** *Obtaining a Clean-Catch Midstream Specimen (Male Patient)* 1. Wash your hands and expose the penis. 2. Retract the foreskin of the penis (if not circumcised). 3. Cleanse the area around the glans penis (tip of the penis) and the urethral opening by washing each side of the glans with a separate antiseptic wipe. 4. Cleanse directly across the urethral opening using a third antiseptic wipe. 5. Void a small amount of urine into the toilet or urinal. 6. Collect the next portion of the urine in the sterile container, filling the container halfway without touching the inside of the container with the hands or the penis. 7. Void the last amount of urine into the toilet or urinal. 8. Place the lid on the container, taking care not to touch the interior surface of the lid. Wipe in your usual manner, redress. Wash your hands. 9. Return the sterile specimen to the place designated by the medical facility.			
Processing a Clean-Catch Urine Specimen			
4. Document the date, time, and collection type.	**10**		
5. Wash hands or use hand sanitizer. Put on the fluid-impermeable lab coat, protective eyewear, and gloves.	**15***		
6. Process the specimen according to the provider's orders. Perform urinalysis in the office or prepare the specimen for transport to the laboratory. If it is to be sent to an outside laboratory, complete the following steps: • Make sure the label is properly completed with the patient's information and the date, time, test ordered, and your initials. • Place the specimen in a biohazard specimen bag. • Complete a laboratory requisition and place it in the outside pocket of the specimen bag. • Keep the specimen refrigerated until pickup.	**15***		
7. Remove gloves, protective eyewear, and lab coat. Dispose of gloves appropriately. Wash hands or use hand sanitizer. Document that the specimen was sent.	**10***		
Total Points	**100**		

Documentation

Comments

CAAHEP Competencies	Step(s)
I.P.11.c. Obtain specimens and perform: CLIA-waived urinalysis	Entire procedure
ABHES Competencies	**Step(s)**
9.d. Collect, label, and process a specimen	Entire procedure
9.e. Instruct patients in the collection of 1) clean-catch midstream urine specimens	3

Procedure 46.3   Assess Urine for Color and Turbidity: Physical Test

Name _____ Date _____ Score _____

Task: To assess and record the color and clarity of a urine specimen.

Equipment and Supplies:
- Patient's record
- Urine specimen
- Centrifuge tube
- Fluid-impermeable lab coat, protective eyewear, and gloves
- White piece of paper with thin black lines drawn on it
- Biohazard waste container

Standard: Complete the procedure and all critical steps in _____ minutes with a minimum score of 85% within two attempts (*or as indicated by the instructor*).

Scoring: Divide the points earned by the total possible points. Failure to perform a critical step, indicated by an asterisk (*), results in grade no higher than an 84% (*or as indicated by the instructor*).

Time: Began_____ Ended_____ Total minutes: _____

Steps:	Point Value	Attempt 1	Attempt 2
1. Wash hands or use hand sanitizer. Put on the fluid-impermeable lab coat, protective eyewear, and gloves.	10*		
2. Mix the urine by gently swirling the specimen.	10		
3. Label a centrifuge tube if a complete urinalysis is to be done.	10		
4. Pour the specimen into a standard-sized centrifuge tube.	10		
5. Assess and record the color.	15*		
6. Assess the turbidity by placing a piece of white paper with fine, dark black print behind the specimen and see if you can see the print: • *Clear*—Able to read through the specimen; no cloudiness • *Slightly turbid*—Can barely see fine lines on white paper through the specimen • *Turbid*—Cannot see fine lines through the specimen at all	15*		
7. Clean the work area and dispose of procedure supplies in the biohazard waste container.	10*		
8. Dispose of gloves. Remove lab coat and protective eyewear. Wash hands or use hand sanitizer.	10*		
9. Document the results in the patient's record.	10		
Total Points	100		

Documentation

Comments

CAAHEP Competencies	Step(s)
I.P.11.c. Obtain specimens and perform: CLIA-waived urinalysis	Entire procedure
ABHES Competencies	**Step(s)**
9 b. Perform selected CLIA-waived tests that assist with diagnosis and treatment 1) Urinalysis	Entire procedure
9.c. Dispose of biohazardous materials	7

Procedure 46.4 Perform Quality Control Measures: Differentiate Between Normal and Abnormal Test Results While Determining the Reliability of Chemical Reagent Strips

Name _____ Date _____ Score _____

Task: To reconstitute a control sample and test the reliability of the urinalysis chemical testing strip.

Equipment and Supplies:
- Chek-Stix Control Strips with reference ranges for urinalysis
- Distilled water
- Capped tube with milliliter markings
- Test tube rack
- Forceps
- Timer
- Urine chemical strips for urine testing
- Color chart for interpreting the chemical strip results
- Fluid-impermeable lab coat, protective eyewear, and gloves
- Biohazard waste container
- Control reference sheet and control flow sheet

Standard: Complete the procedure and all critical steps in _____ minutes with a minimum score of 85% within two attempts (*or as indicated by the instructor*).

Scoring: Divide the points earned by the total possible points. Failure to perform a critical step, indicated by an asterisk (*), results in grade no higher than an 84% (*or as indicated by the instructor*).

Time: Began_____ Ended_____ Total minutes: _____

Steps:	Point Value	Attempt 1	Attempt 2
1. Assemble the equipment and supplies. Record the lot number and the expiration date of the Chek-Stix on the control log sheet.	5		
2. Wash hands or use hand sanitizer. Put on the fluid-impermeable lab coat, protective eyewear, and gloves.	10*		
3. Place a conical tube in a test tube rack and remove the cap.	5		
4. Pour 15 mL of distilled water into the tube.	5		
5. Using forceps, remove one strip from the Chek-Stix bottle. Inspect the strips for mottling or discoloration.	5		
6. Place the strip into the water and tightly cap the tube.	5		
7. Invert the tube for 2 minutes.	5		
8. Allow the tube to sit in the rack for 30 minutes.	5		
9. Invert the tube one time and remove the strip with forceps.	5		
10. Discard the strip in the biohazard waste container. Once reconstituted, the control solution is stable for 8 hours at room temperature.	5*		
11. Perform quality control of the chemical reagent strip by dipping it into the control solution.	5		
12. Read and record the results.	10*		

13. Compare the results with the control reference ranges provided on the Chek-Stix package insert.	**10**		
14. Discard the chemical reagent strip and the control solution in the biohazard waste container.	**5***		
15. Clean up the work area and appropriately dispose of supplies and gloves in a biohazard waste container.	**5**		
16. Remove protective eyewear and lab coat. Wash hands or use hand sanitizer.	**10***		
Total Points	**100**		

Documentation

Comments

CAAHEP Competencies	**Step(s)**
I.P.10. Perform a quality control measure	Entire procedure
II.P.2. Differentiate between normal and abnormal test results	13
ABHES Competencies	**Step(s)**
9.a. Practice quality control	Entire procedure

Procedure 46.5   Test Urine with Chemical Reagent Strips

Name _____ Date _____ Score _____

Task: To perform chemical testing on a urine sample.

Equipment and Supplies:
- Patient's record
- Urine specimen
- Reagent strips
- Timer
- Fluid-impermeable lab coat, protective eyewear, and gloves
- Biohazard waste container

Standard: Complete the procedure and all critical steps in _____ minutes with a minimum score of 85% within two attempts (*or as indicated by the instructor*).

Scoring: Divide the points earned by the total possible points. Failure to perform a critical step, indicated by an asterisk (*), results in grade no higher than an 84% (*or as indicated by the instructor*).

Time: Began_____ Ended_____ Total minutes: _____

Steps:	Point Value	Attempt 1	Attempt 2
1. Wash hands or use hand sanitizer. Put on the fluid-impermeable lab coat, protective eyewear, and gloves.	10*		
2. Check the time of collection, the container, and the mode of preservation.	5		
3. If the specimen has been refrigerated, allow it to warm to room temperature.	5		
4. Check the reagent strip container for the expiration date.	5*		
5. Remove the reagent strip from the container. Hold it in your hand or place it on a clean, dry paper towel. Recap the container tightly.	5		
6. Compare nonreactive test pads with the negative color blocks on the color chart on the container.	5		
7. Thoroughly mix the specimen by gently swirling the container.	5		
8. Following the manufacturer's directions, note the time, dip the strip into the urine, and then remove it.	5		
9. Quickly remove the excess urine from the strip by pulling the back of the strip across the lip of the specimen container and then blotting the edge of the strip on a clean, dry paper towel or the side of the specimen container.	10*		
10. Hold the strip horizontally. At the required time, compare the strip with the appropriate color chart on the reagent container. *Do not touch the strip to the bottle.*	10*		
11. Alternately, the strip can be placed on a paper towel.	5		
12. Read and record the first two results 30 seconds after dipping the strip. Compare the two reagent pads closest to your hand with the bottom two rows of the color chart. Continue reading and recording each row of possible results with its appropriate reagent pad at its designated time.	10*		

13. Clean the work area. If a paper towel was used, dispose of it and the reagent strip in an appropriate biohazard waste container.	**5**			
14. Remove gloves and dispose of appropriately. Remove protective eyewear and lab coat. Wash hands or use hand sanitizer.	**10***			
15. Document the results in the patient's record.	**5**			
Total Points	**100**			

Documentation

Comments

CAAHEP Competencies	**Step(s)**
I.P.11.c. Obtain specimens and perform: CLIA-waived urinalysis	Entire procedure
II.P.2. Differentiate between normal and abnormal test results	12
ABHES Competencies	**Step(s)**
9 b. Perform selected CLIA-waived tests that assist with diagnosis and treatment 1) Urinalysis	Entire procedure
9.c. Dispose of biohazardous materials	13

Procedure 46.6 Prepare a Urine Specimen for Microscopic Examination

Name _____ Date _____ Score _____

Task: To prepare a urine specimen for the provider's microscopic examination to determine the presence of normal and abnormal elements.

Equipment and Supplies:
- Patient's record
- Urine specimen
- Centrifuge tube
- Centrifuge
- Disposable pipet
- Sedi-Stain
- Microscope slide and coverslip
- Microscope
- Permanent marker
- Fluid-impermeable lab coat, protective eyewear or face shield, and gloves
- Biohazard waste container

Standard: Complete the procedure and all critical steps in _____ minutes with a minimum score of 85% within two attempts (*or as indicated by the instructor*).

Scoring: Divide the points earned by the total possible points. Failure to perform a critical step, indicated by an asterisk (*), results in grade no higher than an 84% (*or as indicated by the instructor*).

Time: Began_____ Ended_____ Total minutes: _____

Steps:	Point Value	Attempt 1	Attempt 2
1. Wash hands or use hand sanitizer. Put on the fluid-impermeable lab coat, protective eyewear, and gloves.	10*		
2. Gently mix the urine specimen by swirling the covered specimen container.	5		
3. Pour 12 mL of urine into a labeled centrifuge tube and cap the tube.	5		
4. Place the tube in the centrifuge.	10		
5. Place another tube containing 12 mL of urine or water in the opposite cup.	10*		
6. Secure the lid and centrifuge for 5 minutes or for the time specified for your instrument.	5		
7. Remove the tube from the centrifuge after the instrument has come to a full stop.	5		
8. Pour off the clear supernatant from the top of the specimen by inverting the centrifuge tube over the sink drain while allowing the running water from the faucet to flush the urine down the drain.	10		
9. Turn the tube upright when the supernatant has been decanted, allowing a small amount to return to the sediment on the bottom of the tube without losing sediment down the drain	10		
10. Thoroughly mix the sediment with a drop of Sedi-Stain by grasping the tube near the top and rapidly flicking it with the fingers of the other hand until all sediment is thoroughly resuspended.	10		

11. Transfer 1 drop of sediment to a clean, labeled slide using a clean, disposable transfer pipet. Transfer pipet should be disposed of in a sharps container.	**5**		
12. Place a clean coverslip over the drop and place the slide on the microscope stage. Remove face protection.	**5**		
13. Focus under low power and reduce the light.	**10**		
Total Points	**100**		

Comments

Procedure 46.7   Test Urine for Glucose Using the Clinitest Method

Name _____   **Date** _____   **Score** _____

Task: To perform confirmatory testing for glucose and other simple sugars in the urine using the Clinitest procedure for reducing substances.

Equipment and Supplies:
- Patient's record
- Urine specimen
- Clinitest tablet, glass test tube,* and transfer pipet
- Distilled water
- Test tube rack
- Appropriately sized plastic or metal forceps
- Color chart
- Timer
- Fluid-impermeable lab coat, protective eyewear, and gloves
- Biohazard waste container

*__Note:__ When performing a Clinitest, always use glass test tubes.

Standard: Complete the procedure and all critical steps in _____ minutes with a minimum score of 85% within two attempts (*or as indicated by the instructor*).

Scoring: Divide the points earned by the total possible points. Failure to perform a critical step, indicated by an asterisk (*), results in grade no higher than an 84% (*or as indicated by the instructor*).

Time: Began_____ Ended_____ Total minutes: _____

Steps:	Point Value	Attempt 1	Attempt 2
1. Wash hands or use hand sanitizer. Put on fluid-impermeable lab coat, protective eyewear, and gloves.	10*		
2. Holding a Clinitest transfer pipet vertically, add 10 drops of distilled water and then 5 drops of urine to a Clinitest tube (glass).	5		
3. Place the prepared tube in the test tube rack.	5		
4. Remove a Clinitest tablet from the bottle by shaking a tablet into the bottle cap. **NOTE:** *Do not handle Clinitest tablets with your hands or gloved hands. Always use forceps to transfer the tablet to the test tube.*	10		
5. Using a metal or plastic forceps, pick up the Clinitest tablet from the bottle cap and drop the tablet into the prepared test tube. Recap the container. **NOTE:** *Use caution when performing a Clinitest as the reaction boils. Always use glass test tubes; plastic tubes may melt!*	10*		
6. With the test tube in the rack, observe the entire reaction to detect the rapid pass-through phenomenon, which indicates that the glucose level in the urine is very high.	10		
7. When boiling stops, time exactly 15 seconds and then gently shake the tube to mix the entire contents.	5		

8. Immediately compare the color of the specimen with the five-drop color chart and record your findings.	10*			
9. Record the results.	5			
10. Clean up the work area, dispose of supplies in appropriate waste containers. Remove and discard gloves in a biohazard waste container.	10			
11. Remove fluid-impermeable lab coat and protective eyewear.	5			
12. Wash hands or use hand sanitizer.	10*			
13. Document the results in the patient's record.	5			
Total Points	100			

Documentation

Comments

CAAHEP Competencies	Step(s)
I.P.11.c. Obtain specimens and perform: CLIA-waived urinalysis	Entire procedure
ABHES Competencies	**Step(s)**
9 b. Perform selected CLIA-waived tests that assist with diagnosis and treatment 1) Urinalysis	Entire procedure

Procedure 46.8 Perform a CLIA-Waived Urinalysis: Perform a Pregnancy Test

Name _____ Date _____ Score _____

Task: To perform a pregnancy test on urine using the QuickVue pregnancy test method.

Equipment and Supplies:
- Patient's record
- Urine specimen
- QuickVue test kit
- Fluid-impermeable lab coat, protective eyewear, and gloves
- Biohazard sharps container
- Biohazard waste container

Standard: Complete the procedure and all critical steps in _____ minutes with a minimum score of 85% within two attempts (*or as indicated by the instructor*).

Scoring: Divide the points earned by the total possible points. Failure to perform a critical step, indicated by an asterisk (*), results in grade no higher than an 84% (*or as indicated by the instructor*).

Time: Began_____ Ended_____ Total minutes: _____

Steps:	Point Value	Attempt 1	Attempt 2
1. Wash hands or use hand sanitizer. Put on fluid-impermeable lab coat, protective eyewear, and gloves.	10*		
2. Prepare the testing equipment. Check the expiration date of the kit before proceeding.	10*		
3. Obtain the proper patient specimen (preferably a first morning specimen).	5		
4. Remove the test cassette from the foil pouch.	5		
5. Add 3 drops of urine using the transfer pipet (dropper) that accompanies the kit.	10		
6. Dispose of the pipet in a biohazard sharps container.	10*		
7. Wait 3 minutes and read the test results.	5		
8. Interpret the results as: • *Negative*: A blue control line is next to the letter C; no line is seen next to the letter T. • *Positive*: A blue control line is next to the letter C; a pink line is next to the letter T. • *Invalid*: If a blue line does not appear in the C area, the test is invalid and the specimen must be retested using another kit.	15*		
9. Discard the test cassette in the biohazard waste container, clean up testing area, then remove and discard gloves in a biohazard waste container. Remove lab coat and protective eyewear.	10*		
10. Wash hands or use hand sanitizer.	10*		
11. Document the results in the patient's record as either positive or negative for pregnancy.	10		
Total Points	**100**		

Documentation

Comments

CAAHEP Competencies	Step(s)
I.P.11.c. Obtain specimens and perform: CLIA-waived urinalysis	Entire procedure
ABHES Competencies	**Step(s)**
9 b. Perform selected CLIA-waived tests that assist with diagnosis and treatment 1) Urinalysis	Entire procedure
9.c. Dispose of biohazardous materials	9

Procedure 46.9   Reassure a Patient of the Accuracy of the Test Results

Name _____ Date _____ Score _____

Task: Show empathy and communicate respectfully and professionally with patient. Reassure patient of the accuracy of the test result.

Scenario: Elyse is seeing Jean Burke, NP at WMFM Clinic today. Elyse has been feeling tired and slightly nauseous for the last few weeks. She and her husband use birth control, but her menstrual periods are very irregular. She did a home pregnancy test 2 weeks ago, and it was negative. But she is still feeling poorly. Jean orders a urine pregnancy test. The lab runs a CLIA-waived urine pregnancy test and it is positive. Elyse doesn't believe the result. You need to reassure her the accuracy of the test result.

Directions: Role-play the scenario with a peer. The peer is the patient and you are the medical assistant. Your responses should include a discussion of what was different between the first and second test.

Standard: Complete the role-play in _____ minutes with a minimum score of 100% within two attempts (*or as indicated by the instructor*).

Scoring: Divide the points earned by the total possible points. Met competency: 100% (10 points). Not met competency: 0% (0 points).

Time: Began_____ Ended_____ Total minutes: _____

Affective Behavior	*Directions:* Check behaviors observed during the role-play.					
Respect	**Negative, Unprofessional Behaviors**	**Attempt**		**Positive, Professional Behaviors**	**Attempt**	
		1	**2**		**1**	**2**
	Rude, unkind, disrespectful, impolite			Courteous, polite		
	Unwelcoming, brief, abrupt			Welcoming, took time with the patient		
	Unconcerned with person's dignity			Maintained person's dignity		
	Poor eye contact with patient			Proper eye contact with patient		
	Negative nonverbal behaviors			Positive nonverbal behaviors		
	Other:			Other:		

Empathy	Didn't listen to the patient, interrupted patient; unsupportive, uninterested, or uncaring			Listened to the patient; supportive and caring		
	Did not acknowledge or respond appropriately to the patient's emotional responses; cold, aloof, insensitive, indifferent, or unfeeling			Acknowledged and responded appropriately to the patient's emotional responses; showed sensitivity		
	Failed to reassure patient; did not respond to the patient's concerns			Reassured patient by repeating and responding to the patient's concerns		
	Used language that is hard to understand (e.g., slang, generational terms, medical terminology, too scientific)			Used language that the patient can understand		
	Failed to address the patient's questions; or answers to patient's questions are inappropriate			Answered the patient's questions appropriately		
	Other:			Other:		

Grading		Point Value	Attempt 1	Attempt 2
Does not meet Expectation	• Response was disrespectful and/or lacks empathy. • Student demonstrated more than 2 negative, unprofessional behaviors during the interaction.	0		
Needs Improvement	• Response was disrespectful and/or lacks empathy. • Student demonstrated 1 or 2 negative, unprofessional behaviors during the interaction.	0		
Meets Expectation	• Response was respectful and empathetic; no negative, unprofessional behaviors observed. • More practice is needed for behavior to appear natural and for student to appear comfortable and at ease.	10		
Occasionally Exceeds Expectation	• Response was respectful and empathetic; no negative, unprofessional behaviors observed. • At times student appeared comfortable and at ease; but more practice is needed for behavior to become natural and consistent with a professional medical assistant.	10		
Always Exceeds Expectation	• Response was respectful and empathetic; no negative, unprofessional behaviors observed. • Student's behaviors appeared natural and comfortable. Behaviors are consistent with a professional medical assistant.	10		

Comments

CAAHEP Competencies	Step(s)
II.A.1. Reassure a patient of the accuracy of the test results	Entire role-play

Blood Collection

CAAHEP Competencies	Assessment
I.P.2.b. Perform: venipuncture	Procedure 47.1-47.3
I.P.2.c. Perform: capillary puncture	Procedure 47.4
I.A.2. Incorporate critical thinking skills when performing patient care	Procedure 47.1, 47.2, 47.3
I.A.3. Show awareness of a patient's concerns related to the procedure being performed	Procedure 47.5
III.P.2. Select appropriate barrier/personal protective equipment (PPE)	Procedure 47.1, 47.2, 47.3, 47.4
III.P.10.a. Demonstrate proper disposal of biohazardous material: sharps	Procedure 47.1, 47.2, 47.3, 47.4
III.P.10.b. Demonstrate proper disposal of biohazardous material: regulated wastes	Procedure 47.1, 47.2, 47.3, 47.4
XII.P.2.c. Demonstrate proper use of: sharps disposal containers	Procedure 47.1, 47.2, 47.3, 47.4
ABHES Competencies	Assessment
3. Medical Terminology c. Apply medical terminology for each specialty	Vocabulary Review – A. 1-10, B. 1-10, C. 1-10, D. 1-6
d. Define and use medical abbreviations when appropriate and acceptable	Abbreviations – 1-20
9. Medical Laboratory Procedures c. Dispose of biohazardous materials	Procedure 47.1, 47.2, 47.3, 47.4
d. Collect, label, and process a specimen 1) Perform venipuncture	Procedure 47.1-47.3
d. Collect, label, and process a specimen 2) Perform capillary puncture	Procedure 47.4

VOCABULARY REVIEW

Using the word pool, find the correct word to match the definition. Write the word on the line after the definition.

Amardeep Kaur

Group A

1. The inner bend in front of the elbow ___antecubital___
2. To create a vacuum in a tube, flask, or reaction vessel ___evacuated___
3. Substances that inhibit the growth of microorganisms on living tissue (e.g., alcohol) and are used to cleanse the skin, wounds, and so on ___antiseptic___
4. Infections that are acquired in a healthcare setting ___nosocomial___
5. The most common method of obtaining a blood specimen ___venipuncture___
6. A condition in which the concentration of blood cells is increased in proportion to the volume of plasma ___hemoconcentration___
7. Fainting; a brief lapse of consciousness ___syncope___
8. A device with a slender barrel and needle used to withdraw blood from a vein or artery ___syringe___
9. A device for temporarily constricting blood flow ___tourniquet___
10. The process of acquiring blood from a patient ___phlebotomy___

Word Pool
- phlebotomy
- venipuncture
- syncope
- tourniquet
- evacuated
- syringe
- antecubital
- nosocomial
- hemoconcentration
- antiseptic

Group B

1. The liquid portion of a clotted blood specimen that no longer contains active clotting agents ___Serum___
2. The medical abbreviation for the Latin term *statum*, meaning immediately; at this moment ___STAT___
3. A chemically neutral gel added to evacuated blood tubes that creates a physical barrier between red blood cells and plasma or serum when centrifuged ___Thixotropic gel___
4. The chemical breakdown of carbohydrates (glucose) by enzymes, with the release of energy ___Glycolysis___
5. A substance (i.e., medication or chemical) that prevents clotting of blood ___anticoagulant___
6. One end of the needle shaft is cut at an angle and forms the ___Bevel___
7. A microbiologic procedure where a blood sample is placed in a nutrient medium and held at body temperature to encourage the growth of the infecting bacteria in the laboratory ___Blood culture___
8. The liquid portion of a whole blood sample that has not clotted due to an anticoagulant; liquid portion of blood that contains clotting factors ___Plasma___
9. Substances added to a venipuncture tube to enhance and speed up blood clotting ___clot activators___
10. This type of tube top has the advantage of not splattering blood when the cap is removed from the tube ___hemogard___

Word Pool
- blood culture
- Hemogard
- anticoagulants
- clot activators
- thixotropic gel
- serum
- plasma
- glycolysis
- STAT
- bevel

Group C

1. Obstruction or interruption of normal lymph flow
   lymphostasis
2. Space between the cells _interstitial_
3. The breakdown of red blood cells with the release of hemoglobin
   hemolysis
4. Small blood vessels that connect small arterioles to small venules
   capillaries
5. The bore, or hollow space, inside the needle is called the
   lumen
6. An abnormal buildup of blood in an organ or tissue
   of the body, caused by a leak or cut in a blood vessel
   hematoma
7. Very small, round hemorrhage in the skin or mucous membrane
   petechiae
8. Blood fills small, narrow tubes without the help of suction
   capillary action
9. Lumen size is important and is referred to as the
   gauge
10. The device used to perform a dermal puncture or capillary
    puncture _lancet_

Word Pool
- lumen
- gauge
- hemolysis
- hematoma
- lymphostasis
- petechiae
- interstitial
- capillaries
- lancet
- capillary action

Group D

1. The production of a partial vacuum by the removal of air to force
   fluid into a vacant space _suction_
2. The sole of the foot _plantar_
3. A legal term that refers to the process used to maintain and
   document the history of a specimen _chain of custody_
4. A force acting on an object because of gravity; for example, a
   centrifuge spinning _G-force_
5. To draw off or remove by suction _aspirating_
6. The palm of the hand _palmar_

Word Pool
- plantar
- palmar
- aspirating
- g-force
- chain of custody
- suction

ABBREVIATIONS
Write out what each of the following abbreviations stands for.

1. PPE _Personal Protective Equipment_
2. ASCP _American Society for Clinical Pathology_
3. HBV _Hepatitis B Virus_
4. HCV _Hepatitis C virus_
5. HIV _Human Immunodeficiency Virus_
6. OSHA _Occupational Safety and Health Administration_

7. IAPS _International Academy Of Pelvic Surgery._

8. NCA _Neurocirculatory Asthenia._

9. NPA _Nasopharyngeal Airway_

10. POL _Physician Office Laboratory._

11. CLSI _Clinical Clinical and Laboratory Standards Institute._

12. CBC _Complete Blood Count._

13. EDTA _Ethylene Diamine Tetraacetic Acid._

14. SST _Serum - Seperating Tubes._

15. PST _Paroxymal Supraventricular Tachycardia._

16. PT _Prothrombin Time._

17. APTT _Activated Partial Thromboplastin Clotting Time._

18. FDA _Food And Drug Administration._

19. POCT _Point-of-care testing_

20. PKU _Phenylketonuria._

SKILLS AND CONCEPTS
Answer the following questions. Write your answer on the line or in the space provided.

A. Introduction and Venipuncture Equipment

1. What is the most common specimen tested in the laboratory? _Blood_

2. The bloodborne viruses identified as possible blood-borne pathogen risks are _Hep B_, _Hep C_, and _HIV_.

3. To become a certified phlebotomist, what three activities must be successfully completed?_____
   • Complete course work, preform specific number of witnessed venipuncture and pass a national medical assistant exam.

4. In your own words, define *venipuncture*. _____
   when we use needle to draw blood from a vein.

5. *Syncope* is another term for _Fainting_.

6. What PPE should be worn while performing a venipuncture?_____
   Gloves, lab coat, facemask, eyewear

7. Why should you use a tourniquet during a venipuncture? _It helps locate a vein as well as preventing the venous blood flow out of site._

8. If a tourniquet is left on the arm for more than 1 minute, it increases the possibility of _hemoconcentration_

9. Define *hemoconcentration* in your own words. _When concentration of blood cells increased in proportion number to volume of plasma._

10. Why is 70% alcohol allowed to air dry on the venipuncture site? _The solution is most effective when given time to air dry._

11. Define *blood culture*. _A laboratory test to check for bacteria or other microorganisms in a blood sample._

12. Explain what additional skin preparation is needed for a blood culture venipuncture. _Chlorhexidine needed if someone allergy to iodine._

13. Match the evacuated tube stopper color with the anticoagulant.

Stopper Color		Anticoagulant
_d_	light blue	a. EDTA
_e_	green	b. none
_a_	lavender	c. potassium oxalate and sodium fluoride
_b_	red	d. sodium citrate
_c_	gray	e. heparin

14. Define a *clot activator*. _It promotes blood clotting with glass or silica particles._

15. What is thixotropic gel? _It forms a barrier between blood cells and serum or plasma._

16. What is the difference between plasma and serum? _Plasma contains fibrogen. Serum does not have fibrogen._

17. Why is it important to avoid a short draw when performing a venipuncture? _It can create false results as well as making a test take longer or unable to be performed at all._

B. Order of the Draw

1. Why is there a specific order of the draw? _There is a specific order of draw because it can prevent the carryover of additives from one tube to the next._

2. What is the proper order of the draw? ① Blood culture ② light blue ③ red or royal blue ④ green ⑤ⁿᵈ ⑥ lavender ⑦ Gray.

3. Can you make up a saying to remember the order of the draw? _Sarah's Light Red Glasses Look Gray._

C. Needles and Supplies Used in Phlebotomy

1. Where are phlebotomy needles discarded after a venipuncture? _Biohazard sharps container._

2. Needles have two parts, the ___hub___ that attaches to the vacuum tube needle holder or ___shaft___. The second part of the needle is the ___bevel___, which is the part that penetrates the skin during a venipuncture. The sharp, angled end of the shaft is called the ___syringe___.

3. If a needle has a high gauge number, is the lumen larger or smaller? _Smaller_

4. If the lumen of a needle is too small, it may cause ___hemolysis___, which is a breakdown of RBCs.

5. Describe the features of a needle that make it a Multisample needle. _It permit several samples to be taken with a single puncture, smooth edges help reduce pain._

6. Why are syringes used for venipuncture? _The strong vacuum in a stoppered tube might collapse the vein._

7. Why should blood that has been drawn with a syringe be transferred to evacuated tubes as soon as possible?

Because it will clot quicker

8. Why are butterfly assemblies used for venipuncture? They are used for small veins on the backs of hands in elderly and pa pediatric patients.

D. Needle Safety

1. Is it okay to recap a used phlebotomy needle? Explain your answer. No, It is not Okay to recap because if we try to recap it it may lead to needlestick injury.

2. Read through the box entitled "Protect Against Needlestick Injuries." List four safety measures that should be taken to protect against needlestick injuries.

- select device with safety features.
- Never recap a contaiminated needle except with safety device
- Always dispose used needles.
- Report add plan for safe handling before begin procedure.

3. Describe the four points of postexposure needlestick management.
- Washed area for 10 minutes with soap.
- Report to supervisior.
- Test for HBV, MCV, and HIV.
- Intermin test performed.

E. Routine Venipuncture

1. Why is patient identification such an important step in a routine venipuncture?

To make sure you have the right patient.

2. What four questions should you ask your patient before you start a venipuncture procedure?

① do you have any questions or concerns?
② do you have any speyfic preferenc?
③ were you given any speyfic instruction prior to procedur?
④ have you any complicatons in past from venipuncture?

3. What two antecubital veins should be drawn for venipuncture? _____

   Medial and Cephalic vein.

   _____

   _____

4. Which vein in the antecubital area should not be used for phlebotomy? Explain why. _____

   Basilic veins because they are too close to artery
   and nerves.

5. Why should a tourniquet be tied so that the ends of the tourniquet are pointing upward on the arm?

   So that they do not contaminate the cleansed
   area during veripuncture.

6. When you palpate for a vein, you should use your _____ _index_ _____ finger.

7. What is the maximum time you should leave a tourniquet tied on an arm? _____

   One minute.

8. Once you have cleaned the venipuncture site with alcohol, can you retouch the area? Explain your answer.

   No, we cannot retouch because if we retouch it
   contaminate again.

9. When you reapply the tourniquet, do not have the patient _____ _Clench_ _____ or
   _____ _pump_ _____ their fist. If their fist is relaxed the venipuncture will feel less painful. Visually _____ _relocate_ _____ the vein. _____ _Anchor_ _____ the vein by gently stretching the
   skin downward below the collection site with the _____ _thumb_ _____ of the nondominant hand.
   Smoothly and quickly insert the needle into the vein at about a(n) _15_ -degree angle, depending on
   the depth and position of the vein. The _____ _bevel_ _____ should be facing up.

10. After drawing each tube, they should be gently inverted. Explain why inversion is necessary. _____

    If we cannot do inversion, blood may clot.

11. When the _____ _last_ _____ tube has started to fill, carefully release the
    _____ _tourniquet_ _____. Gently tug on the short portion of the tourniquet and it should just fall open.
    Remove the _____ _tubes_ _____. Cover the venipuncture area with _____ _gauge_ _____,
    then smoothly and quickly remove the _____ _needle_ _____. Once the needle is out of the arm,
    apply _the pressure_ to the site. At the same time, activate the _____ to
    cover the needle. Dispose the entire venipuncture assembly into a(n) _____ _biohazard_ _____ con-
    tainer. Ask the _____ _patient_ _____ to apply direct pressure to the _____ _site_ _____. Do
    not _____ _bend_ _____ the arm.

12. Venipuncture tube labels should contain what patient information? _____

    Patient name, date & time, Phlebotomist Duties.

    _____

13. Explain why you should observe the venipuncture site before putting on a bandage. Describe the process.

    To see there is no more bleeding on that area.

14. What special precautions should be taken with patients who are on anticoagulants? _____

    We need extra gauge and extra pressure.

F. Problems with Venipuncture

1. List the four most common problems that occur with a venipuncture. _____

    hematoma, petechiae, hemoconcentration, hemolysis.

2. Why is blind probing NOT recommended as a phlebotomy technique? Because it can cause nerve damage or nerve injury.

3. List five reasons for specimen rejection that can occur in the laboratory. • Misspelled specimen
    • Insufficient quantity.
    • Defective tube
    • Incorrect tube for the test.
    • hemolysis

G. Capillary Puncture

1. Capillaries connect small ___blood vessels___ and small ___arterioles___.

2. List five reasons why a capillary puncture might be preferable to a venipuncture. • Patient injury less often.
    • If a patient have thin veins.
    • Capillary sampling doesnot risk complications from hematoma.
    • It require less precision
    • Minimises less iatrogenic anemia.

3. Analyte levels are usually the same in capillary and venous blood, with a few exceptions. Which two analytes have higher values in capillary blood than venous blood?

   hemoglobin and glucose

4. The device used to perform a dermal puncture is called a(n) _lancet_.

5. _OSHA_ has directed that lancets must have _retractable_ blades. Safety lancets only puncture once and cannot be _reused_. Lancets are available as _needle_ lancets and _blade_ lancets. Lancets should always be discarded in a(n) _sharp container_ immediately after use.

6. What two containers are used to collect many capillary samples?

   Microcollection tubes and microtainers.

7. Capillary punctures are also done for point-of-care testing. Give an example of two POC tests that use capillary samples.

   Hb A1c, glucose.

8. Infant heelstick samples are used for newborn screening tests known as a(n) _neonatal screening._

H. Routine Capillary Puncture

1. In adults and children (older than 1 year), capillary puncture sites include the _ring_ or _middle_ fingers. Capillary punctures are made on the _palmar_ surface of the finger.

2. Another term for the swirls of a fingerprint is a(n) _whorls_.

3. For infants, a heelstick is done on the _medial_ or _lateral_ areas of the _plantar_ surface of the heel.

4. For capillary punctures, it is important to _massage_ the finger if it is cold to avoid poor blood flow.

5. Why should you wipe away the first drop of blood when performing a capillary puncture?

   You should wipe away first drop to remove tissue fluid.

6. Capillary tubes and microtainer tubes are often put in labeled _tube_ or labeled _zipper-lock_ biohazard bags for transport.

I. Pediatric Phlebotomy

1. Explain why pediatric phlebotomy can be difficult. Pediatric phlebotomy can be difficult because child don't trust anyone and they scared of needles.

2. How can parents or guardians be of help during pediatric phlebotomy? By telling their child previous experience with this procedure. They also emotionally support their child during phlebotomy.

3. When the medical assistant is required to perform pediatric phlebotomy, he/she should remember to:
   - Wear a colorful jacket lab coat.
   - Be truthful about discomfort the child will feel.
   - Provide tokens and praise for laboratory.

J. Handling Specimens After Collection

1. Sample processing may include separation of plasma or serum from red blood cells.

2. A solid clot forms in a tube without anticoagulant in 15 to 60 minutes.

3. Describe how to properly remove serum from a clot tube. Removing the serum from a clot tube requires centrifugation. For thixotropic gel to form a barrier between clot and serum, certain requirements must be met. Tube must be centrifuged at specific g force, time and temperature.

4. Define the term *aspirating* in your own words. Aspirating means remove by suction.

5. The College of American Pathologists (CAP) recommends that whole blood for automated blood counts be refrigerated and tested within ___72___ hours.

6. Define *chain of custody*. _____

   It is a legal document which order when we do test for paternity test.

CERTIFICATION PREPARATION

Circle the correct answer.

1. Which vessel type is most frequently used for phlebotomy?
   a. Artery
   b. Vein *(circled)*
   c. Capillary
   d. Both a and c

2. Fainting, or a brief lapse of consciousness, is the definition of what term?
   a. Syncope *(circled)*
   b. Evacuated
   c. Antecubital
   d. None of the above

3. What type of blood collection procedure should be used for a health screening blood glucose test?
   a. Arterial puncture
   b. Capillary puncture
   c. Venipuncture
   d. All of the above *(circled)*

4. Which colored-stopper tube contains EDTA as an anticoagulant?
   a. Green
   b. Light blue
   c. Gray
   d. Lavender *(circled)*

5. Which blood sample contains clotting factors?
   a. Serum
   b. Plasma *(circled)*
   c. Blood collected in a red-topped tube
   d. All of the above

6. The tourniquet should be removed during a routine venipuncture when
   a. blood starts to flow in the first tube.
   b. the last tube has completed filling.
   c. blood starts to flow in the last tube of the draw. *(circled)*
   d. none of the above.

7. Which vein in the antecubital region should *not* be used for routine venipuncture?
   a. Medial
   b. Cephalic
   c. Basilic *(circled)*
   d. None of the above

8. A substance that prevents clotting of blood is the definition of which term?
   a. Clot activator
   b. Antiseptic
   c. Anticoagulant *(circled)*
   d. Thixotropic gel

9. Which substance listed below is an anticoagulant?
   a. FDA
   b. CBC
   c. ASCP
   d. EDTA *(circled)*

10. The device used to perform a capillary puncture is called a
    a. tourniquet.
    b. lancet. *(circled)*
    c. butterfly assembly.
    d. hematocrit tube.

WORKPLACE APPLICATIONS

1. Maggie is quizzing a medical assistant student about the order of the draw. For each of the tube combinations below, put them in the correct order of the draw.

   a. light blue, green, red _____ light Blue, Red, Green. _____

   b. gray, lavender, green _____ Green, Lavender, Grey _____

   c. gold, gray, green _____ Gold, green, gray, _____

   d. red, light blue, lavender _____ light Blue, Red, lavender. _____

2. Maggie goes to the waiting room to bring back Stella Brown for a capillary puncture. Stella is 9 years old and needs to have a capillary puncture today for red blood cell count. Maggie notices that Stella is anxious and also notices Stella is wearing a necklace with an ice skate charm on it. How can Maggie show awareness of a patient's concerns related to the procedure being performed?

   _____ Maggie De First step Maggie needs to do is to _____ make her calm and tell the truth that she _____ just feel little pinch. _____

3. Maggie will be performing a heelstick on a 3-week-old infant girl. The infant needs to have her bilirubin level checked and the mother is very nervous about her baby having the procedure done. The mother really wants to stay with her baby but doesn't like the sight of blood. How can Maggie help the mother with her concerns and still perform the heelstick that needs to be done?

   _____ By asking their previous experience about this _____ procedure. _____

INTERNET ACTIVITIES

1. Go to the OSHA website, https://www.osha.gov/SLTC/bloodbornepathogens/index.html and read through the OSHA Bloodborne Pathogens Standard fact sheet. Summarize the standard fact sheet in a one-page paper.

2. Using online resources, research the possible complications of a venipuncture. Create a poster presentation, a PowerPoint presentation, or an infographic summarizing your research. Include the following points in your project:
   a. Describe at least five complications of a venipuncture.
   b. How are the complications caused during the venipuncture?
   c. How can complications be avoided?
   d. What equipment should or should not be used to avoid complications?

3. Make a poster or infographic about the order of the draw for phlebotomy. Be ready to share your poster and catch-phrase with the class. Include the following information:
   a. Create a unique saying or catch-phrase to help remember the order of the draw.
   b. Explain how you came up with your saying and why it is memorable to you.
   c. Why is the order of the draw needed for a multiple tube venipuncture?

Procedure 47.1 Perform a Venipuncture: Collect a Venous Blood Sample Using the Vacuum Tube Method

Name _____ Date _____ Score _____

Task: To collect a venous blood specimen by the vacuum tube technique.

Equipment and Supplies:
- Patient's health record
- Provider's order and/or lab requisition
- Vacuum tube needle, needle holder, and proper tubes for requested tests
- 70% isopropyl alcohol wipes
- Gauze
- Tourniquet
- Hypoallergenic self-stick wrap, tape, or bandage
- Permanent marking pen and/or printed labels
- Fluid-impermeable lab coat, protective eyewear, and gloves
- Biohazard sharps container
- Biohazard waste container

Standard: Complete the procedure and all critical steps in _____ minutes with a minimum score of 85% within two attempts (*or as indicated by the instructor*).

Scoring: Divide the points earned by the total possible points. Failure to perform a critical step, indicated by an asterisk (*), results in grade no higher than an 84% (*or as indicated by the instructor*).

Time: Began_____ Ended_____ Total minutes: _____

Steps:	Point Value	Attempt 1	Attempt 2
1. Check the provider's order and/or requisition form to determine the tests ordered. Gather the appropriate tubes and supplies. Put on a fluid-impermeable lab coat.	4		
2. Greet the patient. Identify yourself. Verify the patient's identity with full name, ask the patient to spell the first and last name, and give their date of birth. Explain the procedure to be performed in a manner that is understood by the patient. Answer any questions the patient may have on the procedure. Obtain permission for the capillary puncture.	4*		
3. Wash hands or use hand sanitizer, then put on gloves and protective eyewear.	4*		
4. Ask the patient if he/she has a preference which arm is used for the venipuncture. Have the patient sit with his/her arm well supported in a slightly downward position.	4		
5. Apply the tourniquet around the patient's arm 3-4 inches above the elbow on the patient's preferred arm. The tourniquet should never be tied so tightly that it restricts blood flow in the artery. Tourniquets should remain in place no longer than 60 seconds.	4		
6. Select the venipuncture site by palpating the antecubital space. Use your index finger to trace the path of the vein and to judge its depth. Look at both arms and use your *critical thinking skills* to find the vein that will give you the greatest chance of success for the venipuncture. (*Refer to the Checklist for Affective Behaviors.*)	4*		

7.	Remove the tourniquet and cleanse the site with a 70% alcohol wipe.	4		
8.	Assemble your equipment and supplies on the nondominant side of the patient's arm. The choice of needle size depends on your inspection of the patient's veins. Attach the needle firmly to the vacuum tube holder. Keep the cover on the needle.	4		
9.	Reapply the tourniquet when the alcohol is dry.	4		
10.	Hold the vacuum tube assembly in your dominant hand. Your thumb should be on top and your fingers underneath. Remove the needle sheath.	4		
11.	Grasp the patient's arm with the nondominant hand and anchor the vein with your thumb.	4		
12.	With the bevel up and the needle aligned parallel to the vein, insert the needle at a 15- to 20-degree angle through the skin and into the vein with a quick but smooth motion.	4*		
13.	Hold the assembly in place with the dominant hand, steady through the venipuncture.	4		
14.	Place two fingers on the flanges of the needle holder and use the thumb to push the tube onto the double-pointed needle. Make sure you do not change the needle's position in the vein.	4*		
15.	Allow the tube to fill to its maximum capacity. Remove the tube by placing the fingers at the end of the tube and pushing on the needle holder with the index finger. Do not to move the needle when removing the tube. Immediately after removing the tube from the needle holder, gently invert the tube to mix the additives and the blood.	4*		
16.	Insert the second tube into the needle holder, following the instructions in the previous steps. Continue filling tubes until they are all filled. Gently invert each tube after removing it from the needle holder.	4		
17.	As the last tube begins filling, release the tourniquet. The tourniquet must be released before the needle is removed from the arm.	4		
18.	Remove the last tube from the holder. Place gauze over the puncture site and quickly remove the needle, engaging the safety device.	4*		
19.	Dispose of the entire needle/holder assembly into the sharps container.	4*		
20.	Apply pressure to the gauze or instruct the patient to do so. The patient may elevate the arm but should not bend the elbow.	4		
21.	While the patient is applying pressure to the site, label the tubes with the patient's name, date, time, and your initials, or affix the preprinted tube labels and print your initials and time on the label.	4		
22.	Check the venipuncture site. Make sure bleeding has stopped. Apply a hypoallergenic self-stick wrap, gauze and tape, or bandage.	4		
23.	Disinfect the work area. Dispose of blood-contaminated materials in a biohazard waste container. Remove your protective eyewear and gloves.	4*		
24.	Wash hands or use hand sanitizer.	4*		
25.	Complete the laboratory requisition form and route the specimen to the proper place. Record the procedure in the patient's record.	4		
	Total Points	**100**		

Checklist for Affective Behaviors

Affective Behavior	*Directions:* Check behaviors observed during the role-play.					
Critical Thinking	**Negative, Unprofessional Behaviors**	**Attempt**		**Positive, Professional Behaviors**	**Attempt**	
		1	**2**		**1**	**2**
	Coached or told of an issue or problem			Independently identified the problem or issue		
	Failed to consider alternatives; failed to ask questions that demonstrate understanding of principles/concepts			Willing to consider other alternatives; asked appropriate questions that showed understanding of principles/concepts		
	Failed to make an educated, logical judgment/decision; actions or lack of actions demonstrated unsafe practices			Made an educated, logical judgment/decision and actions reflected principles of safe practice		
	Other:			Other:		

Grading for Affective Behaviors		Point Value	Attempt 1	Attempt 2
Does not meet Expectation	• Response fails to show critical thinking. • Student demonstrated more than 2 negative, unprofessional behaviors during the interaction.	0		
Needs Improvement	• Response fails to show critical thinking. • Student demonstrated 1 or 2 negative, unprofessional behaviors during the interaction.	0		
Meets Expectation	• Response demonstrates critical thinking; no negative, unprofessional behaviors observed. • More practice is needed for behavior to appear natural and for student to appear comfortable and at ease.	4		
Occasionally Exceeds Expectation	• Response demonstrates critical thinking; no negative, unprofessional behaviors observed. • At times student appeared comfortable and at ease; but more practice is needed for behavior to become natural and consistent with a professional medical assistant.	4		
Always Exceeds Expectation	• Response demonstrates critical thinking; no negative, unprofessional behaviors observed. • Student's behaviors appeared natural and comfortable. Behaviors are consistent with a professional medical assistant.	4		

Documentation

Comments

CAAHEP Competencies	Step(s)
I.P.2.b. Perform: venipuncture	Entire procedure
I.A.2. Incorporate critical thinking skills when performing patient care	6
III.P.2. Select appropriate barrier/personal protective equipment (PPE)	3
III.P.10.a. Demonstrate proper disposal of biohazardous material: sharps	19
III.P.10.b. Demonstrate proper disposal of biohazardous material: regulated wastes	23
XII.P.2.c. Demonstrate proper use of: sharps disposal containers	19
ABHES Competencies	**Step(s)**
9.c. Dispose of biohazardous materials	19, 23
9.d. Collect, label, and process a specimen 1) Perform venipuncture	Entire procedure

Procedure 47.2 Perform a Venipuncture: Collect a Venous Blood Sample Using the Syringe Method

Name _____ **Date** _____ **Score** _____

Task: To collect a venous blood specimen using the syringe technique.

Equipment and Supplies:
- Patient's health record
- Provider's order and/or lab requisition
- Syringe with 21- or 22-gauge safety needle
- Vacuum tubes appropriate for tests ordered
- 70% isopropyl alcohol wipes
- Gauze
- Tourniquet
- Safety transfer device to transfer blood from syringe to vacuum tubes
- Hypoallergenic self-stick wrap, tape, or bandage
- Permanent marking pen or printed labels
- Fluid-impermeable lab coat, protective eyewear, and gloves
- Biohazard sharps container
- Biohazard waste container

Standard: Complete the procedure and all critical steps in _____ minutes with a minimum score of 85% within two attempts (*or as indicated by the instructor*).

Scoring: Divide the points earned by the total possible points. Failure to perform a critical step, indicated by an asterisk (*), results in grade no higher than an 84% (*or as indicated by the instructor*).

Time: Began_____ Ended_____ Total minutes: _____

Steps:	Point Value	Attempt 1	Attempt 2
1. Check the provider's order and/or requisition form to determine the tests ordered. Gather the appropriate tubes and supplies. Put on a fluid-impermeable lab coat.	5		
2. Greet the patient. Identify yourself. Verify the patient's identity with full name, ask the patient to spell the first and last name, and give their date of birth. Explain the procedure to be performed in a manner that is understood by the patient. Answer any questions the patient may have on the procedure. Obtain permission for the venipuncture.	5*		
3. Wash hands or use hand sanitizer. Put on gloves and protective eyewear.	5*		
4. Ask the patient if he/she has a preference which arm is used for the venipuncture. Have the patient sit with the arm well supported in a slightly downward position.	3		
5. Apply the tourniquet around the patient's arm 3-4 inches above the elbow on the patient's preferred arm. The tourniquet should never be tied so tightly that it restricts blood flow in the artery. Tourniquets should remain in place no longer than 60 seconds.	5		

6. Select the venipuncture site by palpating the antecubital space. Use your index finger to trace the path of the vein and to judge its depth. Look at both arms and use your *critical thinking skills* to find the vein that will give you the greatest chance of success for the venipuncture. *(Refer to the Checklist for Affective Behaviors.)*	5*		
7. Remove the tourniquet and cleanse the site with a 70% alcohol wipe.	3		
8. Assemble the equipment and supplies on the nondominant side of the patient's arm. Use your *critical thinking skills* to choose the proper syringe barrel size and needle size. This depends on the amount of blood required for the ordered tests and your inspection of the patient's veins.	5*		
9. Attach the needle firmly to the syringe. Pull and depress the plunger several times to loosen it in the barrel while keeping the cover on the needle. The plunger must be pushed in completely after you have loosened in the barrel.	5*		
10. Reapply the tourniquet when the alcohol is dry.	3		
11. Hold the syringe in your dominant hand. Your thumb should be on top and your fingers underneath, the same as in the vacuum tube method. Remove the needle sheath.	3		
12. Grasp the patient's arm with the nondominant hand and anchor the vein by stretching the skin downward below the collection site with the thumb of the nondominant hand.	3		
13. With the bevel up and the needle aligned parallel to the vein, insert the needle at a 15- to 20-degree angle through the skin and into the vein with a quick but smooth motion. Observe for a *flash* of blood in the hub of the syringe.	5		
14. Slowly pull back the plunger of the syringe with the nondominant hand. Do not allow more than 1 mL of head space between the blood and the top of the plunger. Make sure you do not move the needle after entering the vein. Fill the barrel to the needed volume.	5		
15. Release the tourniquet when the proper volume is reached. The tourniquet must be released before the needle is removed from the arm.	5*		
16. Place sterile gauze over the puncture site at the time of needle withdrawal. Then, immediately activate the needle safety device using the syringe hand and apply pressure to the site with the nondominant hand.	5*		
17. Instruct the patient to apply direct pressure on the puncture site with gauze. The patient may elevate the arm but should not bend the elbow.	3		
18. Remove the syringe safety needle and transfer the blood immediately to the required tube or tubes using a safety transfer device. Do not push on the syringe plunger during transfer.	5*		
19. Discard the entire unit in the sharps container when transfer is complete. Gently invert the tubes after the addition of blood.	5*		
20. Label the tubes with the patient's full name, date, time, and your initials or affix the preprinted tube labels and print your initials and time on the label.	3		
21. Check the venipuncture site. Make sure bleeding has stopped. Apply a hypoallergenic self-stick wrap, gauze, or bandage.	3		
22. Disinfect the work area. Dispose of blood-contaminated materials (e.g., gauze and gloves) in the biohazard waste container. Remove your eyewear and gloves.	3		

23. Wash hands or use hand sanitizer.	5*		
24. Complete the laboratory requisition form and route the specimen to the proper place. Record the procedure in the patient's record. Thank your patient and walk him/her to the exit.	3		
Total Points	100		

Checklist for Affective Behaviors

Affective Behavior	Directions: Check behaviors observed during the role-play.					
Critical Thinking	**Negative, Unprofessional Behaviors**	**Attempt**		**Positive, Professional Behaviors**	**Attempt**	
		1	2		1	2
	Coached or told of an issue or problem			Independently identified the problem or issue		
	Failed to consider alternatives; failed to ask questions that demonstrate understanding of principles/ concepts			Willing to consider other alternatives; asked appropriate questions that showed understanding of principles/ concepts		
	Failed to make an educated, logical judgment/decision; actions or lack of actions demonstrated unsafe practices			Made an educated, logical judgment/decision and actions reflected principles of safe practice		
	Other:			Other:		

Grading for Affective Behaviors		Point Value	Attempt 1	Attempt 2
Does not meet Expectation	• Response fails to show critical thinking. • Student demonstrated more than 2 negative, unprofessional behaviors during the interaction.	0		
Needs Improvement	• Response fails to show critical thinking. • Student demonstrated 1 or 2 negative, unprofessional behaviors during the interaction.	0		
Meets Expectation	• Response demonstrates critical thinking; no negative, unprofessional behaviors observed. • More practice is needed for behavior to appear natural and for student to appear comfortable and at ease.	5		
Occasionally Exceeds Expectation	• Response demonstrates critical thinking; no negative, unprofessional behaviors observed. • At times student appeared comfortable and at ease; but more practice is needed for behavior to become natural and consistent with a professional medical assistant.	5		
Always Exceeds Expectation	• Response demonstrates critical thinking; no negative, unprofessional behaviors observed. • Student's behaviors appeared natural and comfortable. Behaviors are consistent with a professional medical assistant.	5		

Documentation

Comments

CAAHEP Competencies	Step(s)
I.P.2.b. Perform: venipuncture	Entire procedure
I.A.2. Incorporate critical thinking skills when performing patient care	6
III.P.2. Select appropriate barrier/personal protective equipment (PPE)	1, 3
III.P.10.a. Demonstrate proper disposal of biohazardous material: sharps	19
III.P.10.b. Demonstrate proper disposal of biohazardous material: regulated wastes	22
XII.P.2.c. Demonstrate proper use of: sharps disposal containers	19
ABHES Competencies	**Step(s)**
9.c. Dispose of biohazardous materials	19, 22
9.d. Collect, label, and process a specimen 1) Perform venipuncture	Entire procedure

Procedure 47.3   Perform Venipuncture: Obtain a Venous Sample with a Safety Winged Butterfly Needle Assembly

Name _____ Date _____ Score _____

Task: To obtain a venous sample accurately from a hand or arm vein using a butterfly needle and syringe.

Equipment and Supplies:
- Patient's health record
- Provider's order and/or lab requisition
- Safety winged (butterfly) needle set
- Syringe of appropriate volume for testing
- Vacuum tubes appropriate for tests ordered
- 70% isopropyl alcohol wipes
- Gauze
- Tourniquet
- Hypoallergenic self-stick wrap, tape, or bandage
- Permanent marking pen or printed labels
- Fluid-impermeable lab coat, protective eyewear, and gloves
- Biohazard waste container
- Biohazard sharps container

Standard: Complete the procedure and all critical steps in _____ minutes with a minimum score of 85% within two attempts (*or as indicated by the instructor*).

Scoring: Divide the points earned by the total possible points. Failure to perform a critical step, indicated by an asterisk (*), results in grade no higher than an 84% (*or as indicated by the instructor*).

Time: Began_____ Ended_____ Total minutes: _____

Steps:	Point Value	Attempt 1	Attempt 2
1. Check the provider's order and/or requisition form to determine the tests ordered. Gather the appropriate tubes and supplies. Put on a fluid-impermeable lab coat.	4		
2. Greet the patient. Identify yourself. Verify the patient's identity with full name, ask the patient to spell the first and last name, and give their date of birth. Explain the procedure to be performed in a manner that is understood by the patient. Answer any questions the patient may have on the procedure. Obtain permission for the venipuncture.	4*		
3. Wash hands or use hand sanitizer. Put on gloves and protective eyewear.	4*		
4. If drawing from the **antecubital region**: ask the patient if they have a preference which arm is used for the venipuncture. Have the patient sit with their arm well supported in a slightly downward position.	4		
4a. If drawing from the **back of the hand**: have the patient place the venipuncture hand over their other, fisted hand with the fingers lower than the wrist.			

5.	If drawing from the **antecubital region**: apply the tourniquet around the patient's arm 3-4 inches above the elbow on the patient's preferred arm. The tourniquet should never be tied so tightly that it restricts blood flow in the artery. Tourniquets should remain in place no longer than 60 seconds.	4		
5a.	If drawing from the **back of the hand**: apply the tourniquet above the wrist just proximal to the wrist bone. Do not apply the tourniquet so tightly that blood flow in the arteries is impeded.			
6.	If drawing from the **antecubital region**: select the venipuncture site by palpating the antecubital space. Use your index finger to trace the path of the vein and to judge its depth. Look at both arms and use your *critical thinking skills* to find the vein that will give you the greatest chance of success for the venipuncture. *(Refer to the Checklist for Affective Behaviors.)*	4		
6a.	If drawing from the **back of the hand**: select a vein on the back of the hand that is prominent, stable, and straight as possible.			
7.	Remove the tourniquet and cleanse the site with a 70% alcohol wipe.	4		
8.	Assemble your equipment and supplies on the nondominant side of the patient's arm. Remove the butterfly device from the package and stretch the tubing slightly. Take care not to activate the needle-retracting safety device accidentally.	4		
9.	Attach the butterfly device firmly to the **syringe**. If using a syringe, make sure to loosen the plunger a few times after the butterfly and syringe are attached. *Note:* The Butterfly assembly can be attached to a needle holder OR a syringe. Make sure the connection is firmly in place.	4		
9a.	If using a **needle assembly**, lay the first tube in the vacuum tube holder and place the unit carefully where it will not roll away.			
10.	Reapply the tourniquet when the alcohol is dry.	4		
11.	Hold the butterfly wings pinched in between your dominant hand thumb and index finger or hold the base of the needle. Remove the needle sheath.	4		
12.	If drawing the **antecubital region**: grasp the patient's arm with the nondominant hand and anchor the vein by stretching the skin downward below the collection site with the thumb of the nondominant hand.	4		
12a.	If drawing from the **back of the hand**: using your thumb, pull the patient's skin taut over the knuckles and anchor the vein.			
13.	With the bevel up and the needle aligned parallel to the vein, insert the needle at a 10- to 15-degree angle through the skin and into the vein with a quick but smooth motion.	4		
14.	If drawing with a **needle holder assembly**: push the blood collecting tube into the end of the holder with your nondominant hand.	4		
14a.	If drawing with a **syringe**: make sure the vacuum you create is slow and steady and that no more than 1 mL of head space exists between the blood and the plunger. Slowly pull back the plunger of the syringe with the nondominant hand. Fill the barrel of the syringe to the needed volume			
15.	Release the tourniquet when the blood appears in the tubing or a *flash* of blood is seen in the hub of the syringe.	4		
16.	Always keep the tube and the holder in a downward position so that the tube fills from the bottom up.	4		

17. Place a gauze over the puncture site and gently remove the needle, engaging the safety device. Dispose of the entire unit in the sharps container.	4			
18. Instruct the patient to apply direct pressure on the puncture site with gauze. The patient may elevate the arm but should not bend the elbow.	4			
19. If drawing with a **syringe**: remove the syringe safety needle and transfer the blood immediately to the required tube or tubes using a safety transfer device. Do not push on the syringe plunger during transfer.	4			
20. Discard the entire unit in the sharps container when transfer is complete. Gently invert the tubes after the addition of blood.	4			
21. Label the tubes with the patient's full name, date, time, and your initials, or affix the preprinted tube labels and print your initials and time on the label.	4			
22. Check the venipuncture site. Make sure bleeding has stopped. Apply a hypoallergenic self-stick wrap, gauze, or bandage.	4			
23. Disinfect the work area. Dispose of blood-contaminated materials (e.g., gauze and gloves) in the biohazard waste container. Remove your eyewear and gloves.	4*			
24. Wash hands or use hand sanitizer.	4*			
25. Complete the laboratory requisition form and route the specimen to the proper place. Record the procedure in the patient's record. Thank your patient and walk them to the exit.	4			
Total Points	100			

Checklist for Affective Behaviors

Affective Behavior	**Directions:** Check behaviors observed during the role-play.					
	Negative, Unprofessional Behaviors	**Attempt**		**Positive, Professional Behaviors**	**Attempt**	
Critical Thinking		**1**	**2**		**1**	**2**
	Coached or told of an issue or problem			Independently identified the problem or issue		
	Failed to consider alternatives; failed to ask questions that demonstrate understanding of principles/concepts			Willing to consider other alternatives; asked appropriate questions that showed understanding of principles/concepts		
	Failed to make an educated, logical judgment/decision; actions or lack of actions demonstrated unsafe practices			Made an educated, logical judgment/decision and actions reflected principles of safe practice		
	Other:			Other:		

Grading for Affective Behaviors		Point Value	Attempt 1	Attempt 2
Does not meet Expectation	• Response fails to show critical thinking. • Student demonstrated more than 2 negative, unprofessional behaviors during the interaction.	0		
Needs Improvement	• Response fails to show critical thinking. • Student demonstrated 1 or 2 negative, unprofessional behaviors during the interaction.	0		
Meets Expectation	• Response demonstrates critical thinking; no negative, unprofessional behaviors observed. • More practice is needed for behavior to appear natural and for student to appear comfortable and at ease.	4		
Occasionally Exceeds Expectation	• Response demonstrates critical thinking; no negative, unprofessional behaviors observed. • At times student appeared comfortable and at ease; but more practice is needed for behavior to become natural and consistent with a professional medical assistant.	4		
Always Exceeds Expectation	• Response demonstrates critical thinking; no negative, unprofessional behaviors observed. • Student's behaviors appeared natural and comfortable. Behaviors are consistent with a professional medical assistant.	4		

Documentation

Comments

CAAHEP Competencies	**Step(s)**
I.P.2.b. Perform: venipuncture	Entire procedure
I.A.2. Incorporate critical thinking skills when performing patient care	6
III.P.2. Select appropriate barrier/personal protective equipment (PPE)	1, 3
III.P.10.a. Demonstrate proper disposal of biohazardous material: sharps	17, 20
III.P.10.b. Demonstrate proper disposal of biohazardous material: regulated wastes	23
XII.P.2.c. Demonstrate proper use of: sharps disposal containers	17, 20
ABHES Competencies	**Step(s)**
9.c. Dispose of biohazardous materials	17, 20, 23
9.d. Collect, label, and process a specimen 1) Perform venipuncture	Entire procedure

Procedure 47.4 Perform a Capillary Puncture: Obtain a Blood Sample by Capillary Puncture

Name _____ Date _____ Score _____

Task: To collect a blood specimen suitable for testing using the capillary puncture technique.

Equipment and Supplies:
- Patient's health record
- Provider's order and/or lab requisition
- Sterile, disposable safety lancet
- 70% alcohol wipes
- Gauze
- Hypoallergenic self-stick wrap, tape, or bandage
- Fluid-impermeable lab coat, protective eyewear, and gloves
- Appropriate collection containers (e.g., capillary tubes, Microtainer tubes)
- Permanent marking pen or printed labels
- Biohazard sharps container
- Biohazard waste container

Standard: Complete the procedure and all critical steps in _____ minutes with a minimum score of 85% within two attempts (*or as indicated by the instructor*).

Scoring: Divide the points earned by the total possible points. Failure to perform a critical step, indicated by an asterisk (*), results in grade no higher than an 84% (*or as indicated by the instructor*).

Time: Began_____ Ended_____ Total minutes: _____

Steps:	Point Value	Attempt 1	Attempt 2
1. Check the provider's order and/or requisition form to determine the tests ordered. Gather the appropriate tubes and supplies. Put on a fluid-impermeable lab coat.	5		
2. Greet the patient. Identify yourself. Verify the patient's identity with full name, ask the patient to spell the last name, and give their date of birth. Explain the procedure to be performed in a manner that is understood by the patient. Answer any questions the patient may have on the procedure. Obtain permission for the venipuncture.	5		
3. Wash hands or use hand sanitizer. Put on gloves and protective eyewear.	10*		
4. Select a puncture site, depending on the patient's age and the sample to be obtained (e.g., palmar side of middle or ring finger of nondominant hand, medial or lateral curved surface of the plantar surface of heel for an infant).	5		
5. Gently rub the finger or have your patient wiggle fingers and open and close hand.	5		
6. Once the finger is warm, clean the site with a 70% alcohol pad and allow it to air dry.	5		
7. Hold onto the patient's finger above the puncture site with your nondominant hand.	5		

8. Hold the safety lancet firmly against the patient's finger and press down on the safety trigger that activates the needle or blade to penetrate the skin. The sharp will then automatically retract into the plastic housing of the lancet.	5		
9. Dispose of the lancet in the sharps container. Wipe away the first drop of blood with gauze	5*		
10. Apply gentle, intermittent pressure to cause the blood to flow freely.	5		
11. Collect the blood samples. Gently squeeze and release the finger two or three times to get a large drop of blood. Touch the capillary tube to the drop of blood. Do not scoop blood from the finger's surface. Fill the capillary to approximately 3/4 full or to the indicated line. Then tip the tube with the presealed end down. When the blood flows down and touches the sealant, hold it for 30 seconds to allow it to seal automatically.	5		
12. Wipe the patient's finger with gauze. Express another large drop of blood in the same way and fill a Microtainer. Do not touch the container to the finger. If more blood is needed, gently squeeze, and release the finger to get another drop. Cap the Microtainer tube when the collection is complete.	5		
13. When collection is complete, apply pressure to the site with gauze. The patient may be able to assist with this step.	5		
14. Select an appropriate means of labeling the containers. Sealed capillary tubes can be placed in a red-topped tube, which is then labeled. Microtainers can be placed in zipper-lock biohazard bags that are subsequently labeled. Follow your institutions procedures for labeling.	5		
15. Check the patient for bleeding and clean the site if traces of blood are visible. Apply a folded gauze square to the puncture site and wrap with hypoallergenic self-stick wrap, tape, or bandage.	5		
16. Disinfect the work area. Dispose of blood-contaminated materials (e.g., gauze and gloves) in the biohazard waste container. Remove your protective eyewear.	5		
17. Wash hands or use hand sanitizer.	10*		
18. Complete the laboratory requisition form and route the specimen to the proper location. Record the procedure in the patient's record.	5		
Total Points	100		

Documentation

Comments

CAAHEP Competencies	Step(s)
I.P.2.c. Perform: capillary puncture	Entire procedure
III.P.2. Select appropriate barrier/personal protective equipment (PPE)	1, 3
III.P.10.a. Demonstrate proper disposal of biohazardous material: sharps	9
III.P.10.b. Demonstrate proper disposal of biohazardous material: regulated wastes	16
XII.P.2.c. Demonstrate proper use of: sharps disposal containers	9
ABHES Competencies	**Step(s)**
9.c. Dispose of biohazardous materials	9, 16
9.d. Collect, label, and process a specimen	Entire procedure

Procedure 47.5   Show Awareness of a Patient's Concern Related to a Procedure

Name _____ Date _____ Score _____

Task: Show awareness of a patient's concern related to a venipuncture.

Scenario: You are a medical assistant working with Dr. Walden, who ordered bloodwork for Sam Brown. Your role includes performing venipuncture when bloodwork is ordered. You obtain the order, greet Sam, identify yourself, verify Sam's identity, and explain what you need to do. You notice that Sam appears to be uncomfortable and restless. Sam states she/he didn't really want the bloodwork done.

Directions: Role-play this scenario with a peer. The peer will play Sam and you are the medical assistant. During the role-play, address Sam's concerns regarding the procedure.

Standard: Complete the role-play in _____ minutes with a minimum score of 100% within two attempts (*or as indicated by the instructor*).

Scoring: Divide the points earned by the total possible points. Met competency: 100% (10 points). Not met competency: 0% (0 points).

Time: Began_____ Ended_____ Total minutes: _____

Checklist for Affective Behaviors

Affective Behavior	Directions: Check behaviors observed during the role-play.					
Awareness	**Negative, Unprofessional Behaviors**	**Attempt** 1	**Attempt** 2	**Positive, Professional Behaviors**	**Attempt** 1	**Attempt** 2
	Rude, discourteous			Pleasant and courteous		
	Disregarded the person's dignity and rights			Maintained the person's dignity and rights		
	Failed to use therapeutic communication techniques (e.g., reflection, restating, clarifying, and summarizing) to verify patient's concerns			Used therapeutic communication techniques (e.g., reflection, restating, clarifying, and summarizing) to verify patient's concerns		
	Nonempathetic behaviors; failed to address patient's concerns			Showed empathy; addressed patient's concerns		
	Failed to clearly and/or professionally address the situation and/or patient's questions/concerns			Clearly and professionally addressed the situation and/or patient's questions/concerns		
	Failed to reassure patient or inappropriately reassured patient			Appropriately reassured patient		
	Negative nonverbal behaviors			Positive nonverbal behaviors		
	Other:			Other:		

Grading for Affective Behaviors		Point Value	Attempt 1	Attempt 2
Does not meet Expectation	• Response fails to show awareness of patient's concerns. • Student demonstrated more than 2 negative, unprofessional behaviors during the interaction.	0		
Needs Improvement	• Response fails to show awareness of patient's concerns. • Student demonstrated 1 or 2 negative, unprofessional behaviors during the interaction.	0		
Meets Expectation	• Response shows awareness of patient's concerns; no negative, unprofessional behaviors observed. • More practice is needed for behavior to appear natural and for student to appear comfortable and at ease.	10		
Occasionally Exceeds Expectation	• Response shows awareness of patient's concerns; no negative, unprofessional behaviors observed. • At times student appeared comfortable and at ease; but more practice is needed for behavior to become natural and consistent with a professional medical assistant.	10		
Always Exceeds Expectation	• Response shows awareness of patient's concerns; no negative, unprofessional behaviors observed. • Student's behaviors appeared natural and comfortable. Behaviors are consistent with a professional medical assistant.	10		

Comments

CAAHEP Competencies	Step(s)
I.A.3. Show awareness of a patient's concerns related to the procedure being performed	Entire role-play

Analysis of Blood

chapter

48

CAAHEP Competencies	Assessment
I.P.10. Perform a quality control measure	Procedure 48.3, 48.7
I.P.11.a. Obtain specimens and perform: CLIA-waived hematology test	Procedure 48.2-48.4
I.P.11.b. Obtain specimens and perform: CLIA-waived chemistry test	Procedure 48.6, 48.7
II.P.2. Differentiate between normal and abnormal test results	Procedure 48.7
VI.P.8. Perform routine maintenance of administrative or clinical equipment	Procedure 48.1
ABHES Competencies	**Assessment**
9.a. Practice Quality Control	Procedure 48.3, 48.7
9.b. Perform selected CLIA-waived test that assist with diagnosis and treatment 2) hematology testing	Procedure 48.2-48.5
9.b. Perform selected CLIA-waived test that assist with diagnosis and treatment 3) chemistry testing	Procedure 48.6, 48.7

VOCABULARY REVIEW

Using the word pool, find the correct word to match the definition. Write the word on the line after the definition.

Group A

1. A cell with uncontrolled growth, rapidly spreading, and doing harm _____
2. A hormone that helps T cells mature and understand their role in the immune system _____
3. Most abundant plasma protein in human blood; it is important in regulating the water balance of blood _____
4. An old or aging cell that can no longer divide and reproduce _____
5. A group of related proteins that functions as antibodies; found in plasma and other body fluids _____
6. A chemical substance produced in an endocrine gland and transported in the blood to a specific tissue, where it applies a specific effect _____
7. The liquid that remains after blood has clotted _____
8. The liquid portion of whole blood _____
9. Special proteins that speed up the chemical reaction in the body _____
10. A measurement of the percentage of packed red blood cells (RBCs) in a volume of blood _____

Word Pool
- enzyme
- hormone
- plasma
- senescent cell
- malignant
- thymosin
- albumin
- immunoglobulin
- serum
- hematocrit

Group B

1. Consistent with the normal function of the body _____
2. The oxygen-carrying pigment of RBCs _____
3. A substance for use in a chemical reaction _____
4. A deficiency of hemoglobin in the blood; accompanied by a reduced number of RBCs, pale skin, weakness, and shortness of breath, among other symptoms _____
5. A small tube or vessel used in laboratory experiments _____
6. A machine that rotates at high speed and separates substances of different densities _____
7. Caused by or involving disease _____
8. A disorder characterized by an abnormal increase in the number of RBCs _____
9. A slender tube attached to or including a bulb, for transferring or measuring small amounts of a liquid, often used in a laboratory _____
10. The layer of white blood cells (WBCs) and platelets that separates the RBCs from plasma in a centrifuged whole blood sample _____

Word Pool
- centrifuge
- buffy coat
- anemia
- polycythemia
- physiologic
- pathologic
- hemoglobin
- microcuvettes
- reagent
- pipet

Group C

1. An increase in number of normal WBCs is a condition called _____

2. A person trained in the nature, function, and diseases of the blood and blood-forming organs; can be a physician, trained laboratory personnel, or researcher _____

3. The study of the form, shape, and structure of an organism or cell _____

4. Pale RBCs; lacking color _____

5. A structure in a cell that contains genetic material and controls the characteristics and growth of the cell _____

6. Describes how compact or concentrated something is _____

7. The cell substance that fills the area between the nucleus and the cell membrane; contains organelles of the cell _____

8. A decrease in the WBC count is called _____

9. Reducing the concentration of a mixture or solution by adding a known volume of liquid _____

10. An immune response against a person's own tissues, cells, or cell parts _____

Word Pool
- autoimmune
- dilution
- hypochromic
- leukocytosis
- leukopenia
- density
- morphology
- hematologist
- nucleus
- cytoplasm

Group D

1. Smaller-than-normal RBCs _____

2. RBCs with a normal amount of hemoglobin are referred to as _____

3. A condition where different sizes of RBCs are present _____

4. RBCs with less-than-normal hemoglobin are referred to as _____

5. A condition where RBCs that have a significant variation in shape _____

6. In many viral infections, stimulated or reactive lymphs are called _____

7. A decreased platelet count is called _____

8. Larger-than-normal RBCs _____

9. An increase in platelets is called _____

10. Normal-sized RBCs _____

Word Pool
- atypical lymphs
- normocytic
- macrocytic
- microcytic
- anisocytosis
- poikilocytosis
- normochromic
- hypochromic
- thrombocytosis
- thrombocytopenia

Group E

1. Another term for blood clot _____

2. Any small abnormal patch on or within the body; deposit of fatty material _____

3. The result of glucose irreversibly binding to the hemoglobin molecules in the RBCs _____

4. A blood transfusion with a person's own blood

   _____

5. Cholesterol travels in the blood as distinct particles containing both lipid and proteins _____

6. Fat in the blood related to caloric intake _____

7. A fat-like substance present in cell membranes; needed to form bile acids, steroid hormones, the coverings of nerves, and some brain tissue _____

8. A condition seen during pregnancy in which the effect of insulin is partially blocked by hormones produced by the placenta

   _____

9. Relating to or resulting from metabolism (the chemical process where cells produce the substances and energy needed to sustain life) _____

10. Test performed to prevent transfusion reactions in patients receiving blood from a donor _____

Word Pool

- compatibility testing
- autologous transfusion
- metabolic
- plaque
- gestational diabetes
- glycosylated hemoglobin
- cholesterol
- thrombus
- triglycerides
- lipoprotein

ABBREVIATIONS

Write out what each of the following abbreviations stands for.

1. POL _____

2. ESR _____

3. CBC _____

4. ALT _____

5. AST _____

6. PT _____

7. RBC _____

8. WBC _____

9. CLIA _____

10. EDTA _____

11. OSHA _____

12. Hct _____

13. Hg _____

14. H&H _____

15. LED _____

16. INR _____

17. WHO _____

18. MC _____

19. MCH _____

20. MCHC _____

21. FBG _____

22. GTT _____

23. FDA _____

24. LDL _____

25. HDL _____

26. T_3 _____

27. T_4 _____

28. TSH _____

29. TRH _____

30. POCT _____

SKILLS AND CONCEPTS

Answer the following questions. Write your answer on the line or in the space provided.

A. Hematology

1. The liquid portion of whole blood is called _____.

2. List the three types of formed elements in whole blood. _____

   _____

3. Where are blood cells made in the body? _____

   _____

4. Where do T cell lymphocytes mature in the body? _____

   _____

5. What hormone helps T cell lymphocytes mature and learn their role in the immune system? _____

   _____

6. Other than the formed elements of blood and water, what other substances make up plasma?_____

    _____

    _____

7. List the plasma proteins found in plasma. _____

    _____

    _____

8. What three nutrients are carried in the plasma? _____

    _____

B. Hematology in the Physician's Office Laboratory (POL)

1. Why is EDTA the preferred anticoagulant for hematology specimens? _____

    _____

2. Define *hematocrit*. _____

    _____

3. Explain how a centrifuge works. _____

    _____

4. What makes up the buffy coat of a centrifuged whole blood sample?_____

    _____

5. Do hematocrit normal values vary depending upon the patient's age and gender?   YES   NO

6. What are two possible causes of a low microhematocrit value? _____

    _____

7. What are two possible causes of a high microhematocrit value? _____

    _____

8. Why is hemoglobin testing done? _____

    _____

    _____

9. Briefly describe how the HemoCue waived hemoglobin analyzer detects hemoglobin. _____

    _____

    _____

10. What factors affect a person's hemoglobin level? _____

    _____

11. The hemoglobin value multiplied by _____ should equal the hematocrit value.

12. Describe an erythrocyte sedimentation rate (ESR). _____

    _____

    _____

    _____

    _____

13. What diseases or disorders may cause an increased ESR value? _____

    _____

    _____

14. Describe what factors may affect the results of an ESR test. _____

    _____

15. What is the most common coagulation test performed in a CLIA-waived POL?_____

    _____

16. Describe the principle of how a PT test works. _____

    _____

17. Why are PT tests done on patient samples? _____

    _____

18. What is another name for a PT test? _____

    _____

19. What is a normal value for a PT/INR? _____

    _____

    _____

C. Hematology in the Reference Laboratory

1. What tests are included in a complete blood count (CBC)? _____

   _____

   _____

2. What is the normal range for an RBC count? _____

3. What are RBC indices?_____

   _____

   _____

4. Why are WBC counts performed on a patient sample? _____

_____

_____

_____

5. What is a normal WBC count? _____

6. What normal conditions may increase a person's WBC count? _____

_____

_____

7. What diseases or disorders increase a person's WBC count? _____

_____

_____

8. Describe a differential and why it is performed on patient samples. _____

_____

_____

_____

_____

9. Why are peripheral blood smears useful as part of a CBC? _____

_____

_____

10. What is a normal platelet count for a healthy person? _____

D. Immunohematology

1. What is another term used for *immunohematology*? _____

2. What are the two major blood antigen systems in the human body? _____

_____

3. Why is blood typing *not* a CLIA-waived test? _____

_____

_____

4. Define *autologous donation.* _____

_____

E. Blood Chemistry in the Physician's Office Laboratory

1. What is the most frequently tested chemical analyte in the blood? _____

2. What conditions can cause elevated blood glucose levels? _____

_____

_____

_____

3. Describe diabetes mellitus. _____

_____

_____

_____

4. Describe hemoglobin A1c testing. _____

_____

_____

_____

5. What factors affect a person's cholesterol level? _____

_____

_____

_____

6. Describe the effect of high LDL cholesterol in the body. _____

_____

_____

_____

_____

7. What is an optimal LDL cholesterol level in the blood? _____

8. How often should adults have their cholesterol levels checked? _____

9. Should patients fast before giving a blood sample for cholesterol testing?   YES   NO

10. What two liver enzymes are indicators of liver damage? _____

_____

11. What two hormones produced by the thyroid gland affect body metabolism? _____

_____

12. Deficient activity of the thyroid gland is also known as _____.

F. Reference Laboratory Chemistry Panels and Single Analyte Testing and Monitoring

1. Describe a chemistry panel._____

_____

_____

_____

2. List three common chemistry panels tested in the laboratory. _____

_____

CERTIFICATION PREPARATION

Circle the correct answer.

1. The liquid that remains after blood has clotted is called
   a. serum.
   b. plasma.
   c. anticoagulant.
   d. none of the above.

2. The formed elements in whole blood are RBCs, WBCs, and
   a. platelets.
   b. senescent cells.
   c. thrombocytes.
   d. both a and c.

3. What is the most abundant protein in human blood?
   a. Immunoglobulins
   b. Fibrinogen
   c. Albumin
   d. Prothrombin

4. The most common anticoagulant used to collect hematology specimens is
   a. EDTA.
   b. heparin.
   c. sodium citrate.
   d. no anticoagulant is needed.

5. The layer of centrifuged blood that contains the WBCs and platelets is
   a. serum.
   b. plasma.
   c. buffy coat.
   d. both a and b.

6. An ESR is used to test for what condition?
   a. A possible heart attack
   b. Uncontrolled asthma
   c. General inflammation
   d. Diabetes mellitus

7. What test is used to monitor patients taking an anticoagulant drug?
   a. PT
   b. INR
   c. ESR
   d. Both a and b

8. What condition is defined as RBCs with different or varied sizes?
   a. Poikilocytosis
   b. Hypochromic
   c. Anisocytosis
   d. Thrombocytosis

9. The term *glycosylated hemoglobin* is described as
   a. low blood sugar.
   b. low iron hemoglobin.
   c. high blood sugar.
   d. sugar-coated hemoglobin.

10. Which two liver enzymes are used to monitor liver function?
    a. ESR and INR
    b. AST and ALT
    c. HDL and LDL
    d. Hct and Hgb

WORKPLACE APPLICATIONS

1. Bella is a 22-year-old female patient who is in to see Dr. Perez today for a routine checkup. One of the tests they performed in the lab was a capillary puncture hemoglobin test. Bella's results were a bit low; her hemoglobin was 10.8 g/dL.

    a. What is the normal hemoglobin range for an adult female?_____

    b. What factors can affect a person's hemoglobin level? _____

    _____

    c. What other test is often run with a hemoglobin level to confirm test results?_____

    _____

2. Anita is reviewing blood typing for a continuing education course she is taking.

    a. If a specimen has only anti-B plasma antibodies, which ABO blood type is the specimen? _____

    b. If a specimen has no plasma antibodies, which ABO blood type is the specimen? _____

    c. If a specimen has a B antigen on their RBCs, which ABO blood type is the specimen?_____

    d. If a specimen has no antigens on their RBCs, which ABO blood type is the specimen? _____

3. Sophie is looking over her lab results for cholesterol testing. Indicate if each result is normal or abnormal.

Cholesterol component	Sophie's result	Normal	Abnormal
Total cholesterol	202 mg/dL		
LDL	104 mg/dL		
HDL	42 mg/dL		

INTERNET ACTIVITIES

1. Using online resources, research the rise in diabetes mellitus type 2 in the United States over the last 50 years. Summarize your findings in a poster or infographic.

2. Using online resources, research hemolytic disease of the newborn (HDN). Create a poster presentation, a PowerPoint presentation, or a written paper summarizing your research. Include the following points in your project:
    a. Describe how a woman becomes sensitized to the Rh antigen.
    b. Describe how HDN is treated.
    c. Describe how RhoGAM works in the body of the Rh-negative mother.

3. Using online resources, research hemoglobin A1c testing for diabetics. Create a poster presentation, infographic, or PowerPoint presentation summarizing your research. Include the following points in your project.:
    a. Describe the principle of hemoglobin A1c testing.
    b. What are normal and abnormal results, and how do they relate to blood sugar?
    c. List and briefly describe two CLIA-waived hemoglobin A1c tests.

Procedure 48.1   Perform Preventive Maintenance for the Microhematocrit Centrifuge

Name _____   Date _____   Score _____

Task: To perform daily, monthly, semiannual, and annual preventive maintenance on a microhematocrit centrifuge.

Equipment and Supplies:
- Microhematocrit centrifuge
- Maintenance logbook
- Utility gloves
- Fluid-impermeable lab coat, eye protection, and gloves
- Disinfectant
- Biohazard waste container

Standard: Complete the procedure and all critical steps in _____ minutes with a minimum score of 85% within two attempts (*or as indicated by the instructor*).

Scoring: Divide the points earned by the total possible points. Failure to perform a critical step, indicated by an asterisk (*), results in grade no higher than an 84% (*or as indicated by the instructor*).

Time: Began_____ Ended_____ Total minutes: _____

Steps:	Point Value	Attempt 1	Attempt 2
Wash hands or use hand sanitizer. Put on fluid-impermeable lab coat, eye protection, and gloves. In all maintenance procedures, gloves are worn under the utility gloves. *Note 1:* These are generic recommendations. Always check the manufacturer's guidelines for specific instructions. *Note 2:* Always unplug the power cord before cleaning or servicing the centrifuge.	10*		
Daily Maintenance 1. Clean the inside of the centrifuge and the gasket with a disinfectant recommended by the manufacturer. Plastic and nonmetal parts may be cleaned with a fresh solution of 5% sodium hypochlorite (bleach) mixed 1:10 with water.	10		
Monthly Maintenance 1. Check the reading device. Misuse and zeroing of the reading devices can result in considerable error. Always use a second simple reading device as a cross-check. Use a ruler or a flat plastic card specially made for this purpose. To use these cards, lay the spun hematocrit tube on the card and align the red cells with a line on the card to obtain the reading.	10		
2. Check the rotor for cracks or corrosion and check the interior for signs of white powder.	10		
3. Record all preventive maintenance in the laboratory logbook.	10		
Semiannual Maintenance 1. Check the gasket for cuts and breaks.	10		
2. Check the timer with a stopwatch to verify timer accuracy.	10		

3.	Perform a maximum cell pack to verify the time required for complete packing by reading a sample after centrifuging and then recentrifuging for 1 minute. The results should be the same. If they are not, perform preventive maintenance and/or call the service technician.	10		
4.	Record all preventive measures in the equipment maintenance log.	5		
Annual Maintenance (or Maintenance Performed as Needed) 1. The centrifuge functions and maintenance verification should be performed by qualified personnel. This includes checking the centrifuge mechanism, rotors, timer, speed, and electrical leads.		10		
2.	Record all professional service calls in the laboratory logbook.	5		
	Total Points	100		

Documentation

Comments

CAAHEP Competencies	Step(s)
VI.P.8. Perform routine maintenance of administrative or clinical equipment	Entire procedure

Procedure 48.2 CLIA-Waived Hematology Testing: Perform a Microhematocrit Test

Name _____ Date _____ Score _____

Task: To perform a microhematocrit test accurately.

Equipment and Supplies:
- Provider's order and/or lab requisition, microhematocrit lab log, patient's health record
- Fresh sample of blood collected in a tube containing ethylenediaminetetraacetic acid (EDTA) anticoagulant (or equipment for fingerstick specimen: lancet, alcohol wipe, gauze, bandage)
- Plastic-coated self-sealing capillary tubes, or plain capillary tubes (blue-tipped)
- Sealing clay (if capillary tubes are not self-sealing)
- Gauze
- Microhematocrit centrifuge
- Fluid-impermeable lab coat, protective eyewear, and gloves
- Biohazard waste container
- Biohazard sharps containers

Standard: Complete the procedure and all critical steps in _____ minutes with a minimum score of 85% within two attempts (*or as indicated by the instructor*).

Scoring: Divide the points earned by the total possible points. Failure to perform a critical step, indicated by an asterisk (*), results in grade no higher than an 84% (*or as indicated by the instructor*).

Time: Began_____ Ended_____ Total minutes: _____

Steps:	Point Value	Attempt 1	Attempt 2
1. Wash hands or use hand sanitizer. Put on fluid-impermeable lab coat, protective eyewear, and gloves.	10*		
2. Assemble the materials needed. ***If the capillary tubes are self-sealing***, fill two tubes by inserting the end opposite the sealed end into the well-mixed EDTA blood sample. When the self-sealing capillary tubes are two-thirds to three-fourths filled, tilt them upright causing the blood sample to flow down the tube and meet the sealant. Continue to hold the tube vertical when the blood contacts the sealant for an additional 15 seconds. ***Alternatively, fill two plain (blue-tipped) capillary tubes*** two-thirds to three-fourths full of a well-mixed EDTA blood sample. When enough blood has filled the capillary tube, tip the blue end of the tube down causing the blood to flow towards the blue tip. Then readjust the tube horizontally while inserting the blue tip of the capillary tube into the clay sealant. Insert the tube as many times as needed to achieve a plug up to the blue band.	5		
3. Wipe the outside of the tubes with clean gauze without touching the wet open end of the tube.	5		
4. Place the tubes opposite each other in the centrifuge with the sealed ends securely against the gasket.	10*		
5. Note the numbers on the centrifuge slots and record the numbers on the log sheet along with the patient's name.	10*		

6.	Secure the locking top, fasten the lid down, and lock it.	**5**		
7.	Set the timer to 3-5 minutes and adjust the speed to 11,000 to 12,000 rpm, as needed.	**5**		
8.	Allow the centrifuge to come to a complete stop. Unlock the outer locking top and then remove the inner lid.	**5**		
9.	Remove the tubes immediately and read the results. If this is not possible, store the tubes in an upright position.	**10**		
10.	Determine the microhematocrit values using one of the following methods: ***Centrifuge with built-in reader using calibrated capillary tubes.*** • Position the tubes as directed by the manufacturer's instructions. • Read both tubes. • The average of the two results is reported. • The two values should not vary by more than 2%. ***Centrifuge without a built-in reader.*** • Carefully remove the tubes from the centrifuge. • Place a tube on the microhematocrit reader. • Align the clay-RBC junction with the zero line on the reader. Align the plasma meniscus with the 100% line. The value is read at the junction of the red cell layer and the buffy coat. The buffy coat is not included in the reading. • Read both tubes. • The average of the two results is reported. • The two values should not vary by more than 2%.	**10***		
11.	Dispose of the capillary tubes in a biohazard sharps container.	**10***		
12.	Disinfect the work area and properly dispose of all biohazardous materials. Remove your gloves, eyewear, and lab coat. Wash hands or use hand sanitizer.	**10***		
13.	Record the results in the Hematocrit Patient Log and document the results in the patient's medical record or the electronic medical record.	**5**		
	Total Points	**100**		

Documentation

Comments

CAAHEP Competencies	Step(s)
I.P.11.a. Obtain specimens and perform: CLIA-waived hematology test	Entire procedure
ABHES Competencies	**Step(s)**
9.b. Perform selected CLIA-waived tests that assist with diagnosis and treatment 2) hematology testing	Entire procedure

Procedure 48.3 Perform CLIA-Waived Hematology Testing: Perform a Hemoglobin Test

Name _____ Date _____ Score _____

Task: To accurately determine the level of hemoglobin present in a blood sample using the HemoCue B-Hemoglobin System.

Equipment and Supplies:
- Patient's health record
- Provider's order and/or lab requisition
- Hemoglobin laboratory log
- HemoCue monitor
- HemoCue microcuvette
- Safety blood lancet
- Alcohol wipes
- Gauze
- Fluid-impermeable lab coat, protective eyewear, and gloves
- Biohazard waste container
- Biohazard sharps containers

Standard: Complete the procedure and all critical steps in _____ minutes with a minimum score of 85% within two attempts (*or as indicated by the instructor*).

Scoring: Divide the points earned by the total possible points. Failure to perform a critical step, indicated by an asterisk (*), results in grade no higher than an 84% (*or as indicated by the instructor*).

Time: Began_____ Ended_____ Total minutes: _____

Steps:	Point Value	Attempt 1	Attempt 2
1. Perform an instrument quality control check by inserting the control cuvette into the instrument. Make sure the reading is within acceptable limits before proceeding.	10*		
2. Wash hands or use hand sanitizer. Put on fluid-impermeable lab coat, protective eyewear, and gloves.	10*		
3. Assemble all equipment and supplies needed.	5		
4. Greet the patient. Identify yourself. Verify the patient's identity with full name, ask the patient to spell the first and last name, and give their date of birth. Explain the procedure to be performed in a manner that is understood by the patient. Answer any questions the patient may have on the procedure. Obtain permission for the capillary puncture.	10		
5. Examine the patient's fingers and choose the site to be used to obtain the blood sample.	5		
6. Clean the site with an alcohol wipe or another recommended antiseptic preparation. Allow the site to air dry.	10		
7. Perform a capillary puncture and wipe away the first drop of blood.	5		
8. Obtain a large drop blood on the surface of the finger.	5		

9.	Touch the microcuvette to the drop of blood. Do not touch the finger. The correct volume is drawn into the cuvette by capillary action. Wipe off any excess blood from the sides of the cuvette.	10		
10.	Place the cuvette in the cuvette holder of the HemoCue sample door, and close the door of the instrument.	5		
11.	Read the result and record it in the lab's hemoglobin log and the patient's health record.	5		
12.	Dispose of biohazardous waste in biohazard waste containers. Turn off the instrument. Properly disinfect the work area.	5*		
13.	Remove gloves and dispose in biohazard waste container. Remove lab coat and protective eyewear.	5		
14.	Wash hands or use hand sanitizer.	10*		
	Total Points	100		

Documentation

Comments

CAAHEP Competencies	Step(s)
I.P.10. Perform a quality control measure	1
I.P.11.a. Obtain specimens and perform: CLIA-waived hematology test	Entire procedure
ABHES Competencies	**Step(s)**
9.a. Practice Quality Control	1
9.b. Perform selected CLIA-waived test that assist with diagnosis and treatment 2) hematology testing	Entire procedure

Procedure 48.4 Perform CLIA-Waived Hematology Testing: Determine the Erythrocyte Sedimentation Rate Using a Modified Westergren Method

Name _____ Date _____ Score _____

Task: Fill a Westergren tube properly and observe and record an erythrocyte sedimentation rate (ESR) obtained by using a modified Westergren method.

Equipment and Supplies:
- Patient's health record
- Provider's order and/or lab requisition
- Erythrocyte sedimentation rate (ESR) laboratory log
- EDTA–anticoagulated blood specimen
- Safety tube decapper (if tubes do not have a Hemogard plastic top)
- Disposable transfer pipet
- Sediplast ESR system (pre-filled Sediplast vial)
- Sediplast rack
- Timer
- Fluid-impermeable lab coat, eye protection, and gloves
- Biohazard waste container
- Biohazard sharps container

Standard: Complete the procedure and all critical steps in _____ minutes with a minimum score of 85% within two attempts (*or as indicated by the instructor*).

Scoring: Divide the points earned by the total possible points. Failure to perform a critical step, indicated by an asterisk (*), results in grade no higher than an 84% (*or as indicated by the instructor*).

Time: Began_____ Ended_____ Total minutes: _____

Steps:	Point Value	Attempt 1	Attempt 2
1. Wash hands or use hand sanitizer. Put on fluid-impermeable lab coat, eye protection, and gloves.	10*		
2. Assemble the materials needed.	5		
3. Check the leveling bubble of the Sediplast rack.	5		
4. Bring the blood sample to room temperature if it has been refrigerated and mix the sample well by gently inverting the tube six to eight times, making sure the tube has no bubbles.	5		
5. Remove the plastic Hemogard stopper on the blood sample by twisting and slowly pushing up on the stopper with your thumbs (or by using a tube decapper on rubber-stoppered blood tubes). Also remove the stopper on the prefilled Sediplast vial.	10		
6. Fill the Sediplast vial with blood to the indicated line using a disposable transfer pipet. Replace the stopper on the prefilled vial and invert it several times to mix. Recap the blood collection tube with its stopper.	10		
7. Insert a Sediplast pipet through the pierceable stopper on the prefilled vial and push down until the pipet touches the bottom of the vial. The pipet automatically draws the blood up and over the zero mark	10		
8. Insert the filled Sediplast pipet and its vial into the Sediplast rack, making sure the vial is vertical.	5		

9.	Note the start time on the ESR log sheet and allow the vial to stand undisturbed for 60 minutes.	**5**		
10.	After 60 minutes, measure the distance the erythrocytes have fallen at the top of the tube. The scale reads in millimeters; each line is 1 mm.	**10**		
11.	Properly dispose of all biohazardous materials. Disinfect the work area. Dispose the plastic Sediplast pipet and its vial into a biohazard sharps container. Remove your gloves, protective eyewear, and lab coat.	**10**		
12.	Wash hands or use hand sanitizer.	**10***		
13.	Record the findings in the lab's ESR log and the patient's health record. Remember—the Westergren ESR is reported in millimeters per hour (mm/hr).	**5**		
	Total Points	**100**		

Documentation

Comments

CAAHEP Competencies	Step(s)
I.P.11.b. Obtain specimens and perform: CLIA-waived chemistry test	Entire procedure
ABHES Competencies	**Step(s)**
9.b. Perform selected CLIA-waived test that assist with diagnosis and treatment 2) hematology testing	Entire procedure

Procedure 48.5   Perform a CLIA-Waived Protime/INR Test

Name _____ Date _____ Score _____

Task: Perform a coagulation test to determine protime/INR using the CoaguChek XS instrument with built-in quality control.

Equipment and Supplies:
- Patient's health record or flow chart
- Provider's order and/or lab requisition
- PT/INR lab log
- Gauze, alcohol wipes, bandage
- CoaguChek XS PT Test monitor
- CoaguChek lancet
- CoaguChek test strip container and code chip
- Package insert or flow chart with directions
- Fluid-impermeable lab coat, protective eyewear, and gloves
- Biohazard waste container
- Biohazard sharps containers

Order: Perform a protime/INR test on Connie Lange STAT.

Standard: Complete the procedure and all critical steps in _____ minutes with a minimum score of 85% within two attempts (*or as indicated by the instructor*).

Scoring: Divide the points earned by the total possible points. Failure to perform a critical step, indicated by an asterisk (*), results in grade no higher than an 84% (*or as indicated by the instructor*).

Time: Began_____ Ended_____ Total minutes: _____

Steps:	Point Value	Attempt 1	Attempt 2
1. Wash hands or use hand sanitizer. Put on fluid-impermeable lab coat, protective eyewear, and gloves.	10*		
2. Assemble the materials needed.	5		
3. If you are using test strips from a new, unopened container, you must change the test strip code chip. The three-number code on the test strip container must match the three-number code on the code strip. To install the code strip, follow the instructions in the Code Chip section of the User's Manual.	10		
4. Place the meter on a flat surface so that it will not vibrate or move during testing.	5		
5. Greet the patient. Identify yourself. Verify the patient's identity with full name, ask the patient to spell the first and last name, and give their date of birth. Explain the procedure to be performed in a manner that is understood by the patient. Answer any questions the patient may have on the procedure. Obtain permission for the capillary puncture.	10*		
6. Examine the patient's fingers and choose the site to be used to obtain the blood sample.	5		

7.	Prepare the site by: • Warming the hand by placing it under the arm, using a hand warmer, and/or washing the hand in warm water. • Have the patient hold his or her arm down to the side so that the hand is below the waist. • Massage the palm of the hand toward the base of the finger and toward the tip until the fingertip has increased color.	**5**		
8.	When you are ready to test, remove a test strip from the container and immediately close the container. Make sure it seals tightly. *Do not open the container or touch the test strips with wet hands or wet gloves.*	**5**		
9.	Insert test strip as far as you can into the meter. This powers the meter ON.	**5**		
10.	Disinfect the finger with an alcohol wipe and allow the finger to air dry. Perform the capillary puncture. If necessary, immediately after lancing, gently squeeze the finger to encourage blood flow.	**5***		
11.	Hold the finger with a blood drop very close to the test strip. Apply one drop of blood to the top or side of the target area and wait until you hear the beep. You must apply a hanging drop of blood to the test strip within 15 seconds of the fingerstick. Do not add more blood. Do not touch or remove the test strip while the test is in progress. The flashing blood drop symbol changes to an hourglass symbol when the meter detects a sufficient sample.	**10**		
12.	The result appears in approximately 1 minute. It may be displayed in three ways: as the International Normalized Ratio (INR); as the protime (PT) in seconds; or as %Quick (a unit used mainly in Europe).	**5**		
13.	Record the result in the lab's PT/INR log and in the patient's warfarin therapy flow sheet and/or electronic health record. Circle any results that do not fall into the Desirable Ranges. You may add comments to the test result about the test conditions or the patient. Identify *critical values* and take appropriate steps to notify the provider.	**5**		
14.	Dispose of all sharps into the biohazard sharps container. Dispose of regulated medical waste into the biohazard waste container. Disinfect the test area and remove your PPE.	**5**		
15.	Wash hands or use hand sanitizer.	**10***		
	Total Points	**100**		

Documentation

Comments

CAAHEP Competencies	Step(s)
I.P.11.a. Obtain specimens and perform: CLIA-waived hematology test	Entire procedure
ABHES Competencies	**Step(s)**
9.b. Perform selected CLIA-waived test that assist with diagnosis and treatment 2) hematology testing	Entire procedure

Procedure 48.6 Assist the Provider with Patient Care: Perform a Blood Glucose Test

Name _____ Date _____ Score _____

Task: To perform a blood test for diabetes mellitus accurately.

Equipment and Supplies:
- Patient's record
- Glucometer
- Glucose test strips
- Lancet and/or autoloading finger-puncturing device
- Alcohol wipes
- Gauze
- Fluid-impermeable lab coat, protective eyewear, and gloves
- Biohazard waste container
- Biohazard sharps containers

Standard: Complete the procedure and all critical steps in _____ minutes with a minimum score of 85% within two attempts (*or as indicated by the instructor*).

Scoring: Divide the points earned by the total possible points. Failure to perform a critical step, indicated by an asterisk (*), results in grade no higher than an 84% (*or as indicated by the instructor*).

Time: Began_____ Ended_____ Total minutes: _____

Steps:	Point Value	Attempt 1	Attempt 2
1. Check the provider's order and collect the necessary equipment and supplies. Perform quality control measures according to the manufacturer's guidelines and office policy.	5		
2. Wash hands or use hand sanitizer. Put on fluid-impermeable lab coat, protective eyewear, and gloves.	5*		
3. Greet the patient. Identify yourself. Verify the patient's identity with full name, ask the patient to spell the first and last name, and give their date of birth. Explain the procedure to be performed in a manner that is understood by the patient. Answer any questions the patient may have on the procedure. Obtain permission for the capillary puncture.	5*		
4. Ask the person to wash his/her hands in warm, soapy water, then rinse them in warm water, and finally dry them completely.	5		
5. Check the patient's middle and ring fingers and select the site for the capillary puncture (both forearm and fingertip testing can be done).	5		
6. Turn on the glucometer. See manufacturer's coding instructions for each individual brand of glucose testing system.	5		
7. The glucometer may be preloaded with test strips (depends on manufacturer). Check the expiration date on the container of test strips.	5		
8. Cleanse the selected site on the patient's fingertip with an alcohol wipe and allow the finger to air dry.	5*		
9. Perform the capillary puncture and wipe away the first drop of blood.	10		
10. Apply a small blood sample (0.5 mL) to the end of the test strip.	5		

11.	Give the patient gauze to hold securely over the puncture site; apply a hypoallergenic bandage or wrap if needed.	**5**		
12.	The glucometer automatically begins the measurement process, and results are obtained in a short period of time.	**5**		
13.	The test result is shown in the display window in milligrams per deciliter (mg/dL) for most glucometers. Read manufacturer's instruction on how the result is displayed. The glucometer will likely turn off automatically.	**5**		
14.	Encourage patients to bring their personal glucometer to the clinic so the provider can review daily averages and previous test results.	**5**		
15.	Discard all biohazardous waste in biohazard waste containers.	**5**		
16.	Clean the glucometer according to the manufacturer's guidelines.	**5**		
17.	Disinfect the work area. Remove your gloves and dispose of them properly.	**5**		
18.	Remove protective eyewear. Wash hands or use hand sanitizer.	**5***		
19.	Record the test results in the patient's health record.	**5**		
	Total Points	**100**		

Documentation

Comments

CAAHEP Competencies	Step(s)
I.P.11.b. Obtain specimens and perform: CLIA-waived chemistry test	Entire procedure
ABHES Competencies	**Step(s)**
9.b. Perform selected CLIA-waived test that assist with diagnosis and treatment 3) chemistry testing	Entire procedure

Procedure 48.7 Perform a CLIA-Waived Chemistry Test: Determine the Cholesterol Level or Lipid Profile Using a Cholestech Analyzer

Name _____ Date _____ Score _____

Task: To perform a Cholestech test for total cholesterol level and/or a lipid panel and accurately report the results.

Equipment and Supplies:
- Patient's health record
- Provider's order and/or lab requisition
- Cholestech analyzer
- Package insert or flow chart with directions
- Optics check cassette
- Test cassettes (provided by Cholestech)
- Level 1 and 2 liquid controls
- Capillary tubes and plungers for fingerstick sample (provided by Cholestech)
- Mini-Pet pipet and pipet tips for venipuncture sample (provided by Cholestech)
- Lancet, gauze, alcohol wipes, bandage for capillary blood, or lithium heparin (green-topped) tube for venous blood
- Safety tube decapper (if tubes do not have a Hemogard plastic top)
- Fluid-impermeable lab coat, protective eyewear, and gloves
- Biohazard waste container
- Biohazard sharps containers

Directions: Perform a total blood cholesterol level or lipid panel on Connie Lange STAT.

Standard: Complete the procedure and all critical steps in _____ minutes with a minimum score of 85% within two attempts (*or as indicated by the instructor*).

Scoring: Divide the points earned by the total possible points. Failure to perform a critical step, indicated by an asterisk (*), results in grade no higher than an 84% (*or as indicated by the instructor*).

Time: Began_____ Ended_____ Total minutes: _____

Steps:	Point Value	Attempt 1	Attempt 2
1. Wash hands or use hand sanitizer. Put on fluid-impermeable lab coat, protective eyewear, and gloves.	10*		
2. Assemble the materials needed.	5		
3. Perform quantitative quality control by performing a calibration check with the optics check cassette. Then test level 1 and level 2 liquid controls if using a new set of cassettes.	5*		
4. Allow refrigerated testing cassettes to come to room temperature (at least 10 minutes before opening).	5		
5. Remove cassette from its pouch and place on flat surface without touching the black bar or magnetic strip.	5		
6. Press RUN, allowing the analyzer to do a self-test; this will be followed by OK on the screen, and then the test drawer will open. The drawer will stay open for 4 minutes while the specimen is prepared.	5		

7.	Perform a fingerstick and collect the capillary blood to the black line of the Cholestech capillary tube with its plunger inserted into the red end of the tube. Or collect the fresh capillary whole blood with the Cholestech Mini-Pet pipet.	**10**		
8.	Place the whole blood sample into the well of the cassette. ***Note:*** The capillary specimen must be in the cassette within 5 minutes of collection.	**10**		
9.	Immediately put the cassette into the drawer of the analyzer and press RUN. ***Note:*** if the drawer has closed, press RUN again to open the drawer and proceed loading the specimen into the drawer, and then pressing to close the drawer.	**5**		
10.	When the test is complete, the analyzer beeps, the screen displays, and then prints out the results.	**5**		
11.	Record the finding in the laboratory log and in the patient's health record.	**5**		
12.	Circle the results that do not fall within the Desirable Ranges column of the following table. Identify *critical values* and take appropriate steps to notify the provider. ***Note:*** See desirable ranges in table below in documentation.	**10**		
13.	Dispose of all sharps in the biohazard sharps container. Place all regulated medical waste into the biohazard waste container. Disinfect test area, remove PPE, and dispose gloves in biohazard waste container.	**10**		
14.	Wash hands or use hand sanitizer.	**10***		
	Total Points	**100**		

Documentation

Attach printed readout, or record results on the electronic chart:

CHOLESTECH LDX REFERENCE RANGE CHART		
TEST	**RESULTS**	**DESIRABLE**
Total cholesterol (TC)	190	<200 mg/dL
HDL cholesterol	50	>40 mg/dL
LDL cholesterol	120	<130 mg/dL
Triglycerides	135	<150 mg/dL
TC/HDL ratio	4.3	≤4.5
Other		
Glucose	80	Fasting: 70-110 mg/dL
		Nonfasting: <160 mg/dL

Comments

CAAHEP Competencies	Step(s)
I.P.10. Perform a quality control measure	3
I.P.11.b. Obtain specimens and perform: CLIA-waived chemistry test	Entire procedure
II.P.2. Differentiate between normal and abnormal test results	12
ABHES Competencies	
9.a. Practice Quality Control	3
9.b. Perform selected CLIA-waived test that assist with diagnosis and treatment 3) chemistry testing	Entire procedure

Microbiology and Immunology

chapter
49

CAAHEP Competencies	Assessment
I.P.2.c. Perform: capillary puncture	Procedure 49.4
I.P.10. Perform a quality control measure	Procedure 49.3, 49.4
I.P.11.d. Obtain specimens and perform: CLIA-waived immunology test	Procedure 49.2 (collection only), 49.3, 49.4
I.P.11.e. Obtain specimens and perform: CLIA-waived microbiology test	Procedure 49.1 (collection only), 49.2 (collection only), 49.3 (perform test only)
II.P.2. Differentiate between normal and abnormal test results	Procedure 49.3, 49.4
II.P.3. Maintain lab test results using flow sheets	Procedure 49.3, 49.4
III.P.2. Select appropriate barrier/personal protective equipment (PPE)	Procedure 49.2, 49.3,4 49.4
III.P.10.a. Demonstrate proper disposal of biohazardous material: sharps	Procedure 49.4
III.P.10.b. Demonstrate proper disposal of biohazardous material: regulated wastes	Procedure 49.2, 49.3, 49.4
XII.P.2.c. Demonstrate proper use of: sharps disposal containers	Procedure 49.4
ABHES Competencies	**Assessment**
9.a. Practice Quality Control	Procedure 49.3, 49.4
9.b. Perform selected CLIA-waived test that assist with diagnosis and treatment 4) immunology testing	Procedure 49.3, 49.4
9.b. Perform selected CLIA-waived test that assist with diagnosis and treatment 5) microbiology testing	Procedure 49.3, 49.4
9.b. Perform selected CLIA-waived test that assist with diagnosis and treatment 6) kit testing	Procedure 49.3, 49.4
d. Collect, label, and process specimens 4) Obtain throat specimens for microbiologic testing	Procedure 49.2 (collection only), 49.3
9.e. Instruct patients in the collection of 2) fecal specimen	Procedure 49.1

VOCABULARY REVIEW

Using the word pool, find the correct word to match the definition. Write the word on the line after the definition.

Group A

1. Substances that inhibit the growth of microorganisms on living tissue _____

2. A large group of microorganisms that are single-celled, lack a nucleus, reproduce asexually, or can form spores; some can cause disease; the most abundant life form on earth

   _____

3. Any chemical agent used on nonliving objects to destroy or inhibit the growth of harmful organisms _____

4. A substance or medication that can destroy or inhibit the growth of bacteria _____

5. Various single-celled fungi, which reproduce by budding and are able to ferment sugars _____

6. Includes living and nonliving pathogens such as bacteria, viruses, fungi, protozoa, parasites, helminths, and prions that can cause disease; also called *infectious particles*

   _____

7. Microorganisms (mostly bacteria and yeast) that live on or in the body; normal microscopic residents of the body

   _____

8. Any of a diverse group of single-celled organisms that include mushrooms, molds, mildew, smuts, rusts, yeasts

   _____

9. Protein substances produced in the blood or tissues in response to a specific antigen; part of the immune system

   _____

10. Any living organism such as bacterium, protozoan, fungus, parasite, or helminth of microscopic size; some definitions include viruses, which are not alive _____

Word Pool

- microorganism
- infectious agents
- antibiotics
- normal flora
- bacteria
- yeast
- antibody
- antiseptics
- disinfectants
- fungus

Group B

1. Any organism that is made up of at least one cell; has genetic material that is not enclosed in a nucleus

_____

2. A reagent or dye used to treat specimens for microscopic examination _____

3. A growth of tiny fungi forming on a substance; often looks downy or furry and is associated with dampness or decay

_____

4. Single-celled organisms that are the most primitive form of animal life; most are microscopic _____

5. Asexual reproduction in single-celled organisms where one cell divides into two daughter cells _____

6. Any single-celled or multicellular organism that has genetic material contained in a distinct membrane-bound nucleus

_____

7. Pertaining to a parasite _____

8. The simplest unit of a chemical compound that can exist, consisting of two or more atoms held together with chemical bonds _____

9. A name consisting of a generic and a specific term

_____

10. A system of names or terms used in science and art to categorize items _____

Word Pool

- protozoa
- parasitic
- binomial
- nomenclature
- prokaryote
- binary fission
- stains
- molecule
- eukaryotes
- molds

Group C

1. Structures inside of the cell that have specific tasks

_____

2. A substance that stimulates the production of an antibody when introduced into the body _____

3. A syringe is used to gently squirt a small amount of sterile saline into the nose and the resulting fluid is collected into a cup

_____

4. A medium used to keep an organism alive during transport to the laboratory _____

5. A glass slide holding a specimen suspended in a drop of liquid for microscopic examination _____

6. When the small airways of the lungs become inflamed because of a viral infection _____

7. Any animal that lacks a spine such as insects, crustaceans, arachnids, and others _____

8. The technique or process of keeping tissue alive and growing in a culture medium _____

9. A process where a specific substance is separated from a group or solution _____

10. The molecules needed for metabolism: carbohydrates, lipids, proteins, amino acids, and nucleic acids _____

Word Pool

- arthropod
- wet mount
- organelles
- macromolecules
- tissue culture
- antigen
- transport medium
- extraction
- nasal washes
- bronchiolitis

Group D

1. Phase when the host recovers gradually and returns to baseline or normal health _____
2. To cultivate an organism (a bacteria) again on a new nutrient surface _____
3. Latin term meaning *in glass*; commonly known as "in the laboratory" _____
4. A liquid substance that dilutes or lessens the strength of a solution or mixture _____
5. Inflammation of the lungs with congestion of the air sacs (alveoli); can be caused by a bacteria or virus

   _____
6. Phase of rapid multiplication of the pathogen; symptoms are very distinct _____

Word Pool
- pneumonia
- acute stage
- convalescent stage
- diluent
- subcultured
- in vitro

ABBREVIATIONS

Write out what each of the following abbreviations stands for.

1. POL _____
2. QA _____
3. CBC _____
4. EM _____
5. CNS _____
6. ARV _____
7. AIDS _____
8. CDC _____
9. WHO _____
10. OSHA _____
11. GPC _____
12. GNB _____
13. MAC _____
14. AFB _____
15. cfu _____
16. C&S _____
17. CLIA _____
18. BAP _____
19. PPE _____

20. KOH _____

21. PG _____

22. O&P _____

23. nm _____

24. CCMS _____

25. GAS _____

26. RSV _____

27. HIV _____

28. EBV _____

29. UTI _____

30. Mono _____

31. DNA _____

32. RNA _____

33. STI _____

SKILLS AND CONCEPTS

Answer the following questions. Write your answer on the line or in the space provided.

A. Introduction

1. Describe the benefits of normal flora. _____

   _____

   _____

2. Describe the term *opportunistic pathogen.* _____

   _____

   _____

3. Explain the benefits of saprophytes. _____

   _____

4. List three examples of infection control practices. _____

   _____

   _____

   _____

B. Classification of Microorganisms

1. List three types of microorganisms. _____

   _____

2. According to binomial nomenclature rules, what two methods are used to emphasize organism names when you are writing?

   _____

   _____

   _____

C. Characteristics of Bacteria

1. Describe why bacteria can reproduce and grow in numbers so quickly. _____

   _____

   _____

2. Describe the differences between Gram-positive cells, Gram-negative cells, and acid-fast cells. _____

   _____

   _____

   _____

3. Describe the different shapes of bacteria: cocci, bacilli, spirilla. _____

   _____

   _____

4. Define the terms of bacterial arrangements below.

   a. Strepto- _____

   b. Diplo-_____

   c. Staphylo-_____

   d. Tetrads_____

   e. Sarcinae _____

5. Define the terms *aerobe*, *anaerobe*, and *facultative anaerobe*. _____

   _____

   _____

   _____

   _____

6. Describe the advantage of bacteria being able to form endospores._____

_____

_____

D. Unusual Pathogenic Bacteria: Chlamydia, Mycoplasma, Rickettsia

1. Briefly describe what makes Chlamydia unusual. _____

_____

_____

2. Briefly describe what makes Rickettsia unusual._____

_____

_____

3. Briefly describe what makes Mycoplasma unusual. _____

_____

_____

E. Pathogenic Fungi

1. Define *mycology*. _____

_____

2. How are fungi transmitted in the environment? _____

_____

3. A superficial fungal infection is often referred to as _____.

4. Define *eukaryote*. _____

_____

5. Fungi include _____ and _____.

F. Pathogenic Protozoa

1. Protozoa are _____-celled parasitic organisms that contain a(n)
    _____. They range in size from microscopic to _____.
    They are present in _____ environments and in bodies of water, such as
    _____ and _____. Protozoa are transmitted through con-
    taminated _____, _____, and _____.
    Some pathogenic protozoa inhabit the _____, whereas others inhabit the
    _____ and _____ tract. Diagnosis usually is based on the
    patient's _____ and _____ and on microscopic examination of
    stool and/or blood.

G. Pathogenic Parasites

1. Define *parasitology*. _____

    _____

2. In a parasitic relationship, the host _____, and the parasite
    _____.

3. What is an arthropod? _____

    _____

H. Pathogenic Helminths

1. List each step in a helminth's life cycle._____

    _____

    _____

2. _____ specimens are commonly examined for parasitic _____
    and _____. The specimen is collected and placed into two vials, each with a(n)
    _____. From these preparations, a(n) _____ slide is made to
    observe moving organisms.

3. What does *O&P* stand for? _____

    _____

I. Pathogenic Viruses

1. Are viruses considered living organisms? _____

    _____

2. Define *capsid*. _____

    _____

3. Viruses are not able to _____ or _____ unless they are in-
    side of a host cell. Viruses have their own _____ but must use the host cell
    _____ and _____ to reproduce and metabolize. Because of the
    absolute need for a host cell, a virus can be considered a(n) _____.

4. Most viral diseases and disorders are diagnosed by detecting specific _____ to the
    virus.

J. Specimen Collection and Transport to the Physician's Office Laboratory (POL)

1. Specimens for microbiology testing must be collected carefully so that contaminating
    _____ are not introduced into the _____.

2. List steps to prevent sample contamination. _____

   _____

   _____

3. List steps to protect yourself from pathogen exposure. _____

   _____

   _____

   _____

   _____

4. Why is patient education/instruction important for samples that are collected at home? _____

   _____

   _____

5. Microorganisms are _____ organisms, so they must be given conditions that ensure their _____. Care must also be taken so that any _____
   in the sample will not _____ and _____ possible
   _____. The type and number of _____ in the sample should
   reflect the type and number of microorganisms at the _____ of collection, at the
   _____ of collection.

6. Define *transport medium.* _____

   _____

7. Most pathogenic organisms prefer _____, approximately. They will remain
   _____ for up to _____ if held at _____ tem-
   perature or _____ temperature.

8. How are humans infected with pinworms? _____

   _____

   _____

9. Describe how pinworm samples are collected from children._____

   _____

   _____

   _____

K. CLIA-Waived Microbiology Testing

1. Often, growing a(n) _____ on a nutrient medium plate is difficult, and it
   takes _____ to grow and _____ the pathogen. A(n)
   _____ demonstrates the presence of the _____ in a specimen
   that is placed in a test kit containing its specific _____. If the pathogen is present, it
   produces a(n) _____ reaction, indicating a(n) _____ result.

2. List the information contained in a package insert._____

_____

_____

_____

3. Strep throat is caused by what microorganism? _____

4. If a throat culture specimen tests negative for Streptococcus with a rapid strep kit, what additional test should be performed?

_____

5. Define *influenza*. _____

_____

6. The specimens that can be used with most rapid influenza A and B tests are:_____

_____

7. What does the acronym *RSV* stand for? _____

_____

8. What conditions are caused by RSV, a major cause of upper and lower respiratory tract infections. It is the major cause of _____ and _____ in children and infants

9. The CLIA-waived rapid direct immunoassay for RSV uses a(n) _____ swab specimen or _____ to detect the virus.

L. CLIA-Waived Immunology Testing

1. Testing done in the immunology laboratory is designed to demonstrate the reaction between a(n) _____ and its specific _____.

2. In the acute stage of a disease, the _____ level is high. During the convalescent stage, the antibody level _____.

3. What is the causative agent (organism) of infectious mononucleosis (Mono)? _____

_____

4. What complications can be seen with Mono?_____

_____

_____

5. What laboratory testing is commonly done when Mono is suspected? _____

_____

_____

6. What is a heterophile antibody? _____

_____

_____

7. *Helicobacter pylori* causes what disease state? _____

_____

_____

8. Briefly describe the principle of an *H. pylori* test._____

_____

_____

9. What is the causative agent of Lyme disease? _____

_____

10. How does a person contract Lyme disease? _____

_____

_____

M. Microbiology Reference Laboratory: Identification of Pathogens

1. What are the four components of a Gram stain? _____

_____

_____

2. What color is a Gram-positive organism?_____

_____

3. What color is a Gram-negative organism? _____

_____

4. An acid-fast stain is used in the identification protocol for what bacteria?_____

_____

5. What are the three components of an acid-fast stain?_____

_____

6. What color is an acid-fast positive and negative organism? _____

_____

7. Inoculating _____ and _____ are used to transfer samples to _____ media or _____ to slides for staining.

8. Define *pure culture*. _____

_____

9. When the organism is in pure culture, _____ and additional
_____ testing can be done to _____ the organism.

10. *Streptococcus pyogenes* is also known as _____ .

11. What are complications of untreated *Streptococcus pyogenes*? _____

_____

_____

12. Referring to a traditional overnight throat culture, the antibiotic disk contains
_____, which prevents the growth of _____. Complete
_____ of the agar around the colonies indicates _____, which
is caused by a(n) _____ produced by *S. pyogenes*. The toxin breaks down the
_____ in the agar, causing the agar to be a(n) _____ color
around the colonies. The presence of _____ and a(n) _____
around the disk indicate that the patient has _____.

13. A(n) _____ inoculating _____ is used to set up urine culture
plates.

14. What does the acronym *cfu* stand for?_____

15. Describe the final cfu results listed below and how they would be interpreted.

- Normal _____

_____

- Borderline _____

_____

- Positive _____

_____

16. Describe why a provider would order culture and sensitivity testing. _____

_____

_____

17. Define the terms *susceptible, resistant,* and *intermediate* as they relate to sensitivity testing.

- Susceptible _____

_____

- Resistant _____

_____

- Intermediate _____

_____

CERTIFICATION PREPARATION

Circle the correct answer.

1. Beneficial microorganisms that are responsible for breaking down organic matter are called
   a. virus.
   b. saprophyte.
   c. acid-fast bacilli.
   d. mycoplasma.

2. What color is a Gram-positive organism?
   a. Baby blue
   b. Pink
   c. Red
   d. Purple

3. A disease-causing organism or agent is the definition for which term?
   a. Normal flora
   b. Opportunistic organism
   c. Pathogen
   d. Microorganism

4. What is a substance that inhibits the growth of microorganisms on living tissue?
   a. Antiseptic
   b. Disinfectant
   c. Antimicrobial
   d. Antifungal

5. If a bacterium is rod-shaped, it is described as
   a. cocci.
   b. spirilla.
   c. bacilli.
   d. spirochete.

6. If an organism is able to live and thrive in the presence of oxygen, it is
   a. an anaerobe.
   b. a facultative anaerobe.
   c. an aerobe.
   d. none of the above.

7. Tiny Gram-negative bacteria that are transmitted by blood-sucking insects are called
   a. chlamydia.
   b. virus.
   c. mycoplasma.
   d. rickettsia.

8. Scarlet fever, rheumatic fever, and glomerulonephritis are all possible complications of an infection with what bacteria?
   a. *Escherichia coli*
   b. *Staphylococcus aureus*
   c. *Streptococcus pyogenes*
   d. *Clostridium difficile*

9. The causative agent for Lyme disease is
   a. *Streptococcus pyogenes.*
   b. Epstein-Barr virus (EBV).
   c. *Helicobacter pylori.*
   d. *Borrelia burgdorferi.*

10. HIV is a
    a. viral infection.
    b. bloodborne pathogen.
    c. condition that is treated with ARV medications.
    d. all of the above.

WORKPLACE APPLICATIONS

1. Laura just collected a throat swab from a 10-year-old boy. He had a fever, sore throat, and white patches on his tonsils. Laura runs a rapid strep test and it is negative. Is there any additional testing that Laura should do? Explain your answer.

_____

_____

_____

_____

_____

2. Susie Cvanshara has an appointment at WMFM clinic today because she is very tired and has swollen lymph nodes in her neck and armpits, a sore throat, and no appetite. She has had these symptoms for 5 days and they are not improving. Jean Burke NP orders a CBC with differential and CLIA-waived Mono test. The Mono test result from the laboratory is positive.

   a. What condition does Susie have? _____

   b. What abnormalities may be seen in Susie's CBC and differential testing?_____

   _____

   _____

3. Laura is reviewing patient microbiology results received from the reference laboratory. She sees a urine culture result for Mrs. Bingley of 54,000 cfu/mL. The provider has now requested sensitivity testing be completed on this culture. Explain what this report means. Why will sensitivity testing be helpful to the provider?

   _____

   _____

   _____

   _____

INTERNET ACTIVITIES

1. Using online resources, research Lyme disease. Summarize your findings in a poster or infographic. Include the following information in your project.
   a. Description of the disease
   b. The causative agent of the disease
   c. Signs and symptoms
   d. Diagnostic procedures including CLIA-waived testing
   e. Treatment

2. Using online resources, research a CLIA-waived HIV test kit. Create a poster presentation, a Power-Point presentation, or a written paper summarizing your research. Include the following points in your project:
   a. Description of the test
   b. Any contraindications for the test
   c. Patient preparation for the test
   d. Principle of the test

3. Using online resources, create a poster or infographic about two types of pathogenic microorganisms. Choose from bacteria, viruses, fungi, protozoa, or parasites. Include the following information in your project:
   a. Size of the microorganism
   b. Common routes of transmission
   c. 5-10 examples of infectious agents for each type of organism
   d. 5-10 examples of disease states for each type of organism

Procedure 49.1 Instruct Patients in the Collection of Fecal Specimens to Be Tested for Ova and Parasites

Name _____ Date _____ Score _____

Task: To instruct a patient in the proper collection of stool for an ova and parasite microscopic examination.

Equipment and Supplies:
- Patient's health record
- Provider's order and/or lab requisition
- Clean, dry container for stool collection
- Two parasitology collection vials*
- Plastic biohazard zipper-lock bag

Note: Several types of preservatives are available. Check with the referral laboratory to make sure the patient is given the proper vials for collection. Preservatives include low-viscosity polyvinyl alcohol (LV-PVA), zinc sulfite polyvinyl alcohol (ZN-PVA), sodium acetate acetic acid formalin (SAF), and 10% neutral buffered formalin.

Standard: Complete the procedure and all critical steps in _____ minutes with a minimum score of 85% within two attempts (*or as indicated by the instructor*).

Scoring: Divide the points earned by the total possible points. Failure to perform a critical step, indicated by an asterisk (*), results in grade no higher than an 84% (*or as indicated by the instructor*).

Time: Began_____ Ended_____ Total minutes: _____

Steps:	Point Value	Attempt 1	Attempt 2
1. Greet the patient. Identify yourself. Verify the patient's identity with full name, ask the patient to spell the first and last name, and give their date of birth. Explain the procedure to be performed in a manner that is understood by the patient. Answer any general questions the patient may have about the collection procedures before you give detailed instructions.	15*		
2. Instruct the patient not to take any antacids, laxatives, or stool softeners before collecting the specimen.	10		
3. Instruct the patient to urinate before collecting the specimen.	10		
4. The patient then collects the specimen. *Adults:* Instruct the patient to defecate into the container provided. Stool cannot be retrieved from the toilet bowl. *Children:* Instruct parents/guardians to loosely drape the toilet rim with plastic wrap and lower the seat. The child should have a bowel movement into the toilet, onto the wrap. Remove the stool using a disposable plastic spoon.	15		
5. Instruct the patient to add stool to the collection container. a. If the stool is formed, use the scoop on the lid of the container to add a large, jelly bean–sized piece of stool to the liquid in the containers b. If the stool is liquid, pour it into the container. c. In both of the previous cases, keep adding the specimen until the liquid preservative in the vial reaches the indicated level on the containers.	10		
6. Instruct the patient to tighten the caps completely and wipe the outside of the vials with alcohol wipes or to wash carefully with soap and water.	15		
7. The vials should be labeled, placed in a biohazard bag with a zippered closure, and transported to the laboratory immediately, if possible. The vials should not be refrigerated.	10		

8. Instruct the patient to wash his or her hands after the specimen collection process.	**15***		
Total Points	**100**		

Documentation

Comments

CAAHEP Competencies	**Step(s)**
I.P.11.e. Obtain specimens and perform: CLIA-waived microbiology test	Entire procedure
ABHES Competencies	**Step(s)**
9.e. Instruct patients in the collection of 2) fecal specimen	Entire procedure

Procedure 49.2 Collect a Specimen for a Throat Culture

Name _____ Date _____ Score _____

Task: To collect a throat culture specimen using sterile technique for immediate testing or for transportation to the laboratory.

Equipment and Supplies:
- Patient's health record
- Provider's order
- Laboratory requisition
- Fluid-impermeable lab coat, face shield, and gloves
- Sterile swab if transporting to a reference laboratory, or sterile swab from the rapid strep test kit if testing patient in POL
- Sterile tongue depressor
- Transport medium
- Biohazard waste container

Standard: Complete the procedure and all critical steps in _____ minutes with a minimum score of 85% within two attempts (*or as indicated by the instructor*).

Scoring: Divide the points earned by the total possible points. Failure to perform a critical step, indicated by an asterisk (*), results in grade no higher than an 84% (*or as indicated by the instructor*).

Time: Began_____ Ended_____ Total minutes: _____

Steps:	Point Value	Attempt 1	Attempt 2
1. Wash hands or use hand sanitizer. Put on fluid-impermeable lab coat.	10*		
2. Gather the materials needed.	5		
3. Greet the patient. Identify yourself. Verify the patient's identity with full name, ask the patient to spell the first and last name, and give their date of birth. Explain the procedure to be performed in a manner that is understood by the patient. Answer any questions the patient may have on the procedure.	10*		
4. Put on face shield and gloves. Position the patient so that the light shines into the mouth.	5		
5. Remove the sterile swab from the sterile wrap with your dominant hand and grasp the sterile tongue depressor with your nondominant hand.	5		
6. Instruct the patient to open the mouth and say "Ah." Depress the tongue with the depressor.	5		
7. Swab the back of the throat between the tonsillar pillars in a figure-8 pattern, especially any reddened, patchy areas of the throat, white pus pockets, purulent areas, and the tonsils; take care not to touch any other areas in the mouth.	10		
8. Place the swab in the transport medium, label it, and send it to the laboratory. If rapid strep testing is requested, return the labeled swab to the laboratory.	10		
9. Dispose of contaminated supplies in the biohazard waste container.	10		
10. Disinfect the work area.	10		

11. Remove your gloves and discard them in the biohazard waste container. Remove face shield.	**5**			
12. Wash hands or use hand sanitizer.	**10**			
13. Document the procedure in the patient's health record.	**5**			
Total Points	**100**			

Documentation

Comments

CAAHEP Competencies	Step(s)
I.P.11.d. Obtain specimens and perform: CLIA-waived immunology test	Procedure is collection only
I.P.11.e. Obtain specimens and perform: CLIA-waived microbiology test	Procedure is collection only
III.P.2. Select appropriate barrier/personal protective equipment (PPE)	1,4
III.P.10.b. Demonstrate proper disposal of biohazardous material: regulated wastes	9,11
ABHES Competencies	**Step(s)**
9.b. Perform selected CLIA-waived test that assist with diagnosis and treatment 5) microbiology testing	Entire procedure

Procedure 49.3   Perform a CLIA-Waived Microbiology Test: Perform a Rapid Strep Test

Name _____ Date _____ Score _____

Task: To perform a rapid strep screening test to assist in the diagnosis of strep throat.

Equipment and Supplies:
- Patient's health record
- Provider's order and/or lab requisition
- QuickVue In-Line Strep A test kit contents, CLIA-waived kit
- 1 extraction solution bottle
- 1 individually packaged test cassette
- 1 individually wrapped sterile rayon swab provided in kit
- 1 positive (+) control swab provided in kit
- Visual flow chart outlining the steps of the test
- Rapid Strep Test Log Sheet (Work Product 49.1)
- Stopwatch or timer
- Fluid-impermeable lab coat, face shield or protective eyewear, gloves
- Biohazard waste container

Standard: Complete the procedure and all critical steps in _____ minutes with a minimum score of 85% within two attempts (*or as indicated by the instructor*).

Scoring: Divide the points earned by the total possible points. Failure to perform a critical step, indicated by an asterisk (*), results in grade no higher than an 84% (*or as indicated by the instructor*).

Time: Began_____ Ended_____ Total minutes: _____

Steps:	Point Value	Attempt 1	Attempt 2
1. Collect all necessary supplies and equipment. Bring all reagents to room temperature. Check the expiration date on the test kit package.	5		
2. Wash hands or use hand sanitizer. *Note:* Before running the first patient test from a new test kit, positive and negative controls must be run using the control swabs provided in the kit. Confirm that both controls reacted correctly and record the control results on the log sheet.	15*		
3. Greet the patient. Identify yourself. Verify the patient's identity with full name, ask the patient to spell the first and last name, and give their date of birth. Explain the procedure to be performed in a manner that is understood by the patient. Answer any questions the patient may have on the procedure. Obtain permission to collect a throat culture.	10*		
4. Put on gloves and face shield or protective eyewear. Collect a throat specimen using the rayon swab provided in the test kit.	10		
5. Remove the test cassette from the foil pouch and place it on a clean, dry, level surface. Using the notch at the back of the chamber as a guide, insert the patient's swab completely into the swab chamber.	5		

6.	Place the extraction bottle between your thumb and forefinger, and squeeze once to break the glass ampule inside the extraction solution bottle. Vigorously shake the bottle five times to mix the solutions. The solution should turn green.	**5**		
7.	Immediately remove the cap on the extraction solution bottle, hold the bottle vertically over the chamber, and quickly fill the chamber to the rim (approximately 8 drops).	**5**		
8.	Remove your face shield. Wait 5 minutes to read the results and record them in the lab log. • *Positive result:* A pink line shows in the T area, indicating the presence of *Streptococcus pyogenes* antigen; a blue line appears in the C area, indicating that the fluid activated the internal control. • *Negative result:* No pink line appears in the T test area; a blue line appears in the C control area, indicating that the internal control worked. • *Invalid result:* The blue control line does not appear next to the letter C at 5 minutes. The test result cannot be reported.	**10**		
9.	Discard all the test materials in the appropriate biohazard waste container.	**10**		
10.	Disinfect the work area. Remove your gloves. Wash hands or use hand sanitizer.	**10***		
11.	Record the test results in the patient's health record.	**10**		
12.	If the test results are negative, a second throat swab should be obtained and sent to the reference laboratory for a throat culture. *Often two swabs are used simultaneously when the sample is initially collected from the throat to prevent the need to recollect a specimen.*	**5**		
	Total Points	**100**		

Documentation

Comments

CAAHEP Competencies	Step(s)
I.P.10. Perform a quality control measure	2
I.P.11.d. Obtain specimens and perform: CLIA-waived immunology test	Entire procedure – perform test only
I.P.11.e. Obtain specimens and perform: CLIA-waived microbiology test	Entire procedure – perform test only
II.P.2. Differentiate between normal and abnormal test results	2
II.P.3. Maintain lab test results using flow sheets	11
III.P.2. Select appropriate barrier/personal protective equipment (PPE)	2, 4
III.P.10.b. Demonstrate proper disposal of biohazardous material: regulated wastes	9
ABHES Competencies	**Step(s)**
9.a. Practice Quality Control	2
9.b. Perform selected CLIA-waived test that assist with diagnosis and treatment 4) immunology testing	Entire procedure
9.b. Perform selected CLIA-waived test that assist with diagnosis and treatment 5) microbiology testing	Entire procedure
9.b. Perform selected CLIA-waived test that assist with diagnosis and treatment 6) kit testing	Entire procedure
9.d. Collect, label, and process specimens 4) obtain throat specimens for microbiologic testing	4

Work Product 49.1   Rapid Strep Test Log Sheet

To be used with Procedure 49.3.

Name _____ Date _____ Score _____

Directions: Complete the documentation

QUALITATIVE CONTROL/PATIENT LOG SHEET

TEST: ___Strep A test___

KIT NAME AND MANUFACTURER: QuickVue In-Line Strep A Test − Quidel

LOT #___12345___   EXPIRATION DATE: ___11/22/20XX___

STORAGE REQUIREMENTS: ___Room Temp___   TEST FLOW CHART ___yes___

DATE	SPECIMEN I.D. (CONTROL/PATIENT)	RESULT (+ OR −)	INTERNAL CONTROL PASSED (Y or N)	CHARTED IN PATIENT RECORD	TECH INITIALS
7/11/20XX	POSITIVE CONTROL	+	Y		LP
7/11/20XX	NEGATIVE CONTROL	−	Y		LP
7/11/20XX	PT ID: 5432	+	Y	✔	LP

Procedure 49.4   Perform a CLIA-Waived Immunology Test: Perform the QuickVue+ Infectious Mononucleosis Test

Name _____ **Date** _____ **Score** _____

Task: To perform and interpret a rapid CLIA-waived test for infectious mononucleosis.

Equipment and Supplies:
- Patient's health record
- Provider's order and/or lab requisition
- CLIA-waived QuickVue+ test kit for infectious mononucleosis and blood collecting supplies
- Package with supplies for 20 tests
- Color-coded bottles of positive and negative controls and the developer
- Test cassette in its foil-wrapped protective pouch
- Alcohol wipes, gauze, and bandage
- Pipets supplied in kit with black line indicating amount of capillary blood to collect
- Lancet
- Timer or wristwatch with sweep second hand
- Fluid-impermeable lab coat, protective eyewear, gloves
- Biohazard waste container
- Qualitative Control/Patient Log Sheet (Work Product 49.2)

Standard: Complete the procedure and all critical steps in _____ minutes with a minimum score of 85% within two attempts (*or as indicated by the instructor*).

Scoring: Divide the points earned by the total possible points. Failure to perform a critical step, indicated by an asterisk (*), results in grade no higher than an 84% (*or as indicated by the instructor*).

Time: Began_____ Ended_____ Total minutes: _____

Steps:	Point Value	Attempt 1	Attempt 2
1. Remove the test kit from the refrigerator and allow the reagents to warm to room temperature. Check the expiration date of the kit.	5		
2. Wash hands or use hand sanitizer. Put on the fluid-impermeable lab coat.	10*		
3. Before running the first patient test from a new test kit, run the positive and negative liquid controls provided in the kit to see whether they react correctly. Record your control results on the log sheet.	10*		
4. Greet the patient. Identify yourself. Verify the patient's identity with full name, ask the patient to spell their first and last name, and give their date of birth. Explain the procedure to be performed in a manner that is understood by the patient. Answer any questions the patient may have on the procedure.	10		
5. Put on gloves and protective eyewear. Remove the test device from its protective pouch, and label it with the patient's identification.	5		
6. Disinfect the patient's finger with an alcohol wipe. Allow it to air dry and then perform a capillary puncture.	5*		
7. Wipe away the first drop of blood and then fill the disposable pipet provided in the kit to the calibration mark with capillary blood. (See Chapter 47 for proper blood collection methods.)	10		

8. Dispense all the blood from the capillary tube into the "Add" well of the testing device. (Or, if you are using venous blood, transfer a large drop from the venous whole blood specimen using the longer capillary pipet provided in the kit.)	**5**		
9. Hold the developer bottle vertically above the "Add" well and allow 5 drops to fall freely.	**5**		
10. Read the results at 5 minutes. Note: The "Test Complete" box must be visibly colored by 10 minutes. • *Positive result:* A vertical line in any shade of blue forms a plus sign in the "Read Result" window, along with a blue "Test Complete" line. Even a faint blue plus sign should be reported as a positive. • *Negative result:* No vertical blue line appears, leaving a minus sign in the "Read Result" window, along with a blue "Test Complete" line. • *Invalid result:* After 10 minutes, no line is seen in the "Test Complete" window, or a blue color fills the "Read Result" window. If either of these is noted, the test must be repeated with a new testing device. If the problem continues, request technical support.	**10**		
11. Properly dispose of biohazardous waste material in the proper container and disinfect the work area.	**10**		
12. Remove your gloves and protective eyewear. Wash hands or use hand sanitizer.	**10***		
13. Document the patient's result and the control sample results in the lab logs and in the patient's health record.	**5**		
Total Points	**100**		

Documentation

Comments

CAAHEP Competencies	Step(s)
I.P.2.c. Perform: capillary puncture	6, 7
I.P.10. Perform a quality control measure	2
I.P.11.d. Obtain specimens and perform: CLIA-waived immunology test	Entire procedure
II.P.2. Differentiate between normal and abnormal test results	2
II.P.3. Maintain lab test results using flow sheets	2, 13
III.P.2. Select appropriate barrier/personal protective equipment (PPE)	2, 5
III.P.10.a. Demonstrate proper disposal of biohazardous material: sharps	11
III.P.10.b. Demonstrate proper disposal of biohazardous material: regulated wastes	11
XII.P.2.c. Demonstrate proper use of: sharps disposal containers	11
ABHES Competencies	**Step(s)**
9.a. Practice Quality Control	2
9.b. Perform selected CLIA-waived test that assist with diagnosis and treatment 4) immunology testing	Entire procedure
9.b. Perform selected CLIA-waived test that assist with diagnosis and treatment 6) kit testing	Entire procedure

Work Product 49.2   Qualitative Control/Patient Log Sheet
To be used with Procedure 49.4.

Name _____ **Date** _____ **Score** _____

Directions: Document the patient's result and the control sample results on the log.

QUALITATIVE CONTROL/PATIENT LOG SHEET

TEST: _____ Mononucleosis Rapid Test _____

KIT NAME & MANUFACTURER: QUICK VUE+ Infectious Mononucleosis Test -QUIDEL

LOT # _____ 12345 _____   EXPIRATION DATE: _____ 11/22/20XX _____

STORAGE REQUIREMENTS: _ Refrigerator _   TEST FLOW CHART _ yes _

DATE	SPECIMEN I.D. (CONTROL/PATIENT)	RESULT (+ OR −)	INTERNAL CONTROL PASSED (Y or N)	CHARTED IN PATIENT RECORD	TECH INITIALS
7/11/20XX	POSITIVE CONTROL	+	Y		LP
7/11/20XX	NEGATIVE CONTROL	−	Y		LP
7/11/20XX	PT ID: 5432	−	Y	✔	LP

Skills and Strategies

CAAHEP Competencies	Assessment
X.C.9. List and discuss legal and illegal applicant interview questions	Skills and Concepts – J. 6; Certification Preparation – 7

ABHES Competencies	Assessment
10. Career Development a. Perform the essential requirements for employment, such as resume writing, effective interviewing, dressing professionally, time management, and following up appropriately	Procedure 50.1-50.6
b. Demonstrate professional behavior	Procedure 50.5, 50.6
c. Explain what continuing education is and how it is acquired	Certification Preparation – 10; Internet Activities – 3

VOCABULARY REVIEW

Using the word pool on the right, find the correct word to match the definition. Write the word on the line after the definition.

Group A

1. Allowing the listener to recap and review what was said
   _____

2. Rewording a statement to check the meaning and interpretation; also shows you are listening and understanding the speaker
   _____

3. The ability to communicate and interact with others; sometimes referred to as *soft skills* _____

4. Websites where employers post jobs; can be used by job seekers to identify open positions _____

5. Putting words to the patient's emotional reaction, which acknowledges the person's feelings _____

6. The act of working with another or other individuals
   _____

7. Allows the listener to get additional information
   _____

8. Exchange of information among others in your field
   _____

9. Being worthy of honor and respect from others
   _____

10. To have a deep awareness of another's suffering and the desire to lessen it _____

Word Pool
- job boards
- summarizing
- networking
- dignity
- paraphrasing
- interpersonal skills
- reflecting
- compassion
- collaboration
- clarification

Group B

1. A resume format that focuses on the person's employment history; useful when seeking employment in the same field as the education or experience _____

2. The most recent item is on top and the oldest item is last
   _____

3. A resume format that lists a person's abilities and skill sets and also includes the employment history _____

4. To read and mark corrections _____

5. Simulated; intended for imitation or practice
   _____

6. A resume format that is customized to a unique job posting
   _____

7. A person's abilities, skills, or expertise in an area
   _____

8. Return offer made by one who has rejected an offer or a job
   _____

Word Pool
- combination resume
- targeted resume
- counteroffer
- skill set
- reverse chronologic order
- proofread
- chronologic resume
- mock

ABBREVIATIONS
Write out what each of the following abbreviations stands for.

1. CPR _____

2. CMA _____

3. BLS _____

4. AAMA _____

5. RMA _____

6. AMT _____

7. CCMA _____

8. NHA _____

9. NCMA _____

10. NCCT _____

11. HIPAA _____

SKILLS AND CONCEPTS
Answer the following questions. Write your answer on the line or in the space provided.

A. Understanding Personality Traits Important to Employers

1. What traits help new employees blend with the existing staff? _____

   _____

   _____

2. List four interpersonal skills that are important for new employees to have._____

   _____

   _____

3. Describe effective verbal and nonverbal communication. _____

   _____

   _____

4. List four traits of effective nonverbal communication._____

   _____

   _____

5. Describe why listening to others is important._____

   _____

6. Describe five ways a person can demonstrate professionalism. _____

_____

_____

_____

_____

B. Assessing Your Strengths and Skills

1. Describe four personality traits you have and list the "evidence" to support your claim. _____

_____

_____

_____

2. Define *technical skills* and give two examples. _____

_____

_____

3. List at least four technical skills you possess and indicate where you developed each skill. _____

_____

_____

4. Define *transferable job skills*. _____

_____

5. List at least two transferable skills that you have and indicate where you developed each skill. _____

_____

_____

_____

_____

C. Developing Career Objectives

1. Identify career objectives for yourself. Answer the following questions.

   a. What area and skills did you enjoy in class and/or in practicum? _____

   _____

   b. Where do you want to be in 5 years? _____

   _____

c. Where do you want to be in 10 years? _____

_____

d. What additional skills do you need to get where you want to go? _____

_____

e. Based on these answers, describe at least two goals you have for yourself. _____

_____

_____

D. Identifying Personal Needs

1. Identify your personal needs by answering the following questions.

   a. Do you need a specific wage and/or benefits? If so, describe your needs. _____

   _____

   b. Do you need specific hours? If so, describe the hours. _____

   _____

   c. How far are you willing to travel? _____

   _____

   d. Do you have a reliable mode of transportation?_____

   _____

   _____

E. Finding a Job

1. Name four credential examinations for medical assistants._____

   _____

   _____

   _____

2. Describe the difference between facility job boards and public job boards. _____

   _____

   _____

3. List four possible job search methods you can use in your area. These can include job boards, newspapers, and so on.

   _____

   _____

F. Developing a Resume

1. What is the purpose of a resume? _____

    _____

    _____

2. List three types of resumes and describe why each is used. _____

    _____

    _____

3. Describe information found in the education section of a resume._____

    _____

    _____

4. Describe the work experience information required for all three types of resume. _____

    _____

    _____

5. How many years of employment history should be included in the resume? _____

6. What information should be included for certifications? _____

    _____

    _____

7. Describe how to create a visually appealing resume. _____

    _____

    _____

    _____

    _____

G. Developing a Cover Letter

1. What is the goal of a cover letter?_____

    _____

    _____

2. What two things can be done to help identify errors in a cover letter? _____

    _____

    _____

    _____

3. What specific position information should appear in the cover letter? _____

_____

_____

H. Completing Online Profiles and Job Applications

1. What are the advantages of online profiles over paper applications for both the applicant and the employer?

_____

_____

_____

2. Describe four types of information required for online profiles and paper applications._____

_____

_____

_____

_____

3. Describe the professional way to obtain references. _____

_____

_____

4. List three types of people that should be included on the reference list._____

_____

_____

I. Creating a Career Portfolio

1. Describe the purpose of a career portfolio._____

_____

_____

2. Describe materials you could include in a career portfolio._____

_____

_____

_____

_____

J. Job Interview

1. What are the four things a job seeker must do to prepare for an interview?_____

    _____

    _____

    _____

2. Why is it important to research the facility prior to the interview? _____

    _____

3. Describe what your interview attire would be like. _____

    _____

4. List six items to bring to an interview. _____

    _____

    _____

    _____

5. Explain how you would answer this question during an interview: "Tell me about yourself." _____

    _____

    _____

6. List six topics that might be discussed during an interview. For each topic, provide a legal and illegal question that addresses the topic. Use the book examples as a guide and come up with your own questions.

    _____

    _____

    _____

    _____

    _____

7. How should a person treat a phone interview? _____

    _____

    _____

8. Just prior to the interview starting, list three things an interviewee should do._____

    _____

    _____

9. Discuss the importance of good eye contact during an interview. _____

_____

_____

_____

10. Describe the importance of sending a thank-you note after an interview. _____

_____

_____

_____

K. You Got the Job!

1. Describe five ways a medical assistant can be successful in a new job. _____

_____

_____

_____

_____

2. Describe the 180-degree style performance appraisal. _____

_____

_____

_____

_____

3. Describe the 360-degree style performance appraisal. _____

_____

_____

_____

_____

4. When leaving a job, how soon should you give notice? _____

_____

CERTIFICATION PREPARATION

Circle the correct answer.

1. _____ means to have a deep awareness of another's suffering and a desire to lessen it.
   a. Interpersonal skills
   b. Reflecting
   c. Compassion
   d. Dignity

2. "Communicates well" is a _____.
   a. technical skill
   b. personality trait
   c. transferable job skill
   d. both a and b

3. What is the best and most effective way to find employment?
   a. Checking job boards and newspaper ads
   b. Using the school career placement office
   c. Networking and checking job boards
   d. Using employment agencies

4. Which is the most popular type of resume that is used when people are seeking employment in the same field as their education or experience?
   a. Reverse chronologic
   b. Chronologic
   c. Combination
   d. Targeted

5. What is true regarding the header in the resume and cover letter?
   a. The information should appear on all pages of the cover letter and resume
   b. Contains the person's name and mailing address
   c. Contains a phone number and a professional email address
   d. All of the above are true

6. Which item is typically presented in a reverse chronologic order on a resume?
   a. Education information
   b. Work experience
   c. Skills
   d. Both a and b

7. What is an illegal interview question?
   a. "Are you eligible to work in this state?"
   b. "Who looks after your children when you work?"
   c. "Are you able to work 8 AM to 3 PM on the weekends?"
   d. "Have you ever been convicted of a federal offense?"

8. Form _____ is the Employee's Withholding Allowance Certificate.
   a. W-3
   b. W-2
   c. I-9
   d. W-4

9. Form _____ is the Employment Eligibility Verification Form.
   a. W-3
   b. W-2
   c. I-9
   d. W-4

10. What is the importance of continuing education for a medical assistant?
    a. Helps with keeping updated and current
    b. Needed to maintain a certification or registration
    c. Important for professional development
    d. All of the above

WORKPLACE APPLICATIONS

1. Select six interview questions from Figure 50.8 and write a response for each question. Your answer should be at least five sentences in length.

   _____

   _____

   _____

   _____

   _____

   _____

   _____

   _____

2. During an interview, Michelle was asked her age. Michelle knew this was not a legal interview question. If you were in this situation, how would you respond?

   _____

   _____

   _____

INTERNET ACTIVITIES

1. Using appropriate online resources, research one of the four national certification exams:
   - Certified Medical Assistant (CMA) through the American Association of Medical Assistants (AAMA)
   - Registered Medical Assistant (RMA) through the American Medical Technologists (AMT)
   - Medical Assistant Certification (CCMA) through the National Healthcareer Association
   - Medical Assistant (NCMA) through the National Center for Competency Testing (NCCT)

   In a PowerPoint, poster, or paper, address the following points:
   a. List the credential and the sponsoring agency
   b. Describe the exam (e.g., number of questions, coverage of topics, time limit)
   c. Describe the registration process
   d. Describe the requirements for maintaining the credential (e.g., continuing education, fees, retaking the exam)

2. Using online resources, identify four potential job openings that interest you. Describe each position in a brief paper and provide the websites for the openings.

3. Using online resources, identify two resources for continuing education for medical assistants. Briefly describe the resources and list the websites.

4. Using online resources, identify 8-10 potential job postings that interest you.

Procedure 50.1   Prepare a Chronologic Resume

Name _____   Date _____   Score _____

Task: Write an effective resume for use as a tool in obtaining employment.

Equipment and Supplies:
- Computer with word processing software and a printer
- Current job posting
- Resume paper
- Paper and pen

Standard: Complete the procedure and all critical steps in _____ minutes with a minimum score of 85% within two attempts (*or as indicated by the instructor*).

Scoring: Divide the points earned by the total possible points. Failure to perform a critical step, indicated by an asterisk (*), results in grade no higher than an 84% (*or as indicated by the instructor*).

Time: Began_____   Ended_____   Total minutes: _____

Steps:	Point Value	Attempt 1	Attempt 2
1. Apply critical thinking skills as you create a list of the personality traits (wanted by employers), technical skills, and transfer job skills that you possess. Also write down your career goal(s).	5		
2. Using the current job posting, identify the required and recommended qualifications and credentials needed for the position.	10		
3. Using the computer with word processing software, create a professional-looking header for your document. Include your name, address, telephone number(s), and email address. Select an appropriate font style for your name and a smaller font size for your contact information.	10		
4. Create a section header for "Education." For the learning institution(s) you attended, list the school's name, city and state, degree obtained, or coursework successfully completed, and the year. Include any additional educational information, such as grade point average (GPA), awards, and practicum information.	10		
5. Create a section header for "Healthcare Experience" and/or "Work Experience." Provide details about your work experience, including the facility's name, city and state, title of your position, start and end date (month and year), and job duties. The job duties must start with an active verb using the appropriate tense (e.g., a past job would have past tense verbs and a current job would include present tense verbs).	10		
6. Create a section header for "Special Skills" and list your special language skills, computer proficiencies, and other unique skills you possess that relate to the position.	10		
7. Create a section header for "Certifications and Credentials" and list the active credentials and certifications you have. Include the title of the certification, awarding agency, and the expiration date.	10		
8. All information on the resume needs to appear in reverse chronologic order (newest information is on top). Work experience should include both the start and end month and year.	10		

9.	The resume needs to look professional and interesting. Utilize font styles (e.g., bold, underline, italic) to emphasize important words and phrases. Use professional-looking bullets to list job duties and other information. Use keywords from the posting throughout the resume.	**15***		
10.	Proofread the resume. Correct any spelling, grammar, punctuation, or sentence structure errors you find. If time allows, have another person review the resume and use the feedback to revise your resume.	**10**		
	Total Points	**100**		

Comments

ABHES Competencies	Step(s)
10.a. Perform the essential requirements for employment, such as resume writing, effective interviewing, dressing professionally, time management, and following up appropriately	Entire procedure

Procedure 50.2   Create a Cover Letter

Name _____ Date _____ Score _____

Task: Write an effective cover letter that will accompany the resume.

Equipment and Supplies:
- Computer with word processing software and a printer
- Current job posting
- Resume paper
- Pen

Standard: Complete the procedure and all critical steps in _____ minutes with a minimum score of 85% within two attempts (*or as indicated by the instructor*).

Scoring: Divide the points earned by the total possible points. Failure to perform a critical step, indicated by an asterisk (*), results in grade no higher than an 84% (*or as indicated by the instructor*).

Time: Began_____ Ended_____ Total minutes: _____

Steps:	Point Value	Attempt 1	Attempt 2
1. Using the job posting, read through the job description. With a pen, circle the position requirements and the key phrases.	5		
2. Using the computer with word processing software, create a professional-looking header in the document's header that matches your resume header. Include your name, address, telephone number(s), and email address.	10		
3. Type the date in the correct location using the correct format. Have one blank line between the date line and the last line of the letterhead.	10		
4. Type the inside address using the correct spelling, punctuation, and location for the information. Leave 1 to 9 blank lines between the date and the inside address, depending on the location of the body of the letter.	10		
5. Starting on the second line below the inside address, type the salutation using the correct format. Use a colon after the person's name.	10		
6. Type the message in the body of the letter using the proper location and format. There should be a blank line after the salutation and between each paragraph. The message should be clear, concise, and professional. Use proper grammar, punctuation, capitalization, and sentence structure.	10		
7. The first paragraph should contain the title and number of the job posting. The middle paragraph(s) should summarize your strengths and include key phrases from the posting. The final paragraph should discuss your availability for an interview. The body should end with an expression of gratitude to the reader.	10		
8. Type a proper closing, leaving one blank line between the last line of the body and the closing. Use the correct format and location.	10		
9. Type the signature block using the correct format and location. There should be four blank lines between the closing and the signature block.	10*		
10. Spell-check and proofread the document. Check for proper tone, grammar, punctuation, capitalization, and sentence structure. Check for proper spacing between the parts of the letter.	10		

11. Make any final corrections. Print the document on resume paper and sign the letter or email the document to your instructor or employer.	**5**		
Total Points	**100**		

Comments

ABHES Competencies	**Step(s)**
10.a. Perform the essential requirements for employment, such as resume writing, effective interviewing, dressing professionally, time management, and following up appropriately	Entire procedure

Procedure 50.3   Complete a Job Application

Name _____   Date _____   Score _____

Task: Complete an accurate, detailed job application legibly to secure a job offer.

Equipment and Supplies:
- Pen
- Application form
- Information regarding your past education, job experiences, and the skill sets you have developed (e.g., computer skills, keyboarding speed)
- Contact information for former supervisors and references
- Current resume

Standard: Complete the procedure and all critical steps in _____ minutes with a minimum score of 85% within two attempts (*or as indicated by the instructor*).

Scoring: Divide the points earned by the total possible points. Failure to perform a critical step, indicated by an asterisk (*), results in grade no higher than an 84% (*or as indicated by the instructor*).

Time: Began_____ Ended_____ Total minutes: _____

Steps:	Point Value	Attempt 1	Attempt 2
1. Read the entire job application before completing any part of the document.	5		
2. Refer to your information on past jobs, education experiences, and skill sets you have developed as you complete the application. Answers to the questions need to be accurate and honest.	45		
3. Use proper grammar, sentence structure, punctuation, spelling, and capitalization. Handwriting should be legible to the reader.	15		
4. Do not leave any space blank. Answer each question on the document. If the question does not apply, write "not applicable."	10		
5. Do not write "See resume" anywhere on the document.	5		
6. Include information on the application that exhibits dependability, punctuality, teamwork, attention to detail, a positive work ethic and initiative, the ability to adapt to change, a responsible attitude, and use of technology.	10		
7. Sign the document and date it.	5		
8. Proofread the document and make sure none of the information conflicts with the resume.	5		
Total Points	100		

Comments

ABHES Competencies	Step(s)
10.a. Perform the essential requirements for employment, such as resume writing, effective interviewing, dressing professionally, time management, and following up appropriately	Entire procedure

Work Product 50.1   Job Application

To be used with Procedure 50.3.

Name _____   **Date** _____   **Score** _____

WALDEN-MARTIN
FAMILY MEDICAL CLINIC
1234 ANYSTREET | ANYTOWN, ANYSTATE 12345
PHONE 123 123 1234 | FAX 123 123 5678

APPLICATION FOR EMPLOYMENT

Walden-Martin Family Medical Clinic is an equal opportunity employer and upholds the principles of equal opportunity employment. It is the policy of Walden-Martin Family Medical Clinic to provide employment, compensation and other benefits related to employment based on qualifications and performance, without regard to race, color, religion, national origin, age, sex, veteran status or disability, or any other basis prohibited by federal or state law. As an equal opportunity employer, Walden-Martin Family Medical Clinic intends to comply fully with all federal and state laws, and the information requested on this application will not be used for any purpose prohibited by law. Disabled applicants may request any needed accommodation. Please complete this application using ink, answer all questions completely, and sign the application.

Date: _____

Name: (First, Middle Initial, Last) _____

Social Security No.:_____   Phone: _____

Address:_____

City, State, Zip: _____

Have you been previously employed by Walden-Martin Family Medical Clinic?
☐ Yes ☐ No

If "Yes", when and job title?

How did you learn of the position for which you are applying?

☐ Newspaper/Print Advertisement ☐ Friend/Relative ☐ Employment Agency
☐ Job Service

☐ Radio/TV Advertisement ☐ Clinic Staff Person Name:

EMPLOYMENT DESIRED

Position(s) applied for: _____

☐ Full-time ☐ Part-time (If "Part time", number of shifts/hours desired _____)

Date available to start: _____   Salary requested: _____

PERSONAL HISTORY

Are you a United States citizen or do you have an entry permit which allows you to lawfully work in the U.S.? ☐ Yes   ☐ No
    If applicable, Visa Type: _____   Immigration No.: _____

Are you at least 18 years old?   ☐ Yes   ☐ No

Are you ineligible to be employed with an AnyState licensed health care entity as a result of being found guilty by a court of law for abusing, neglecting, or mistreating individuals in a health care related setting?   ☐ Yes   ☐ No
    If "Yes," please explain: _____

Are you able to perform all of the duties required by the position for which you are applying, without endangering yourself or compromising the safety, health, or welfare of the patients or other staff member? ☐ Yes   ☐ No
    If "No," please explain:_____

EDUCATION

	Name, City, State	Graduation Date	Course of Study/ Degree Obtained
High School:			
College:			
Other:			

LICENSURE/CERTIFICATION/REGISTRATION

Type of Certification, License or Registration	Agency/State	Registration Name

List any special skills or qualifications which you possess and feel are relevant to health care and the position for which you are applying.

_____

_____

_____

_____

_____

MILITARY SERVICE

From: _____   To: _____

Branch: _____

Duties: _____

Did you receive any specialized training? ☐ Yes   ☐ No
If "Yes", describe: _____

EMPLOYMENT HISTORY

Please give accurate and complete information. Start with present or most recent employer.
May we contact and communicate with your present employer? ☐ Yes   ☐ No

Employer:		Phone:	
Address:		**Supervisor:**	
Employed	Start: Month/Year: _____ Ended: Month/Year: _____	**Hourly Pay:**	Start: _____ Ended: _____
Position title and responsibilities:			
Reason for leaving:			

Employer:		Phone:	
Address:		**Supervisor:**	
Employed	Start: Month/Year: _____ Ended: Month/Year: _____	**Hourly Pay:**	Start: _____ Ended: _____
Position title and responsibilities:			
Reason for leaving:			

Employer:		Phone:	
Address:		Supervisor:	
Employed	Start: Month/Year: _____ Ended: Month/Year: _____	Hourly Pay:	Start: _____ Ended: _____
Position title and responsibilities:			
Reason for leaving:			

Employer:		Phone:	
Address:		Supervisor:	
Employed	Start: Month/Year: _____ Ended: Month/Year: _____	Hourly Pay:	Start: _____ Ended: _____
Position title and responsibilities:			
Reason for leaving:			

REFERENCES

Names of co-workers (no relatives) you have worked with and whom we may contact for a reference.

Name:	
Address:	
Phone:	
Job Title:	

Name:	
Address:	
Phone:	
Job Title:	

Name:	
Address:	
Phone:	
Job Title:	

Please read the following statements completely and carefully before you sign your name.

The Applicant HEREBY CERTIFIES that the answers given on this Application For Employment, including any statements or answers provided by the Applicant during interview, are true and correct. The Applicant fully authorizes Walden-Martin Family Medical Clinic to contact any references, past and present employers, persons, schools, law enforcement agencies and any other sources of information which may be relevant to the Applicant and this Application For Employment. It is understood and agreed that any misrepresentation, false statement, or omission by the Applicant will be sufficient reason for rejection of the Application For Employment or for dismissal from employment at any time, without recourse or liability to Walden-Martin Family Medical Clinic.

I have read, understand and agree to the above statement.

Sign: _____

Date: _____

Procedure 50.4   Create a Career Portfolio

Name _____   Date _____   Score _____

Task: Create a custom portfolio that provides potential employers evidence of your skills and knowledge as a medical assistant.

Equipment and Supplies:
- Three-ring binder or folder
- Plastic sleeves for the three-ring binder
- Dividers with tabs for the three-ring binder
- Current resume and cover letter
- Documents providing evidence of your skills and knowledge (e.g., transcripts, job and practicum evaluation forms, practicum skill checklist, projects completed in school, letters of recommendation, copies of certifications [e.g., CPR card])

Standard: Complete the procedure and all critical steps in _____ minutes with a minimum score of 85% within two attempts (*or as indicated by the instructor*).

Scoring: Divide the points earned by the total possible points. Failure to perform a critical step, indicated by an asterisk (*), results in grade no higher than an 84% (*or as indicated by the instructor*).

Time: Began _____ Ended _____ Total minutes: _____

Steps:	Point Value	Attempt 1	Attempt 2
1. Group documents in a logical manner, putting similar documents together. Identify the arrangement for the portfolio. An arrangement could include cover letter and resume, education section (e.g., transcript, practicum evaluation form and skills checklist, awards), prior job-related documents (e.g., evaluations), reference letters, and work products (e.g., projects you created in your medical assistant program).	25		
2. Insert one document per plastic pocket. Place all documents in plastic pockets.	15		
3. Neatly write the topic area on the tab of the dividers. Insert the tabbed dividers in the binder or folder.	15		
4. Place all documents in the binder or folder behind the correct divider. Place your cover letter and resume in the front of all the other documents.	15		
5. Create a table of contents to identify the tabbed areas.	15		
6. After the portfolio is assembled, review the entire portfolio to ensure it looks professional and the documents provide positive support of your skill set and knowledge.	15		
Total Points	100		

Comments

ABHES Competencies	Step(s)
10.a. Perform the essential requirements for employment, such as resume writing, effective interviewing, dressing professionally, time management, and following up appropriately	Entire procedure

Procedure 50.5 Practice Interview Skills During a Mock Interview

Name _____ Date _____ Score _____

Tasks: Project a professional appearance during a job interview and to be able to express the reasons the medical assistant is the best candidate for the position.

Equipment and Supplies:
- Current job posting
- Resume
- Cover letter
- Interview portfolio (optional)
- Application (optional)
- Interviewer
- Mock interview questions

Standard: Complete the procedure and all critical steps in _____ minutes with a minimum score of 85% within two attempts (*or as indicated by the instructor*).

Scoring: Divide the points earned by the total possible points. Failure to perform a critical step, indicated by an asterisk (*), results in grade no higher than an 84% (*or as indicated by the instructor*).

Time: Began_____ Ended_____ Total minutes: _____

Steps:	Point Value	Attempt 1	Attempt 2
1. Wear interview-appropriate attire and be groomed professionally.	15		
2. Portray a professional image by shaking hands firmly prior to the start of the interview. Ensure that each interviewer has a copy of your resume and cover letter. Refrain from nervous behaviors (e.g., saying "um", tapping a pen or your foot) during the interview.	10		
3. Answer introductory questions by providing only professional information. This may include information about your education, experience, and career goals.	10		
4. Answer interview questions with open, honest, and positive responses. Completely answer questions, provide information or examples, and do not answer in single sentences or with limited responses.	25		
5. Use key words from the job posting when answering the interview questions.	10		
6. Ask the interviewer two to three appropriate questions about the facility or the position.	20		
7. Express interest in the job and politely complete the interview by shaking hands and thanking the interviewer for the opportunity for the interview.	10		
Total Points	100		

Comments

ABHES Competencies	Step(s)
10.a. Perform the essential requirements for employment, such as resume writing, effective interviewing, dressing professionally, time management, and following up appropriately	Entire procedure

Procedure 50.6   Create a Thank-You Note for an Interview

Name _____ Date _____ Score _____

Task: Create a meaningful thank-you note to be sent after the interview process.

Equipment and Supplies:
- Computer with word processing software and a printer
- Job description
- Contact name from interview

Standard: Complete the procedure and all critical steps in _____ minutes with a minimum score of 85% within two attempts (*or as indicated by the instructor*).

Scoring: Divide the points earned by the total possible points. Failure to perform a critical step, indicated by an asterisk (*), results in grade no higher than an 84% (*or as indicated by the instructor*).

Time: Began_____ Ended_____ Total minutes: _____

Steps:	Point Value	Attempt 1	Attempt 2
1. Using word processing software, compose a professional letter using the business letter format. Include all of the required elements in the letter. Use correct spacing between the elements.	30		
2. Emphasize the particulars of the interview in the body of the letter.	20		
3. Include positive information you wish you had covered in the interview.	20		
4. Create a message that is concise and to the point.	20		
5. Proofread the letter and make any revisions as needed. Sign and send the thank-you note.	10		
Total Points	100		

Comments

ABHES Competencies	Step(s)
10.a. Perform the essential requirements for employment, such as resume writing, effective interviewing, dressing professionally, time management, and following up appropriately	Entire procedure